D1568675

Textbook of Administrative Psychiatry

New Concepts for a Changing Behavioral Health System

Second Edition

Editorial Board

Textbook of Administrative Psychiatry

New Concepts for a Changing Behavioral Health System

Second Edition

Edited by

John A. Talbott, M.D.
Robert E. Hales, M.D., M.B.A.

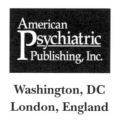

American Psychiatric Publishing, Inc.

Washington, DC
London, England

Copyright © 2001 American Psychiatric Publishing, Inc.
ALL RIGHTS RESERVED

Manufactured in the United States of America on acid-free paper
04   03   02   01   4   3   2   1
Second Edition

American Psychiatric Publishing, Inc.
1400 K Street, N.W.
Washington, DC 20005
www.appi.org

Library of Congress Cataloging-in-Publication Data
Textbook of administrative psychiatry : new concepts for a changing behavioral health
system / edited by John A. Talbott, Robert E. Hales.—2nd ed.
    p. ; cm.
    Includes bibliographical references and index.
    ISBN 0-88048-745-3 (alk. paper)
        1. Mental health services—United States—Administration. 2.
    Psychiatry—Practice—United States. I. Talbott, John A. II. Hales, Robert E.
        [DNLM: 1. Mental Health Services—organization & administration—United States. 2.
    Psychiatry—organization & administration—United States. WM 30 T3555 2001]
    RA790.6 .T49 2001
    362.2'068—dc21
                                                                                                00-047539

British Library Cataloguing in Publication Data
A CIP record is available from the British Library.

Contents

SECTION I
Overview of the Evolving
Behavioral Health System

Michael A. Freeman, M.D., D.M.H., Section Editor

SECTION IV
New Concepts for a
Changing Behavioral Health System
Judith H. Browne, R.N., M.S.N., Section Editor

Contributors

Boris M. Astrachan, M.D.
Distinguished Professor of Psychiatry, Department of Psychiatry, University of Illinois at Chicago, Chicago, Illinois

Alan A. Axelson, M.D.
Chief Executive Officer and Medical Director, InterCare Psychiatric Services, Pittsburgh, Pennsylvania

Michael J. Bennett, M.D.
Associate Clinical Professor of Psychiatry, Harvard Medical School, Boston, Massachusetts

Jonathan F. Borus, M.D.
Chairman, Department of Psychiatry, and Psychiatrist-in-Chief, Brigham and Women's Hospital, Boston, Massachusetts

Judith H. Browne, R.N., M.S.N.
Executive Vice President, Business Development, FHC Health Systems (including OPTIONS Health Care, Alternative Behavioral Systems [ABS], and FirstLab), Norfolk, Virginia

Simon H. Budman, Ph.D.
President and Founder, Innovative Training Systems, Newton, Massachusetts

Mantosh Dewan, M.D.
Professor and Chair, Department of Psychiatry and Behavioral Sciences, State University of New York Upstate Medical University, Syracuse, New York

Lisa Dixon, M.D., M.P.H.
Associate Professor, Department of Psychiatry, University of Maryland School of Medicine, Baltimore, Maryland

John P. Docherty, M.D.
Chief Executive Officer and President, Comprehensive Neuroscience; Adjunct Professor, Department of Psychiatry, Weill Medical College, Cornell University, White Plains, New York

Catherine M. Donovan, B.S.
Quakertown, New Jersey

Joseph A. Flaherty, M.D.
Professor and Head, Department of Psychiatry, University of Illinois at Chicago, Chicago, Illinois

Michael A. Freeman, M.D., D.M.H.
Founder, Behavioral Healthcare Tomorrow National Dialogue Conference; Founding Editor in Chief, *Behavioral Healthcare Tomorrow*, Mill Valley, California

Franklyn L. Giampa, Ph.D.
Regional Vice-President, Correctional Medical Services, Okemos, Michigan

Paul F. Giannandrea, M.D.
Assistant Professor of Psychiatry, Department of Psychiatry, University of Maryland School of Medicine, Baltimore, Maryland; former Lt. Commander, Medical Corps, U.S. Navy

Linda S. Godleski, M.D.
Chief, Mental Health and Behavioral Medicine, Department of Veterans Affairs Medical Center; Associate Professor, Department of Psychiatry and Behavioral Sciences, University of Louisville School of Medicine, Louisville, Kentucky

Howard Goldman, M.D., Ph.D.
Professor, Department of Psychiatry, University of Maryland School of Medicine, Baltimore, Maryland

Gary L. Gottlieb, M.D., M.B.A.
Professor of Psychiatry, Harvard Medical School; Chairman, Partners Psychiatry and Mental Health System, Massachusetts General Hospital, Boston, Massachusetts

Thomas S. Gunnings, Ph.D.
Emeritus Professor of Psychiatry, Department of Psychiatry, Michigan State University, East Lansing, Michigan

Robert E. Hales, M.D., M.B.A.
Professor and Chair, Department of Psychiatry, University of California, Davis, School of Medicine; Director, Behavioral Health Center, UC Davis Health System; Medical Director, Sacramento County Mental Health Services, Sacramento, California

Michael F. Hogan, Ph.D.
Director, Ohio Department of Mental Health, Columbus, Ohio

Wendy Holt, M.P.P.
Senior Associate, Dougherty Management Associates, Lexington, Massachusetts

F. Joseph Hullett, M.D.
Vice President, Medical and Clinical Operations, Value Options Western Region, Long Beach, California

Eugene A. Kaplan, M.D.
Professor and Chair Emeritus, Department of Psychiatry and Behavioral Sciences, State University of New York Upstate Medical University, Syracuse, New York

Debra L. Klamen, M.D., M.H.P.E.
Associate Professor of Psychiatry and Assistant Dean for Preclerkship Curriculum, Department of Psychiatry, University of Illinois at Chicago, Chicago, Illinois

Teresa L. Kramer, Ph.D.
Assistant Professor and Associate Director, Center for Outcomes Research and Effectiveness (CORE), University of Arkansas for Medical Sciences, Little Rock, Arkansas

Susan G. Larson, M.D., M.P.A.
Northern Virginia Psychiatric Group, Fairfax, Virginia; Chief of Staff, National Capital Area Health Care System; former Captain, Medical Corps, U.S. Navy

Arthur Lazarus, M.D., M.B.A.
Vice President and Corporate Medical Director, Behavioral Health, Humana Inc., Louisville, Kentucky; Professor of Psychiatry, MCP Hahnemann University School of Medicine, Philadelphia, Pennsylvania

Jeremy A. Lazarus, M.D.
Associate Clinical Professor of Psychiatry, University of Colorado Health Sciences Center, Denver, Colorado

Harriet P. Lefley, Ph.D
Professor of Psychiatry and Behavioral Sciences, University of Miami School of Medicine, Miami, Florida

Benjamin Liptzin, M.D.
Professor and Deputy Chair of Psychiatry, Tufts University School of Medicine, Boston, Massachusetts

John Manring, M.D.
Associate Professor of Psychiatry and Director of Residency Training, Department of Psychiatry and Behavioral Sciences, State University of New York Upstate Medical University, Syracuse, New York

David McDuff, M.D.
Associate Professor of Psychiatry, Department of Psychiatry, University of Maryland School of Medicine, Baltimore, Maryland; Lt.Colonel, Medical Corps, U.S. Army Reserve

Bentson H. McFarland, M.D., Ph.D.
Professor of Psychiatry, Public Health and Preventive Medicine, Oregon Health Sciences University; Adjunct Investigator, Kaiser Permanente Center for Health Research, Portland, Oregon

Robert D. Miller, M.D., Ph.D.
Professor of Psychiatry and Director, Program for Forensic Psychiatry, Colorado Health Sciences Center, Denver, Colorado; Adjunct Professor of Law, University of Denver College of Law, Denver, Colorado; Director of Research and Education, Institute for Forensic Psychiatry, Colorado Mental Health Institute at Pueblo, Pueblo, Colorado

Kenneth Minkoff, M.D.
Medical Director, Arbour-Choate Health Management, Acton, Massachusetts; Clinical Assistant Professor of Psychiatry, Harvard University, Cambridge, Massachusetts

Carol T. Mowbray, Ph.D.
Professor and Associate Dean for Research, University of Michigan School of Social Work, Ann Arbor, Michigan

David P. Moxley, Ph.D.
Professor and Interim Associate Dean, Wayne State University School of Social Work, Detroit, Michigan

Deborah C. Nelson, Ph.D.
Vice President, Quality Management and Improvement, Beacon Health Strategies, Woburn, Massachusetts

Michael T. O'Mahoney, Ph.D.
Clinical Director, Cancer Wellness Center, Northbrook, Illinois

Fred C. Osher, M.D.
Associate Professor and Director, Center for Behavioral Health, Justice, and Public Policy, Department of Psychiatry, University of Maryland School of Medicine, Baltimore, Maryland

David Pollack, M.D.
Associate Professor of Psychiatry, Family Medicine, and Public Health and Preventive Medicine; Associate Director, Public Psychiatry Training Program, Oregon Health Sciences University, Portland, Oregon

Susan Ridgely, M.S.W., J.D.
Senior Policy Analyst, RAND Health, Santa Monica, California

James E. Sabin, M.D.
Clinical Professor of Psychiatry, Harvard Medical School; Director, Ethics Program, Harvard Pilgrim Health Care, Boston, Massachusetts

Jose M. Santiago, M.D.
Corporate Medical Officer, Carondelet Health Network, Tucson, Arizona

Pamela M. Senesac, R.N., M.S., S.M.
Project Director, Clinical Programs, Harvard Pilgrim Health Care, Wellesley, Massachusetts

Ian A. Shaffer, M.D.
Principal, Ian A. Shaffer and Associates, Reston, Virginia

Steven S. Sharfstein, M.D.
President and Chief Executive Officer, Sheppard Pratt Health System, Towson, Maryland; Clinical Professor of Psychiatry, University of Maryland, Baltimore, Maryland

Miles F. Shore, M.D.
Bullard Professor of Psychiatry, Harvard Medical School, Boston, Massachusetts; Visiting Scholar, Kennedy School of Government, Cambridge, Massachusetts

Derri L. Shtasel, M.D.
Clinical Associate Professor of Psychiatry, Harvard Medical School, Boston, Massachusetts; Clinical Director, Psychiatry and Mental Health, North Shore Medical Center, Salem Hospital, Salem, Massachusetts

Gregory E. Simon, M.D., M.P.H.
Center for Health Studies, Group Health Cooperative, Seattle, Washington

Robert I. Simon, M.D.
Clinical Professor of Psychiatry and Director, Program in Psychiatry and Law, Georgetown University School of Medicine, Washington, DC

G. Richard Smith, M.D.
Professor of Psychiatry, Professor of Medicine, and Director of Centers for Mental Health Care Research, Department of Psychiatry and Behavioral Sciences, University of Arkansas for Medical Sciences, Little Rock, Arkansas

Brett N. Steenbarger, Ph.D.
Assistant Professor, Department of Psychiatry and Behavioral Sciences, and Director, Student Counseling, State University of New York Upstate Medical University, Syracuse, New York

Anne Stoline, M.D.
Courtesy Staff Psychiatrist, Sheppard Pratt Health System, Towson, Maryland

Richard C. Surles, Ph.D.
Senior Vice President and Executive Director, Division of Medical Information Technology, Comprehensive Neuroscience, White Plains, New York

Carole Szpak
Director of Communications, National Association of Psychiatric Health Systems, Washington, DC

John A. Talbott, M.D.
Professor of Psychiatry, Department of Psychiatry, University of Maryland School of Medicine, Baltimore, Maryland

Allan Tasman, M.D.
Professor and Chair, Department of Psychiatry and Behavioral Sciences, University of Louisville School of Medicine, Louisville, Kentucky

Robert Vadnal, M.D.
Private practice, Colorado; former Chief, Mental Health and Behavioral Medicine, Department of Veterans Affairs Medical Center; former Associate Professor, Department of Psychiatry and Behavioral Sciences, University of Louisville School of Medicine, Louisville, Kentucky

Mark Vanelli, M.D., M.H.S.
Management Consultant, Braun Consulting, Boston, Massachusetts

Laura Van Tosh
Consultant, Van Tosh Consulting, Silver Spring, Maryland

V. Susan Villani, M.D.
Medical Director, Kennedy Krieger School Programs, Kennedy Krieger Institute; Assistant Professor of Psychiatry, Johns Hopkins School of Medicine, Baltimore, Maryland; former Director, Child and Adolescent Psychiatry, Sheppard Pratt Health System, Towson, Maryland

Jonathan S. Wald, M.D., M.P.H.
Associate Director, Clinical Systems Research and Development, Partners Healthcare System, Inc., Chestnut Hill, Massachusetts

Donald H. Williams, M.D.
Professor of Psychiatry, Michigan State University, East Lansing, Michigan

Daniel Yohanna, M.D.
Medical Director, Stone Institute of Psychiatry; Assistant Professor, Northwestern University Medical School, Chicago, Illinois

Introduction

Michael A. Freeman, M.D., D.M.H.

The challenge of introducing the definitive textbook on psychiatric administration at the beginning of the twenty-first century is a daunting one. Like illustrations of the future rendered by artists long ago, the use of books to anticipate the nature of psychiatry and administration may simply be a way of recasting the outgoing metaphors of today into a future that never arrives.

Books may soon be obsolete and replaced by byte-sized interactive infopaks delivered just in time on-line. Similarly, psychiatry as we know it may be headed for the blending blades of the behavioral healthcare new-speak, newthink Osterizer. Finally, administration itself may become an obsolete discipline in the brave new world of empowered and resourced front-line process owners who manage themselves in re-engineered and flattened virtual organizations. So, does it even make sense to write a book about psychiatric administration?

Yes, and this is it. The book you are about to read is the defining statement of the field at the moment, and each section and chapter has been carefully developed to provide today's psychiatric managers and administrators the resources and information they need to succeed in the next few years. Skills required for effectiveness beyond this time horizon may be different as wave after wave of so-called disruptive technologies continue to restructure virtually every aspect of mental health and addiction treatment financing, services, and management.

The hegemony of psychiatry within the behavioral healthcare field has eroded. Our contemporary market recognizes a new discipline, behavioral healthcare, as the all-encompassing field that bridges mental health, addiction treatment, employee assistance, child and family services, social and rehabilitative wraparound services, and behavioral medicine in the primary care setting. To begin a meaningful discussion of the future of psychiatric administration, we must recognize that in the world of healthcare financing and services, the mind is being reconnected to the brain, the brain is being reconnected to the rest of the body, and the net impact of mental health and addictive disorders is being appreciated and addressed in the workplace, the community, and the general medical sector.

As the behavioral healthcare enterprise, and those who are entrusted to manage it, enter the twenty-first century, our mission and mandate remain unchanged: to improve the mental health status and mental health–related quality of life, and to reduce the impact of mental illness and addictive disorders, within individuals and defined populations. However, the choice of methods used to achieve these aims, and the policy framework that is most likely to enable the behavioral health-care field to produce the greatest social benefit, are uncertain. Who will have jobs within the new frame-work, and what those jobs will be, is even less clear.

Psychiatric Administration— Past

The familiar context for modern psychiatric adminis-tration was established in the early 1960s, when the Kennedy administration implemented its community mental health and mental retardation program. Under psychiatric leadership, the community mental health movement structured a plausible and optimistic policy agenda for behavioral healthcare in the United States. Psychiatrists and other professionals entrusted with the stewardship of the field were able to implement new fi-nancing methods and service delivery systems with con-fidence. Remaining state psychiatric hospitals comple-mented new community-based services. Many of these were also managed by psychiatric administrators.

The community mental health movement has come and gone, contributing a rich legacy to succeed-ing generations of organized behavioral healthcare sys-tems (Ray and Finley 1994). A new paradigm, resulting in the need for this book, is emerging largely from the marketplace rather than from the type of sweeping fed-eral legislation that propelled change in the 1960s. The next policy and service delivery framework will be driv-en by these marketplace phenomena, such as managed care, information systems, and consumer empower-ment. The impact of these "disruptive" financing meth-ods, service delivery systems, and technologies is not yet fully understood.

Psychiatric Administration— Future

The first section of this book establishes our current sit-uation with an overview of the field. The remainder of this volume, Sections II–VI, is structured around five central issues to be faced by psychiatric administrators during this period of restructuring in mental health and addiction treatment financing and services. Taken together, these issues represent the framework of de-bate that will guide the evolution of our field and the

uncharted territory on which new behavioral health-care road maps will be drawn.

Core competencies are addressed in Section II. A set of outstanding psychiatric administrators outline or-ganizational theories, leadership requirements, plan-ning models, and information system solutions that work in today's environment. New models of program evaluation and quality management, and innovations in training and human resource development, are also addressed.

Section III addresses the challenge of delivery sys-tem configuration and integrated service delivery. As an acknowledgment that the days of fragmented cost-based or fee-for-service provider settings are over, this section outlines the emerging infrastructure and ad-ministrative challenges of integrated delivery for men-tal health and addiction treatment services. Clearly there will be important roles for psychiatric administra-tors within these systems. This section addresses estab-lishing and maintaining behavioral provider networks and related competencies required for effective opera-tions. Staffing, capitation contracting, and capitated service delivery all fall within this spectrum. Managing outcomes and providing culturally competent services while ensuring confidentiality of increasingly comput-erized medical records are covered as well.

What are the human resource consequences of such dramatic changes? Section IV addresses the new roles that are emerging for behavioral healthcare pro-fessionals. Within that context, the section reviews not only the changing roles of the psychiatrist, administra-tor, and mental health clinician but also the changing roles of consumers and their families. These changes are a key trend in our evolving approach to service de-livery. Consumer empowerment and participation in treatment planning and personal health management will emerge as hallmarks of the consumer-focused healthcare systems of the future, which our markets currently aspire to create.

As fragmentation gives way to integration and as old roles give way to new ones, the traditional settings within which services are rendered must also change. Section V provides a comprehensive overview of behav-ioral healthcare in its current form. This model will re-main largely intact for a few years. Included in the fam-ily of today's behavioral health systems are general medical hospitals, private psychiatric hospitals, the Vet-erans Administration and military services, county mental health departments, child and family service agencies, and community mental health centers. Also included are newer members of this family such as health maintenance organizations (HMOs), physician-hospital organizations, and behavioral group practices. The type of behavioral healthcare portrayed in this section encompasses settings where psychiatric administrators actually work. It does not include the mental health chat rooms of America Online and the emerging consumer-focused world of delivering behavioral health services, for which no Current Procedural Terminology (CPT) code exists in cyberspace rather than in licensed settings.

The legal and ethical challenges faced by psychiatric administration within these new environments and systems are overwhelming. Innovation, science, and the marketplace are running well ahead of the legal and bioethics communities in this regard. Consequently, this volume concludes in Section VI with an important overview of ethics, criminal law, prisons, and civil law issues that pertain to psychiatric administration as we know it today and as we anticipate it tomorrow.

Psychiatric Administration— Reconsidered

Psychiatric administrators currently hold positions in settings that were not even contemplated at the time the last edition of this volume was published. These new environments include online interactive therapeutic communities, interactive consumer information and self-care information companies, work/life companies, and employee assistance programs. They also include the consolidated and institutionalized health maintenance organizations (HMOs) and single-specialty health plans known today as MBHOs (managed behavioral healthcare organizations), as well as the expansive regional integrated delivery systems that now own and operate many of the psychiatric health facilities that formerly functioned independently when the health care system was more fragmented.

The challenges of change and change management are touched upon in every section of this book. When we begin our journey through the chapters that follow, it is incumbent on us to remember that one of our core competencies as psychiatric administrators must be the

ability to welcome and manage change. Once perched at the precipice of society—peering over the edges of the world from a comfortable vantage point behind the couch—psychiatry is now deeply embedded within the fast-paced, technology-enabled socioeconomic setting, which does not tolerate phobia very well.

The six sections of this volume are geared to the real world in which the psychiatric administration of today and tomorrow takes place. In addition to familiar hospitals, clinics, treatment centers, and community mental health centers, these settings include the home of the consumer, reached through the Internet; the workplace, reached through the work/life and employee assistance program; the primary care office, reached through integrated disease-management programs; and the community, reached through new and innovative integrated service delivery systems.

Continuous rapid change can provoke both excitement and fear. Mastering the fear and building upon the excitement will be necessary for the psychiatric administrator of today and tomorrow, because the administrator is frequently required to be the leader of the change process—the skillful skipper who guides the ship through the permanent white water of today's health care environment. Readers of this book are often called upon to identify new opportunities, incorporate clinical and management innovations, redesign organizations and work functions, adjust to new reimbursement models, and find improved ways to meet the needs of people with mental and addictive conditions.

Volume editors John A. Talbott, M.D., and Robert E. Hales, M.D., M.B.A., along with the section editors, the chapter authors, and American Psychiatric Publishing, are proud to bring you this relevant and currently definitive textbook of administrative psychiatry. We are certain that you will benefit from studying this volume.

References

Ray CG, Finley JK: Did CMHCs fail or succeed? Analysis of the expectations and outcomes of the community mental health movement. Administration and Policy in Mental Health 21:4, 1994

❖ Section I ❖

Overview of the Evolving Behavioral Health System

Michael A. Freeman, M.D., D.M.H., Section Editor

Introduction

Michael A. Freeman, M.D., D.M.H.

As the behavioral healthcare enterprise, and those who are entrusted to manage it, enters the twenty-first century, many professionals in the field express a bewildering sense of disorientation. Our mission and mandate remain unchanged: to improve patients' mental health status and mental health–related quality of life and to reduce the effect of mental illness and addictive disorders on individuals and defined populations. However, the choice of methods used to achieve these aims and the policy framework that is most likely to enable the behavioral healthcare field to produce the greatest social benefit are uncertain. Who will have jobs within the new framework, and what those jobs will be, are even less clear.

In the 1960s, when the community mental health movement structured a plausible and optimistic policy agenda for American behavioral healthcare, professionals entrusted with the stewardship of the field implemented new financing methods and service delivery systems with confidence. As today's clinicians, clinician executives, and policymakers alike grapple with the behavioral healthcare challenges faced at the beginning of the new millennium, the next policy framework will once again be driven by disruptive technologies, financing methods, and service delivery systems, whose effects are not yet fully understood (Ray and Finley 1994).

Disruptive Technologies

During the 1990s, a pattern of industrial failure and consolidation, accompanied by massive economic dislocation and layoffs of high-wage, highly skilled employees, has been indelibly etched on the surface of American sensibilities. Harvard Business School Professors Joseph Bower and Clayton Christensen pointed out that Xerox allowed Canon to create the small copier market, Sears eroded as Wal-Mart gained dominance, and IBM and Digital imploded as bootstrap competitors introduced personal computers that made mainframes irrelevant (Bower and Christensen 1995). In a similar manner, the academic behavioral healthcare establishment, the public behavioral healthcare infrastructure, and the commercial behavioral healthcare provider segments face dramatic erosion and, in some instances, have collapsed as managed care plans, integrated delivery systems, and virtual healthcare services have made their core products and operations obsolete.

Why? Extending the logic applied to other industrial sectors, established enterprises that focus on making incremental improvements in operations that are working for the moment may lack the capacity, incentives, or willingness to respond to and incorporate disruptive technologies that can completely undermine the fundamental premises on which the organization relied to add value to its customers.

Several disruptive technologies have had an effect on the behavioral healthcare field simultaneously. For example, the explosive growth of knowledge in behavioral neuroscience and central nervous system pharmacy has made possible a new and better set of diagnostic and therapeutic methods that render much of the pre-existing delivery system obsolete. As a consequence of these disruptive technologies, most conditions that formerly required inpatient hospitalization can now be managed in outpatient settings. In the short-term future, genetic screening and other methods may make it possible for many of these conditions to be detected before an index episode has occurred, and health management strategies may supplant illness management strategies to improve patients' functioning and further reduce episode-driven healthcare use.

Leaders in other industrial segments are learning that they must be true to their customers, not their factories. In today's competitive global economy, senior executives are called on to identify emerging technologies that are likely to restructure their operations or their markets and then to commercialize these disruptive technologies rapidly to continue serving their established customers and to develop new markets (Bower and Christensen 1995). *Investment in disruptive technology is typically unappealing to established enterprises for which the status quo is working and for which the cost structure established by previous investments in existing technologies makes rapid change difficult.* For this reason, the U.S. psychiatric hospital industry (nonprofit and for-profit), which had so much capital invested in the "brick and mortar" that was required for inpatient care, failed to adjust rapidly when a disruptive technology called *managed care* altered the structure of the hospital market during the 1980s and 1990s. Industry erosion with local pockets of collapse and significant economic dislocation resulted.

Mental illness and addictive disorders will not be eradicated any time soon. However, the advent of powerful new financing systems and clinical tools will dramatically improve the ability of the healthcare establishment to render preventive and therapeutic care—if we embrace and harness disruptive technologies instead of restraining them. As we enter the twenty-first century, behavioral healthcare policymakers would be well advised to create market incentives (not regulations) that foster the development and deployment of the most promising of the emerging disruptive technologies to improve the mental health of individuals and

defined populations and to minimize the consequences of mental and addictive disorders.

Value-Based Purchasing Methods

With luck, behavioral healthcare markets of the near future will likely be dominated by consumers who seek value in return for their investment in health care, including mental health and addiction treatment. However, in the absence of an ability to prove value, healthcare consumers will make purchasing decisions based on price. The price-driven purchasing scenario would most likely lead to an incessant continuation of the current downward price pressure experienced by mental health providers and an enterprise-wide death spiral driven by the vast oversupply of mental health clinicians, facilities, health plans, and delivery systems of all kinds.

Value-based purchasing methods can be applied by a new generation of healthcare purchasing agents—the aggregated purchasing pool. Larger than the Fortune 500 "jumbo account" of the commercial marketplace, joint purchasing groups, variously referred to as *business coalitions, healthcare purchasing cooperatives,* and *health purchasing alliances,* are actively translating overall health policy objectives of the constituencies they represent into specifications for the healthcare and behavioral healthcare products they purchase in the open marketplace (Keller 1995; Torchia 1994). Both public and private purchasers leverage their purchasing power through this approach.

One consequence of this new approach to purchasing is the rapid consolidation of the healthcare and the behavioral healthcare marketplace. Economies of scale must be realized if health plans and delivery systems are to remain solvent within the context of reduced funding.

A second, and more promising, consequence is the use of value-based strategies in selecting and renewing healthcare vendors. Standardized measures (report cards) are increasingly used to establish the comparative value of the behavioral healthcare service or delivery system. These methods go beyond current concepts of efficacy and effectiveness to measure performance indicators, such as accessibility and patient satisfaction, as well as impact indicators, such as change in individual and population health status and health-related quality of life per dollar expended (Stephenson and Findlay 1995).

These methods will make consultants, epidemiologists, health economists, and consumers, rather than physicians, the arbiters of value and quality. Data obtained from claims, accreditation agencies, and outcomes measurement systems allow this new generation of health system evaluators to manipulate benefit plan designs and purchasing criteria in order to produce desired results, including cost containment and value enhancement(s) (Umland 1995). In disrupting the former quality ownership structure, the consultants, epidemiologists, health economists, and consumers that judge and guide the acquisition of quality in the emerging value-based purchasing infrastructure promise to incorporate direct and indirect cost measurement, satisfaction, and outcome data into benefit plan designs and incentive systems that yield the best results within.

Disease Management Programs

Value-based purchasing strategies are made possible by the advent of Internet-based consumer health management functionality, organized systems of care, and long-term disease management programs. These disease management programs are disruptive technologies that enable healthcare purchasers to measure total (direct and indirect) cost and outcomes per treated case as an alternative to price per episode, or price per intervention, as the indicator of success within specific disease categories such as depression and schizophrenia (Zalta et al. 1994). Total cost per treated case will decrease as acute episodes, and costly utilization, are prevented and managed.

Various new technology-supported approaches are emerging to prevent or reduce morbidity and the need for acute care. Referred to as *health management, demand management,* and *disease management* systems, these programs integrate self-care, population care methods, early identification and treatment, patient education, pharmacotherapy, and medical care into a patient-centered healthcare protocol (Docherty 1996; Sclar 1995). All of these methods make the current, episode-driven approach to care obsolete. With the general aim of "compressing the morbidity curve" so that acute episodes are prevented as much as possible, and postponed when they cannot be prevented, delivery systems designed to provide excellent acute care will become increasingly ill-matched to emerging healthcare needs.

Of even greater potential import, current advances in gene mapping and in utero detection of predisposition to a widening array of diseases may have unanticipated, or at least unplanned-for, consequences for the behavioral healthcare field and other healthcare systems. What will happen when parents can learn that the embryo they carry is predisposed to a psychiatric condition? Parents who carry a fetus that may develop Down syndrome or sickle cell anemia already have this op-

tion, and the results are instructive for the behavioral healthcare field.

Alternative Services and Service Delivery Systems

Capitated, Computerized, Guideline-Driven Managed Care Systems

Capitation and other new approaches to healthcare financing create incentives for delivery systems, held accountable for defined populations, to invest in prevention and promotion programs that will reduce demand for and use of healthcare in the long run by improving and sustaining health status. Until now, achieving this goal has been elusive. However, the advent of modern information technology, Internet-based consumer health information, computerized medical records, large-scale relational databases, and validated practice guidelines permits previously identified objectives to be achieved (Maloney 1996). The application of competitive financial incentives that motivate consumers to choose their health plan or delivery system on the basis of projected long-term satisfaction and outcome, coupled with consumer empowerment and value-based purchasing strategies used by consolidated commercial and public purchasers, will accelerate the evolution of these systems.

The current growth of information-driven integrated delivery systems is fueled by the new ability to use electronically captured outcomes data to drive clinical process redesign (Bologna and Feldman 1995). Evidence-based approaches to clinical process improvement (Handley and Stuart 1994), resulting in clinical road maps (Teeter and Johnson 1994) that allow disease management systems to be installed within health plans and integrated delivery systems, further remove the mental health clinician from making subjective, moment-to-moment healthcare service decisions. Further accentuating this trend are automated systems for monitoring psychiatric patients (Hunkeler et al. 1995) and computerized artificial intelligence programs that apply expert systems technology to case management and direct clinical care situations (Brown and Kornmayer 1996).

Interactive, Multimedia, Virtual Therapeutic Devices and Services

Although the shift to integrated delivery systems that use disease-management rather than episode-based care is challenging, the future technology horizon promises to be even more disorienting. A whole new generation of interactive and multimedia technologies will make it possible to dramatically redesign and virtualize the process by which healthcare services are delivered. Rather than requiring the patient to come into the environment of the health plan and the provider, it will become increasingly possible to move the healthcare system into the environment of the patient and to make it available on demand. The Celebration Healthcare System in Orlando, Florida, was designed with this concept in mind and installed interactive home health workstations in each house in the community it serves to facilitate the transition to this new model of "virtual healthcare system" (Bezold 1994).

Interactive computer programs already make cognitive therapy available at home, and managed behavioral health plans are now offering a variety of Web-based interactive patient education and "coaching" programs to their members through the Internet. Movie director Steven Spielberg recently launched "Starbright World," a real-time, on-line, interactive virtual playground for severely ill children. This application of virtual reality in real medical settings connects children's hospitals around the country through a system that replaces some current behavioral healthcare functions championed by play therapists and consultation-liaison psychiatrists. Mental health clinicians already have begun to use virtual reality headsets to help patients with acrophobia reduce their fear of heights through graded exposure exercises (Rothbaum et al. 1995). Telemedicine services that use interactive video systems make psychiatric diagnosis and treatment planning available in remote locations (Baer et al. 1995). Medical self-care CD-ROM and Internet products enjoy vast popularity, and interactivity allows for the automation of many behavioral healthcare service functions that were formerly provided by people. Interactive, multimedia, virtual technology applications in healthcare, and in behavioral healthcare, have a significant potential to reduce costs, improve patient satisfaction, expand access, and improve outcomes.

Toward a Twenty-First-Century Behavioral Healthcare Enterprise

At the end of the nineteenth century, Sigmund Freud proposed that mental health could be equated with the ability to work and to love. As we enter the new millennium, these concepts have been replaced by more measurable objectives such as functioning at one's highest level in the workplace, the family, and the community and enjoying the highest achievable behavioral health-related quality of life. Fortunately for the poets among us, love has not yet been operationalized and quantified. However, it is understood that having loved ones remains a compelling behavioral health objective because such relationships serve as a powerful protective factor against morbidity and mortality from many causes and therefore confer a "medical offset effect."

When paradigms change, stakeholders in the previous paradigm risk losing their stake in the paradigms that follow. The behavioral healthcare field has entered a period of multiple simultaneous paradigm shifts. Within this context, the challenge for administrators and managers is to resist the temptation to obstruct the implementation of disruptive technologies in response to the urgent need to not be displaced. As the experience of other industrial sectors has shown, disruptive technologies will be implemented anyway. Today's behavioral healthcare leaders are uniquely positioned to guide the implementation and orchestration of these technologies, so that the entire behavioral healthcare enterprise can evolve in the direction it should go rather than where it otherwise may. In this way, we can deploy disruptive technologies to assist our efforts to achieve the overarching ideal of sustaining healthy people in a healthy world (McNerney et al. 1992) within an outcomes-driven context of quality and accountability in behavioral healthcare (O'Kane and Rickel 1995).

References

Baer L, Cukor P, Jenike MA, et al: Pilot studies of telemedicine for patients with obsessive-compulsive disorder. Am J Psychiatry 152(9), 1995

Bezold C: Mental health services in the 21st century: challenges and vision (editorial). Behavioral Healthcare Tomorrow 3(5):88, 1994

Bologna NC, Feldman MI: Using outcomes data and clinical process redesign: improving clinical services. Behavioral Healthcare Tomorrow 4(6):59–64, 1995

Bower JL, Christensen CM: Disruptive technologies: catching the wave. Harvard Business Review, January–February, 1995

Brown GS, Kornmayer K: Expert systems restructure managed care practice: implementation and ethics. Behavioral Healthcare Tomorrow 5(1):31–34, 1996

Casano K: Multimedia interactive video program as adjunct to cognitive therapy. Psychiatric Times, November 1995

Docherty IP: Disease management strategy: initiative links pharmaceutical and mental health data. Behavioral Healthcare Tomorrow 5(1):51–53, 1996

England MJ: Perspective: mental health care: buyers take the lead. Business & Health, January 1991

Handley MR, Stuart ME: An evidence-based approach to evaluating and improving clinical practice: guideline development. HMO Practice 8(1), 1994

Hunkeler EM, Westphal JR, Williams M: Developing a system for automated monitoring of psychiatric outpatients: a first step to improve quality. HMO Practice 9(4), 1995

Keller J: Business coalition initiatives related to behavioral healthcare purchasing and quality improvement. Behavioral Healthcare Tomorrow 4(4):49–52, 1995

Lewis PH: Virtual spaces find a niche in real medicine. The New York Times, June 1995

Maloney WR: How information systems are opening the way for integrated healthcare (editorial). Behavioral Healthcare Tomorrow 5(1):76, 1996

McNerney W, Bezold C, Lec DR, et al: Healthy People in a Healthy World: The Belmont Vision for Health Care in America. Alexandria, VA, Institute for Alternative Futures, 1992

O'Kane ME, Rickel ALJ: Quality and accountability as imperatives in managed behavioral healthcare. Behavioral Healthcare Tomorrow 4(5):79–80, 1995

Ray CG, Finley JK: Did CMHCs fail or succeed? Analysis of the expectations and outcomes of the community mental health movement. Adm Policy Ment Health 21(4), 1994

Rothbaum BO, Hodges LI, Kooper R, et al: Effectiveness of computer-generated (virtual reality) graded exposure in the treatment of acrophobia. Am J Psychiatry 152(4):626–628, 1995

Sclar D: Disease state management: an overview for the managed care pharmacist. Drug Benefit Trends, August 1995

Stephenson GM, Findlay S: Hedis: almost ready for prime time. Business & Health, March 1995

Teeter DF, Johnson RE: The roadmap for clinical quality. HMO Practice 8(1), 1994

Torchia NI: How twin cities employers are reshaping health care by forming an integrated system of care. Business & Health, February 1994

Umland B: Behavioral healthcare benefit strategies of self-insured employers. Behavioral Healthcare Tomorrow 4(6):67–72, 1995

Zalta E, Bichner H, Henry M: Implications of disease management in the future of managed care. Medical Interface, December 1994

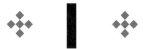

The Private Sector

History, Current Status, and Future Implications

Gary L. Gottlieb, M.D., M.B.A.

Derri L. Shtasel, M.D., M.P.H.

The nearly 250-year evolution of private sector psychiatric services in the United States reflects critical changes in American society, the development of general health services delivery, and the emergence of scientific methods in clinical practice (Alexander and Selesnick 1966; Grob 1994; Romano 1994). During the twentieth century, these elements have been influenced remarkably by changes in mechanisms of payment for healthcare services (Goldman and Frank 1990; Gottlieb 1996). Interactions among social need and tolerance, science, prevailing government policy, and economic imperatives have determined the current status of private sector psychiatric services. Not unlike in the general health services sector, these factors created a large, capital-rich, and institutionally based system of psychiatric services delivery (Starr 1984). The reconfiguration and rationalization of services that we are experiencing now has devalued some of those roots, creating upheaval in the private sector and imperiling some of its venerable history. As in the past, however, economic factors and scientific advances are catalyzing innovation, encouraging entrepreneurial activity and the application of new

scientific methods. An understanding of the historical context of private sector psychiatric services is essential to deriving opportunity from the perceived challenges of the current and future marketplace.

Eighteenth and Nineteenth Centuries

Private sector psychiatry was born in a colonial America fraught with economic uncertainty and built on the shoulders of European religious oppression (Alexander and Selesnick 1966; Grob 1994; Perloff 1994). The relatively mysterious nature of medical and behavioral disorders and an absence of successful interventions drove colonial Americans, like their European counterparts, to hide, isolate, or imprison psychiatrically ill people. However, the unpleasant conditions in public almshouses, prisons, and cellars of private homes became increasingly socially unacceptable (Thompson 1994). Focused on the social injustice and inhumanity of this care, members of the Religious Society of Friends, who helped to found the Pennsylvania Hospital in 1752, included care of the insane as a critical component of the medical services provided in America's first general hospital (Bell 1980; Deutsch 1949). While mentally ill patients continued to be treated with shackles and other forms of severe mechanical restraint, a more humane approach to care was adopted. Benjamin Rush's leadership brought only modest improvement to treatment at Pennsylvania Hospital. Although he endorsed improved staff, activity programs, and isolation of more violent patients, corporal punishment and mechanical restraints remained the mainstays of treatment (Binger 1966; Thompson 1994).

Moved by the atrocities of Bedlam and similar European institutions, William Tuke became the architect of the era of "moral treatment" (Grob 1994; Perloff 1994). Through his leadership in the development of the York Retreat in England and the adaptation of moral treatment to the American Friends Asylum in Philadelphia, Pennsylvania, the private sector became the foundation for radical change in psychiatric care. Environmental approaches to treatment, including the use of open spaces, inviting grounds, and rehabilitation programs and the elimination of extreme methods of restraint or punishment, characterized a group of pioneering private psychiatric hospitals founded in the first half of the nineteenth century. These include the McLean Asylum of Massachusetts in Boston, Bloomingdale Asylum in New York City, the Hartford and Brattleboro Retreats in New England, Sheppard and Enoch Pratt Hospital in Baltimore, Maryland, and the Institute of Pennsylvania Hospital in Philadelphia.

A design for humane conditions for psychiatric treatment, replicated in public and private institutions throughout the United States, was derived from Thomas Kirkbride's creation of the Pennsylvania Hospital for the Insane, later to become the Institute of Pennsylvania Hospital (Romano 1994). The introduction of an environment that could support the notion of moral treatment at a time when few, if any, rational somatic interventions were available set the stage for the construction of large asylums for people with mental illness. Leadership of the private sector, and its commitment to humane approaches to care, helped to fuel Dorothea Dix's movement to improve services in the public sector (Thompson 1994). Her efforts led to government investment in state-sponsored hospitals to care for indigent people with mental illness. Care in private sector institutions was limited to those with the ability to pay or, in some cases, to members of the Quaker community (Perloff 1994).

The parallel development of the general health services system encouraged the growth of large institutions with substantial infrastructure. Epidemics of infectious disease in the late eighteenth and nineteenth centuries created the need for large urban hospital centers to provide isolation and supportive care to afflicted individuals (Starr 1984). Increasingly, private sector psychiatric services and asylums developed with emerging general hospital services. For example, like the Pennsylvania Hospital (and the later Institute), the McLean Asylum of Massachusetts and the Massachusetts General Hospital were founded simultaneously. The mission of caring for both the sick and the insane garnered increasing support.

Early Twentieth Century

The growth of state-funded psychiatric institutions was ultimately accompanied by a deterioration in care and a general hopelessness about outcome (Deutsch 1949; Grob 1994). Despite an explosion of science in pathology, infectious disease, and management of medical illnesses, institutional psychiatric care had made little progress. Within the profession, the pressure was increasing to reintegrate psychiatric services with general healthcare and to exploit the emerging emphasis on medical education and science to advance psychiatric treatment.

In 1902, the first psychiatric unit in a general hospital was opened in Albany, New York. Unlike its freestanding counterparts, the ward was used to care for more acute or transitory conditions. The marriage of medical science and psychiatric treatment was further reinforced in 1906, through the opening of the first university hospital for the treatment of psychiatric disorders at the University of Michigan. The academic nature of private psychiatric care became mainstream when, in 1912, Adolph Meyer became the director of the newly established Henry Phipps Clinic at the Johns Hopkins School of Medicine in Baltimore, Maryland (Grob 1994). These events changed the nature of private psychiatric care and continued to reinforce the growth of large institutions. These efforts were strengthened by an evolving vernacular of psychiatric medicine and science. A growing descriptive phenomenology and categorization of illness led by Emil Kraepelin and Eugen Bleuler and Freud's influence in the introduction of psychoanalytic approaches to care began to transform private sector psychiatric services in freestanding and general hospital settings. Large inpatient facilities were enhanced by outpatient and community clinics fostered by the therapeutic optimism associated with new science (Bell 1980; Grob 1994; Thompson 1994).

From 1918 through the 1930s, various somatic interventions showed some effectiveness in controlling behaviors, particularly in violent patients. Both general hospital and freestanding psychiatric facilities availed themselves of new technologies, including hypoglycemic therapy, pharmacological convulsive therapy, electroconvulsive treatment, and psychosurgery (Alexander and Selesnick 1966). These interventions allowed some patients with very long hospital stays to return to less supervised or community settings. The advent of these treatments forced private sector psychiatry to become more focused on acute care. Over the course of the early to mid–twentieth century, freestanding institutions became more heterogeneous: they continued to provide asylum for those with persistent illnesses but began to offer treatments associated with more favorable outcomes, creating more patient turnover and shorter lengths of stay.

Mid–Twentieth Century

As the public sector began to flourish through a mental hygiene movement that expanded the continuum of available mental health services to include ambulatory care, aftercare, and social services, the private sector enjoyed the growth of private practice psychiatry and psychology (Deutsch 1949; Grob 1994; Thompson 1994). Simultaneously, World War II moved psychiatry into the mainstream of public consciousness: psychiatrists participated in the screening process for draftees in the U.S. Selective Service system, the prevalence of new-onset psychoses in people of military induction age became obvious to authorities, and the importance of stress as a contributor to neuropsychiatric illness became evident throughout society. The ability of psychiatry to ameliorate some of the symptoms of mental illness and return soldiers to the battlefield or safely home inspired Congress to enact the National Mental Health Act in 1946 (Romano 1994).

The National Mental Health Act provided funding for psychiatric education and research. The act instantaneously expanded the magnitude of private sector psychiatric services. The development of a vast academic infrastructure moved general hospital psychiatry to the forefront and enhanced freestanding psychiatric hospitals and programs. The number of trained psychiatrists in the community increased from approximately 2 per 100,000 population in the 1930s to about 14 per 100,000 in the early 1990s (Romano 1994). This allowed for the expansion of private practice, access to psychiatrists in community and academic general hospitals, and demand for psychiatric inpatient beds.

A tension between the growth of psychoanalysis as a treatment approach and the evolution of neuropharmacology grew with the funding of the National Institute of Mental Health and the National Institutes of Health. Controversies regarding treatment grew as rapidly as treatment options. While evidence of the demonstrable efficacy of psychiatric treatments was slowly increasing, huge variations in practice among psychiatrists and psychologists created worrisome doubts among general healthcare providers, the public, and newly influential entities, health insurance companies (Gottlieb 1989).

The availability of indemnity insurance for catastrophic medical illness started to grow through the organized labor movement of the early twentieth century. However, employment-based insurance did not grow remarkably until the advent of the community-rated Blue Cross Blue Shield plans in the late 1930s and 1940s (Starr 1984). During and after the Depression, health insurance helped to consolidate some of the hospital resources that were available and to make more expensive care available to most individuals and families. Because of insurers' fear of the need for open-ended, long-term care for chronic disabilities, psychiatric care and treatment of tuberculosis were excluded from private insurance programs. In 1954 Blue Cross Blue Shield plans nationally shifted their policies to include acute treatment for psychiatric disorders, particularly in general hospital settings (Sharfstein 1990). This reinforced active treatment for acute illness and spawned the development of inpatient psychiatric services in small and mid-sized hospitals and large academic medical centers. Combined with the growth of electroconvulsive therapy use and the advent of antipsychotic and antidepressant treatments in the 1950s and lithium carbonate in the mid-1960s, general hospital settings became the dominant location of acute inpatient care (Goldman et al. 1987).

Over the course of the 1960s, insurance coverage for psychiatric services proliferated through the growth of commercial indemnity insurance companies. Simultaneously, training and research resources available from the National Institute of Mental Health and infrastructure investment provided by the Hill-Burton Act and tax-free financing fueled the growth of a large private sector delivery system, dominated by psychiatric care in general hospital settings (Goldman et al. 1987; Grob 1994). The availability of acute care in general hospital psychiatric services and the optimism associated with active psychiatric treatments eroded the length of stay in freestanding psychiatric hospitals. As the demand for greater efficiency and acuity of care in freestanding hospitals increased and the number of commercial payers grew, an increasing number of proprietary, investor-owned psychiatric hospitals emerged (Dorwart and Schlesinger 1988; McCue and Clement 1993; Salmon 1985). Commercial and Blue Cross policies limited the number of days and episodes of treatment covered annually or in a beneficiary's lifetime, but access to insurance increased hospital admissions and days substantially (Redick et al. 1996).

Reimbursement for acute psychiatric services expanded markedly in 1965. On July 1, 1966, under Title XVIII of the Social Security Act, the federal government launched Medicare as a social insurance program first designed to provide medical care benefits for people older than 65 (Gottlieb 1996). In 1972 the program was expanded to include younger disabled people. Medicare improved access to private psychiatric services for a huge segment of the American population. Medicare's retrospective cost-based reimbursement design encouraged the development of resource-intensive services. It also reimbursed a portion of capital outlays and debt service, reinforcing the growth of infrastructure. However, Medicare's relatively discriminatory benefit design encouraged the use of general hospital psychiatric services over freestanding psychiatric hospitals: the lifetime benefit for freestanding hospital care was limited to 190 days (Goldman et al. 1987; Gottlieb 1996).

Deinstitutionalization of psychiatric patients from state-run facilities led to numerous older and disabled people eligible for Medicare with newfound insurance for acute psychiatric services. The private sector rapidly readied itself to provide more intensive services for shorter durations. General hospitals and freestanding psychiatric facilities developed specialty programs for older adults to attract Medicare funding to their services. Cost-based reimbursement made general hospital psychiatric services attractive to private hospital administrators because overhead, debt service, and capital costs could be captured. Services catering to employed people and their families with Blue Cross and commercial insurances made operating margins easily achievable (American Psychiatric Association 1986; Goldman et al. 1987; McCue and Clement 1993; Redick et al. 1996).

In 1965 Congress also enacted Medicaid. This social insurance program was designed to pay for medical care for indigent Americans through a state and federal matching program (Gottlieb 1996). The introduction of Medicaid had several effects on private sector psychiatry: Medicaid precluded federally funded reimbursement for psychiatric services in so-called institutions for the mentally disabled. Therefore, most states prevented Medicaid beneficiaries from receiving reimbursement for their care in freestanding psychiatric facilities. However, Medicaid did reimburse psychiatric care provided in general hospitals and the long-term care of medically indigent people (American Psychiatric Association 1986). Therefore, private sector nursing homes became the beneficiaries of substantial Medicaid funding for deinstitutionalized psychiatric patients who were disabled and in need of intermediate or skilled nursing supervision. States could shift their costs from state-funded hospitals to Medicaid-funded nursing homes, which were approximately 60% supported by the federal government (Goldman et al. 1986).

The explosion of available indemnity insurance changed the nature of private sector psychiatric services. Long-term psychiatric patients who could pay for their services stayed in private freestanding psychiatric hospitals. Freestanding hospitals also provided acute, short-term care for patients with Medicare, Blue Cross, and commercial indemnity insurances. Medicaid patients were not accepted in these settings because of the institutions for the mentally disabled exclusion (except in some states where state governments paid the federal share).

General hospital psychiatric services became the mainstay of acute psychiatric treatment, serving all payers. By 1981, general hospitals received about 63% of all Medicare expenditures for psychiatric services, and they were responsible for about 35% of all inpatient episodes of psychiatric care (Goldman et al. 1987). Ambulatory psychiatric services expanded greatly, and the number of psychiatrists and psychologists in private practice grew extensively. However, insurance coverage for these services was generally unavailable or limited to levels far below those generally required for even the most short-term care (Sharfstein et al. 1993).

Private sector nursing homes became new sites for the care of severely and persistently mentally ill people, largely through the Medicaid system (Goldman et al. 1986). Inasmuch as people with dementia no longer had access to state psychiatric facilities, substantial evidence began to emerge that nursing homes were becoming the de facto long-term psychiatric facilities for the older adults of the late twentieth century (Burns et al. 1988).

Late Twentieth Century

The simultaneous expansion of indemnity insurance and science and technology fueled enormous growth in national healthcare expenditures. As the proportion of gross domestic product attributable to healthcare expenditures grew, policymakers and employers became increasingly concerned with the economic effects of healthcare inflation (Sharfstein et al. 1993). Coupled with massive reductions in personal and business taxes, the earliest acts of the Reagan administration included substantial reform to hospital payments under Medicare (Gottlieb 1996).

The Tax Equity and Fiscal Responsibility Act of 1982 (TEFRA) was an effort to convert the cost-based retrospective reimbursement incentives of the Medicare system to a more efficient prospective payment system. TEFRA emphasized cost containment, providing limits for inpatient hospital operating costs. The prospective payment system is based on a discharge classification system that uses diagnosis-related groups (DRGs) to cluster patients who presumably require similar care. Under TEFRA, hospitals are paid a predetermined amount for each case consistent with the assigned DRG, independent of the actual costs incurred. Therefore, payment is an incentive for efficient use of resources. If patients use extraordinary resources or require prolonged inpatient care, they are classified as "outliers," and Medicare provides additional payments but at a rate considerably less than the actual cost (English et al. 1986; Frank and Lave 1985; Gottlieb 1996).

Fourteen of the DRGs apply to discharges related to treatment of psychiatric and substance abuse disorders. Concerns about the ability of DRGs to predict resource consumption for psychiatric disorders accurately led to DRG exemption for freestanding psychiatric hospitals and for distinct general hospital psychiatric units. The treatment of psychiatric patients in "scatter" beds on general medical and surgical units is reimbursed through the DRG system (English et al. 1986; Goldman et al. 1987; Gottlieb 1996).

Most psychiatric services continue to be paid retrospectively by Medicare. However, TEFRA modified and limited these reimbursements. Medicare reimbursement for treatment in psychiatric sites is capped at a target rate established for each facility based on resource use during a base year (the first full fiscal year of operation after October 1, 1983). If the per-case cost exceeds the target rate, the hospital must absorb the loss. If the cost is less than the TEFRA rate, the hospital receives an incentive, retaining 50% of the difference up to 5% of the target rate.

TEFRA exemptions created the opportunity for general hospitals to continue to retain a cost-based reimbursement service in psychiatry while developing greater efficiencies for their nonpsychiatric services. Although foresight inspired the development of a better continuum of psychiatric resources, investment in the broad spectrum of ambulatory services was more limited than in general healthcare.

Through the 1980s, the increase in funding available through equity funding for for-profits and debt financing, especially for nonprofits, provided for infrastructure expansion supported by continued Medicare cost-based reimbursement (Goldman et al. 1987; Redick et al. 1996). Equity markets fueled the expansion of investor-owned psychiatric and for-profit general hospital chains (Dorwart and Schlesinger 1988; McCue and Clement 1993; Salmon 1985). The growth of these chains created efficient service delivery and national negotiating clout for purchasing and contracting.

Federal legislation continued to prioritize reduction of available resources and slowing of healthcare inflation. The Omnibus Budget Reconciliation Act of 1987 (OBRA-87) (Public Law 100-203) and its nursing home reform provisions curtailed accessibility of nursing homes to people with active psychiatric diagnoses. This act created a series of regulations to improve active treatment of psychiatric symptoms in nursing home settings and to control the use of psychotropic agents. The Omnibus Budget Reconciliation Act of 1989 (OBRA-89) (H.R. 3299 Report 101-386) expanded the outpatient benefit for psychiatric services under Medicare, eliminating the annual dollar limit for outpatient mental health services and allowing direct reimbursement for psychologists and social workers. However, OBRA-89 developed a uniform fee schedule for all Part B Medicare providers and curtailed annual growth in these fees. OBRA-89 also limited the fees that could be charged to Medicare beneficiaries by providers who did not participate in the Medicare program.

These changes in government reimbursement policies fueled much more dramatic private sector approaches to reduce healthcare expenditures. The most extreme of these outcomes was a national transition from indemnity insurance to even greater controls to resource consumption through managed care. Although provisions to encourage employers to offer health insurance through health maintenance organizations (HMOs) were enacted in 1972, a major migration to managed care did not accelerate notably until the early 1990s (Iglehart 1992). Diminished access to psychiatric care through the use of intensive precertification of services and utilization review accelerated in the late 1980s and early 1990s (Sharfstein et al. 1993).

The increase in these controls had many effects. The percentage of commercial health insurance premiums attributable to behavioral health services declined from approximately 6.1% in 1988 to 3.1% in 1996 (Hay Group 1998). The demand for inpatient services diminished, and the reduction in inpatient admissions was exaggerated by decreased lengths of stay. Private sector psychiatric services expanded the availability of ambulatory, partial hospital, in-home, and services in residential facilities to substitute for inpatient care and to provide rapidly accessible aftercare. However, total outpatient encounters also have decreased (Hay Group 1998). Excess capacity is particularly acute in general hospital inpatient services, in which lower pricing is inadequate to offset high overhead costs. Increased penetration of managed care among Medicare recipients has reduced the proportion of cost-based reimbursed episodes of care (Redick et al. 1996). Private sector academic health centers have endured substantial negative effects from reduced reimbursement as indirect and direct medical education reimbursements are threatened by substitution of managed care for Medicare, Blue Cross, and Medicaid (Iglehart 1994, 1998a).

The marketplace clout of vast for-profit managed care organizations has driven down revenues derived from inpatient services (Frank et al. 1995; Hay Group 1998; Ma and McGuire 1998). The size of for-profit psychiatric chains has grown, and their dominance in freestanding private psychiatric service delivery has increased through access to less expensive capital and economies of size and geography (McCue and Clement 1993). Additionally, vertical integration of for-profit

psychiatric services with for-profit managed care organizations has enhanced their market strength. Nonprofit freestanding psychiatric hospitals, hampered by higher cost structures, debt service, and mission-driven values (McCue and Clement 1993), have had difficulty in their ability to compete; institutions that are more than a century and a half old have been downsized, acquired, and closed.

New models of care have begun to emerge. Larger academic health systems that continue to have local market share dominance have been able to sustain some stability in pricing. The growth of managed Medicaid has made freestanding psychiatric services more accessible to indigent populations, and their programs can be partnered with community mental health providers to provide a continuum of more efficient resources for severely and persistently mentally ill people. In larger systems of care, vertical integration of service delivery and insurance risk is allowing psychiatric services to be "carved in," integrating behavioral health with medical-surgical benefits. This may allow the traditional relationships among primary care physicians, psychiatrists, and other specialists to remain intact. In this scenario, private sector psychiatry has the advantage of becoming closer to the mainstream of general healthcare. It has the potential to show its benefits to primary care through greater accessibility and potential cost offsets to general medical conditions.

The private healthcare delivery sector has been scrutinized carefully by government law enforcement agencies regarding appropriateness of treatment, provider-induced demand, and fraud and abuse in the Medicare program (Iglehart 1998b). Increasing federal vigilance and regulatory changes have created internal compliance programs that include behavioral healthcare. The more intensive regulatory environment has stemmed the growth of alternative treatment activities, including Medicare-funded partial hospital and in-home services.

Medicare payment reform, intended to balance the federal budget, has reduced payment for psychiatric services disproportionately. A maximum TEFRA limit set at approximately the 75th percentile of national rates was imposed for the first fiscal year starting after October 1, 1997. Also, incentive payments were eliminated for providers whose costs are below their limit (Hospital Association of Pennsylvania 1997). These changes were not phased in and, therefore, had to be absorbed by providers instantaneously. These changes likely will create further disincentives for general hospitals to maintain their psychiatric programs. They also will imperil freestanding psychiatric facilities, particularly nonprofits, whose higher cost structure benefited from higher TEFRA limits.

Simultaneously, the Healthcare Financing Administration granted waivers to numerous states to allow Medicaid populations to be fully managed; outcomes have been variable. However, they have been universally successful in reducing total inpatient days and overall prices (Ma and McGuire 1998). Although these programs have improved accessibility to freestanding psychiatric services where traditional Medicaid had been proscriptive, pricing in state-run carve-out programs is generally below the costs of urban academic health systems that provide the bulk of this care. Similarly, state and federal welfare reform has increased the proportion of uninsured people who do not have demonstrable disability. These reforms affect people with mental illness and substance abuse disorders who often have difficulty proving their inability to work. The burden of this uninsured population threatens nonprofits and large urban centers required to provide their care (Olfson and Mechanic 1996).

The Future

Recent changes in social policy and advances in science suggest that the capital infrastructure required to provide psychiatric care will be less intensive. Private psychiatric resources have the opportunity to thrive because their specialty focus allows innovation and flexibility responsive to the needs of the populations that they must serve. As the current managed cost environment shifts to greater management of care, private psychiatric services that are integrated with large systems can provide holistic care with incremental efficiency.

Mainstream health services must have instantaneous access to psychiatric resources:

- Psychiatric services must be located on site or adjacent to primary care.
- Psychiatric programs must be totally accessible to crisis services in the community and in the general hospital.
- Psychiatrists must reach out into acute and general medical populations in general hospitals, nursing homes, and community health centers.
- Psychiatrists must provide an integrated continuum of services that is managed to the least restrictive

alternative but most appropriate level of care for a given level of acuity of illness.

Integration with general health services provides the opportunity for prevention. Prevention can evolve through new models of employee assistance programming, primary healthcare, and outreach.

The private sector provides the perfect opportunity for flexible partnering. Public and private partnerships will enhance the quality of technology and labor force accessible to traditionally public sector programs. Academic partnerships will reinvent the classroom to teach future providers, and they will create health services and clinical, epidemiological, and translational research opportunities. Both kinds of partnerships will allow psychiatric programs to become beta sites for government and private sector demonstration programs.

On behalf of the public, policymakers must determine how to allocate tax dollars and tax-shielded healthcare premium dollars. For-profit insurers, managed care companies, and hospital systems have become the objects of regulation and investigation (Iglehart 1998b). The public is increasingly concerned about the effects of the pressures imposed by publicly traded companies on healthcare quality and moral values. Increasing regulation will make the market less attractive to for-profit insurers, inhibiting growth and share price.

A future in the service of the populations that we must serve and our values as providers depend on the expansion of research on service delivery and population needs. Much of the erosion in expenditure for behavioral health services has resulted from long-standing fears of the "moral hazard" associated with insurance for psychiatric care (Sharfstein 1990). Moral hazard suggests that providers or beneficiaries will use insurance benefits because of dishonesty, lack of judgment, or an innate desire to maximize personal welfare. We have expected for too long that people will have access to psychiatric services because they are "necessary," without evidence of the outcomes of our efforts. We must continue to invest in prospective research that advances access to state-of-the-art somatic treatments and psychotherapies while confirming their effectiveness in the community and in settings that are relevant to the needs of society.

Moral treatment was the genesis of private sector psychiatry. A research agenda and policy mandate that supports quality services and the least restrictive alternative for appropriate care is the moral imperative for our future.

References

Alexander FG, Selesnick ST: The History of Psychiatry. New York, Harper & Row, 1966

American Psychiatric Association, Office of Economic Affairs: The Coverage Catalog. Washington, DC, American Psychiatric Association, 1986

Bell LV: Treating the Mentally Ill From Colonial Times to the Present. New York, Praeger, 1980

Binger C: Revolutionary Doctor: Benjamin Rush, 1746–1813. New York, WW Norton, 1966

Burns BJ, Larson DB, Goldstrom ID, et al: Mental disorders among nursing home patients: preliminary findings from the National Nursing Home Survey Pretest. Int J Geriatr Psychiatry 3:27–35, 1988

Deutsch A: The Mentally Ill in America: A History of Their Care and Treatment From Colonial Times. New York, Columbia University Press, 1949

Dorwart RA, Schlesinger M: Privatization of psychiatric services. Am J Psychiatry 145:543–553, 1988

English JT, Sharfstein SS, Scherl DJ, et al: Diagnosis related groups and general hospital psychiatry: the APA Study. Am J Psychiatry 143:131–139, 1986

Frank RG, Lave JL: The psychiatric DRG's: are they different? Med Care 23:1148–1155, 1985

Frank R, McGuire TG, Newhouse JP: Risk contracts in managed mental health care. Health Aff (Millwood) 14:50–64, 1995

Goldman HH, Frank RG: Division of responsibility among payors, in Mental Health Policy for Older Americans: Protecting Minds at Risk. Edited by Fogel BS, Furino A, Gottlieb GL. Washington, DC, American Psychiatric Press, 1990, pp 85–95

Goldman HH, Feder J, Scanlon W: Chronic mental patients in nursing homes: reexamining data from the National Nursing Home Study. Hosp Community Psychiatry 37:269–272, 1986

Goldman HH, Taube CA, Jencks SF: The organization of the psychiatric services system. Med Care 25 (9, suppl):S6–S21, 1987

Gottlieb G: Diversity, uncertainty and variations in practice: the behaviors and clinical decision making of mental health care providers, in The Future of Mental Health Services Research (DHHS Publ No ADM-89-1600). Edited by Taube CA, Mechanic D, Homan AA. Washington, DC, U.S. Government Printing Office, 1989, pp 225–251

Gottlieb GL: Financial issues, in Comprehensive Review of Geriatric Psychiatry—II, 2nd Edition. Edited by Sadavoy J, Lazarus LW, Jarvik LF, et al. Washington, DC, American Psychiatric Press, 1996, pp 1065–1085

Grob GN: The Mad Among Us: A History of the Care of America's Mentally Ill. New York, Free Press, 1994

Hay Group: Health Care Plan Design and Cost Trends—1988 Through 1997. Document prepared for the National Association of Psychiatric Health Systems, Association of Behavioral Group Practices and National Alliance for Mentally Ill, 1998

Hospital Association of Pennsylvania (HAP): HAP Analysis of House, Senate and Budget Agreement on Medicare Budget Proposals, 1997. Document prepared by Hospital Association of Pennsylvania, 1997

Iglehart JK: Health policy report: the American health care system. N Engl J Med 327:1467–1472, 1992

Iglehart JK: Rapid changes for academic medical centers. N Engl J Med 331:1391–1394, 1994

Iglehart JK: Medicare and graduate medical education. N Engl J Med 338:402–407, 1998a

Iglehart JK: Pursuing health care fraud and abuse (editorial). Health Aff (Millwood) 17:6, 1998b

Ma CA, McGuire TG: Costs and incentives in a behavioral health carve-out. Health Aff (Millwood) 17:53–69, 1998

McCue MJ, Clement JP: Relative performance of for-profit psychiatric hospitals in investor-owned systems and non-profit psychiatric hospitals. Am J Psychiatry 150:77–82, 1993

Olfson M, Mechanic D: Mental disorders in public, private, non-profit and proprietary general hospitals. Am J Psychiatry 153:1613–1619, 1996

Perloff CB: The Asylum: The History of Friends Hospital and the Quaker Contribution to Psychiatry. Philadelphia, PA, Friends Hospital, 1994

Redick RW, Witkin MJ, Atay JE, et al: Highlights of organized mental health services in 1992 and major national and state trends, in Center for Mental Health Services: Mental Health United States, 1996 (DHHS Publ No SMA 96-3098). Edited by Manderscheid RW, Sonneschein MA. Washington, DC, U.S. Government Printing Office, 1996, pp 90–111

Romano J: Reminiscences: 1938 and since (c. 1990). Am J Psychiatry 151 (6, sesquicentennial suppl):83–89, 1994

Salmon JW: Profit and health care: trends in corporatization and proprietization. Int J Health Serv 15:395–418, 1985

Sharfstein SS: Payment for services: a provider's perspective, in Mental Health Policy for Older Americans: Protecting Minds at Risk. Edited by Fogel BS, Furino A, Gottlieb GL. Washington, DC, American Psychiatric Press, 1990, pp 97–107

Sharfstein SS, Stalin AM, Goldman HH: Psychiatric care and health insurance reform. Am J Psychiatry 150:7–18, 1993

Starr P: The Social Transformation of American Medicine. New York, Basic Books, 1984

Thompson JW: Trends in the development of psychiatric services, 1844–1994. Hosp Community Psychiatry 45:987–992, 1994

❖ 2 ❖

The Evolving Behavioral Health System: The Public Sector

Past, Present, and Future

Lisa Dixon, M.D., M.P.H.
Susan Ridgely, M.S.W., J.D.
Howard Goldman, M.D., Ph.D.

The role of the public sector in organizing, financing, and delivering alcohol, drug, and mental health (ADM) services is changing dramatically. In this chapter we review key aspects of the past and present role of the public sector in providing care for persons with mental illness and discuss important questions for the future. Although the public sector has assumed the clear role of funding care for the poor and persons with severe mental illness, this history reveals a gradual blurring of the public sector/private sector dichotomy in how these services are organized and provided. Psychiatric administrators must understand all of these historical trends in order to lead their institutions successfully into the future.

In this chapter we focus primarily on the funding and delivery of services for adults with severe and persistent mental illness, with some discussion of addiction services. Categories of publicly funded behavioral healthcare beneficiaries that are beyond the scope of this chapter include child mental health and child welfare, criminal justice, mental retardation and developmental disability, and Medicare.

The public cost of providing behavioral healthcare services is considerable, demanding the focus of psychiatric administrators. According to estimates prepared by Frank and associates (1994) for President Clinton's Health Care Reform Task Force, the annual direct costs for ADM services in 1990 were $42.4 billion. Public expenditures derive from state and local government general revenues (almost 28%), Medicaid (19%; a combination of 44% state funds and 56% federal dollars), and federal funds for Medicare, the Department of Veterans Affairs, and the ADM Block Grant (9%). In the general healthcare sector, the state contribution is greater, and the federal share is smaller.

The range and variety of financing mechanisms and the functional differentiation of the ADM services system have made the development of comprehensive mental healthcare financing policy challenging for any psychiatric administrator. The recent attempt at sweeping national healthcare reform (and within it mental healthcare reform) failed. The states now have center stage in attempts to implement public sector managed care Medicaid programs (Ridgely and Goldman 1996).

The Past

People with mental illnesses were cared for at home before the early nineteenth century development of a specialized system of services. Some received care in cell-like accommodations in general hospitals or welfare institutions. As more poor people with mental illnesses were detected, private asylums were gradually unable to meet the demand and need for care. The number of public asylums increased, involving almost every state by the time of the Civil War (Grob 1973). At the turn of the twentieth century, state governments enacted a series of care acts codifying into law the states' fiscal responsibility for mentally ill people (Grob 1983). This produced a sharply demarcated two-tier system of care in which private hospitals provided care to those who could afford it, and public hospitals cared for all the rest.

The introduction of health insurance began to break down the barriers between the public and the private sectors. For the first time in the 1950s, insurance benefits included coverage for inpatient services for ADM disorders. The number of private sector behavioral healthcare service providers thus expanded. Simultaneously, the federal government developed Veterans Administration neuropsychiatric hospitals and began to reimburse for care rendered in psychiatric units in general hospitals. Categorical funding from the government also provided resources to build, staff, and operate community mental health centers (CMHCs) throughout the United States (Ridgely and Goldman 1996).

The organization and financing of healthcare for the poor and the elderly were restructured in 1965 with the passage of Medicare and Medicaid legislation. These public insurance programs facilitated the gradual blurring of distinction between public sector and private sector providers. Through these programs, the federal and state governments jointly paid for medical care of Medicaid and Medicare enrollees in the private sector.

Medicare and Medicaid did not eliminate the two-class system but in its place created a partially hybrid-

ized elaborate mixture of services. The public sector continued to provide a safety net for the poor and for patients who depleted private sector insurance benefits. This was particularly relevant for difficult or treatment-resistant patients who required extended hospital stays. Public systems thus maintained a special and important role in the acute and long-term care of the indigent, involuntarily committed, and severely disabled (Lave and Goldman 1990; Taube et al. 1990). Furthermore, Medicare and Medicaid, like other types of insurance, had no incentives for providers to contain costs and set up relatively arbitrary benefit limits for ADM services.

In the 1960s, while Medicaid and Medicare became entrenched as payers for ADM services in the public and private sectors, the federal government continued to fund construction and staffing grants for CMHCs. Stimulated by President Kennedy's Mental Retardation Facilities and Community Mental Health Centers Act of 1963, this was a period of significant federal oversight of community mental health policy, with the federal government essentially bypassing state mental health authorities to directly fund mental health centers in local communities.

In 1972 President Nixon declared the CMHC program a "demonstrated success" and decided that federal funding should be phased out and that local and private sources should be found to fund continued CMHC development. When Congress disagreed, the president attempted to impound the congressional appropriations for new CMHCs (Foley and Sharfstein 1983).

President Carter appointed a President's Commission on Mental Health to review the status of mental healthcare in the nation and to create specific recommendations for federal action. The 1978 report resulted in the development of the Mental Health Systems Act (MHSA) submitted to the Congress in 1979. A comprehensive review by the U.S. Department of Health and Human Services led to the development of a National Plan for the Chronically Mentally Ill.

Where did this federal effort lead? President Reagan's defeat of President Carter led to a so-called new federalism and the trend toward increasing the power and authority of the states throughout government. The MHSA was repealed, and the National Plan was not widely disseminated. However, several incremental changes resulted. First, a small categorical program, the Community Support Program, funded throughout the 1980s, fostered the innovative service development and coordination of mental health and support services in local communities envisioned by the MHSA, albeit on a much smaller scale. Second, in 1986 Congress enacted legislation requiring each state to develop and implement a statewide plan for local community-based systems of care for people with severe mental illnesses (Koyanagi and Goldman 1991; Ridgely and Goldman 1996; Turner and TenHoor 1978). Despite these surviving elements of the national vision, control and authority over ADM services remained at the state level as this era ended.

A final important historical trend in both the public and the private sectors is the major shift in the patterns and locus of care. From 1955 to 1975, outpatient episodes increased more than ten-fold, whereas the rate of inpatient episodes in specialized psychiatric settings remained steady. As is described in more detail later in this chapter, the locus of inpatient care also has changed from the state mental hospital to psychiatric units in general hospitals, CMHCs, and private psychiatric hospitals. The number of residents in state inpatient facilities declined from 560,000 in 1955 to 77,000 in 1995 (Bachrach 1996). From 1970 to 1992 the number of state hospitals decreased from 310 to 273 (Witkin et al. 1996). This trend is accelerating; more state psychiatric hospitals have been closed in the first half of the 1990s than in the 1970s and 1980s combined. Changes in treatment methods, patterns of practice, legal decisions on the civil rights of patients, and the financing of care provided the incentives for outpatient care to expand (Goldman et al. 1983; Ridgely and Goldman 1996).

The Present

State Mental Health Agency

Psychiatric administrators now must recognize that state mental health agencies are the principal organizational structure for funding the administration of mental health services in the public sector. The location of the state mental health agencies within state government is shown in Table 2–1.

These state mental health agencies are undergoing tremendous change. According to the National Association of State Mental Health Program Directors Research Institute, 17 of 46 (37%) state mental health agencies were reorganized between 1994 and 1996. In six states, the state mental health agency was relocated within state government. In seven states, funding for

TABLE 2–1. Location of state mental health agencies (SMHAs) within state government

Number of states	Location of SMHA
17	Department of Human Services
11	Independent mental health agency
4	Department of Health
1	Department of Institutions
9	Other department (e.g., Health and Human Services)

Source. Adapted from National Association of State Mental Health Program Directors Research Institute: Preliminary 1996 SMHA Profiles. Information supported under contract CMHS-SAB-96-0003 from Center for Mental Health Services/Substance Abuse and Mental Health Services Administration (CMHS/SAMHSA). www.rdmc.org/nri/Default.htm

the administration of services for other disabilities was moved into or out of the state mental health agencies.

The number of persons who have received services funded or operated by state mental health agencies is uncertain. Table 2–2 shows the total number of persons who received ambulatory, residential, and hospital care services during fiscal year 1995 in states responding to a National Association of State Mental Health Program Directors Research Institute survey. If we focus on ambulatory services and assume that the 24 states that did not respond to the survey had the same average number of persons receiving services as the responding states, almost 6 million people would have received a state mental health agency ambulatory service in fiscal year 1995.

These services are provided within the context of a variety of programs for persons with severe mental illness and other comorbidities. Table 2–3 shows the types of specialized treatment services funded by various states for special needs populations.

Public Sector Challenge

These numbers reflect the tremendous challenges faced by the public sector in financing the care of persons with severe mental illnesses. Despite the best efforts of the state mental health agencies, people with severe mental illnesses are poorly served in many publicly financed mental health systems. Most communities have ADM systems that lack comprehensive service alternatives, coordination of care among various mental health and social service providers, and continuity of care (especially between inpatient and ambulatory

TABLE 2–2. Number of persons receiving ambulatory, residential, and hospital care services from state mental health agencies in fiscal year 1995

	Ambulatory services		Residential services		Hospital care services	
	Average daily census	Unduplicated clients served	Daily census	Unduplicated clients served	Average daily census	Unduplicated count of adults with severe mental illnesses who received any mental health services
Total	94,867	3,045,819	36,794	366,503	64,827	1,212,015
Average	6,776	117,147	1,314	14,660	1,621	34,629
Median	4,590	36,380	385	2,106	1,087	17,792
Responses	14	26	28	25	40	35

Source. Adapted from National Association of State Mental Health Program Directors Research Institute: Preliminary 1996 SMHA Profiles. Information supported under contract CMHS-SAB-96-0003 from Center for Mental Health Services/Substance Abuse and Mental Health Services Administration (CMHS/SAMHSA). www.rdmc.org/nri/Default.htm

TABLE 2–3. Specialized services offered by state mental health agencies

Type of individuals for whom service is provided	No. of states providing services	No. of states not providing services	Responding states providing services (%)
Persons with substance abuse	15	30	33
Persons with dual diagnosis: mental illness and substance abuse	21	24	47
Persons with dual diagnosis: mental illness and mental retardation	8	37	18
Persons with HIV	3	42	7
Persons with developmental disability	19	26	42
Elderly clients	23	22	51
Persons with personality disorders	5	40	11
Persons with mental illness/ medical disorders	6	39	13

Source. Adapted from National Association of State Mental Health Program Directors Research Institute Preliminary 1996 SMHA Profiles. Information supported under contract CMHS-SAB-96-0003 from Center for Mental Health Services/Substance Abuse and Mental Health Services Administration (CMHS/SAMHSA). www.rdmc.org/nri/Default.htm

settings). People with severe mental illnesses suffer most in these inadequate systems because they need a variety of medical and supportive services provided in a coordinated fashion. This ideal has been expressed by the Substance Abuse and Mental Health Services Administration as the need to develop a community support system capable of substituting community for institutional care (Stroul 1986). Without the development of community support systems, the shift of the locus from institutional to community care results in people with severe mental illnesses being unemployed and financially dependent, living in substandard housing or being homeless, lacking appropriate supervision and medical-psychiatric care, and not having recreational and social opportunities (Stroul 1986).

Some have argued that state mental health agencies and Medicaid systems should be responsible only for financing the provision of medical care and not for funding other social and rehabilitative wraparound services such as housing and vocational services. However, in the desire to create substitutes for institutional care, others have recognized that the "total institution" provided for these various aspects of a person's life (shelter, food, clothing, structured activities, medical care, therapy, and rehabilitation). Several studies support the necessity of these medical and nonmedical interventions in creating community alternatives that can substitute for expensive inpatient and other institutional (i.e., jail) care.

In addition to the need to provide a comprehensive set of services is the recognition that, for at least some patients with severe mental illness, community care must be prolonged and intensive. Insurance and healthcare plans that reimburse acute episodes of brief therapy may be insufficient to finance long-term care services required to maintain community tenure. The costs of maintaining a suicidal, dangerous, noncompliant, or treatment-refractory client in the community are very different from the costs of maintaining compliant, treatment-responsive consumers (Taube and Goldman 1989). Furthermore, alcohol and other drug abuse may be substantially related to dangerousness and treatment noncompliance among people with severe mental illnesses (Ridgely et al. 1987). As many as 50% of the people with severe mental illnesses have co-occurring substance use disorders (Regier et al. 1990).

Many of these problems in systems of care are rooted in the characteristics of the mental health organization and financing system. Because most service delivery systems are made up of "independent, autonomous organizations each able to maintain itself through access to diverse resources" (Greenly 1992), there has been little movement toward the development of integrated service delivery systems in the public ADM sector. Minor systems innovations (such as the development of joint planning and the institution of case management programs) have not been sufficient to change fragmented provider practice patterns and resulting costs. Even larger-scale innovations, such as local mental health authorities developed under the auspices of the Robert Wood Johnson Foundation Program on Chronic Mental Illness, varied in their ability to integrate funding sources and exercise control over the distribution of funding and the regulation of the direct provision of services (Goldman et al. 1994).

Few local mental health authorities achieved significant control over the two major sources of state ADM

financing: the state mental hospital budget and Medicaid, which are addressed in turn below (Goldman et al. 1990). The rapid state of flux of these entities is striking. The evidence suggests, however, that some degree of centralized control is possible.

State Mental Hospitals

States continue to spend a reported $7 billion annually on state mental hospitals (National Association of State Mental Health Program Directors 1997). The historical decline in the number of state hospitals and state hospital patients has preceded the current dramatic alterations in roles, management, and financing of state hospitals. State hospital closure is part of a larger reorganization effort occurring in 76% of the states (National Association of State Mental Health Program Directors 1997). Other states are downsizing hospitals, closing wards, reconfiguring one or more hospitals, and consolidating hospitals. These changes have been accompanied by a reduction in the relative amount of state-controlled dollars being spent on inpatient versus community-based services, as shown in Table 2–4.

State hospitals are also undergoing privatization. Fifteen states are attempting privatization by contracting out the operation and management of 66 hospitals (National Association of State Mental Health Program Directors 1997). Table 2–5 shows the components of services currently privatized or in which privatization is planned.

In addition to privatization, states are giving community mental health programs some control over budgets and use of state psychiatric hospitals. Community-based programs serve as a gatekeeper for entry into state psychiatric hospitals (29 states) and receive financial incentives or rewards to reduce state psychiatric hospital use (13 states) (National Association of State Mental Health Program Directors 1997).

Bachrach (1996) characterized the 77,000 patients currently residing in state psychiatric hospitals as being old long-stay patients, new long-stay patients, and short-stay patients. The long-stay patients may be difficult to discharge, and the current changes in state psychiatric hospital management and financing raise questions about how these individuals will be cared for in the future.

Medicaid

Public spending for Medicaid totaled $142 billion during fiscal year 1994. Of that total, approximately $61

TABLE 2–4. Percentage of state mental health agency expenditures on community-based vs. hospital services

	FY81	**FY83**	**FY85**	**FY87**	**FY90**	**FY93**
State mental hospital	63	60	60	58	53	49
Community mental health center	33	35	37	39	43	49

Note. FY = fiscal year.
Source. Adapted from National Association of State Mental Health Program Directors Research Institute: Preliminary 1996 SMHA Profiles. Information supported under contract CMHS-SAB-96-0003 from Center for Mental Health Services/Substance Abuse and Mental Health Services Administration (CMHS/SAMHSA). www.rdmc.org/nri/Default.htm

TABLE 2–5. Privatization of state hospitals

Maintenance and support	10 states contracted	AL, AZ, DE, MD, ND, OR, PA, TN, TX, VA
	5 states planned	GA, KS, NJ, PA, TX
Direct patient care	4 states contracted	IL, MD, OR, VA
	3 states planned	AZ, DC, IL
Medical/physician services	5 states contracted	AL, DE, MD, OK, VA
	2 states planned	AZ, NY
Entire state hospital	1 state	KY
Contracted management to a managed care company	2 states	NE, OR

Source. Adapted from National Association of State Mental Health Program Directors Research Institute: Preliminary 1996 SMHA Profiles. Information supported under contract CMHS-SAB-96-0003 from Center for Mental Health Services/Substance Abuse and Mental Health Services Administration (CMHS/SAMHSA). www.rdmc.org/nri/Default.htm

billion was spent by states, surpassing state expenditures for higher education for the first time in 1993 (General Accounting Office 1995a; Monack 1995). This level of expenditure has focused states' attention on comprehensive Medicaid reform, including the introduction of managed care.

Before the introduction of managed care, Medicaid was essentially an open-ended voucher program. Medicaid recipients were covered for a defined set of health services (ambulatory, hospital, and long-term care) and could choose their own providers; reimbursement was made on a fee-for-service basis, although at below-market rates. Fee-for-service structures provided incentives to provide more care and, at least theoretically, to provide quality care because recipients were free to change providers at will (Frank and Goldman 1989).

Fiscal pressures have been the chief impetus for states to adopt managed care programs. Although historically costs for Medicaid have exceeded estimates, Medicaid expenditures by states have skyrocketed since 1980. States had found ways to increase the federal dollars coming into their Medicaid systems while controlling their own outlays by creating schemes to use other

state dollar commitments as state matching dollars. Unfortunately for the states, the federal government began to recognize and discourage these matching schemes.

Since the 1981 passage of the Omnibus Budget Reconciliation Act, more states have been experimenting with managed care systems. Nationwide, as of June 1998, just under 54% of the 31 million Medicaid recipients were enrolled in some form of managed care. In the same year, the Health Care Financing Administration reported a total of 52 mental health carve-out plans in 18 states (Health Care Financing Administration 1998).

Waivers

The chief mechanism by which states have implemented managed care systems within their state-financed Medicaid populations is through 1115 (Research and Demonstration) and 1915(b) (Medicaid Managed Care) waivers. These waivers provide mechanisms that allow states to waive requirements in the Medicaid law to develop innovations in the financing and delivery of services to Medicaid recipients.

Of note, the status of state psychiatric hospitals under these waivers is variable. In some cases, the state psychiatric hospitals are included in the benefit package (five states for the 1115 waiver, four states for the 1915(b) waiver). In other states, psychiatric hospitals are outside the benefit package (one state for the 1115 waiver, seven states for the 1915(b) waiver). Various other arrangements also have been made (National Association of State Mental Health Program Directors 1997).

Managed Care

Managed care is now the general term used to describe a variety of arrangements in healthcare financing, organization, and delivery in which an entity other than the direct treating physician is managing or overseeing payment for necessary, appropriate, and authorized medical services. The possibility of applying managed care principles to public sector Medicaid programs has excited many advocates. The potential to enhance ADM care is clear: an end to arbitrary benefit limits as a strategy to manage costs, the development of comprehensive continua of care (in place of the current inpatient/outpatient dichotomy), the development of innovative new service approaches, the use of capitated financing to improve efficiencies, and so forth. The risks of managed care are also clear—a financial incentive to undertreat rather than to overtreat and an intrusion into the doctor-patient relationship.

Types of Programs

The best, and perhaps most profitable, way to provide mental health services has raised many questions for managed care companies. The *carve-in* approach integrates mental healthcare in general health financing and services. The *carve-out* model segregates the mental health benefit and service delivery system from general healthcare. Most state systems have opted for the carve-out approach for Medicaid populations. States were wary of the limited experience health maintenance organizations (HMOs) had in providing care for persons with severe mental illnesses. Furthermore, state mental health authorities also wanted to maintain as much control as possible over their expenditures. Integration might mean a loss of resources for persons with severe mental illnesses (Essock and Goldman 1995).

According to the Intergovernmental Health Policy Project (1995), among the 16 states with approved or pending Health Care Financing Administration 1115

waiver requests, the most common approach is to offer acute but limited mental health and/or addiction benefits to all Medicaid recipients but to carve out people with more intense mental health and addiction needs, to be served either by the state mental health agency or addiction authority or under a contract with a private managed behavioral healthcare organization (General Accounting Office 1995b).

Arguments for carving out include the increased likelihood that evaluation of competing vendor proposals will focus more on mental health criteria for medical necessity and appropriateness of care, that adequate resources will be devoted to providing mental health and addiction care, and that a wider range of specialized behavioral healthcare providers will be available in a carved-out plan (Petrila 1996). On the other hand, carve-outs may be inefficient and isolate mental health from general healthcare. This is a particular concern for individuals with severe mental illness who also are likely to have comorbid physical health disorders (Bartsch et al. 1990; Koran et al. 1989). Carve-outs also may perpetuate the stigma of mental illness and institutionalize the notion that severe mental illness is not a medical problem (Petrila 1996). An additional question is whether drug and alcohol treatment is paired with mental health and carved in or carved out. Given the range of organizational forms of carved-out and carved-in behavioral health benefits and services and the fundamental nature of the questions about each, a better understanding of their effect on access, cost, and outcomes is essential for public purchasers.

In the context of discussions of managed care, and especially with the focus on cost containment, people with severe mental illness may be exceedingly vulnerable because of their complex needs (including the need for social service supports as well as medical-psychiatric services) and their need for ongoing care over long periods. What is problematic is that some of the needed services fall beyond the definition of medical necessity approved in some managed care plans.

Additionally, many people with severe mental illnesses are vulnerable to the managed care systems designed and financed by public purchasers because they may lack the opportunity to negotiate on their own behalf like consumers in a marketplace. The definition of *medical necessity*, and the specification of types and quality of services to be provided, and rate structures are determined by public purchasers including the Medicaid authority and administered by public or private managed care organizations, well outside of the reach of the potential consumers of services. Yet these public purchasers determine the amount, type, and quality of services available to the public sector consumer.

Effective consumer choice also depends on the ability of consumers to observe and make judgments about services and their ability to opt out of managed care programs that they perceive are not meeting their needs (Frank and Goldman 1989). Many public purchasers require managed care systems to lock in consumers for 6 months to 1 year, making these managed care systems potentially less responsive to market pressures.

Outcomes

Early experience with public purchasing strategies that aim to reduce Medicaid expenditures by using managed care has illustrated some dangers. Public purchasers specify and select managed care plans that have great potential for achieving short-term savings at the expense of longer-term costs and putting vulnerable target populations at risk. Mechanic et al. (1995), in a review of the current state of the art in behavioral managed healthcare, warned that quality of care will depend, not on the existence of managed care per se, but rather on the specific incentive structures, the network of providers, the utilization reviewers, and the overall responsiveness of the managed care organization.

Beyond theoretical effects, some research has suggested caution in applying some managed care strategies used in the general health sector to behavioral healthcare for people with severe mental illness. One of the chief concerns in the application of managed care principles to public Medicaid systems (especially in the care of people with severe mental illness) has been the fear that HMOs are particularly unsuited to provide the long-term community treatment that many people with severe mental illness require (Christianson and Osher 1994; Taube et al. 1990). The Rand Health Insurance Experiment in the late 1980s suggested that patterns of mental healthcare within HMOs were different from patterns of care in fee-for-service systems, with the probability of receiving some mental health services about the same but a with much lower average number of visits (Wells et al. 1986). Also of significance, HMOs did not provide the range of nonmedical and supportive services that many people with severe ADM disorders need to avoid hospitalization. Taube and his colleagues (1990) suggested, from an overview of HMO experience in Wisconsin and Minnesota, that people with severe mental illnesses are gradually excluded

from HMOs over time, returning to public mental health systems at an additional public cost. However, a 1989 survey suggested that 54% of the HMOs surveyed provided their ADM services through contracts or subcontracts with ADM specialty providers rather than within their own service structures (Wainstock 1993).

A recent comprehensive review of the literature suggested that managed care principles can be applied to ADM treatment and can produce significant cost reductions, generally through reduced rates of hospitalization (Mechanic et al. 1995). However, these authors cautioned that current research is insufficient to draw definitive conclusions about the likely effect of specific forms of managed care, and others also have noted the lack of a consensus in the ADM field about what constitutes a good outcome of managed behavioral healthcare (Wells et al. 1986).

Several Medicaid behavioral healthcare demonstration projects are ongoing across the United States, although many of the waiver programs and evaluations are just under way. These demonstration programs differ greatly in scope and sophistication, with few states having sufficient evaluation resources. Some materials on the programs and evaluations have been compiled by the Evaluation Center (Evaluation Center@HSRI 1995). Among the waiver programs in Arizona, Iowa, Massachusetts, Ohio, Oregon, Tennessee, and Washington, only Massachusetts has provided a detailed report on the effect of adopting and implementing a managed care program for addiction and mental health services (Callahan and Shepard 1994).

The Massachusetts waiver was granted in 1992 and covers 370,000 lives. The evaluation report concluded that the managed care plan for addiction and mental health services provided an overall estimated cost savings of 22% (although there were differential savings across addiction and mental health services and across enrollment groups—Supplemental Security Income [SSI] and Aid to Families with Dependent Children/Temporary Assistance for Needy Families [AFDC/TANF]). The plan was also found to provide a slight increase in access (although there was considerable variability) and an improvement in quality (as measured by a provider survey on readmission rates). The report also noted a number of unavoidable weaknesses in design and caveats in interpreting the findings.

In summary, state Medicaid expenditures were out of control as a result of the cost-shifting behavior of the states themselves. The need to contain costs in both health and mental health has stimulated the financing of various managed care approaches that encompass an enormous variety of specific financial, regulatory, and organizational arrangements. Whether to blend funds for general health with those for addiction and mental health treatment within one plan or to maintain separate fund pools to finance specialized mental health services is a fundamental decision in the design of these programs.

The Future

The major question about the future of the public sector is its very existence as a provider of care beyond serving as an informed purchaser and providing funds for services to be delivered and managed by the private sector. Societal pushes to shrink government, the requirements of managed care, and the willingness of the private sector to provide these services all suggest a redefined role for the public sector. A challenge for the public sector will be to create efficient and effective ways to plan, purchase, and oversee and to ensure that private sector care managers and service providers are accountable. Ultimately, the public sector provider community may become a shadow of its past, if the private sector can effectively assume managed care and service delivery functions. By contrast, the public sector likely will assume an important role as value- and quality-based purchasers of both medical and rehabilitative or wraparound services required by people with severe and persistent mental and addictive disorders.

References

Bachrach LL: The state of the state mental hospital in 1996. Psychiatr Serv 47:1071–1078, 1996

Bartsch D, Shern D, Feinberg LE, et al: Screening CMHC outpatients for physical illness. Hosp Community Psychiatry 41:35–38, 1990

Callahan J, Shepard D: Evaluation of the Massachusetts Medicaid Mental Health/Substance Abuse Program. Waltham, MA, Heller School for Advanced Studies in Social Welfare, Brandeis University, 1994

Christianson J, Osher F: HMOs, health care reform and persons with serious mental illness. Hosp Community Psychiatry 45:898–905, 1994

Essock S, Goldman H: States' embrace of managed mental health care. Health Aff (Millwood) 14:34–44, 1995

Evaluation Center@HSRI: Medicaid Managed Mental Health Care Program and Evaluation Materials From Participating States. Cambridge, MA, Evaluation Center@HSRI, 1995

Foley HA, Sharfstein SS: Madness and Government: Who Cares for the Mentally Ill? Washington, DC, American Psychiatric Press, 1983

Frank R, Goldman H: Financing care of the severely mentally ill: incentives, contracts, and public responsibility. Journal of Social Issues 45:131–144, 1989

Frank R, McGuire T, Regier D, et al: Paying for mental health and substance abuse care. Health Aff (Millwood) 13(1):337–342, 1994

Freund D, Hurley R: Medicaid managed care: contribution to issues of health reform. Annu Rev Public Health 16:473–496, 1995

General Accounting Office: Medicaid: Restructuring Approaches Leave Many Questions (GAO/HEHS-95-103). 1995a

General Accounting Office: Medicaid: Spending Pressures Drive States Toward Program Reinvention (GAO/HEHS-95-122). Washington, DC, Government Printing Office, 1995b

Goldman H, Adams N, Taube C: Deinstitutionalization: the data demythologized. Hosp Community Psychiatry 34:129–134, 1983

Goldman H, Morrissey J, Ridgely MS: Form and function of mental health authorities at RWJ Foundation Program Sites: preliminary observations. Hosp Community Psychiatry 41:1222–1230, 1990

Goldman H, Morrissey J, Ridgely MS: Evaluating the Robert Wood Johnson Foundation Program on Chronic Mental Illness. Milbank Q 72:37–47, 1994

Greenly JR: Neglected organization and management issues in mental health systems development. Community Ment Health J 28:371–384, 1992

Grob G: Mental Institutions in America: Social Policy to 1875. New York, Free Press, 1973

Grob G: Mental Illness and American Society, 1875–1940. Princeton, NJ, Princeton University Press, 1983

Health Care Financing Administration: Medicaid Managed Care Enrollment Report: Summary Statistics as of June 30, 1998. Baltimore, MD, Health Care Financing Administration 1998

Intergovernmental Health Policy Project: Medicaid Managed Care and Mental Health: An Overview of Section 1115 Programs. Washington, DC, Georgetown University, 1995

Koran L, Jox HC, Marton KI, et al: Medical evaluation of psychiatric patients, 1: results in a state mental health system. Arch Gen Psychiatry 46:733–740, 1989

Koyanagi C, Goldman H: Quiet success of the national plan for chronic patients. Hosp Community Psychiatry 42:899–905, 1991

Lave JR, Goldman HH: Medicare financing for mental health care. Health Aff (Millwood) 9:5–18, 1990

Mechanic D, Schlesinger M, McAlpine D: Management of mental health and substance abuse services: state of the art and early results. Milbank Q 73:19–55, 1995

Monack D: Medicaid and managed care: opportunities for innovative service delivery to vulnerable populations. Behavioral Healthcare Tomorrow 4:191–223, 1995

National Association of State Mental Health Program Directors Research Institute: Preliminary 1996 SMHA Profiles, 1997. Available on line at: www.rdmc.org/nri/Default.htm

Petrila J: Ethics, money and the problems of coercion in managed behavioral health care. Saint Louis University Law Journal 40:359–405, 1996

Regier DA, Farmer ME, Rae DS, et al: Comorbidity of mental disorders with alcohol and other drug abuse: results from the Epidemiologic Catchment Area (ECA) study. JAMA 21:2511–2518, 1990

Ridgely MS, Goldman HH: Putting the failure of national health care reform in perspective: mental health benefits and the "benefit" of incrementalism. Saint Louis University Law Journal 40:407–435, 1996

Ridgely MS, Goldman H, Talbott J: Chronic Mentally Ill Young Adults With Substance Abuse Problems: Review of the Literature and Creation of a Research Agenda. Baltimore, MD, University of Maryland School of Medicine, Mental Health Policy Studies Program, 1987

Stroul B: Models of Community Support Services: Approaches to Helping Persons With Long-Term Mental Illness. Rockville, MD, NIMH Community Support Program, 1986

Taube CA, Goldman HH: State strategies to restructure state psychiatric hospitals—a selective review. Inquiry 26:1237–1241, 1989

Taube C, Goldman H, Salkever D: Medicaid coverage for mental illness. Health Aff (Millwood) 9(1):1–18, 1990

Turner J, TenHoor W: The NIMH Community Support Program: pilot approach to a needed social reform. Schizophr Bull 4:319–348, 1978

Wainstock EJ: How HMOs can effectively manage mental health services in the 1990s. Adm Policy Ment Health 21:15–26, 1993

Wells KB, Manning W, Benjamin B: Use of outpatient mental health services in HMO and fee-for-service plans: results from a randomized controlled trial. Health Serv Res 21:453–474, 1986

Witkin MJ, Atay J, Manderscheid RW: Trends in state and county mental hospitals in the U.S. from 1970 to 1992. Psychiatr Serv 47:1079–1081, 1996

❖ Section II ❖

Core Administrative Psychiatry Concepts

Miles F. Shore, M.D., Section Editor

Introduction

Miles F. Shore, M.D.

Among industrialized nations, the United States is alone in linking health coverage to employment. This connection came about during World War II when wage controls made it impossible to offer increased salaries to attract workers, and profits were capped by excess-profits taxes. This situation made it both expedient and financially feasible to offer healthcare as an attractive benefit. Since then, the financing and delivery of healthcare have been tied to the fortunes of American industry. Because industry's successes and failures are felt directly by healthcare institutions and providers, it is understandable that any discussion of the administration of mental health programs must begin by reviewing the massive restructuring of industrial activity in this country.

Although change has been the way of the world since Adam and Eve were forced to vacate the Garden of Eden, since the 1970s the pace and the scope of change of industrial organizations worldwide have assumed startling dimensions. The movement of capital from banks to financial markets has placed in the hands of financial managers great power to influence corporate behavior. Because of the almost-instantaneous transfer of information, capital can be moved swiftly across national boundaries, seeking maximum return on investment. For the first time, U.S. industry is in direct competition with industries in countries where costs are lower and the quality of work may be equal or better. The result has been massive restructuring of inefficient, poorly managed U.S. companies as top management sought to increase productivity, market share, and shareholder value (Useem 1996).

The traditional industrial organization, with a hierarchical, bureaucratic structure, pioneered by General Motors in the 1930s, is being replaced by new models of organization that are better suited to these tumultuous times. In their heyday, companies such as General Motors relied on a command-and-control style of leadership, were vertically integrated to produce most of the components of their products, and used their labor force to amortize massive capital investment in heavy machinery that was the key to production. Employees expected jobs for life and advancement through an equitably administered seniority system; in return, they identified with the organizational culture, generating loyalty that might extend through two or three generations and generally was not in conflict with union membership that negotiated working conditions and benefits. This model was well suited to a stable market dominated by a few large companies, with competition that was restrained and demand that was relatively predictable over the long haul (Pottruck 1996; Sumantra and Bartlett 1995).

The current marketplace is very different. Driven by new technology, and responding to the urgent demands of capital markets, competition has been unleashed, even in major industries. Poorly performing companies lose market share and go bankrupt if they are not restructured, acquired, or taken over. Organizational flexibility is required to respond to the competition, plan new products, and keep up with new technology that is the key to success. As U.S. manufacturing moves to other countries, it is replaced by service organizations and entirely new industries in which human capital—the knowledge and technical expertise of individual workers—replaces machinery as the key to market share. Even in established industries, the dominant role of advanced technology means that intelligence, creativity, and the assumption of responsibility are demanded of the work force (Jensen and Fagan 1996).

Vertical integration is replaced by horizontal integration and strategic alliances, at times with competitors. Networks of companies are assembled around specific projects to capitalize on unique expertise. Organizational boundaries tend to be permeable, planning timelines are short, teams focus on specific projects replacing departments, and "learning organizations" instill a culture that increases the value of human capital by fostering new skills and new expertise.

The conditions of employment have changed. The volatility of the corporate environment means that a job for life is no longer the expectation. Workers expect to move from company to company as economic conditions change. Advancement is through the personal acquisition of skills rather than through corporate seniority and titles. The psychological contract between the organization and the individual is built around personal growth; the new obligation to enhance personal employability replaces the traditional obligation to provide guaranteed employment. The conditions of employment also involve the devolution of responsibility to employees rather than continued deference to managerial authority (Pottruck 1996).

To the extent that health benefits are provided as a condition of employment, these changes in the organization of industrial activity have secondary effects on health and mental health services. From the point of view of employers, health benefits are considered as wages and thus are a significant component of labor costs. Consequently, companies seeking to compete successfully must scrutinize carefully what they spend on healthcare. Oligopsony—the dominance of a market by a few large buyers—is characteristic of health-

care to the extent that large companies purchase healthcare for their employees in large amounts. The leverage of these large purchasers has a major influence on determining the price and the quality (i.e., the value to their employees) of what they pay for health and mental health services. These private purchasers have been joined in their quest by public agencies seeking demonstrated value in response to the demands of taxpayers to reduce the cost of government. For health and mental health administrators, the result has been to challenge the core concepts of administration, the role of administrators, and, profoundly, the role of professionals who provide the services.

A host of new core concepts also has been introduced to the lexicon of administration. These concepts include the assumption of risk, the use of population-based services, and the measurement of quality. The new healthcare environment includes, for perhaps the first time, intense competition in seeking market share, a customer orientation, the marketing of programs, and close attention to the determination of variable and fixed costs among various components of business. Downsizing, corporate restructuring, mergers, strategic alliances and acquisitions, and antitrust must be on the administrator's radar screen.

In one way, the organization of health and mental health services is well ahead of our industrial counterparts. Our organizations have traditionally placed great responsibility and autonomy on members of the staff because of their professional status. In fact, the administrative challenge (some might say "nightmare") has been to coordinate the activities of highly skilled, highly independent professionals. Health and mental health organizations have been necessarily driven by new technology, and they have been required to provide a learning environment directed to the improvement of professional practice. The administrative style of healthcare organizations has long been consensus-building rather than command and control (Quinn et al. 1996).

However, healthcare, including mental healthcare, is very different from most other industries in that a great deal of the work has been done by solo practitioners with little connection to one another, accountable primarily to their own professional standards and, in the case of psychotherapists in private practice, isolated from health or mental health institutions. A major challenge to the delivery of mental health services is the pressure from managed care to turn this cottage industry into a more organized activity. Although the mechanism is cost containment, the most significant change is related to accountability. Professional accountability is being supplemented by the need for external accountability to the system of care represented by the managed care organization or professional corporation that must assume financial risk and ensure quality.

The chapters that follow in this section provide a useful guide to the altered administrative concepts and conditions that now form the core of psychiatric administration. The keys to the present administrative environment include

- Managing adaptive change
- Providing vision to generate commitment to organizations that cannot ensure stability or longevity
- Adopting new technology to support rather than interfere with clinical practice
- Sustaining professional standards, while adding organizational accountability for quality and the cost of care
- Expanding the learning environment of mental health organizations to integrate the new knowledge necessary to function in a radically altered, constantly changing environment
- Assisting clinicians to function effectively in organizations

In Chapter 3, Docherty, Surles, and Donovan provide an overview of organizational theory that has evolved as the nature of work, technology, and social forces has changed the relationship of workers to the means of production.

In Chapter 4, Shore and Vanelli discuss the varied roles of leaders in the new environment, but note that even in such altered circumstances, the core attributes of leadership—vision and strategic competence—are of central importance.

As Santiago notes in Chapter 5, planning takes on totally different dimensions in such a rapidly changing, unpredictable environment; it must be short-term, be contingent, and provide for programmatic flexibility in the face of constant change.

The demand for more explicit attention to quality has altered the structure of health organizations and created a new profession that is essential for modern mental healthcare. In Chapter 6, Nelson, Senesac, and

Holt describe the principles that are essential to carry out a quality improvement program that is real and not window dressing.

In Chapter 7, Steenbarger, Kaplan, Dewan, Manring, and Budman describe the vast implications for training in the current administrative environment. Career administrators must learn new skills and, in particular, must be prepared for constant change and learning. Significantly, as these authors point out, all clinicians must now be trained in concepts and skills that were once the province of professional administrators.

For many years the medical director has played a key role in institutions, functioning between the chief executive officer, charged with the overall responsibility for the organization, and the clinical staff, responsible for the delivery of care. In Chapter 8, Pollack and Minkoff describe the feature of this role by using the medical director in the community mental health center as the model but updated in terms of the new demands of various institutional forms.

The altered conditions of the new market environment, as well as the pace of change, place heavy demands on psychiatric administrators. With such demands goes the excitement of participating in a conceptual revolution that must succeed, because to fail will be to ensure the demise of whatever institution is unable to adapt (Levinson 1993).

References

Jensen M, Fagan P: Capitalism isn't broken. Wall Street Journal, March 29, 1996, p 10

Levinson H: Why the behemoths fell: distinguished contributions to psychological practice lecture. Presented at the American Psychological Association, Toronto, Ontario, Canada, August 20, 1993

Pottruck D: Strategies for avoiding the rush toward downsizing: growth, leadership, technology, business and change. Vital Speeches of the Day 62(24):752–755, 1996

Quinn J, Anderson P, Finkelstein S: Making the most of the best. Harvard Business Review 74:71–80, 1996

Sumantra G, Bartlett C: Changing the role of top management. Harvard Business Review 73:86–96, 1995

Useem M: Investor Capitalism: How Money Managers Are Changing the Face of Corporate America. New York, Basic Books, 1996

❖ **3** ❖

Organizational Theory

John P. Docherty, M.D.
Richard C. Surles, Ph.D.
Catherine M. Donovan, B.S.

The healthcare system in the United States is in a period of profound change. The broad social movement referred to as healthcare reform, focused on the goals of rationalizing cost, improving quality, and enhancing access to care, is requiring and stimulating radical and fundamental changes in the structure of the American healthcare system. The possibility of this reform derives from three forces: 1) rapid development of new knowledge and information and the potential to rapidly transfer that information, 2) the increasing importance of the service sector in American economic life, and 3) the development of new organizational forms, concepts, and theories.

The development of new organizational structures and designs is now a major characteristic of contemporary business life, and the healthcare enterprise has begun to participate fully in such organizational change and experimentation. Thus, the understanding of organizational structure and design is of increasing interest to the healthcare administrator. In this chapter we provide a basic overview and introduction to organizational theory. We review the history and evolution of modern organizational theory and introduce some of

the key concepts and approaches that characterize the newer forms of and efforts at organizational design.

Definition of *Organization*

The definition of *organization* has changed and evolved as our understanding of the components operating within an organization has developed. Examples of definitions include

- A system of "division of labor in which each member performs certain specialized activities that are coordinated with the activities of other specialists" (Mott 1965, p. 14)
- "[T]he shape energy takes when the human beings who make up an enterprise blend their collective skills" (Johansen and Swigart 1994, p. 13)
- "[A] small number of people with complementary skills who are committed to a common purpose, performance goals, and approach for which they hold themselves mutually accountable" (Katzenbach and Smith 1993, p. 21)

These definitions highlight the importance and the role of a common objective or goal as a motivating factor within the organization, but they do not address the environment in which the organization exists. Another definition focuses on not only the internal environment but also the inherent link of an organization to its external environment:

- "[A] set of relationships that are persistent over time. One of the functions of an organization, of any organism, is to anticipate the future, so that those relationships can persist over time. ...[A]n organization's reason for being, like that of any organism, [is] to help the parts that are in relationship to each other, to be able to deal with the change in the environment" (Flower 1995, p. 36)

History of Organizational Theory

Interest in the study of organization was stimulated by the Industrial Revolution, during which a movement occurred away from the independent craftsman to workers collected together in a setting to facilitate mass production. Mass production was first studied and popularized, in 1776, by Adam Smith (1995), who had analyzed the practices of an established pin factory. This particular factory employed a group of people who were responsible for making pins. However, instead of these employees serving as generalists, each solely responsible for the fabrication of a pin, these workers were specialists. Different employees had a particular task for which they had developed a depth of knowledge and skill. The combination of the individual tasks led to the production of the final pin. The observation of this successful approach was the genesis of Smith's concept of a *division of labor* as originally explained in *Wealth of Nations* in 1776. Smith found that dividing labor based on a specialization in task increased productivity by a factor of hundreds. Ten employees in the pin factory were capable of making "upwards of forty-eight thousand pins in a day. But if they had all wrought separately and independently, and without any of them having been educated as to this peculiar business, they certainly could not each of them have made twenty, perhaps not even one pin in a day" (Hammer and Champy 1993, p. 12). Smith's concept of a division of labor formed the conceptual basis for a powerful administrative approach to reducing cost, increasing productivity, and maximizing profits.

Stage I: Classical Theory

The introduction of the machine into industry furthered business's capacity to achieve new levels in mass production. The power of Smith's observation and concept served as an ideal organizational companion to this technical revolution and its goal of mass production. The concept of a division of labor served as the driving force behind the modern study of organizations and their design and structure. Theorists began to study the four components that made up the concept of a division of labor: 1) hierarchy of authority, 2) span of control, 3) centralization versus decentralization, and 4) specialization of function or task. As theories of organizations evolved throughout the contemporary era these components were conceptualized in varying ways (Table 3–1). Each of the theories, from the classical theories of Taylor (1911) and Fayol (1949) to the neoclassical work of Mayo (1933) and McGregor (1960), contributed to or elaborated on these four components (Figure 3–1).

Hierarchy of Authority

A hierarchy of authority is the system of rules and regulations that determine the line of communication and control within the company. In a true hierarchical system the line of communication from the upper level to lower levels provides a method of relaying directives to subordinates. The line of communication from the subordinates to supervisors is established primarily for reporting. The particular axis through which control is exercised can determine the organizational structure. Organizational structures based on different axes include the functional organization, the product organization, and the matrix organization.

Functional Organization

A functional organization is one in which specialization of tasks defines the hierarchy of authority. Each area of specialization is separated into its own department with a supervisor possessing extensive experience in that area of specialty. This separation allows for functions to remain centralized and avoids the uncomfortable and often unproductive hypothetical situation of an indi-

TABLE 3–1. Components of division of labor

Theory	Specialization	Hierarchy of authority	Centralization vs decentralization	Span of control
Classical	High	Rigid	Centralized	Narrow
Neoclassical	High/low	Loose	Decentralized	Wide
Contemporary	Low	Loose	Decentralized	Wide

vidual with a background in marketing, for example, becoming the supervisor of the engineering department.

The line of authority is clear within a functional organization. Directives originate in one centralized position and are communicated to the supervisors of each subdepartment and through these supervisors to the staff employees within the department. These employees report to one supervisor who in turn reports to one central supervisor. As Figure 3–2 illustrates, a distinct separation exists between the hierarchy of authority for different specializations. This separation does not foster, and can in fact inhibit, communication between areas and supervisors. This weakness in the design restricts the coordination of efforts between departments, resulting in the organization becoming less responsive to change within its operating environment.

Product Organization

Organizations that are constantly adapting to their environments are more likely to use a product organization design. This design allows the organization to continually change the size and scope of its business practices without outgrowing its own structure. A product organization is departmentalized into distinct product groups. These groups exist as distinct self-contained units, with each unit dedicated to the production of a specific product or group of products. The members within any given group represent different functional specializations.

Each product group may have representatives from finance, research and development, marketing, legal, implementation, and so on (Figure 3–3). These representatives are not responsible for reporting to a functional supervisor. For example, there is no vice president of marketing with authority over the marketing representatives working in different product groups. The members of a given product group report to one

supervisor, the product group manager.

A downside of the product organization is a replication in resources. For example, having research and development run concurrently in different product groups may require a duplication of expensive equipment and personnel. Many successful product organizations are able to maintain a product group design while also centralizing a few departments that can then serve the different product groups. Another obstacle is a restriction in the opportunities for advancement within the company, which inhibits the company's ability to attract and retain talented employees (Organizational Structure and Design 1995).

Matrix Organization

The matrix organization overcomes one of the weaknesses of the product organization by offering employees a clear line of advancement while still dedicating distinct groups to different projects. Matrix organizations use dual authority, in which an employee is assigned to work with a particular project manager who has authority for the work produced within the project team, while at the same time a functional department head or vice president has functional authority over the same employee (Figure 3–4). For example, although a member of the marketing department may report to a particular project manager regarding final changes to the ad campaign for that manager's project, the vice president of marketing still has authority over the employee's work.

The matrix organization is frequently employed in healthcare organizations in which employees have two distinct lines of reporting: 1) to the unit or program manager and 2) to the discipline chief. This organizational design can be sabotaged if an adequate level of coordination and cooperation among the project managers and functional supervisors does not exist. Although the complications of dual authority are clear, a matrix design has a number of advantages. By mandating that the lines of communication

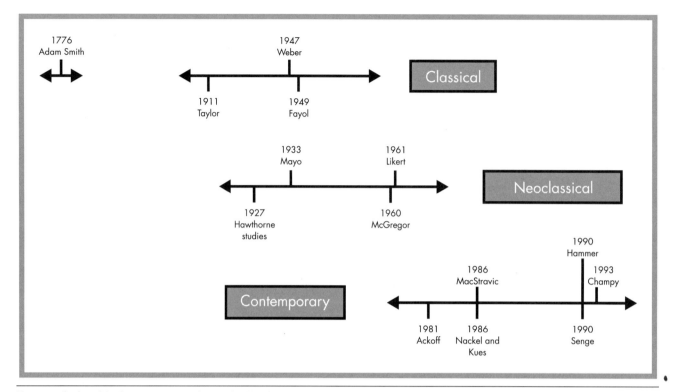

FIGURE 3–1. Modern progress of organization.

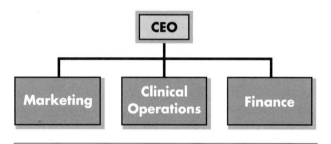

FIGURE 3–2. Functional organization.

between departments remain strong, the matrix organization overcomes the communication weaknesses of the functional organization. This enhanced communication forces program supervisors to become aware of and receptive to the perspectives of different specializations in order to facilitate the interaction between areas of expertise on behalf of a given project.

Major Theorists

Several major figures have contributed prominently to thinking on the hierarchy of authority. Classical theory had its genesis in the work of Max Weber (1947), who formulated the concept of a bureaucracy. Weber's initial vision of a bureaucracy was an organization charac-

terized by clear rules and lines of authority, in which all decisions were made and implemented through a chain of command. Weber's initial principles regarding a strict hierarchy of authority were at the foundation of Frederick Taylor's (1911) theory of scientific management. Taylor believed that to enhance the functioning of such an organization an employee must be carefully chosen for a given specialization, specifically trained for that particular task, and placed appropriately in the organization's hierarchy under the tight control of a suitable supervisor. The structure of authority was also a critical component in Henri Fayol's (1949) classical organizational theory. Fayol stated that it would be most efficient to have strict rules regarding the distribution of control and power within the organization.

Span of Control

Span of control refers to the types of employees over whom a manager has authority. Positions that are given control over a narrow range of subordinates, regardless of how many such employees there may be, are considered to have a narrow span of control. As the types and categories of subordinates reporting to a particular manager increase the span of control becomes

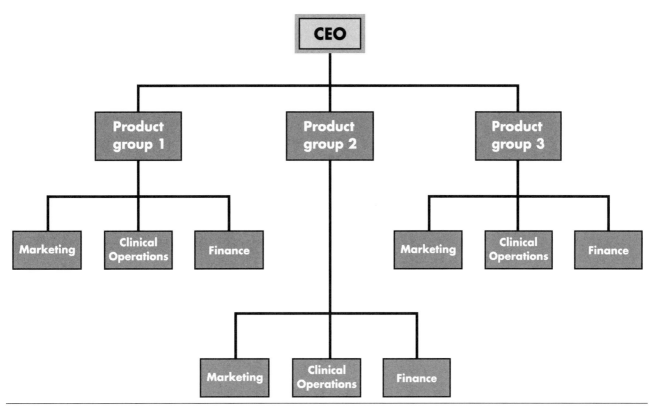

FIGURE 3–3.   Product organization.

wider, while the manager's ability to supervise the efforts of each employee decreases. Organizations in which the span of control is considered narrow are termed tall organizations. Organizations in which the span of control is wide are referred to as flat organizations.

The classical theorists embraced a vision of the organization in which managers or supervisors had tight control of the subordinates in their charge. Based on Taylor's and Fayol's theories, this vision results in organizations having a tall overall structure. This structure emphasizes the importance of a hierarchy of authority and the need to closely supervise employees performing specialized tasks. With the neoclassical movement, as described later in this chapter, a move occurred from tall to flat structures.

Centralization Versus Decentralization of Decision Making

A centralized decision-making structure is one in which the power to make decisions lies with a small number of upper-level executives and ultimately with one centralized figure. In a decentralized organization, the power to make decisions is delegated to all levels of the organization. Decentralization is intended to create a state of affairs in which the individuals who carry out the decisions are the same individuals who make them.

Classical theory did not perceive benefits in a decentralized organization because of the perception of basic human nature implicit in classical theory. Douglas McGregor (1960), of the neoclassical movement, observed that mistrust of human nature prohibited Fayol from incorporating a decentralized system of decision making in the classical theory of the organizational structure. Classical theory held that basic human nature was one of laziness, little desire to work, and low drive to accomplish more than the bare minimum necessary to survive. The neoclassical theorist Rensis Likert (1961) argued that only through the participation of employees in the decision-making process is it possible to substantially enhance the organization's performance. Decentralization of decision making throughout the different levels of the organization, Likert's *System 4*, encouraged not only participation of the employees but also a sense of trust in the competence of all employees (Likert 1961).

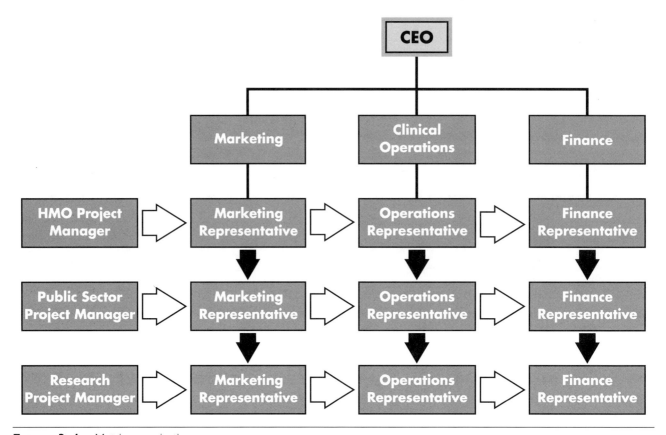

FIGURE 3–4. Matrix organization.

Specialization

Based on Adam Smith's original principles in *Wealth of Nations,* specialization refers to a division of the whole process of production into the most elementary components or tasks, with the sequential completion of the entirety of tasks leading to the finished product. Once each task has been extracted from the whole process, an employee can be assigned to that particular task and receive training in the most efficient manner to complete the task. The employee then becomes a specialist at the given task and, through the repetition of the process and the training initially received, eventually becomes an efficient mechanism. According to Smith, specialization saves the time normally wasted in the transition between different tasks when one employee is responsible for all phases of production.

Taylor's theory of scientific management further enhanced the understanding of specialization. His time-method studies were begun to determine the "one best way" to perform a given task. The theory of scientific management illustrates the focus on specialization that involved the employee as an extension of the machine. This principle met with a great deal of resistance from the labor force, because it took insufficient consideration of the *human factor.* However, its short-term impact on production was indisputable (Lichtman and Hunt 1971).

Summary

Early theory relied heavily on a "mechanical" model and emphasized the value of a rigid hierarchy of authority, a narrow span of control, a centralized system of decision making, and a high degree of specialization. As these mechanistic theories were implemented throughout industry, there was a noticeable difference between the theoretical model and the working of the model within any given corporation. The models conceived of organizations as finely tuned machines working at constant maximum capacity. Increasingly, however, it became clear that there was a "noise" in this machine, the human factor. The progressive recognition of the human factor led organizations to adopt more complicated models.

Stage II: Neoclassical Theory

Previous theoretical models had made considerable efforts to ensure that the employee would enhance the output of the highly efficient machine. With the introduction of the human relations movement by Elton Mayo (1933), concentration was shifted to the study of the individual in the organization. The human relations movement focused on social factors, such as treatment by management and relationships among colleagues, and not economic factors, as the driving forces behind human behavior in an organization. Mayo based much of his work on the results of the famous Hawthorne studies of 1927 (Roethlisberger and Dickson 1939). The Hawthorne research team worked with Western Electric to determine the ideal conditions to bring productivity to capacity level. This end was approached through a series of trials in which the level of lighting in the factory work area was adjusted. The results of the study indicated that work performance was altered in all trials, not only the trials in which the light level was enhanced but also those trials in which the light was diminished to near hazardous working conditions. The level of work performance remained elevated for a number of weeks following the study but declined to previous levels by the time of follow-up testing. The research collected during these studies suggested that the attention of the research team, the relationships of the employees, and employee motivation, rather than an ideal work condition (e.g., lighting, comfort, temperature), altered the observed level of work performance (Roethlisberger and Dickson 1939).

McGregor's work was also one of the seminal contributions to understanding the role of psychological variables in the effective functioning and design of an organization. McGregor argued that the classical theory view of human nature as lazy and unambitious, *Theory X* as he referred to it, directly contradicted actual human nature, which is such that individuals seek out responsibility and have an innate desire to achieve success. McGregor's *Theory Y* is indicative of the neoclassical approach to organizational design and management. *Theory Y* encourages managers to place decision-making capabilities with their subordinates, empowering them to become personally involved in the organization's goals by increasing their participation level (McGregor 1960). This idea of decentralizing authority within the organizational structure is the key contribution of the neoclassical approach, which emphasizes employee satisfaction as integral to the organization's success.

Stage III: Contemporary Theory

It would be fair to say that we have now entered a period of true paradigm change in the field of organizational theory (Kuhn 1996). The search for a new paradigm on which to base organizational theory has several determinants:

- The limits of the division of labor as a generative concept for new models of organizational theory development have been reached. Promising new hypothetical forms of organization are not readily derived from the concept.
- The amount of "fixing" that classical theory requires in order to accommodate the human factor has reached a level of complication that renders new theory development within the classical-neoclassical framework cumbersome and inefficient.
- Fundamental changes in information processing and communications technology have brought about revolutionary shifts in 1) the role and skill level required of the worker, 2) the ability of the organization to cope with increasingly rapid and continuous change, 3) the demand for product customization, and 4) relative industry sector dominance with disproportionate growth in service industries.

A host of new organizational theories have been developed to generate new models to help business cope more effectively with this dramatically altered environment (Figure 3–5). Many of these models radically invert the values of the classical models of organization. For example, re-engineering seeks efficiency through the unification of labor rather than the division of labor (Hammer and Champy 1993), and other theories place the management of human capital as central to the organization and locate the noise in the physical and other conditions that interfere with maximum productivity and creativity of this human capital. Four currently popular and illustrative examples of contemporary theory are re-engineering, the learning organization, the circular organization, and product-line management.

Re-engineering

Re-engineering brings the concept of unification of labor to fruition. Hammer and Champy (1993) define re-engineering as "fundamental rethinking and radical redesign

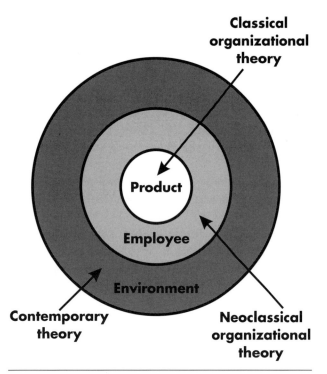

FIGURE 3–5. Evolution of organizational theory.

of business processes to achieve dramatic improvements in critical, contemporary measures of performance, such as cost, quality, service, and speed" (p. 32).

Re-engineering begins with a clear statement of ultimate business objectives, critical thinking, and, if necessary, radical redesign to achieve the best way of accomplishing objectives (Hammer and Champy 1993). Re-engineering is not an examination of ways to improve a particular process or task. The goal of re-engineering is not to make processes faster but rather to determine, first, if the processes are necessary to meet the company's objectives (Hammer 1990).

The revolutionary nature of re-engineering is its fundamental reversal of Smith's original concept of a division of labor. Responsibility for production is moved from a collection of specialists or departments into the hands of one process team aimed at accomplishing a specific objective. An immediate advantage is that these teams are able to avoid miscommunication and error resulting from the previous cumbersome handoff from one department to the next in the transition between different stages of a project. This process of unifying across departmental boundaries is called horizontal compression. In addition, the process approach eliminates the necessity of linear sequencing in the performance of the particular tasks in a given process. Overcoming this linear sequencing significantly

decreases the delay between the start of a process and the customer receiving the finished product (Hammer and Champy 1993).

Empowering a process team means that decisions that typically halted production while being considered by middle and upper management supervisors have been transferred to the process teams (Hammer 1996). This change in decision-making authority is called a vertical compression of the traditional hierarchy of authority.

Hallmark is a company that was able to achieve benefits from re-engineering. The unification of labor into integrated product teams cut the time it took for new products to go from conception to market by over 60% (Hammer and Champy 1993).

The process orientation of re-engineered corporations allows for the transition from the age of mass production to one of mass customization. Re-engineering suggests that each process team or group of process teams be specially designed to handle a particular situation or market. This approach enables an organization to respond more readily to fluctuations in the environment.

The Learning Organization

The learning organization has been defined by Peter Senge as "an organization that is continually expanding its capacity to create its future" (Senge 1990, p. 14). The five disciplines that make up a learning organization include 1) personal mastery, 2) mental models, 3) team learning, 4) a shared vision, and 5) systems thinking. The last discipline, systems thinking, pulls together the first four components, resulting in an efficient organization. These disciplines are founded in an attempt to capitalize on human nature.

The idea of *personal mastery* is based on the "journeys" that have been undertaken to clarify and actualize our individual visions, determine where we actually are, and progressively close the gap between the vision and the reality.

Efforts to achieve an organization's vision can be hampered by *mental models,* which are preconceived frameworks of perception. Teams within the organization are encouraged to acknowledge these images and to openly communicate them to each other. Through this communication these models are exposed, enabling organizations to grow from their very existence.

Communication regarding the mental models leads to the third discipline of the learning organization, *team learning.* Team learning emphasizes the importance of dialogue and discussion among members of a team and recognizes the differences between team members. Senge (1990) identifies dialogue as open and creative exploration of the issues involved in a decision, and discussions as a constant bombardment of ideas and the necessary defense of each perspective leading to decision making. The goal of the learning organization is to promote alignment of the efforts of all team members.

Alignment of energies within a team and ultimately within the entire organization is possible only through a *shared vision*. The shared vision of any organization is founded in the unique visions of each individual. The learning organization prevents the shared vision of any given company from being the vision of one central figure that everyone else simply abides for 8 hours a day (Senge 1990). Furthermore, a company's shared vision cannot simply be a statement that is arbitrarily decided behind closed doors; it must be examined constantly and modified as necessary by all members of the company.

The fifth discipline, *systems thinking*, is at the foundation of the learning organization. Systems thinking overcomes the boundaries of the classical and neoclassical theorists, who examined separate components of the organization and placed them in a static structure. Systems thinking recognizes a much more dynamic process involving constant adaptive organizational change derived from a self-connecting feedback process that provides necessary information to learn from mistakes and develop better adaptational forms (Senge 1990).

Circular Organization

The circular organization is characterized by a very specific focus on the organization's environment and includes the clients and patients in the planning process. This highly interactive planning is achieved through a system of advisory boards, which are integrated in the organization's hierarchy of authority.

In healthcare facilities the lower tier of advisory boards are oriented toward a particular service or program. For example, a specific service board would include the staff and former patients of an outpatient eating disorder program. The head of the program would serve as the chair of the advisory board. The advisory boards on the next tier are commonly oriented to particular units. Continuing along the lines of the example, a specific unit board would be that of adult psychiatric services. The chairs of the independent services boards (e.g., eating disorders, chemical dependency) would serve as the board members of the unit board.

The head of the outpatient eating disorder program then serves as the chair of the service board and as a contributing board member of the unit board. The chair of the unit board, who then becomes a member of the corporate steering committee, is the head of the unit, in this case, adult psychiatry. In this manner all the boards interact with one another throughout the various levels of the organization (Ackoff 1981). The management of the circular organization is data based and requires education of all members of a board regarding the use of data to evaluate the need for change in processes and to verify the effects of implemented changes (Lartin-Drake et al. 1996). The design of a circular organization facilitates the participation of all employees and accentuates the importance of the contributions of human capital to the company's progress.

Decentralized problem solving is also integral to the circular organization. Its intent is to enable organizational change and procedural change to affect every level of the company. The interactive boards encourage an examination of every procedure at every level within the corporation or facility. The circular organization is designed to meet the demands of the competitive healthcare market, specifically the need for continuous service improvement and useful distinctive innovation.

Product-Line Management

Product-line management is an organizational strategy aimed at unifying an organization across functional lines and allowing the organization to adapt to a rapidly changing environment. Product-line management is "the organizational structure, management control systems, and delivery strategies for healthcare services structured around case types or major clinical services" (Nackel and Kues 1986, p. 109). The three components that contribute to the development of a product-line management strategy are planning, management, and marketing.

Planning

An organization first determines what product lines to develop. Each of these product lines then becomes a distinct business unit, which is considered a cost center. The business unit manager is responsible for the management of, and profit and loss associated with, that product. Executive-level employees are responsible for considering the impact of the inclusion or exclusion of a particular product line on the successful functioning of existing product lines (MacStravic 1986). For example, eliminating a chemical dependency treatment business unit may adversely affect the use of the psychiatric product line. Although the chemical dependency business unit may not be profitable in its independent existence within the facility, the exclusion of that unit could decrease or even eliminate the profitability of the inpatient psychiatric business unit. Therefore, decisions regarding the development or elimination of business units must be determined by a corporate examination of the interaction of all business units and a thorough analysis of the organization's objectives.

Management

Decision making is decentralized in a product-line management model. Decision making is the responsibility of the manager of each business unit. The manager is accountable for the planning, profits, utilization, marketing, and actual delivery of service of that particular product line (Patterson and Thompson 1987).

Marketing

The structure of a product-line management organization places a great deal of importance on the ability to market each product line. The ability to market distinct product lines can establish a facility as a center of excellence in a given field and distinguish that facility from all others.

Summary

The four newer theories discussed in this section are representative of developments in organizational theory that are pertinent to the problems facing healthcare today. Coupled with an understanding of basic organizational theory, these new developments provide a source of ideas and methods to aid the psychiatric administrator in more effectively helping his or her organization to adapt to the challenging contemporary environment.

References

Ackoff RL: Creating the Corporate Future. New York, Wiley, 1981

Fayol H: General and Industrial Management. London, Pittman, 1949

Flower J: The structure of organized change: a conversation with Kevin Kelly. The Healthcare Forum Journal 38:1995

Greenberg J, Baron RA (eds): Organizational structure and design, in Behavior in Organizations, 5th Edition. Englewood Cliffs, NJ, Prentice-Hall, 1995, pp 576–601

Hammer M: Reengineering work: don't automate, obliterate. Harvard Business Review, July/August 1990, p 104

Hammer M: Beyond Reengineering: How the Process-Centered Organization Is Changing Our Work and Our Lives. New York, HarperBusiness, 1996

Hammer M, Champy J: Reengineering the Corporation: A Manifesto for Business Revolution. New York, HarperBusiness, 1993

Johansen R, Swigart R: Upsizing the Individual in the Downsized Organization: Managing in the Wake of Reengineering, Globalization, and Overwhelming Technological Change. New York, Addison-Wesley, 1994

Katzenbach JR, Smith DK: The Wisdom of Teams: Creating the High-Performance Organization. New York, HarperBusiness, 1993

Kuhn TS: The Structure of Scientific Revolutions, 3rd Edition. Chicago, University of Chicago Press, 1996

Lartin-Drake JM, Curran C, Gillis-Donovan J, et al: Improving the quality of health services organization structure by reengineering: circular design and clinical case impact in an academic medical center. Am J Med Qual 11:151–158, 1996

Lichtman CM, Hunt RG: Personality and organization theory: a review of some conceptual literature. Psychol Bull 76:271–294, 1971

Likert R: New Patterns of Management. New York, McGraw-Hill, 1961

MacStravic RS: Product-line administration in hospitals. Health Care Manage Rev 11:35–43, 1986

Mayo E: The Human Problems of an Industrialized Civilization. London, Macmillan, 1933

McGregor D: The Human Side of Enterprise. New York, McGraw-Hill, 1960

Mott PE: A definition of social organization, in The Organization of Society. Englewood Cliffs, NJ, Prentice-Hall, 1965, pp 13–37

Nackel JG, Kues IW: Product-line management. Systems and strategies. Hospital and Health Services Administration 31:109–123, 1986

Patterson DJ, Thompson KA: Product line management: Organization makes the difference. Healthcare Financial Management 41:66–72, 1987

Roethlisberger FJ, Dickson WJ: Management and the Worker. Cambridge, Harvard University Press, 1939

Senge PM: The Fifth Discipline: The Art and Practice of the Learning Organization. New York, Doubleday, 1990

Smith A: An Inquiry into the Nature and Causes of the Wealth of Nations, 11th Edition. London, Pickering, 1995

Taylor FW: Scientific Management. New York, Harper & Row, 1911

Weber M: Theory of Social and Economic Organization. New York, Oxford University Press, 1947

❖ 4 ❖

Leadership

Miles F. Shore, M.D.
Mark Vanelli, M.D., M.H.S.

Both leadership and management are essential for organizations, but they are different. In a dictionary, a *leader* is defined as "a person who by force of example, talents, or qualities of leadership plays a directing role, wields commanding influence or has a following in any sphere of activity or thought." A *manager* is "one that conducts business or household affairs with discreet frugality and care" (Webster's 1976). Leadership implies guidance from a position out front, whereas management carries the connotation of hands-on. It is said that leaders know the right thing to do, and managers know how to do it right. Although leadership can be separated from management conceptually, in most cases, individuals with organizational responsibilities must be able both to lead and to manage.

Leadership is a ubiquitous topic in the business literature. Seminars and workshops on leadership are a major industry, and leadership consultants have thriving practices. But leadership has been conspicuously absent in the training of health and mental health professionals. Until very recently, clinical training prepared health professionals primarily to serve individual patients. As a result, in clinical professions, leaders have tended to rise through the ranks and find leadership training in places other than professional schools.

As health and mental health services become organized into systems of care, at least some clinicians must accept leadership roles to preserve the core values of healthcare organizations. This change is currently taking place. Leadership training increasingly is being explicitly adapted for health professionals. Programs for physicians to earn degrees in business administration, health policy and management, and public administration are proliferating. And the special characteristics of leadership demanded by organizations of professionals are being identified and studied (Beckham 1995; Quinn et al. 1996).

Tasks of Leadership

The structure of all organizations is changing dramatically as information and knowledge become the equivalent of capital investment in the previous industrial era. The hierarchical, bureaucratic structure of traditional organizations is giving way to a much more horizontal structure. Command and control leadership working through formally constituted departments is being replaced by a more consensual style with much more emphasis on human capital and the application of knowledge, and with accountability pushed downward to small teams that are responsible for the conduct of work (Bartlett and Ghoshal 1995).

Organizational structure relying on tight boundaries is giving way to what some have termed the *boundaryless organization,* in which departments may be replaced by task groups assembled around specific technology applied to particular projects (Arthur and Rousseau 1996). This project focus may cause the corporation to merge temporarily with other organizations, even with competitors, to work on projects that require novel skills or highly specialized technology.

Despite these changes in organizations, leadership remains essential, and the fundamental requirements for leadership are relatively unchanged. As Heifitz (1994) pointed out, the role of leadership in organizing the behavior of a collection of disparate individuals into activities that are adaptive in solving human problems has an evolutionary basis. The complexity of tasks requires a system of accountability to some central point. Rapid change continues to require direction. Most of all, the values of the organization need to be personified in leadership to elicit the crucial organizational identification that is required for cohesive activity.

The fundamental purpose of all organizations is perpetuation—to survive and grow (Levinson 1981). To do so requires a convincing assessment of the problems facing the organization, a strategy for solving those problems, and the commitment of the participants to work with the leader to accomplish the plan. The leader's task is to identify the problems that threaten survival by scanning the external environment, to develop a strategic plan for solving the problems, and to enlist the support of everyone in the organization. Thus, vision is essential but not sufficient; leaders must have strategic competence. And they must have followers; they cannot do it alone.

In the new healthcare organizations, psychiatric leaders must be comfortable in supporting the activities of teams and in functioning in leadership roles in teams of professionals in which the professional expertise of each member is recognized, supported, and included to enhance the work. In some settings, leaders may need to be comfortable with the exercise of informal power to challenge processes that do not work, inspire a shared vision of change, lead by example, empower subordinates, and reward desired behaviors and values (Kouzes and Posner 1995).

Tools of Leadership

Managerial Alliance

The first essential tool of leadership is what Levinson termed the *managerial alliance.* It is formed by the identification of the members of the organization with the values that are personified by the leader in doing his or her job. This identification is the "glue" that binds the organization together. The values that are crucial are not trivial but instead reflect the larger purposes of the organization that make people proud to be there. A highly publicized example of organizational values expressing larger purposes was the decision at Johnson & Johnson to remove Tylenol from the shelves as soon as poison was found in packages that had been tampered with. The decision was made by a middle manager who knew immediately that the Johnson & Johnson creed was to put patient safety ahead of profits, and he acted accordingly, without needing to consult higher management. Levinson termed these organizational values the *transcendent purposes,* the "why we are here" that people later look back on with satisfaction. They are what add precious meaning to the years of our lives, that one inevitably unrenewable resource. They are the answer to the questions "What makes you proud to work at this place?" and often "What makes this place different from other similar places?"

The individual counterpart of these transcendent organizational purposes is the ego ideal—the characteristics and values to which we personally aspire. The connection between the ego ideals of individuals and the transcendent purposes of the organization forms the bond in healthy organizations so that participation in the activities of the organization makes the workers feel good about themselves. The violation of this bond leads to organizational ill health that manifests itself in corrosive cynicism, unproductive conflict, and implacable mistrust of leadership.

By far, the most important transcendent purpose in health and mental health organizations is commitment to the care of patients. That patients come first is a powerful motivation for dedication to the task; it is highly valued and remarkably resistant even to poor working conditions—noncompetitive salaries, poor supervision, cosmetically inadequate facilities, difficult working hours, and inadequate funding. In some instances, it even restrains greed. Closely allied is the service ethic that "values performance above reward" (Brandeis 1914/1986). Violation of dedication to patient care by dishonesty, abuse of trust, incompetent practice, or exploitation typically results in swift action on the part of others in the organization regardless of the status hierarchy. This explains the observation that "whistle blowers" may be of lower professional or occupational status, because the culture of service to patients pervades healthcare organizations and may override the hierarchy.

The leader must understand the terms of the managerial alliance, particularly the nature of the organizational values. The leader must affirm these on every possible occasion through frequent articulation and by his or her behavior. If patient care is the overriding organizational value, then the leader must appear on the clinical units and, if possible, make rounds. The leader also should take some care of patients, if feasible, either on an ongoing basis or on-call. More important, the leader must ensure that as resources are allocated among patient care, research, and training, patient care receives some preferential treatment. The leader should seize every opportunity to reinforce the values through special awards, systemic performance appraisal, and reminders on special occasions, such as the beginning of the budget year and the academic year.

Psychological Contract

The second indispensable tool of leadership is the *psychological contract* (Levinson 1962; Rousseau 1995). Organizations differ in many ways that affect the kinds of individuals that are attracted to employment. Banks need employees who pay close attention to procedural reliability and exhibit conservative attitudes and behavior to reassure customers that their money is in safe hands. In return for compliance with such a sedate culture, banks offer employees a quiet atmosphere, regular hours, defined benefits, and relative job security. In contrast, software companies that sell the products of creativity require unconventionality and original thinking. Their employees may, unpredictably, stay up all night working at their computers and work inhuman hours for weeks to meet deadlines. If a software offering fails, they may be laid off with little notice. In return, they can dress casually at work, play volleyball in the middle of the morning to harness their restlessness and stimulate their creativity, and move from company to company without being considered unstable or culturally deviant. Needless to say, the kinds of people who feel comfortable working in a bank would be vastly out of place in a software company and, most emphatically, vice versa.

Psychological contracts are inexplicit but powerful cultural agreements that reflect both the nature of the work to be performed and the organizational values. As a set of mutual expectations between leadership and subordinates, the psychological contract is a significant component of the managerial alliance. It is important to emphasize that a contract implies obligations on both parties—the leader and the followers. Violation by either side leads to a breakdown of organizational structure and the emergence of behavior that may be destructive for the organization and highly distressing to individuals. A classic example is the citywide distress in Rochester, New York, when Eastman Kodak, which had promised jobs for life in its psychological contract with employees, for the first time in the 1980s was forced to lay off some of its work force.

All of the mental health professions have psychological contracts; the contract is particularly clear in psychiatry. Young people choose medical careers with the expectation that they will have to excel as students, work hard for very low pay as interns and residents, and continue to place their obligations to patients and the enhancement of their skills above other considerations. In return, they expect to have important careers marked by great professional autonomy, enjoy high status and respect in their communities, and be comfortable financially for the rest of their lives. The rage that most physicians currently feel at the incursions of managed care reflects the violation of almost every one of the rewards that are included in this agreement.

Leaders must be sensitive to the terms of the psychological contract, reinforce it, and avoid violating it, if possible. In difficult times, violation may be inevitable. In that case, the contract must be renegotiated in terms of the new reality. Such renegotiation requires careful consideration of the managerial alliance and the organizational values. In modern organizations, it may be necessary to have different psychological contracts with different groups of workers; contracts with permanent workers inevitably will be very different from those with temporary or part-time employees. The plethora of new employment arrangements—job sharing, part-time work, seasonal work—require elaborate and flexible expectations between employer and employed (Pottruck 1996; Rousseau 1995; Strebel 1996).

Strategic Competence

Strategic competence is the third essential tool of leadership. Not too long ago, the marketplace within which psychiatric leaders functioned was relatively sedate. There was competition, but its excesses were restrained. In the 1980s strong advocacy by the mental health community increased health insurance coverage for mental healthcare. That inpatient care could be delivered at a very low cost made it possible for private psychiatric hospitals in less-regulated states to charge substantial rates, generating a comfortable margin with 50%–60% occupancy. If a patient's insurance coverage ran out, he or she could be transferred to the public sector for care in community mental health centers or state hospitals. In the public sector, competition was largely among state agencies vying for human services dollars and among institutions struggling to stretch their budgets by "turfing" patients to other facilities.

With the advent of health reform and the unleashing of market forces, competition has taken on new intensity. Now, healthcare organizations must be aware of their strategic position and must constantly adjust their strategy to maximize their competitive edge. Margins are much smaller so that solvency requires close calculation of fixed and variable costs by service component, as well as the pricing of services (too high may be unacceptable to purchasers; too low may fail to cover costs). If the organization is managing risk, financial disaster can come from many quarters—mistakes in the assessment of risk in setting capitation rates (misjudging the complexity of the care required), not taking advantage of new clinical technology or information system support, and not acquiring adequate reinsurance or other coverage for catastrophic losses. Added to these considerations is the state of the industry, with the possibility of acquisitions, consolidations, and strategic alliances as avenues to perpetuation. These issues are very new on the agenda of psychiatric leaders.

Porter (1991) suggested that two questions are involved in strategic thinking: 1) What is the structure of the industry in which you are functioning? 2) What is your own organization's relative position in the industry? The answers to these two questions require an assessment of the following five forces of competition that, in Porter's view, determine the degree of profitability in any industry:

1. *The character of the rivalry among the competing companies.* Vicious competition makes an industry less attractive and less profitable than if the competition is more subdued and genteel. Industries that focus on service and image are more profitable than those that are preoccupied with price-cutting. In a current example, the relentless reduction of per member per month prices has reduced margins so that now some managed care companies are using improved quality of service as a new competitive strategy.

2. *The threat of new entrants to the field.* If it is easy for others to enter the business, adding capacity and cutting prices, then it will be less profitable. The managed care revolution has seen numerous start-up companies, some of dubious qualifications and tactics, enter the field and drive down prices and quality. This is possible because managed care companies require relatively low initial capital costs, and an oversupply of providers makes it possible to acquire expertise relatively inexpensively.

3. *The threat of substitute services or products.* Profits for a particular service will drop if alternatives are available. The growth of intensive case management, intensive outpatient treatment, and partial hospitalization have made it difficult for traditional psychiatric inpatient services to be profitable or, in some cases, to survive.

4. *The bargaining power of suppliers.* In healthcare, what appears to be a surfeit of hospital beds and health professionals has eroded their bargaining power as "suppliers" and contributed to the profits of the managed care industry.

5. *The bargaining power of buyers.* In healthcare, the concentrated purchasing power of large self-insured companies, Medicare, and state Medicaid agencies has created market-driven healthcare reform, with managed care as its vehicle. The result is that funds that used to be paid to healthcare providers are now being diverted as savings to the purchasers of care and profits to the managers of care. This is a classic case of "oligopsony," in which a market is dominated by a few purchasers who wield disproportionate influence because they buy such large amounts. The bargaining power of buyers *is a major determinant of the ability to set prices that produce profits.*

Porter (1991) makes the point that these five competitive factors can be influenced by a leader sufficiently agile and imaginative to choose modes of adaptive competition; doing so may, in some cases, reshape the industry. Even without changing the industry, an organization may be positioned strategically to gain competitive advantage. Porter noted two basic varieties of competitive advantage: 1) to have consistently lower costs than your competitors and 2) to reduce the scope of your operation to occupy a particular niche in the market. At times, it may be possible to define a position that does both. For instance, in behavioral healthcare, organizations specializing in intensive case management or residential treatment may offer care for persons with serious mental disorders that is both lower cost and not available from larger organizations that offer more comprehensive services. According to Porter, the mistake to be avoided is to try a little of several strategies. Thus, being "stuck in the middle" does not lead to profits because successful strategies demand trade-offs; low cost is typically inconsistent with high quality, and vice versa.

In the new behavioral healthcare environment, competition is intense, and the consequences of strategic missteps may be fatal. Although strategic vision based on organizational values is essential, without strategic competence, the result may be disastrous.

Management of Change

The fourth essential tool of leadership is *management of change*. Because perpetuation of the organization requires adaptation to a constantly shifting environment, the leader is responsible for the initiation and management of organizational change. In steady economic environments, in businesses that rely on stability and order, or in those that enjoy market dominance, managing change may be less salient. In unstable, rapidly shifting environments, managing change may be the leader's most important concern. This issue is highly relevant for psychiatric leaders because of the current volatility of healthcare in general and behavioral healthcare in particular.

The basic model of change management is the normal grief reaction, defined first by Lindemann (1944) in the aftermath of the Coconut Grove nightclub fire in Boston, Massachusetts, in the mid-1940s. He described a sequence of denial of the loss ("perhaps my daughter went to another club"); reactions of hostility to those who are trying to help ("leave me alone; you can't understand how I feel; your daughter did not die"); disruption of normal activity with emotional numbing; then, gradual awareness of the loss ("at times, it seems as if she is still alive"); acceptance of the loss if the process of gradual awareness is successful; followed by a return to normal activities that may include some compensations or substitutes for what has been lost.

As we know from clinical work, the essence of this psychological process is the loosening of emotional attachments from the original object in order to invest in new objects. This is the "grief work." That this work is necessary in any process of change is captured by the slogan "all change is loss." It accounts for the fact that even changes for the better may be painful and involve considerable emotional work. The best example of this particular counterintuitive phenomenon is the emotional upsets experienced by persons who are promoted. Even if the new job involves higher salary and increased status and is the culmination of lifelong ambition, it is not uncommon to observe sleep loss, depression, and difficulty in organizing activities because the person must abandon ties to familiar associates, familiar places, and activities and invest in the unfamiliar accouterments and relationships of the new position. These reactions may be more pronounced if, as is often the case, the new position is also more complex and demanding.

Organizational change involves similar adjustments on the part of the people throughout the organization. The current turmoil over downsizing, re-engineering, mergers, and acquisitions offers numerous examples of the emotional cost of these changes, many of which add a measure of helplessness and loss of control to the emotional reality of loss. Frequently, the leader, as the interpreter of the environment, must stimulate change to adapt to external conditions that threaten organizational perpetuation. In that case, the leader's role is both as a threat and a consoler in the face of threat. Not surprisingly, a thriving industry exists to assist leaders in managing organizational change involving such a complicated role.

The leader's task is to conduct a normal grieving process by describing the reality without hedging but acknowledging frequently and with feeling the pain involved for everyone in the organization. It is no exaggeration to say that the leader must be the chief mourner, putting into words and expressing for the whole organization the pain that the individual members are feeling. Thus, in the case of downsizing, the leader must say as often as possible that downsizing is a terrible thing that is destructive to the organization and devastating for individuals. As that is said, the reality of the need to downsize must be affirmed to assist individuals in facing the reality through repetition. A fatal error is to offer reassurance that "it really isn't so bad; in fact, in the end, it may be all for the best." Such attempts to gloss over the pain are typically met with cynicism, anger, or outright rebellion. Creating an alliance with the members of the organization around mutual acknowledgment of the pain is the first step toward resolution and a return to organizational health.

The leader must work with key members of the organization to develop a guiding coalition to lead the change process (Kotter 1996). Developing a strategic vision, based on the transcendent purposes of the organization, is the next, and perhaps most crucial, step. It is unlikely that any substantial change is possible unless it can be seen as furthering the core organizational values. The means of realizing the values may have to be changed, but the values must remain intact, or the organization will fracture. Kotter (1996) outlined an elaborate process for achieving organizational change involving eight steps to promote and anchor changes within the organizational culture. He rightly noted that if change is of major proportions, and if it is to last, the process will take at least 5–8 years.

Allocation of Time

The fifth essential tool of leadership, perhaps the most basic of all, is the *allocation of time.* How leaders allocate their time among the various possible tasks that demand attention is the "final common pathway" of leadership effectiveness. What leaders actually do in order to add value is determined by the nature of the organization. A comprehensive study of leadership approaches found that in successful companies, leaders adapted their approach to the needs of the company rather than adopting a leadership style that suited their own personalities (Farkas and Wetlaufer 1996). The needs of the company were defined by the state of the industry; was it growing or mature? Were there many competitors, and were they strong or weak? What was the state of technology in the industry? What were the organization's assets in terms of employees and capital, and what was its competitive position?

The study identified five different approaches to leadership, based on the situation of the company:

1. The *strategic approach* was adopted by leaders who concentrated on developing a long-term strategy for the survival of the corporation into the distant future. These leaders spent 80% of their time on external affairs—assessing the competition, customers, new technology, and market trends. They attended much less to internal matters, such as financial systems or staff recruitment.
2. The *human assets approach* was adopted by leaders who felt that the strategy would be taken care of by the units of the business closest to the customers. They focused on enhancing the organizational culture through the quality of employees. They

spent their time identifying new hires, doing performance appraisal, and mapping the careers of the incumbent personnel.
3. The *expertise approach* involved the leader enhancing competitive advantage by selecting and disseminating areas of expertise throughout the organization. These leaders spent their time studying new technology, assessing the state of the competitors' technological prowess, and conferring with engineers and customers about these innovations.
4. The *box approach* required detailed surveillance of errors and exceptions, as well as detailed specification of procedures and policies. It was appropriate for companies whose success depended on providing customers with a reliable and risk-free experience. Consequently, these leaders focused on internal organizational controls to ensure predictability of product or performance.
5. The *change approach* was chosen when the nature of the business demanded constant reinvention. These leaders spent most of their time creating a culture that embraced change by meeting with employees, suppliers, and customers. They rewarded aggressiveness and independence in their employees.

The authors of this study noted that over the life of the corporation, the emphasis among these five leadership approaches might well change as the business environment changed. Certainly, in the current psychiatric administration, an openness to change, as well as use of the box approach at the service level to ensure reliability of patient care, must be emphasized. Human assets are always important in service industries such as healthcare, and expertise also is essential because of the growing role of technology to improve the quality of care. Psychiatric administrators must, thus, strike a balance among these five approaches to leadership.

Psychiatrists as Leaders

Because leadership involves understanding people and maintaining thoughtful interpersonal relationships, it is logical to imagine that psychiatrists, who are trained in the conduct of special relationships, might be specially fitted for these roles. That expectation is only partially valid. Psychiatry, as a specialty of medicine, attracts certain kinds of people, and training for clinical practice involves concepts and procedures that are specific to the consulting room. Neither the psychological contract to which would-be psychiatrists respond nor the concepts useful in the consulting room are automatically transferable to the corner office (Shore 1991).

Psychiatrists, especially those who are attracted to psychotherapeutic practice, must be comfortable with their own passivity in order to listen and be empathically responsive to patients. Passivity, however, may be a fatal handicap for leaders. Organizations demand action—thoughtful action to be sure, but action nonetheless—sooner rather than later. The leader who cannot step forward to take charge, decide, and launch a course of action will create great anxiety in the organization. Furthermore, the leader must ensure that resources are allocated fairly in terms of the values and strategic requirements of the organization and that overly aggressive, manipulative, or irresponsible members of the organization are held to account. Passivity in carrying out these functions will quickly erode morale, and the organization will drift.

Psychiatrists are trained clinically to seek the latent meaning of events, to foster the expression of feelings, and to allow for the unfolding of intrinsic patterns of behavior. Transferred intact to the leadership role, those clinical habits can be highly destructive. Leaders who spend too much time searching for latent meanings may be avoiding the need for actions. Fostering abreaction and catharsis by the staff can produce a kind of addiction that displaces forward motion that is essential for survival. Personnel in mental health organizations are naturally attracted to introspection, to a search for the latent meaning of events, to emotional expression, and to dialogue. At times, they seem to show a kind of "patient envy," seeking to substitute the role of patient for the role of caregiver. The leader must gently refocus such tendencies, so that time and energy can be devoted to useful work that advances the purposes of the organization by contributing to its perpetuation and growth.

Some concepts of dynamic psychiatry, such as transference, are highly useful to leaders. Transference-like distortions of reality in organizations reflect the normal human tendency to find meaning in random events. Many people prefer to settle on a plot to explain events that actually reflect confusion and happenstance. Most believe that the leader is the leading plotter, hatching schemes whose content, interestingly enough, typically reflects the character styles of those who prefer such conspiratorial explanations. Some of these individuals, caught in a geodetic web of oedipal triangles, see organizational events as a series of power contests with the administration. Others, under the sway of sibling rivalry, have difficulty delegating tasks to subordinates unless they can arrange for them to fail. And they are certain that the leader is stealing their best ideas and giving them to others who are preferred by the leader. The leader must understand such distortions and deal with them by frequent reality checks conveyed to the staff. Apologies for one's errors as a leader, constant clarification of the reasons for decisions, and an open process in which others participate may help to dispel mysteries that stimulate unrealistic and potentially destructive fantasies.

Narcissism is another concept that can usefully be transferred from clinical practice to the leader's armamentarium. Professional organizations are meritocracies made up of individuals who have invested an enormous amount in their own training. These individuals are internally driven to live up to high standards, and they function in a professional culture in which self-esteem is based on those internal standards and the judgment of their peers. This provides fertile soil for high performance but also the persistent danger of narcissistic injury. Personal standards that exceed what is possible, intrusions on personal space or professional prerogatives, and criticism that is not offered in sufficiently tactful terms all may precipitate hurt feelings and lead to conflict.

Being sufficiently attuned to narcissistic injury is extremely useful in understanding personnel problems in professional organizations. Heinz Kohut (1985), whose theories of personality development and therapy rested on understanding the subtle vicissitudes of narcissism, once said that he began to appreciate the importance of narcissism in public affairs during his organizational work at the Chicago Institute for Psychoanalysis and the American Psychoanalytic Association. Although he said it in the midst of battles over his theories, this was no sly jab at his antagonists. Instead, he was making the point that it is in organizational affairs that narcissism is revealed in its infinite variety of constructive and destructive possibilities. This is particularly true in the case of organizations made up of creative, productive people.

The selfobject, a key construct in Kohut's theory, refers to people or things that are reacted to emotionally as if they were part of oneself. Leaders who doubt the usefulness of this concept will change their mind if they attempt to reduce the size of someone's office or reassign the person to a more inconvenient parking spot. The corollary of this observation is that usually beneath anger lie hurt feelings, however well concealed.

The leader must give regular feedback about performance. Such appraisal is typically more honored in the breach than the observance because supervisors fear that they will injure the person's self-esteem. In fact, lack of feedback generates the common complaint in organizations, "no one here cares about what I do until I screw up." Performance appraisal is an opportunity, above all, to provide narcissistic gratification; it reflects genuine interest in the subordinate's work and is an opportunity to connect the individual with the organization and reinforce the organizational values. It is also, of course, an opportunity to identify areas that need improvement, but that should be secondary to the positive reinforcement. And the offer of assistance in improving performance is actually a way of affirming the managerial alliance based on the high standards of the individual being evaluated. Of course, the appraisal should be personal, should focus on critical incidents, and should have as its basis a coherent and specific job description that includes expected behaviors. It definitely should not involve the numerical systems of appraisal that are mechanical, impersonal, and usually destructive to self-esteem because the qualities and performance meriting the top grades in such quantitative schemes could honestly be fulfilled by no human being (Levinson 1976). The appraisal of performance is the primary means of disseminating the organizational culture; as such, it is one of the key functions of leadership.

Finally, the leader must be aware of the potential for organizations to regress. Leaders must devote constant thought and energy to limiting regression in order to get work done. In psychoanalytic psychotherapy, regression is facilitated by reducing the structure of the therapeutic encounter and encouraging the patient to forgo, temporarily, the conventions of usual conversation in order to "say whatever comes to mind" (i.e., to free associate). Bion (1961) demonstrated dramatically what happened when groups were experimentally deprived of their conventional assumptions about expected behavior. He found that the members' behavior deteriorated into regressive longings to be taken care of, wishes to flee the situation, and bitter anger at the leader. Groups in such unstructured situations could not possibly do useful work because of these regressive reactions.

The point of leadership is that it is important to provide structure through a variety of means. The organizational chart, often considered the plaything of obtunded bureaucrats, actually serves an important psychological function in countering regression by providing a reality check regarding reporting relationships, duties and expectations, and the larger structure of the organization. In the case of the new boundaryless organizations, built of more fluid relationships, structure may be provided by clear definitions of projects, products, and time lines; the membership of task-oriented teams; and particularly who is accountable for organizing the work. Meetings of committees or task groups must be tightly organized, with clear definitions of membership, expectations for attendance, formal agendas, and strict adherence to starting and ending times. Roberts Rules of Order (Robert 1990), read as a psychological treatise, provides a set of guidelines to prevent group regression. In early versions, it even called for persons in groups to address one another with civility (i.e., limit regressive emotional expression).

New Demands on Leadership

The changes taking place in the health and mental health systems can be characterized in many ways. Among the most prominent are a shift from primarily intraprofessional accountability for quality of care to the addition of external accountability to consumers and to corporate structures. Another shift is increased reliance on technology to reduce practice variability, provide access to research developments, and monitor the quality of individual provider practice (Shore 1997). From the practitioner's viewpoint, these changes spell more organization but probably not in the old model of corporate structure. Rather, groups of practitioners that can accept risk likely will be organized through technology and will be supported by administrative functions in their interactions with patients and other parts of the human services system.

In these new systems, leadership will be required to perform the following functions: 1) defining the vision, the culture, and the psychological contract for participants in the organization; 2) determining the direction of change, conducting the process of change, and allocating human and financial resources to support the process; and 3) marshaling the resources and providing the conditions for productive work. Careful attention to the efficient allocation of capital, the assumption and management of risk, and a strong commitment to continual change are required.

Experience from industry suggests strongly that there is little to be gained from fighting these tectonic changes in the organization of health and mental healthcare. Industries and companies that clung too strongly to their old ways, dismissed criticism, looked internally for accountability, invested in overcapacity, and did not keep up with new technology were doomed to failure (Levinson 1993). Perpetuation, the fundamental task of organizations, demands much more from leaders. To participate in these creative and exciting but demanding times is at once the burden and the privilege of leadership and requires both technical mastery and vision and courage to succeed.

References

Arthur M, Rousseau D: The Boundaryless Career: A New Employment Principle for a New Organizational Era. Oxford, England, Oxford University Press, 1996

Bartlett C, Ghoshal S: Changing the role of top management: beyond systems to people. Harvard Business Review 73:132–142, 1995

Beckham J: Crafting the new physician executive. Physician Executive 21:3–5, 1995

Bion W: Experiences in Groups and Other Papers. London, Tavistock, 1961

Brandeis L: Business—a profession (1914). Modified by Samuel O. Their, in Familiar Medical Quotations. Edited by Strauss M. Boston, MA, Little, Brown, 1986, pp 457–458.

Farkas C, Wetlaufer S: The ways chief executive officers lead. Harvard Business Review 74:110–122, 1996

Heifitz R: Leadership Without Easy Answers. Cambridge, MA, Harvard University Press, 1994, pp 49–66

Kohut H: Self Psychology and the Humanities. New York, WW Norton, 1985, p 51

Kotter J: Leading Change. Cambridge, MA, Harvard Business School Press, 1996

Kouzes J, Posner B: The Leadership Challenge. San Francisco, CA, Jossey-Bass, 1995

Levinson H: Organizational Diagnosis. Cambridge, MA, Harvard University Press, 1962

Levinson H: Appraisal of *what* performance? Harvard Business Review 54:1–7, 1976

Levinson H: Executive: The Guide to Responsive Management. Cambridge, MA, Harvard University Press, 1981, p 17

Levinson H: Why the behemoths fell: psychological roots of corporate failure. Presented at the Distinguished Contributions to Psychological Practice Lecture, American Psychological Association, Toronto, Ontario, August 20, 1993

Lindemann E: Symptomatology and management of acute grief. Am J Psychiatry 101:141–148, 1944

Porter M: Know your place: how to assess the attractiveness of your industry and your company's position in it. Inc., September 1991, pp 90–93

Pottruck D: Strategies for avoiding the rush toward downsizing. Vital Speeches of the Day 62(64):752–755, October 1, 1996

Quinn J, Anderson P, Finkelstein S: Making the most of the best. Harvard Business Review 74:71–80, 1996

Robert H (ed): The Scott, Foresman Roberts Rules of Order, Newly Revised, 1990 Edition. Glenview, IL, Scott Foresman, 1990

Rousseau D: Psychological Contracts in Organizations: Understanding Written and Unwritten Agreements. Thousand Oaks, CA, Sage, 1995

Shore M: Administration and the third ear, in Administrative Issues in Public Mental Health: New Directions for Mental Health Services. Edited by Keill S. San Francisco, CA, Jossey-Bass, 1991, pp 19–29

Shore M: A lesson in history, circa 2047 (editorial). Am J Psychiatry 154:307–311, 1997

Strebel P: Why do employees resist change? Harvard Business Review, May/June 1996, pp 86–92

Webster's Third New International Dictionary. Springfield, MA, G & C Merriam, 1976

❖ 5 ❖

Planning

Organizational Responses to Uncertainty in Unstable and Complex Environments

Jose M. Santiago, M.D.

Planning has been described as looking forward to create a road map for the organization to follow in positioning itself over a specific time span. A vision of the future is useful to the organization to guide the configuration of its components, its mixture of human resources, and management of its finances and its investments and to measure its successes or failures. In a stable market environment, long-range planning is a cyclical, low-frequency activity that assumes that change will be slow and predictable as it steers the organization toward the fulfillment of its mission. Predicting the future requires data-based understanding of the current situation and the ability to make educated guesses that enable accurate extrapolations into the future. When these conditions are present, market trends may be anticipated and the organization may be positioned to compete successfully in the market. That is no longer the case in healthcare.

In today's rapidly evolving healthcare environment, changes occur at a moment's notice and without any warning. The sale of a large insurance or provider network can bring to the local market a new vision, new management policies, and a different style of operation. These Wall Street–driven transactions, so common as managed care evolves in both the public and the private sectors, are typically arranged quietly in corporate boardrooms and result in abrupt, disruptive changes that are difficult to predict or prepare for (Frank et al. 1995). In the public sector, legislative and executive initiatives may turn state programs over to private enterprises, making long-term planning by public agencies obsolete in a few months (Austin et al. 1995; Crowell et al. 1995). Furthermore, in such unstable conditions, healthcare leaders must concentrate on the daily tasks of operational and financial problems with little time for engaging, even sporadically, in long-term planning (Alexander et al. 1995; Johnson 1995; McCool 1995). Moreover, reliable data on which planning depends are not available, prediction is perilous, and the result is that long-range planning becomes an exercise in futility.

To survive in this new and uncertain environment, a new concept of planning is required (Burton et al. 1995). Rather than attempting to reduce uncertainty, an experimental approach to planning has been proposed as more adapted to the current play of market forces (Deprez and Horton 1996; Handy 1993; Hudson 1995). This concept involves systematic risk-taking in which different options and possibilities are investigated and tested. The results of these trials are constantly monitored. Failures are rejected, and successes are pursued. Risk is mitigated through partnerships or alliances and through diversification rather than specialization. The critical element in planning becomes sequential decision making rather than the forecasting of scenarios. Attempts to assess future data and possibilities are not discarded, but "on a walk into a fog, a light is not much use—you have to stop and feel your way" (Handy 1993, p. 369). Flexibility, quick response, and constant adjustments of direction are highly valued skills for modern managers.

Established assumptions in organizational theory are challenged by the need to find new planning frameworks to deal with uncertainty (Handy 1993). Traditional wisdom is that concentration and specialization improve efficiency, that hierarchy is inevitable, and that employees are a variable cost rather than a fixed asset. Although it is not possible in this chapter to examine all of these assumptions, an example may suffice to illustrate the need to challenge those that have a significant effect on planning. A classic assumption of the market economy is that a company is the property of its shareholders. Now, an individual's or a group's financial portfolio contains so many different shares that a sense of ownership of any one company is diluted. Furthermore, the input of millions of shareholders into an organization they do not control, or even really consider their own, is unrealistic. In principle, boards of directors represent a community of shareholders (or "stakeholders" in the case of not-for-profit organizations), but the current tendency is to reduce the number of board members and to focus on the value to the organization of their expertise in finances, management, or planning rather than their representation of the shareholders.

A more useful concept is to consider the organization as accountable to a community of individuals or groups, each in a different role. For example, the shareholders as a source of capital are entitled to adequate return on their investment. Customers are entitled to less expensive and better products. Governmental entities are entitled to returns in the form of employment for their citizens and other community benefits, as well as tax payments. Employees (including management) have a right to wages and, in some cases, a share of the profits or surplus. Accounting for the fulfillment of benefits to the community is different from planning for benefits for a particular interest group. The benefits to each of these constituent groups must be considered in planning for the future of any organization.

Modern, flexible approaches to planning mean that the planning function must be continuous and therefore become a constant feature of the ongoing operations of the organization. It thus becomes part and parcel of the management of the organization rather than being a separate function. In the description that follows, it will, at times, be difficult to separate the planning function from the familiar functions of leadership—assessment of the competitive environment, attention to customer needs, creation of a vision, steady concern for managing change, attention to cost and processes of quality assurance, education of the work force, refinement of products, and continuous reassessment of competitive advantage.

The Planning Process: Systems Thinking

The first consideration in planning is to understand the organization as a system in which interconnected components have a positive or negative effect on the overall efficiency and effectiveness of the whole (Senge 1990). Each component of a system is continuously affected by the other components in feedback loops.

Simply put, the healthcare organization targets a particular customer in a community and develops a vision of the mission of the organization based on the customer's needs. A process is then developed to deliver the necessary services. Objectives must be identified and action plans developed to meet them. Procedures must be specified to measure the degree of success in achieving these objectives, and there must be feedback based on results to improve the process of care on a continuing basis. Fixing the responsibility for improvement on an individual, or even better, on a team, is necessary in order to decentralize the quality improvement process, even though it challenges the traditional hierarchical model of organization. A graphic illustration of such a system of care is given in Figure 5–1.

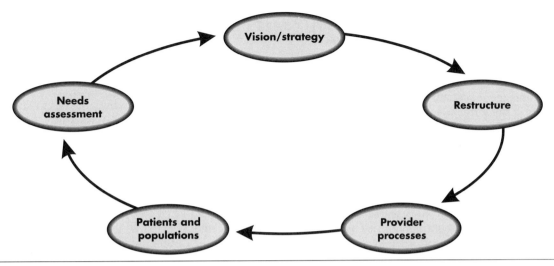

FIGURE 5–1. Cycle of improvement process.

The system is a closed loop that is set up to respond constantly to the following questions:

- What are we trying to do?
- What changes can we make to improve our performance?
- How will we know that we have accomplished our goals?

Four major methods are required to implement this form of planning:

1. Constant review of the vision
2. Constant control of the process
3. Constant analysis of the results of the process
4. Constant redesign of the process, if necessary

Creating a Vision

A vision of the future that is consistent with the organization's philosophy, its mission, and its capabilities must be created. The development and communication of the vision consists of several elements:

- A thorough knowledge of the organizational values, philosophy, mission, and definition of quality
- An accurate and comprehensive understanding of demand in the market and of SWOT (strengths, weaknesses, opportunities, and threats) analyses
- The elaboration of a statement that clearly states the intent of the vision
- The means to communicate effectively the vision to the system's components
- The ability to adjust the vision to maintain the em-

ployees' support while continuing to respond to the demands of the market

The following two examples will illustrate how a strategic plan can be developed and implemented as well as modified in a real setting. The examples are drawn from the public and the private sector.

The Southwestern State Experiment to Change a System of Care

In a southwestern state a small group of individuals planned for major reform of the public sector mental health system. Because no one had appointed them to lead the system or to manage policy, they knew that they did not control the key characteristics and variables. They nevertheless mapped out a strategy to implement changes with only partial control of the system (a county agency), in a climate of great uncertainty for the future and resistance to change.

The first step was to create a vision based on certain values. Seriously mentally ill individuals had been neglected by state programs and deserved a higher priority. The state system not only planned for them poorly but also favored higher-functioning patients at their expense through restricted access, poor service delivery, inadequate treatment and rehabilitation methods, and low funding. The new vision, based on the small reform group's understanding of the needs of seriously mentally ill persons, proposed a patient-centered system that facilitated access and long-term commitment, did not reject patients, and let "the dollars follow the individual patient," thus favoring the seriously mentally ill.

Although the state system subscribed officially to these values, its operations failed to support them. A SWOT analysis by the would-be reformers revealed clearly that the current system had great weaknesses and that there were great threats to change. These included external threats from funding sources such as the federal government and internal threats such as fierce resistance to change by the providers who viewed reform as having serious consequences for their customary operations. However, political opportunity in the form of bipartisan support by the leadership of the state legislature was determined to change the system to deal with a successful class action suit triggered by the reform group.

Backed by this political support, the reformers mounted, over the 6-month legislative session, an intensive and extensive campaign to disseminate their vision and an action plan to implement it. As noted, this approach was opposed strenuously by the provider community whose members launched a vigorous, effective political campaign to defeat the initiative. Only family member groups lent their support to the reform movement. The reformers knew that eventually the opposing provider groups would wear down the legislative leadership and defeat the initiative. As a response to this reality, the strategy in the field, contrary to classic long-term planning, was to modify the proposal into a pilot project, targeting the areas of the state that were assessed as most likely to accept the reforms, and to fund the proposal from new money, thus sparing the traditional vested interests.

A Private Sector Integrated Health System Responds Proactively to Managed Care

In the private sector, a system of comprehensive healthcare in the South decided to learn from the rest of the United States and prepare for managed care with effective tools. The needs were fourfold:

1. Serve the healthcare needs of a defined population, consisting of 30% of the market area, which was an entire state.
2. Have a dedicated set of providers to create a continuum of care.
3. Manage the care.
4. Manage the cost.

The system, a large, not-for-profit organization, decided to create a statewide integrated delivery network (IDN) to deal with these four challenges (Miller 1996). The vision of a statewide IDN was then shared with all the necessary participants (e.g., physicians, hospitals, allied health professionals). A SWOT analysis showed that all the necessary components existed in most of the state except the southern third, which happened to be a particularly important area. The discussions and communications throughout the organization included those who controlled most, if not all, of the internal variables. The challenge was to cover the southern portion of the state

and get support for the IDN from the physicians, two variables that were external to the system.

Objectives of the Organization

If the vision is to become a reality, it must be translated into a set of specific objectives related to key characteristics of the operations of the organization. Typically, these are quality, cost, partnerships and strategic alliances, production (i.e., the delivery of healthcare), education of the management and employees (the so-called learning organization), and organizational values (e.g., providing care that is uncompensated) (Senge 1990).

The objective of achieving quality may be to improve clinical outcomes (decrease mortality and morbidity) or to improve certain processes such as credentialing. A focus on cost will examine indicators such as percentage of charges discounted, intensity of care, and frequency of encounters, all of which have cost consequences. Measuring variables such as patient days per thousand, average length of stay, and costs of delivering various components of care may be important. These variables interact in complex ways. For example, simply decreasing length of stay does not affect cost unless the intensity of the care given also decreases (doing the same very expensive tests in a shorter time only saves the room-and-board costs of a hospitalization). The other objectives must be similarly analyzed. Referring to Figure 5–1, each of the components above can be conceptualized as responding to a market demand and are also subject to continuous reappraisal.

The Public Sector Example

In the public sector experiment cited earlier in this chapter, the objectives proposed by the reform group could be summarized as follows: increased funding, creation of a capitated financing mechanism (to tie these resources to the individual and make "cherry-picking" difficult), creation of continuous treatment teams, creation of regional control and oversight, and, finally, creation of an evaluation agency to measure the quality of the process and outcomes and report them to elected officials. The detailed proposal by the reform group specified the following objectives:

- *Quality:* Continuous treatment teams, for example, represent the redesign of a previous delivery system that had been a traditional combination of outpatient and inpatient services, leading to great expenses for mediocre outcomes for many seriously mentally ill persons (Olsen 1995).

- *Cost:* Capitation was proposed as a means to achieve greater flexibility and efficiency, tie resources to the individual patient, and reduce "cherry-picking"; it was not intended, primarily, to reduce costs.
- *Processes:* The services delivered to seriously mentally ill patients emphasized more life functioning skills and medical intervention rather than therapy. Evaluation also would allow a more outcome-based (or evidenced-based) approach to care (Bennett 1996; Chandler 1996; Goldner and Bilsker 1995).

The Private Sector Example

The private sector IDN vision for a southern state focused on the same objectives:

- *Quality:* By creating a streamlined and integrated system, quality could be enhanced, variability of practice decreased, and outcomes improved.
- *Cost:* Improving quality reduces costs or, in some cases, justifies costs as contributing to long-term outcome. This is true particularly if the aim of the system is to manage disease states over the long term rather than simply immediate costs in the short term. This is the essence of the "disease management" strategy.
- *Processes:* The terms and conditions defining the health insurance benefit determine how employees acquire insurance, pay for it, access and receive care, and are offered prevention and primary care. These elements of the benefit are aimed at improving the system's processes.

All of the components of the health service organization and all of the individuals in it should be able to articulate the objectives identified by senior management. A clear knowledge of these objectives allows the components of the organization to be aligned with one another and achieve synergy. It reflects understanding of the overarching values of the organization—"what we are collectively trying to accomplish." Implementation of action plans to achieve the objectives is the most important measure of the organizational capability.

Implementation Strategy

Having established a vision in the context of systems thinking, and having set specific objectives, the next step for organizational leadership is to outline an implementation strategy (Scholtes 1996).

The first step consists of identifying a coordinating council. This council will be responsible for several

decisions, guided by the vision and objectives identified by senior management:

1. Select processes for improvement.
2. Charter process teams responsible for improvement in specific areas.
3. Establish indicators (outcomes) and thresholds (targets).
4. Support and analyze improvement activities.
5. Support education of management and employees (the learning organization) (Senge 1990).
6. Report to senior management (includes medical staff and boards).

Selecting the processes for improvement requires a specific methodology based on relevant variables. A basic principle is that an organization can deploy its improvement resources on, at most, only four or five projects. Selecting these projects requires establishing a hierarchy of importance based on customer needs and organizational priorities. The criteria include attention to cost-benefit considerations, risk, and visibility. Identifying which areas have a major effect on the organization's ability to deliver the right care at the right price is key to the selection process.

Once the coordinating team has chosen specific projects based on a ranking of priorities, teams must be assigned the task of analyzing and improving the selected processes. The members of these teams are preferably a selected group of individuals who are directly involved in the processes and who have a certain degree of expertise in addition to familiarity with actual operations.

Next, indicators are identified that reflect measurements of outcomes. The indicators can be a mixture of final and intermediate outcomes. Examples are rates of medication compliance and rates of remission for depressed individuals. Adding to the complexity is the need to monitor related indicators to assess the degree to which they are affected by the targeted key indicators. The rate and severity of antidepressant side effects would be an example of related indicators to monitor in addition to the rates of recovery from depression. Excessive morbidity as an intended consequence of the primary treatment modality must be tracked and analyzed.

Each indicator requires a threshold to quantify the improvement. The word *threshold* is preferred to the word *target* for two reasons: 1) targets tend to be static and 2) targets tend to imply a final point to be reached. In contemporary healthcare, targets shift constantly. For example, the ideal per member, per month premium to be charged for psychiatric services is subject to constant revision depending on market forces. Furthermore, improvement efforts must exceed targets if possible. Lowering the incidence of suicide in an elderly population to match national figures is a worthy objective. But achieving a lower than benchmark rate should be the goal; no suicides at all in a population should be the target. A 10% suicide rate might be acceptable as a threshold (i.e., a minimally acceptable rate to be improved on if possible). The goal is to avoid a mind-set in the team that "improvement" has a limit.

The coordinating council also must support and analyze improvement activities. As the process/improvement teams gather data, draft flowcharts, and do other analyses, the coordinating team offers expertise and adds to the process team's quality improvement work. The coordinating council also must deploy an educational effort to ensure that all members of the organization continue to add to their "human capital" by acquiring further technical expertise.

The five steps in the implementation phase can be summarized as follows: choice of a process to improve, analysis of the major key characteristics, flowchart of the process for each key characteristic, identification of the key variables that affect the outcomes, and drafting of alternatives to remove the barriers to higher performance.

Finally, the coordinating council reports to senior management the results of the process team's work. Once the project is complete and has received the approbation of the coordinating team, the senior management team must review and analyze the results to incorporate them into any revision of the original mission.

The Public Sector Example

The coordinating team in the public sector case was the same group that formulated a vision of improvements for the seriously mentally ill population. The selection of an area for improvement was based on their expertise and an analysis of the needs of that population. The coordinating council identified financing, continuity of care, and governance as key outcomes to be focused on. The team proposed capitated financing to ensure that resources were expended on behalf of those for whom they were allocated. Continuous treatment teams were proposed for continuity of care. Finally, regionalization was proposed to deal with governance, a key characteristic in a state with wide variation between distant, large urban areas and vast, sparsely populated areas. The mental health delivery system was analyzed,

financially and clinically, and key variables were identified to measure success. These included, for example, the rate of seriously mentally ill patients unattached to any treatment or support system and the percentage of the allocated resources that actually were spent on the *seriously mentally ill* population.

The legislation authorizing the pilot projects called for feedback to the executive and legislature to measure the effect of the reform. The result over a period of several years was an incremental series of changes in the system of care that, together, documented success:

1. Integration of state and county programs and funding
2. Continuous treatment teams for all seriously mentally ill patients
3. Prioritization of the seriously mentally ill population in the system
4. Increased financial allocations and capped funding to providers for seriously mentally ill patient populations
5. Regionalization of governance and planning

The Private Sector Example

The private sector IDN underwent a similar process. A team of experts was assembled that represented expertise in employer and employee needs, financing of healthcare, medical staff cultures and practices, quality management, and legal issues. Several objectives were assigned to this team, or coordinating council:

- Improvement in quality of care as measured by clinical indicators
- Adaptation to prospective payment and successful management of risk
- Creation of successful partnerships, particularly with physicians
- Creation of an organizational culture that was built on a learning environment

After analyses were done, the following key characteristics were proposed to achieve a competitive advantage for the organization:

- Creation of joint ventures with physicians rather than attempts to employ them or control them
- Creation of triple-option insurance products (health maintenance organization, preferred provider organization, indemnity) to offer employers choices in benefit construction

- A statewide approach to healthcare with maximal local (regional) governance whenever possible
- Emphasis on primary care with active recruitment of primary care physicians
- Emphasis on four key variables: 1) responsibility for the healthcare delivery of a specific population in the market area, 2) establishment of a comprehensive network of providers, 3) management of care, and 4) management of costs
- Creation of a statewide affiliation of mental health providers to establish a partnership with healthcare providers rather than a mental health carve-out; this approach is based on recent findings that appear to make a compelling case that capitated contracts result in savings because of reduced medical costs. Rather than carving out mental health services from global capitation contracts, this approach focuses on reintegration into the healthcare fold. It directly challenges the view of mental health as a "soft science," a double-digit inflation service, and a necessary but unwelcome service area. Instead, risk-sharing partnerships with mental health providers can lead to decreased costs, rising profits, and better health and mental health outcomes (Goldberg 1995; Lazarus 1995a, 1995b; "Partner with behavioral health providers," 1997).

The result was the creation of a statewide health maintenance organization in partnership with a large group of physicians; the creation of four physician hospital organizations (PHOs) to create decision-making (contracting) organizations in joint ventures with physicians (more than 2,000) regionally; the creation of regional primary care physician groups; and the creation of a statewide management service organization to deliver practice management services to primary care physicians.

The result of this redesign was a system that led to a successful presence in the managed care market for the joint ventures. The indicators of outcome included a rapidly increasing enrollment into the health maintenance organization and a multiplication of contracts with the physician hospital organizations.

The difficulties encountered reflected the profound differences in cultures between healthcare administrators, insurance organizations, and physician groups. Distrust, resistance to change, and different definitions of values and priorities led to many stormy discussions, false starts, barriers, and increasing animosity. To deal with these problems that profoundly affected the key outcomes, the coordinating council

fostered several programs to improve physician satisfaction with integrated systems of care by increasing their governance of the systems (Gillies et al. 1993; Shortell et al. 1996; Schreter 1995):

- The creation of an independent practice association
- The appointment of a majority of physicians to the governing boards of the different organizations. Physicians were appointed by the hospital organization to board seats reserved for administrators and as an addition to the maximum allowable elected physicians on boards (as required by the federal government on the governance of such organizations). The importance of joint governance resides in the ability of physicians to participate in the clinical and financial decisions rather than being controlled by corporate organizations.
- Capitalization of primary care practices and of other physicians' joint ventures
- Active participation by physicians in utilization management and quality definitions, including, for example, practice guidelines

This private sector example also illustrates the use of feedback loops and the ability of organizational planning to respond flexibly to rapidly changing variables. When the physician group, co-owners of the health maintenance organization, decided on a different vision for their organization, they quickly disengaged themselves from the partnership. In response, the coordinating council implemented a fallback strategy. Alternative partners were sought, and the system was modified to adjust to the changing environment and to preserve vision and objectives. This kind of rapid, flexible response is required as we learn more about the limitations of integration in healthcare (Executive Chartbook 1996; Robinson 1996).

Planning in the new, volatile environment is thus a continuous cycle of vision and identification of objectives, elaboration of strategies to implement action plans, appointment of teams to improve processes, and analysis of results to realign vision and objectives with changing market conditions.

Summary

Planning processes in stable environments consist of outlining a strategic goal and identifying the financial, operational, clinical, human resources, legal, and other critical data and extrapolating to predict future trends. Activity is then deployed to reduce uncertainty and achieve the goal.

In markets in which the penetration of managed care has created turbulence, inability to predict the future is a constant condition with which administrators must learn to deal. To do so, an experimental approach to planning must be adopted, which involves sequential decision making rather than long-term scenario painting. One may need to launch risky programs to determine the best way to proceed in the face of continuing uncertainty. In any case, planning can no longer be a separate function but must be incorporated in the standard day-to-day operations of the organization.

To carry out this approach to planning requires a search for valid data on the population to be served, the needs of the purchasers of care, and the resources of the organization in meeting those needs. Specific steps must be taken to translate these data into a vision and a set of objectives for the organization. A panel of experts within the organization, a quality coordinating council, must be charged with carrying out a process of continual improvement of the program. This quality coordinating council must assign specific improvement tasks to process teams that report results to the coordinating council. Finally, the organizational governance team must support the initiative, review the results of the improvement process, and modify the vision and objectives based on the outcome of the internal process as well as the continuous assessment of market trends.

References

Alexander JM, Zuckerman HS, Pointer DD: The Challenges of Governing Integrated Health Care Systems. Health Care Manage Rev 20(4):69–81, 1995

Austin MJ, Blum SR, Murtaza N: Local-state government relations and the development of public sector managed mental health care systems. Adm Policy Ment Health 22(3): 203–215, 1995

Bennett MJ: Is psychotherapy ever medically necessary? Psychiatr Serv 47:966–970, 1996

Burton GD, Oviatt BM, Kallas-Burton L: Strategic planning in hospitals: a review and proposal. Health Care Manage Rev 20(3):16–25, 1995

Chandler D: Client outcomes in two model capitated integrated service agencies. Psychiatr Serv 47:176–180, 1996

Crowell A, DelliQuardi T, Austin M: Planning for managed mental health services in Los Angeles. Adm Policy Ment Health 22(3):217–245, 1995

Deprez RD, Horton SL: Community health status and service needs assessment: an analytic tool in a changing health care delivery system. Journal of Hospital Marketing 10(2):117–128, 1996

Executive Chartbook: strategies for steering your integrated delivery system. Hosp Health Netw 70(8): 82, 1996

Frank RG, McGuire TG, Newhouse JP, et al: Risk contracts in managed mental health care. Health Aff (Millwood) 14(3):50–62, 1995

Gillies RR, Shortell SM, Anderson DA, et al: Conceptualizing and measuring integration: findings from the Health Systems Integration Study. Hospital and Health Services Administration 38(4):467–489, 1993

Goldberg RJ: Psychiatry and the practice of medicine: the need to integrate psychiatry into comprehensive medical care. South Med J 88:260–267, 1995

Goldner EM, Bilsker D: Evidence based psychiatry. Can J Psychiatry 40:97–101, 1995

Handy C: Understanding Organizations. New York, Oxford University Press, 1993

Hudson T: Choose your tomorrow. Hosp Health Netw 69(16):38–40, 1995

Johnson RL: Commentary on "The challenges of governing integrated health care systems." Health Care Manage Rev 20(4):82–87, 1995

Lazarus A: Economic grand rounds: the role of primary care physicians in managed mental health care. Psychiatr Serv 46:343–345, 1995a

Lazarus A: Preparing for practice in an era of managed competition. Psychiatr Serv 46:184–185, 1995b

McCool BP: Commentary on "The challenges of governing integrated health care systems." Health Care Manage Rev 20(4):88–90, 1995

Miller RH: Health system integration: a means to an end. Health Aff (Millwood) 15(2):92–106, 1996

Olsen DP: A treatment-team model of managed mental health care. Psychiatr Serv 46(3):252–255, 1995

Partner with behavioral health providers to boost your capitation. Capitation Management Report 4(1):5–8, 1997

Robinson JC: The dynamics and limits of corporate growth in health care. Health Aff (Millwood) 15(2):155–167, 1996

Scholtes PR, Joiner BL, Streibel BJ: The Team Handbook, 2nd Edition. Madison, WI, Oriel, 1996, pp 3–1 through 3–32, 5–1 through 5–64

Schreter RK: Economic grand rounds: earning a living: a blueprint for psychiatrists. Psychiatr Serv 46:1233–1235, 1995

Senge PM: The Fifth Discipline, The Art and Practice of the Learning Organization. New York, Doubleday, 1990

Shortell SM, Gillies RR, Anderson DA, et al: Remaking Health Care in America: Building Organized Delivery Systems. San Francisco, CA, Jossey-Bass, 1996

❖ 6 ❖

Continuous Quality Improvement

Principles of Implementation in Behavioral Healthcare

Deborah C. Nelson, Ph.D.

Pamela M. Senesac, R.N., M.S., S.M.

Wendy Holt, M.P.P.

In this chapter we describe an approach to quality assurance in healthcare organizations relying on intrinsic management initiatives, and we depict practical ways to make the requirements of continuous quality improvement (CQI) work for behavioral health professionals and organizations. We describe the lessons learned in implementing CQI in managed care organizations and suggest how they can be applied to other behavioral healthcare organizations. We conclude with three examples of CQI in action.

Purchasers and others responsible for the quality of healthcare have long relied on credentialing, complaint and grievance procedures, retrospective chart reviews, and critical incident investigation to ensure minimum levels of quality in service delivery. In the new managed care environment, healthcare organizations are shifting from retrospective methods to concurrent and/or prospective approaches. Similarly, purchasers are reorganizing the management of provider networks to enhance the quality and efficiency of service delivery. This approach to CQI involves

- Improving performance by reducing variation in key processes
- Identifying and incorporating better clinical practices within and across healthcare organizations
- Measuring provider performance against baselines and benchmarks
- Emphasizing that healthcare dollars purchase results, not processes

Parameters of CQI

CQI calls for the systematic, coordinated actions of all staff and departments within an organization for the purpose of planning and implementing incremental, ongoing improvements. *Quality* is defined as meeting or exceeding the expectations of the purchasers and the consumers of healthcare services. *Quality of care* is defined as the degree to which services consistent with current professional knowledge are responsive to customer needs and increase individuals' health status, including both the ability to function and a sense of well-being. A CQI program should enable the organization to provide quality at a reasonable cost.

CQI focuses on doing the right thing, the right way, the first time rather than repairing the damage after the fact. It is an operational management philosophy, not a quality control mechanism. With a CQI approach, everyone in the organization is responsible for knowing his or her customers and their needs and for delivering services and products that exceed the customers' requirements.

CQI focuses on increasing efficiency, enhancing performance and outcomes, improving the bottom line, and ensuring the satisfaction of customers. W. Edwards Deming, a pioneer in quality improvement, observed that problems reside more frequently with the process than with the people (Deming 1986). Thus, with CQI, the strategy is to "fix the problem, not to blame." The purpose of a CQI approach is to use a management process to solve problems in the workplace continually and thereby to increase credibility with customers.

The practical benefits that CQI brings to an organization or individual practitioner are (Grossman 1991; Lynn 1991; Maine 1991)

- Enhanced understanding of customers' needs and alignment of processes to support those needs
- Improved quality (increased efficiency, effectiveness, and satisfaction)
- Decreased risk of liability
- Facilitation of radical change when the status quo has lost its competitive edge
- Assurance that all staff are on the same team, working toward common goals
- The use of data or information to effect change

A Brief History of CQI and the Application of CQI Techniques to Healthcare

The ideas of W. Edwards Deming revolutionized Japan's automobile industry in the 1950s by convincing the Japanese business community that it could compete with the rest of the world on the basis of quality (Deming 1986). In less than one generation, the image of Japanese goods was changed from the symbol of inferior, undependable products to the standard setter of reliability and state of the art technology. Belatedly, in the 1980s, Deming's ideas were adopted in the United States as American industries faced for the first time the challenges that Japan had overcome decades earlier.

Deming's key concepts (Deming 1986) include the following:

- Improvement is a continuous process.
- Management is responsible for creating an environment that promotes improvement in all processes.
- Employees closest to the day-to-day operations must be involved in improving them.
- Management should focus on long-term relationships with suppliers and on long-term financial success (not just short-term profits).
- An organization's goal should be to delight customers by identifying and exceeding their needs.

Healthcare and other service industries began to adopt Deming's concepts in response to the increasing competition, rising cost, and declining quality in healthcare. Physicians functioning in administrative and clinical leadership capacities increasingly play an essential role in CQI by joining forces with other practitioners to improve quality and meet the requirements of accreditors and purchasers (Jones 1990). The concept of variation and the use of statistical tools come naturally to medical professionals trained to use data and the scientific method in their daily practice.

In healthcare, traditional quality assurance methods relied on process measures such as the completion of records or appropriate referrals to specialists. The tenets of CQI, while building on traditional measures of quality assurance, take a different approach, as outlined in Table 6–1.

Implementing a Quality Management Plan

Quality management is the coordinated and comprehensive framework for the measurement and continuous improvement of processes and outcomes on behalf of customers. A *quality management program* is made up of quarterly or annual plans, including the processes for review of those plans; it incorporates the principles of CQI, and it involves everyone in the organization in the CQI process.

All healthcare providers need a system or model to identify customers' needs, measure their own current performance, assess what services they are currently providing and what outcomes they are producing, and

TABLE 6–1. Quality assurance and continuous quality improvement

	Quality assurance	Continuous quality improvement
Time frame	Retrospective	Prospective
Personnel	Quality assurance department	All staff, especially those closest to the day-to-day operation
Process	Focuses on defects and minimal acceptable standards	Builds quality in at the beginning Uses data to improve processes to prevent defects Establishes new performance targets as bell curve of quality is shifted in direction of improved quality
Training	Quality assurance department staff	All staff, including (especially) top management
Customer orientation	Focuses on end user	Focuses on prospective identification of customer needs Focuses on customer/supplier functions, both internal and external to organization
Role in organization	A program	A management philosophy
Methods	Reports occurrences of adverse events Tracks risk management indicators	Uses statistical techniques to identify causes and validate proposed solutions A systematic search for best opportunities for improvement in all business operations Uses a form of the scientific method (called plan, do, check, act process) to define problems and aim focused interventions at those problems
Focus	Product	Process and product

systematically improve those areas most tied to customer requirements. Similarly, those who purchase or consume services are increasingly asking for data on quality of services. A successful quality improvement program must yield true value as well as understandable data that are useful for consumers and purchasers as well.

A number of models exist that can improve any organization's ability to respond to customer expectations. The model presented here is based on the plan, do, check, act (PDCA) cycle, which was described by Deming (1986) and Walton (1986). Most models incorporate the PDCA process, so what matters most is to choose a model that fits a given organization's learning style, culture, and needs, whether the entity is a physician practice, a purchaser of care, or a managed care organization. Figure 6–1 is an example of a CQI model.

CQI Model

Plan

Tempting as it may be to jump into CQI, the improvements and the momentum gained are likely to be short-

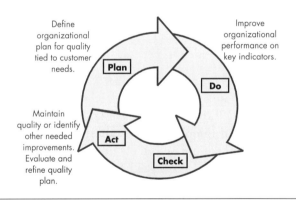

FIGURE 6–1. Example of a continuous quality improvement (CQI) model based on plan, do, check, act (PDCA).

lived without the creation of an infrastructure for quality. A key component in improving healthcare is to take the time to *plan* the organization's approach to quality. Planning includes the following steps:

1. Assessment of current strategic performance and associated planning activities

2. Determination of the key indicators by which relative success will be measured
3. Comprehensive review of existing structures of care or service delivery, including administrative and support functions
4. Assessment of observed gaps or redundancies in service delivery
5. Learning about better practices achieved by other organizations (a process called *benchmarking*)

Most important, planning includes an assessment of current and desired customers and an identification of their requirements, with a focus on what is most important. Customers can include internal customers, end consumers of services, purchasers such as state Medicaid agencies or private employers, managed care companies, and the public at large. Healthcare delivery systems most likely to thrive in the current constantly changing environment are those that identify the various types of customers and stakeholders and establish or refine processes to meet their expectations. Once such expectations are identified, the responsibility for meeting those expectations must be assigned, with time frames and with identification of the indicators by which success will be measured.

Do

The *do* phase of the quality improvement process is about making the changes determined to be important in the plan phase.

Check

The *check* phase of the quality improvement process assesses how well the services delivered in the do phase accomplished the objectives established in the plan phase. If the plan phase centers on the key indicators by which relative success will be measured, the check phase involves comparing actual performance relative to those indicators.

Act

In measuring the quality of any given product or service, differences between what is actually observed and what was expected are likely. In the *act* phase, the organization seeks to maintain the goals achieved in the do phase or analyzes why action taken in the do phase did not meet goals and then designs alternative approaches.

Steps for Improving Quality

In the previous section we described a high-level or macro approach to the PDCA process. Organizations typically use a similar PDCA format to guide the actual improvement process. This is true whether it is individuals or teams of people chartered by management to create improvements. If teams are employed, they need to be oriented to the purpose of CQI, trained in the CQI process itself, and deployed as a team with a precise statement from management staff describing the problem area needing improvement, why it is important, and when the improvement needs to be accomplished. Teams are usually composed of four to seven staff members, customers, or other stakeholders and meet for a time-limited period. During this period, the team should periodically meet formally with the quality council (or similar entity composed of management staff) to review findings and recommendations and to receive further direction.

Teams should have a leader who has been intensively trained in CQI, and frequently another person assists the leader in facilitating that team's process. To ensure that management is committed to the project, one manager from the quality council should formally be assigned to meet with the team leader and the facilitator, offering direction and allocating time or monetary resources, serving as a liaison with the quality council or other managers, and celebrating team successes.

An example of a typical PDCA problem-solving process is summarized in Table 6–2.

Tips for Implementing a CQI Plan

Develop a Multiyear Strategic Plan

That quality is not achieved in a day is captured by the Japanese word *kaizen*, which implies a spirit of incremental improvement and the celebration of small successes. Implementers must begin with *kaizen* in mind, knowing that it will take 3–5 years for a quality plan to be completely implemented and for the culture of quality to be fully integrated in the organization. However, a well-implemented CQI program can produce results and a mood of change that staff and customers can discern in the initial weeks or months. Listed below are some tips for enhancing the culture of quality in a healthcare organization.

TABLE 6–2. Example of a PDCA (plan, do, check, act) six-step problem-solving process

Plan

1. Identify and define the problem.
   Who is involved? What is the precise nature of the problem? When does it occur? Where? What is current performance? Desired performance as defined by customers?
2. Hypothesize root causes of the problem. Verify that they are likely causes.
3. Plan an implementation strategy.
   Who will do what, by when? How will the strategy for implementing proposed solutions be monitored?

Do

4. Implement a solution strategy.

Check

5. Analyze the results.

Act

6. Act on the results.

Obtain Visible, Sincere Commitment From Top Management

Without management support, CQI is likely the very first initiative to be discontinued in an organization. The commitment applies to both the process of CQI and the resources required to implement the process. Complete implementation of CQI requires multiple annual cycles and the training of a significant portion of staff. A half-hearted attempt may be worse than none at all because it will signal to staff that attention to quality is not the core enterprise of the organization.

Create an Oversight Structure

A quality management council, responsible for the establishment and maintenance of the organization-wide CQI effort, is an important structure to establish. The council should include management staff from each department to supply a clear statement of the problem and direction for the quality improvement teams. A coordinating committee, consisting of a director of quality management and any departmental quality managers serving as lead persons in the quality effort who can be responsible for the day-to-day processes of quality planning, control, and improvement, also may be established. The actual application of such a staffing model in a managed behavioral health setting is described elsewhere (Nelson et al. 1995).

Identify Customers and Suppliers

Customers and suppliers are identified in relation to the function they perform in a specific process. Thus, one unit in an organization may function as both a customer and a supplier in relation to other internal units or external organizations. For example, network providers can be both suppliers and customers: supplier of the services purchased, customer of a managed care organization's claims payment system, supplier of data about service, and customer of a managed care organization's provider profiling efforts.

Dedicate Staff and Other Resources to the CQI Effort

CQI may not be a full-time job, but it has to be someone's job and a clearly designated function of the organization. A member of the executive staff must have the ultimate responsibility for the CQI effort. Additionally, quality must be seen as everyone's job, not just those in the "quality" department or those serving on problem-solving teams.

Allocation of time for line staff to take part in quality activities is also required. Supervisors and staff must be assisted in making CQI initiatives a priority, or they will fail to achieve the improvements that customers require. Practical experience suggests that 3 hours/week are required for staff participating as members of quality improvement teams, and 6 hours/week are typical for leaders and facilitators.

Organizations should strongly consider accelerating their improvement cycles. If a project is important enough to be solved, it is important enough to be a priority. If busy staff cannot regularly free the time needed to meet weekly and/or if the problem is pressing enough to need rapid improvement, a 3-day intense effort may provide a solution to the problem in less total time than 6 months of weekly 1-hour meetings.

Employ Adequate Data Collection and Management Information System Capabilities

CQI requires current data and the capacity to manipulate that data—a serious challenge for many human services organizations. A management information system is helpful, but systems do not need to be complicated to yield important information about core processes and products of an organization. Many organizations are already collecting the data that they need to improve processes or outcomes.

Provide Training

Those involved in the problem-solving effort must have the necessary tools. If an organization's management agrees on the tactical benefits to implementing CQI, everyone must know what this means to the organization, its staff, its suppliers, and its customers. The strength of the improvement cycle is found not only in management commitment but also in the involvement of subject matter experts. Subject matter experts are those individuals with important roles in performing the specific process or product deemed in need of improvement. They should be oriented to CQI tools and techniques and trained in a valid problem-solving process.

As an organization begins to implement CQI, it will find that managers assume a variety of positions about whether a quality initiative is needed. Senge et al. (1994) identified this as a common impediment in CQI implementation and list managers' five orientations toward quality, fitting into a continuum (Table 6–3). It can be useful to assess where managers are on the continuum and to address what training or supports may be needed to modify managers' attitudes.

Prioritize

In a process designed to be comprehensive and implemented systemwide, setting an overly ambitious agenda is a common mistake. CQI contains methods to help set priorities for improvement that can help the quality council focus on the most important issues to the organization's customers. If an issue is not important to satisfying or delighting customers (internal or external), it does not merit the organization's improvement effort.

Define Precisely the Problem to Be Solved

When a quality council engages a team of subject matter experts, it should either provide or closely oversee the development of a precise problem statement to ensure that improvement initiatives are conducted in a time- and resource-effective manner. Precise statements typically address *who* is involved in the problem (e.g., in a behavioral health domain, does the problem to be solved involve all patients or just those who are disabled and psychotic?), *what* is the problem (e.g., 30-day readmission rate is at 25%), *when* it is a problem (e.g., the last two quarters have seen the rate jump to 25% from the mid-teens), *where* it is a problem (e.g., statewide or just certain inpatient hospitals?), *why* it is important for the organization to address this problem (e.g., because it is a key concern of consumers, purchasers, and our own organization in terms of quality and cost), and the *delineation of present versus desired performance* (e.g., 25% is the current rate, and the quality council expects to see an initial drop to 18% during the next full quarter). Teams should be provided with a charter that informs them of their mission, problem statement, any parameters on time or money to improve the problem, and deadlines for reaching expected milestones in the six-step problem-solving process.

TABLE 6–3. Continuum of managers' orientations toward quality

Status	Attitudinal statements
Status quo	Quality is not an issue here. Our products, employees, and service are fine.
Quality control	Quality means we monitor and inspect. People are accountable for what they do.
Customer service	Quality means listening to customers at every opportunity. It is known that problems will occur, but all efforts will be made to keep customers satisfied.
Process improvement	We use quality techniques and tools such as reengineering, bar graphs, and control charts to monitor and reduce variation in our processes or products. Staff members and quality improvement teams help us constantly improve how we operate.
Continuous quality	Quality is a paradigm shift in how work is planned, how work is carried out, how individuals inside and outside the organization collaborate, how resources are used, and how progress and success of the organization are evaluated. All staff work together to operate a "seamless" system aimed at satisfying customers. Processes are efficient and effective. The system incorporates elements of quality control, customer service, and process improvement.

Source. Adapted from Senge et al. 1994.

Develop Useful Documentation

Each team should document its work so that it can accurately identify successful and unsuccessful approaches. This allows the organization to learn from the experiences of its problem-solving teams. Many organizations use storyboards, which are a traditional graphical method of demonstrating progress in following the problem-solving process and creating improvements. The most effective storyboards make the improvement process come alive, allowing the organization to take credit for gains made. Many organizations find storyboards helpful to

- Communicate progress, live and as it happens, to all stakeholders.
- Monitor the team's progress in its plan; many teams find it helpful to bring the storyboard to each team meeting to keep focused, to aid in keeping the storyboard current, and to avoid duplicating documentation.
- To allow everyone to have the opportunity to participate, post the storyboard publicly and invite comment.

Ensure Regular, Ongoing Communication

Teams should regularly report back to the quality council. Experience shows that this feedback loop keeps teams directed and, if necessary, refocused and reenergized. The feedback from others helps to identify opportunities for improvement, allows techniques that work to be shared, and helps teams to maintain a broader perspective. Additionally, it is helpful for teams operating simultaneously within an organization to occasionally share their process and data with other teams. Use of storyboards or newsletters is helpful to share the process and the results with the organization at large as well as with outsiders. The feedback of these entities is more objective, and they are apt to have less investment in solutions grounded in the status quo.

Manage With Facts for Quality

CQI is fundamentally based on accurate information. Teams are challenged to move beyond anecdotal information by gathering facts, verifying them, and thinking about what they mean. Do the facts affect customers? Do the data have any surprises? Where is the largest opportunity for improvement? Is this the wrong issue? Organizations acculturated in quality soon become adept at spotting and avoiding "factoids," which often look like facts but are not grounded in data.

Invest in Technical Assistance

An initial time-limited investment in competent technical support can ensure that everyone, especially senior managers, receives training and the opportunity to "become a believer in CQI." Such an investment can help an organization to realize some quick successes and sustain the momentum of a CQI plan.

Measure What You Need to Manage

Indicators are measures of aspects of services or products that are important to customers. An organization that is quality-centered uses indicators to track how well it is doing in its processes and outcomes that are important to its customers. Quality-centered organizations establish key objectives tied to satisfaction of customers and identify associated indicators; then they track these indicators on an ongoing basis and, if needed, implement improvement strategies to close gaps between present performance and desired performance. It is critical to align the organization's measurement system with the strategy and tactics of the organization as well as its mission and values. Managing by indicators and facts rather than by anecdotes becomes contagious. Tracking and making visible key indicators maximize an organization's ability to satisfy customers or consumers.

Start With Success

The initial phase of a CQI program will be scrutinized intently, and the early conclusions drawn by staff or observers may foster or hamper further developments. It is critical to choose an initial project that is both significant and achievable. Management information system development is an important component of CQI implementation; because data are critical to timely success, the program selected should be consistent with the resources available. Table 6–4 elaborates this theme with suggestions on aligning measurement activities of the organization with the needs of the organization.

Solve Implementation Problems

Analysis of quality management implementation in a variety of healthcare organizations suggests that common problems occur in sustaining a viable quality management program. These problems are summarized in Table 6–5, along with some proposed solutions.

TABLE 6–4. Key suggestions on aligning measurement activities with the needs of the organization

---

Coordinate measurement with the mission and values of the organization.

Avoid measuring too many things. Focus on the few significant issues.

Involve stakeholders (e.g., purchaser, consumer) in designing the quality measurement system. Start by measuring and improving factors central to customers (internal or external).

Start seeing some success early. Initial projects should be focused.

Develop precise problem statements as an aid to measurement and improvement.

Show results in a graphic and compelling way to get everyone involved.

Understand basic statistics (for instance, that averages do not tell the whole story and that indicators of dispersion of data are important too). Stratify data (e.g., look for differences by sex, by diagnosis, and by program). As the data are stratified, analysis of outliers in both directions often adds important information (understanding where and why good performance is occurring is as important as understanding more about problematic performance).

Gather data from multiple perspectives and multiple sources.

Use measures for which reliability and validity of information can be determined.

Be wary of overinterpretation of data, especially new data. Disseminate the information and invite comment in an open, nonjudgmental atmosphere. Especially with sensitive issues such as provider profiles, *discuss* the data with various stakeholders before interpreting the data or arriving at conclusions or action steps.

Use information gathered to improve things! If the data are not going to be used, question whether they need to be collected.

TABLE 6–5. Common implementation problems and possible proposed solutions

---

Common implementation problems	Possible proposed solutions
Quality management program is costing more than expected.	A cost-benefit analysis outlines the value received for the investment made. *Revisit the value equation:* What other costs have been reduced by decreasing waste, rework, or redundancy? *Note.* If an organization's efforts have been historically underfunded, the initial effort (additional staff and training) may require a significant financial investment that exceeds initial savings in other areas.
Quality management program is isolated from the rest of the organization's key activities.	Post a storyboard in a key location. Invite comment. Schedule regular presentations at staff meetings to keep everyone involved. Avoid identifying staff solely as "quality" staff—quality should be everyone's job.
Management information system is taxed by the need to produce data (or, little or no management information system capabilities).	Make the best use of already available data; an organization is unlikely to have everything it wants or needs. Many organizations find that the management information system is taxed because new teams "request everything." Educate data consumers to develop strategies to use limited management information system resources efficiently.
Outcomes measurement initiated as part of a quality management program is not helpful to direct care staff or useful in a continuous quality improvement framework.	Involve consumers and the direct care staff who are subject matter experts as team members to get their perspective on the problem. If standardized assessment tools are to be implemented, use the information to write treatment plans and evaluate, with consumers, how treatment is progressing.
Management staff differ in their "buy-in" of the value of implementing continuous quality improvement.	Determine whether disparate views of quality, or lack of understanding of the value of organizational continuous quality improvement implementation, may exist. Reorientation or training may be helpful. Some managers may need to move on to another organization if they cannot be part of the continuous quality improvement implementation and maintenance.
Quality improvement teams or quality improvement studies are not producing results or are taking too long.	Think out of the box: do a blitz 2-day effort, meet more than once a week or for longer than an hour, or work out of the office for a day. Revisit the problem and address a more feasible goal.

CQI in Action: Three Examples

Various problems in the provision of healthcare are amenable to improvement by CQI. These may include excessive readmissions, inadequate telephone access, long wait times for appointments, inadequate service to those who do not speak English as a first language, and limited services for persons with dual diagnoses of substance abuse and mental retardation. In this section, we describe three examples of the use of CQI in addressing service delivery problems in a managed behavioral healthcare organization.

Example 1: Reducing Variability Among Providers in Discharge Planning for Children and Adolescents

In the **plan** phase of this project, data indicated an unacceptable level of variation among hospital-based programs in length of stay, quality of care, and readmission rates. A problem-solving team empowered by the quality council used a specially designed assessment tool to collect data on a random sample of several hundred charts of children and adolescents discharged from network facilities at Time 1. This study identified discharge planning as an area requiring immediate attention in every treatment setting because of its apparent relation to high readmission rates and an inadequate number of days in the community. Solutions were then implemented. A second large random sample of charts was reviewed with the same assessment tool at Time 2, about a year later.

The initial assessment at Time 1 found an unacceptable level of variation in several key performance areas for hospitals. These data were shared with stakeholders who suggested that the team focus on improving one of those key indicators: the degree to which certain kinds of information were available at the time of discharge.

The specific data identified as lacking were

- Medication history, including indications, target symptoms, and side effects
- Behavioral management recommendations
- A schedule of aftercare appointments and needs, with notification of the managed care organization if these services were not available in a timely fashion within the outpatient network
- Documentation of family involvement

As a corrective action, taken in the **do** phase of the process, the team communicated with network providers about the importance of discharge documentation and articulated discharge documentation specifications to them through a variety of written reminders and face-to-face meetings. Compliance with this standard became one of several annual performance measures against which providers were evaluated by the managed care organization's network managers.

At Time 2, several improvements had occurred for hospitals, with some of these facilities showing significant improvements, as indicated in Figure 6–2.

By analyzing the performance of successful facilities, the team identified the best practice models that appeared related to better outcomes. These included the use of protocols that required

- Meetings with aftercare providers on the day of discharge to discuss and pass on aftercare recommendations
- Routine follow-up with children and families to ensure that aftercare services had been secured

The team showcased these better practices in various learning forums attended by other providers.

The substantive gains resulting from this **do** phase were maintained in the **check** phase. In the **act** phase, the team took steps to help the providers maintain their gains. The team identified some additional, "next step" areas needing improvement, based on the findings in Time 2, including tying discharge processes to outcomes such as readmission and functional improvements.

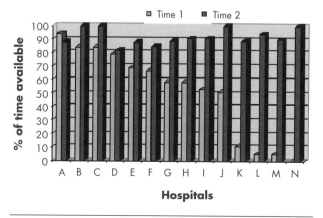

FIGURE 6–2. Discharge information available at discharge for hospitals.

Example 2: Using Satisfaction Data to Improve Quality

Many organizations measure consumer satisfaction and show high satisfaction ratings to their boards of directors or purchasers. Organizations that go no further miss an important opportunity to use their satisfaction data to improve quality of care. The process involves the further step of analyzing their data to answer the following questions:

1. What can be learned about consumers who are not satisfied? Average satisfaction ratings often disguise a bimodal distribution. A great deal can be learned from those who are dissatisfied.
2. What are the predictors of high satisfaction? What can be learned from profiling the clients who are "delighted" with services?
3. What are the predictors of dissatisfaction? These often differ from the predictors of satisfaction.
4. What segments of the population are underrepresented in the results? Focus groups may be helpful to elicit the views of those individuals.
5. What management actions can be taken to address these issues, and how can the results be incorporated into a PDCA process? It is important to use satisfaction survey items that deal with concrete issues that can lead to administrative action. For example, low ratings on "My telephone calls are answered quickly" are easier to act on than "The clinic is responsive."

In one illustrative satisfaction survey, the instrument was constructed by consulting knowledgeable consumer informants and focus groups to develop questions that reflected the live concerns of consumers. The survey was administered according to accepted sampling techniques, and the answers were factor analyzed to identify the underlying components of consumer satisfaction. One of these was the degree to which consumers felt that the staff involved them in a collaborative effort to reach their goals. The performance of six outpatient clinics on this factor is illustrated in Figure 6–3.

The results were shared with each clinic without identifying any other clinic. The data were discussed in a CQI mode; that is, focusing on improving the systems rather than assigning blame. The providers were particularly interested in the degree of variation among clinics: How could one clinic obtain a 92% satisfaction rat-

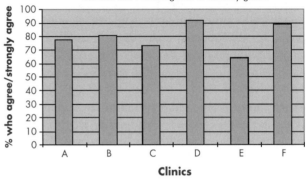

FIGURE 6–3. Results for six clinics on the collaborative factor in consumer satisfaction.

ing with this question but another clinic obtain only 64% satisfaction? Building on this curiosity, "quality forums" were established in which providers could share with one another their approach to increasing consumer involvement in the process of care. This approach stimulated better practice so that on remeasurement a year later, many of the clinics had improved their ratings on this factor.

Example 3: Network Management—An Approach to Quality Improvements in a System of Care

With the privatization of many public services, including especially health services, state agencies have been called on to develop new capabilities as contract managers. Medicaid agencies in particular are in the process of evolving from claims-paying agencies to contract management agencies, conducting a sophisticated procurement process involving the preparation of requests for proposals (RFPs), managing bidder's conferences, selecting a successful vendor, and then, through intensive monitoring, holding that vendor responsible for delivering the service. This has led to a new focus on the value received for the expenditure of public funds. This new approach to vendor management is fully consistent with quality management principles that are intrinsic to the efficient operation of health service systems.

Healthcare purchasers are becoming increasingly value driven and assertive about the need to show better outcomes and processes of care. Often, this demand takes the form of performance requirements for managed care organizations and providers alike, so that a whole system of care is focused on the same goals.

Healthcare purchasers tend to focus on similar clusters of performance requirements, summarized by Oss (1996) as follows:

- Quality of clinical services (e.g., readmission rates, links to outpatient appointments from inpatient settings, improved functioning)
- Administrative efficiency (e.g., wait times, access to care, telephone access, claims accuracy, and timeliness of payment)
- Consumer satisfaction (e.g., consumer or family member satisfaction survey data or frequency and type of appeals)
- Financial performance (e.g., utilization, cost per covered life, penetration rate)
- Cost-shifting considerations (e.g., shifts to medical or pharmacy sector)

Purchasers increasingly use benchmarks to rate provider performance. Benchmarks represent a desirable level of performance achieved by providers serving similar clientele. Benchmarking data are often shared with providers in the format of provider profiles. With provider profiling efforts, the performance of providers or provider organizations is evaluated as stronger or weaker than that of peers on various measures. Table 6–6 illustrates one example of profiling of acute residential treatment programs serving adolescents.

Table 6–6 makes it possible to compare the performance of the facility being profiled with the statewide average of all similar facilities on total discharges, average length of stay, 5-day ambulatory care rate, and readmission rate for all cases and for cases stratified by disabled aid category, for children in custody, and for all other aid categories.

These profiles were reviewed by the managed care organization (MCO) in meetings with unit managers. As with satisfaction data, providers were receptive and quite fascinated by data that allowed them to see how they compared with others. The atmosphere established in the meetings was on learning and exploring, not on blame. On the basis of the meeting, the MCO and the unit determined priorities for improvement and/or correction, set performance goals within a specific time frame, and identified the actions the facility would take to achieve the goal. The MCO summarized the goals and actions in writing and monitored compliance.

Profiling also may provide useful comparative clinical data. For example, one MCO's first outpatient profile identified a number of providers showing similar treatment patterns for people with major depression and those with adjustment disorders. In clinics where treatment for these two disorders was not well differentiated, clinic managers investigated to 1) determine whether diagnoses were accurate and 2) identify treatment patterns for each diagnostic group. For instance, were persons with major depression consistently referred for medication assessment? Were persons with adjustment disorders referred to short-term focused psychotherapies? Although extremely important, provider profiling remains controversial because of limitations in the data (e.g., reliability or validity of measures selected, heavy reliance on administrative measures over clinical or outcomes measures), which limit the ability to generalize (Blumenthal 1996; Brook et al. 1996; Dickey 1996; Eisen and Dickey 1996).

The emphasis on performance specifications and benchmarking will likely become even more important in the future. Healthcare purchasers and consumers alike are demanding value for their healthcare dollar. Implementation of CQI in healthcare systems can deliver that value.

Conclusion

Many healthcare organizations have implemented CQI to some extent but have not realized the full benefits of this powerful management tool. It is important to bear the following benefits in mind:

- Consumers have better healthcare outcomes and improved access to a broader range of services or providers.
- Purchasers e.g., HMOs, employers) serve consumers more efficiently and more effectively.
- Provider organizations improve their capacity to compete successfully, deal with subcapitation, improve local delivery systems, and maximize their efficiency.
- The public experiences cost-effective healthcare and outcomes.

These multiple benefits should provide powerful motivation for modern healthcare organizations to commit the funds and human resources to develop effective CQI programs.

TABLE 6–6. Results for outpatient provider profiling

Example of mental health acute residential treatment profile

Provider: Community acute residential treatment program for children
Provider number: Blank
Region: Blank
Time period: Calendar year 1999
Population: Adolescents (13–18 years)

Utilization	All diagnoses			Disabled aid category			Children in custody category			Other aid category		
	Provider performance (%)	State average (%)	SD	Provider performance (%)	State average	SD	Provider performance (%)	State average	SD	Provider performance (%)	State average	SD
Total number of discharges	61.0	22.0	26.3	3.0	3.6	3.0	31.0	11.5	11.5	27.0	11.9	14.0
Average length of stay (days)	10.7	12.0	3.8	9.3	8.0	2.0	10.7	12.3	3.7	11.0	12.3	9.7
Quality	Provider performance (%)	State average (%)	SD	Provider performance (%)	State average (%)	SD	Provider performance (%)	State average (%)	SD	Provider performance (%)	State average (%)	SD
5-day ambulatory care rate	37.7	35.8	30.3	33.3	36.0	18.1	28.7	28.4	23.7	37.0	33.5	31.0
Mental health readmission rate	16.4	14.2	24.1	0.0	8.0	10.3	22.6	15.2	26.9	11.1	14.4	11.5

Note. 5-day ambulatory care rate = percentage of discharged patients attending an outpatient appointment within 5 days; mental health readmission rate = percentage of discharged patients readmitted to a 24-hour mental health facility within 30 days; standard deviation (SD) = the number of points in 1 standard deviation. Provider performance greater than ±1 SD statistically exceeds or falls below the state average.

References

Blumenthal D: Quality of health care—what is it? N Engl J Med 335:891–894, 1996

Brook RH, McGlynn EA, Cleary PD: Quality of health care, part 2: measuring quality of care. N Engl J Med 335:966–970, 1996

Deming WE: Out of the Crisis. Cambridge, MA, MIT Center for Advanced Engineering Study, 1986

Dickey B: The development of report cards for mental health care in outcomes assessment in clinical practice, in Outcomes Assessment in Clinical Practice. Edited by Sederer L, Dickey B. Philadelphia, PA, Williams & Wilkins, 1996, pp 156–160

Eisen SV, Dickey B: Mental health outcome assessment: the new agenda. Psychotherapy 33:181–199, 1996

Grossman JH: Emerging medical quality management support systems for hospitals, in Health Care Quality Management for the 21st Century. Edited by Couch JB. Tampa, FL, American College of Physician Executives, 1991, pp 237–252

Jones FG: Continuous quality improvement (CQI): solution to QA shortcomings? J S C Med Assoc 86(11):593–596, 1990

Lynn ML: Deming's quality principles: a health care application. Hospital and Health Services Administration 36:1, 1991

Maine LL: Application of Deming's principles to health care. Dynamics in Health Care 3:1, 1991

Nelson DC, Hartman E, Ojemann PG, et al: Outcomes measurement and management with a large Medicaid population: a public-private collaboration. Behavioral Healthcare Tomorrow 4(3), 1995

Oss M: Evaluating public behavioral health programs: possible performance indicators and their implications for evaluating changes in the public sector. Open Minds, February 1996

Senge PM, Kleiner A, Roberts C, et al: The Fifth Discipline Fieldbook: Strategies and Tools for Building a Learning Organization. New York, Doubleday, 1994

Walton M: The Deming Management Method. New York, Putnam, 1986

❖ **7** ❖

Training in Administrative Psychiatry

Current Challenges

Brett N. Steenbarger, Ph.D.
Eugene A. Kaplan, M.D.
Mantosh Dewan, M.D.
John Manring, M.D.
Simon H. Budman, Ph.D.

Changes in healthcare finance and delivery have had a profound effect on the mental health specialties, with significant implications for psychiatry. In response to the prospect of a diminishing demand for psychiatrists in the managed marketplace, proposals have been advanced to redefine psychiatry in relation to medicine overall, and specifically in relation to primary care (AADPRT Task Force 1999; Lieberman and Rush 1996; Shore 1996; Weiner 1994). In this chapter we explore some of the challenges facing psychiatry and potential responses available both through the training of general psychiatrists in the principles of administration and through the training of administrative specialists.

The Shifting Health Care Environment and Its Implications

There is little question that managed healthcare has made sharp inroads into the professional landscape. Approximately three-quarters of all Americans who receive insurance through an employer are covered by a managed plan (Foster Higgins 1997), which is approximately the same proportion of insured Americans enrolled in managed behavioral health plans (OPEN MINDS 1999a). In the public sector, 42 states (including the District of Columbia) operated some form of behavioral healthcare by the year 2000, up from only 14 in 1996 (OPEN MINDS 1999b). In all, more than 62 million Americans are currently enrolled in employee assistance programs (EAPs), three-quarters of which are administered by managed behavioral healthcare firms (OPEN MINDS 2000).

Although recent research suggests that specialty management of mental health services can be effective in reducing costs for benefits purchasers (Grazier et al. 1999), concerns have been voiced concerning the quality of these services. Health plan members with substance use and severe emotional disorders are significantly more likely to disenroll from managed healthcare plans than are other patients (Gresenz and

Sturm 1999), suggesting that benefit limits and/or restrictions on use adversely affect individuals with chronic needs. The extension of managed care to the public sector has also heightened concerns about forced treatment of individuals with major mental illnesses. In one California survey, half of hospitalized patients with a severe emotional disorder indicated that they would never voluntarily seek outpatient assistance, given their poor experience with the healthcare system (Dorman 1998). Accreditation bodies such as the National Commission for Quality Assurance (NCQA) now apply standards to managed behavioral healthcare organizations, challenging administrators to balance the priorities of cost containment and service quality.

Challenges to Academic Psychiatry

Because the formal training of administrative psychiatrists largely occurs in academic medical centers, the challenges faced by these institutions will necessarily affect the development of leaders within the profession (Borus 1992). Meyer (1993) identified several sources of crisis in academic psychiatry, including these:

- A general decline in research dollars directed to academic medical centers
- A decline in outpatient reimbursement rates, reducing the ability of departments to fund clinician teachers
- A decline in inpatient use, undermining the traditional funding base for most departments
- A reduction in the autonomy of departments within integrated practice plans

Meyer and Sotsky (1995) reviewed these developments and concluded that psychiatry "confronts serious structural disadvantages" (p. 70), including sharp budgetary cutbacks in public sector psychiatric services, which have served as a cradle for training programs. Riba and Carli (1996) added that the fate of academic departments of psychiatry is inextricably linked with that of academic medical centers. This is troublesome, they explain, because academic medical centers are typically located in intensely competitive urban markets, where they provide approximately half of all unreimbursed care in the country. Adding to the problem is continued pressure to divert resources within academic

medical centers to the training of primary care physicians, leaving departments of psychiatry vulnerable even within their own institutions (Medical Education Committee Group for Advancement of Psychiatry 1999; Meyer 1993; Meyer and Sotsky 1995).

With the increasing management of Medicaid services and the credentialing mandates imposed by accreditation bodies, the inclusion of psychiatric residents in the emerging healthcare system is uncertain (National Committee for Quality Assurance 1996; Sparer 1997). Cutbacks in Medicaid enrollments and reductions in the use of mental health services leave academic departments of psychiatry with the difficult choice of either joining the fray in competing for managed private and public sector business or possibly losing the patient base needed to sustain training functions. Indeed, the growth in the number of academic managed behavioral healthcare organizations (Tobias 1998) suggests that administrative psychiatrists will not be able to avoid the financial realities of economic healthcare reform.

The Quality Revolution: Implications for Training

To appreciate the implications of these trends for the training of administrative psychiatrists, it is necessary to recognize the heightened pressure that managed care organizations are facing from benefits purchasers with respect to the optimization of cost and quality. Through accreditation bodies such as NCQA, employers and state governments are demanding that managers of care demonstrate programs of data-based quality improvement, high levels of access to and availability of care, research-based practice guidelines, and system-wide programs of prevention and education (Steenbarger et al. 1996). This is a challenging undertaking, requiring ethical sensitivity to both clinical and research values (Beutler 2000).

It is also an expensive undertaking, and not one within the capability of professionals in solo or small group practices (Budman and Steenbarger 1997). Now responsible for quality as well as cost containment, managed care organizations are experiencing the need to form far-reaching collaborations with large practitioner groups, which have the resources to provide 24-hour access, extensive geographic coverage, and quality assessment. These large multispecialty systems of care (Sharfstein and Schreter 1999) also command sufficient patient flows to spread the risk associated with prepaid financing, such as case rates (fixed reimbursements for diagnosis-related groups) and subcapitation (per-member per-month reimbursements to cover a defined set of needs for a covered population).

Such developments suggest that success in the marketplace will depend on the ability of organizations to produce "focused factories" (Herzlinger 1996) that can sustain ever improving levels of efficiency and effectiveness through the redesign of care systems and the redeployment of scarce resources. This means delivering services cost-effectively, not just cheaply (Sturm and Wells 1995).

This multispecialty coordination of cost containment and quality improvement was observed by Budman and Steenbarger (1997) in their study of successful behavioral health practices. Among those practices, the redesign of clinical care to achieve accountability brought seismic changes in both practice patterns and administrative structures. Specifically, fragmented clinical services were replaced by team-based, multidisciplinary programs of care. These integrated psychotherapy, psychopharmacology, social supports, education, and prevention. More advanced versions of such collaborative care found clinical interventions informed by information systems that track patient progress against internal benchmarks and protocols, allowing the elements in the treatment blend to be varied according to patient need. Such a delivery system has many of the qualities of a learning organization, in which individual practice occurs within the context of highly autonomous teams (Senge 1990).

In this environment, training in administrative psychiatry must provide psychiatrists with the information and skill sets necessary to function as managers of the new focused factories. The trickle down of financial risk and quality mandates to provider organizations ensures that trainees will need to be able to manage their own care. *Administrative psychiatry, in that sense, is not merely a specialized discipline, but an activity that must be internalized by practicing psychiatrists.* The ability to collect timely information about patient care and manage resources and outcomes on the basis of empirically validated knowledge is no longer the sole responsibility of a designated psychiatrist-administrator. It is becoming an integral part of routine service delivery.

As Borus (1992) observed, administrative psychiatry has been challenged to compete for the attention of residents and experienced professionals, many of

whom view it as uncreative and bureaucratic when compared to clinical work. Indeed, psychiatric residents tend to rate administrative activities among those with the least educational value (deGroot et al. 2000). In the current healthcare marketplace, however, new and vital roles are emerging for the administrative psychiatrist.

Training in Administrative Psychiatry

Talbott (1992) identified several issues affecting training in administrative psychiatry, including these:

- Changes in patient demography
- Refinements in the diagnostic system
- Increases in consumer participation in health service planning and implementation
- Integration of care delivery systems
- Scientific advances and service innovations
- Managed care
- The trend toward subspecialization

These developments affect both the content and the process of training, because they require psychiatrists to function dually as financial and clinical administrators. Are training programs up to the challenge? Although a number of programs have introduced training innovations (Borus 1992; Sharfstein and Schreter 1999), several factors conspire to suggest that further progress may need to be made:

- *The service delivery structures embedded in residency training do not necessarily mirror those that will be faced by future psychiatrists.* Meyer and Sotsky (1995) pointed out that the Residency Review Committee in Psychiatry imposes educational mandates that do not adequately prepare graduates for the rigors of the practice world. They propose, for example, that rotations on inpatient services—currently recommended to extend for a minimum of 12 months—might be replaced by experiences in following up patients across the care continuum.
- *The clinical skills introduced during residency often do not mirror those demanded in the marketplace.* Mohl (1995) noted that although the Residency Review Committee requires that training programs cover knowledge and skills within both the psychosocial and biological domains, trainees often are not exposed to the

collaborative integration of those domains. For example, the current Program Requirements for Residency Training in Psychiatry (Residency Review Committee for Psychiatry 2000) mandate "sufficient experiences" in "the major types of therapy" (p. 19). These, however, could easily leave trainees unable to integrate these therapies in a time-effective way to divert patients from hospital settings and effect their rapid integration into communities on hospital discharge (Budman and Gurman 1988; Steenbarger and Budman 1996).

- *Residents lack the ethics training essential to the development of administrative psychiatrists.* Talbott (1992) observed that psychiatric administrators must be grounded in their professions, given the frequent tension between financial and clinical administrative mandates. Interestingly, however, the majority of residents experience an ethical dilemma for which they feel unprepared, and a significant proportion of training programs lack formal course work in ethics (Roberts et al. 1996). Nearly 70% of the residents surveyed expressed a desire for course work in ethical issues surrounding the financial coverage of patients' needs. It is difficult to imagine that administrative psychiatrists can be adequately trained without problem-based exposure to the thorny dilemmas that accompany the management of care (Beutler 2000; Schnapp et al. 1996).

- *Essential skills in administrative psychiatry must be modeled by faculty instructors and supervisors.* Lazarus (1996) has called managed care "psychiatry's internecine war" (p. 403), noting the tremendous resistance within the profession to the loss of autonomy yielded by utilization management efforts. This resistance is especially acute in academic settings, which have been long-standing bastions of autonomy and individualism. As a result, faculty members are likely to teach, supervise, and practice in ways that do not mirror the demands of the current practice world, leaving graduating residents unprepared for the rigors that await them (Gabbard 1992; Sabin 1993).

The crux of the challenge is that *demands to contain the costs of care and document service and treatment effectiveness require new levels of expertise from administrative psychiatrists.* Training programs that are dominated by inpatient rotations, individual treatment conducted in the absence of cost and quality considerations, and training experiences that fail to programmatically integrate

therapies for the severely mentally ill will provide a poor foundation for cultivating the next generation of mental health administrators.

Responses to the Challenges of Training

Administrative psychiatry has traditionally embraced skill domains in program development, management, legal and ethical issues, and evaluation (Talbott et al. 1992). There is increasing awareness, however, that the demands of a changed healthcare environment are adding to the administrative mandates of psychiatrists (Sharfstein and Schreter 1999). In an especially thought-provoking presentation, Sabin and Borus (1992) outlined a set of proposals for mental health teaching and research in managed care. Specifically, they identified six skills that are necessary in the current training of psychiatrists:

1. *Individual practice management.* Psychiatrists must learn how to balance treatment needs and process incoming needs across their caseloads, without resorting to "all of my openings are filled."

2. *Collaborative program development.* Training programs must consist of more than aggregations of isolated clinicians practicing under the same roof. The programs must inform residents of the programmatic ways in which needs can be addressed across treatment episodes through the integration of community, psychosocial, and biological services.

3. *Ethical analysis.* Professionals are constantly faced with resource allocation problems, juggling the needs of patients with scarce funds and staffing. Clinicians need decision support tools that are sensitive to the ethical challenges inherent in juggling multiple—and sometimes conflicting—values.

4. *Advocacy.* Managed care systems can be large, intimidating entities that mystify both patients and providers. Psychiatrists must learn how to advocate for patient needs within their systems while maintaining effective working relationships within those systems.

5. *Promotion of development.* Psychiatrists must be grounded not only in the identification and treatment of disorders but in the prevention of disease

and in early intervention with expectable life distress (Budman and Gurman 1988). From the perspective of the benefits purchaser, the goal is to maintain optimal health and productivity.

6. *Broad repertoire of methodologies.* The psychiatrist must be able to blend a variety of somatic and psychosocial interventions into time-effective, empirically grounded programs of treatment that promise clinical and cost effectiveness (Budman and Steenbarger 1997).

Opportunities for training in administrative psychiatry can be woven into standard rotations, as well as obtained through focused electives (Borus 1992; Sharfstein and Schreter 1999). For example, managed care issues can be incorporated into clinical supervision through a role playing of interactions with a care manager. We sometimes prod residents to reflect upon how treatment would be undertaken if a patient came to therapy with a tightly managed insurance benefit. This can provoke stimulating—and somewhat anxiety-provoking—dialogues about the judicious and ethical allocation of resources and the ways in which individual, group, and biological therapies can be blended to achieve time effectiveness. Such an approach fits well with the educational interests of psychiatric residents, who rate direct observation and supervision among their most valued training activities (de Groot et al. 2000).

Administrative training can become a dedicated focus of residency programs also. For more than 30 years the Department of Psychiatry at SUNY Upstate Medical University in Syracuse, New York, has maintained a unique 2-month, half-time rotation in administrative psychiatry in the third year of training. Under the tutelage of the director of the inpatient service at University Hospital, the administrative residents create, review, and modify protocols and policies that enhance clinical care. Clinically, they are responsible for all admissions to the unit, learning in the process to judge the appropriateness of referrals for admission, monitor the unit milieu, and balance the complex clinical and administrative needs of the system. By actively participating in all unit administrative meetings, the administrative resident is afforded a hands-on experience with the blending of managerial, clinical, and economic needs in an integrated healthcare setting. The program has introduced hundreds of residents to administrative psychiatry and has inspired a number of them to make careers in administration, including one commissioner of mental health for New York State and a number of hospital and program directors.

Training the Administrative Psychiatrist

We have emphasized that administrative responsibilities have increasingly become a reality for practicing psychiatrists. Changes in the finances and delivery of healthcare are especially reshaping the work of psychiatrists specializing in administration. The analysis by Budman and Steenbarger (1997), drawn from observations of successful integrated practices, suggests that the emerging administrative psychiatrist must fill several roles simultaneously. These include clinical (Steenbarger et al. 1996), financial (Budman and Steenbarger 1997), and organizational administration (Sharfstein and Schreter 1999). An interesting report from Sperry et al. (1997) indicates that the introduction of data-based management of clinical and financial functions requires broad-based changes in the structure and culture of practice organizations. This places a unique burden of team-building responsibilities on administrative psychiatrists, who must create and maintain bridges within and outside their organizations.

If we were to summarize in a phrase the single most important demand faced by the new generation of administrative psychiatrists, it would be the ability to manage conflict. The need to oversee cost and quality creates potential conflicts between administrators and clinical staff; the ratcheting demands of healthcare purchasers and managed care organizations create potential conflicts between payers and clinical organizations; and the emergence of multidisciplinary practice structures fuels potential turf conflicts among mental health professionals. It is the unique responsibility of the administrative psychiatrist to address these conflicts and channel their energy productively.

How might we train the next generation of administrative psychiatrists to handle these conflicts? Perhaps the first step is to ensure that administrative psychiatrists are trained at clinical sites that are themselves well administered. A training site that does not assess the quality of its own work teaches implicitly that accountability with respect to quality is not essential. Similarly, a site that does not address responsible cost containment through an evidence-based integration of research and practice conveys an attitude that research is irrelevant to the management of care (Steenbarger et al. 1996).

The administratively informed training clinic will look much like a collaborative multispecialty group practice, with experiences in administration continually woven into the delivery of services (Budman and Steenbarger 1997). Among its more prominent features might be an inclusion of evidence-based triage and utilization guidelines in treatment planning; participation within programmatic, multidisciplinary programs of care; and the collection of outcome and satisfaction data to guide quality improvement and refine existing care protocols. Integrating these elements into the basic policies and procedures of clinic operation and making them explicit topics in clinical supervision send a strong message to residents that administration is a fundamental professional activity.

Other intensive administrative experiences can be created through dedicated electives. Trainees might be directly exposed to the financial, marketing, and human resources management of training sites as an introduction to mental health business administration. Training experiences in administration, such as the aforementioned rotation at the SUNY Upstate Medical University, might be expanded into programmatic tracks or fellowships to allow advanced trainees to participate in the clinical, financial, and organizational management of training sites. Administrative positions within the department thus become central *teaching* positions, facilitating the mentoring of residents.

The spirit in which this is undertaken is all-important. If the effort results in an oppressive imposition of a managed care bureaucracy on residents, dissatisfaction and recruitment problems are sure to follow. If, conversely, the experiences empower trainees to learn how to manage their own care, demonstrate the value of their work, and market themselves more effectively, they will be deeply appreciative, and their response will help to invigorate educational activities.

Clearly, however, such changes pose a particular challenge for residency training faculty. Surveys suggest that managed care organizations are not willing to pay premiums for services delivered at academic medical centers, and among both managers and faculty, "traditional patterns of academic training are perceived to be inimical to fostering the prudent management of patients" (Culbertson 1996, p. 868; Gold 1996). If faculty can face this unpleasant reality, their creation of well-administered training sites can generate opportunities for the development of administrative psychiatrists and help to secure the economic future of training programs.

Summary

Coalitions of public and private sector benefits purchasers have driven a mandate for accountability with respect to the quality and cost of mental health services. This, in turn, has shifted care from solo practice sites to multispecialty practices that have the resources to share financial risk and develop needed information systems. The practice world faced by general psychiatrists will require that the administrative knowledge and skills necessary for navigating the shoals of cost and quality become core competencies addressed by training programs. Moreover, new financial and administrative structures will require administrative psychiatrists to serve as clinical, financial, and organizational leaders. Training for these roles can best be accomplished by developing well-managed training sites and clinics that will attract needed referral flows and directly involve residents in administrative experiences and challenges.

References

AADPRT Task Force on the Quality of Residency Programs: The quality of psychiatric residency: the assessment of programs and options for distributing psychiatric residents in the service of health care reform. Academic Psychiatry 23:61–70, 1999

Beutler LE: David and Goliath: when empirical and clinical standards of practice meet. American Psychologist 55:997–1007, 2000

Borus JF: Training, in Textbook of Administrative Psychiatry. Edited by Talbott JA, Hales JA, Keill SL. Washington, DC, American Psychiatric Press, 1992, pp 179–206

Budman SH, Gurman AS: Theory and Practice of Brief Therapy. New York, Guilford, 1988

Budman SH, Steenbarger BN: The Essential Guide to Group Practice in Mental Health. New York, Guilford, 1997

Culbertson RA: How successfully can academic faculty practices compete in developing managed care markets? Academic Medicine 71:858–870, 1996

DeGroot J, Tiberius R, Sinai J, et al: Psychiatric residency: an analysis of training activities with recommendations. Academic Psychiatry 24:139–146, 2000

Dorman R: Left behind: the seriously mentally ill in the managed care era. Behavioral Healthcare Tomorrow 7(6):12–14, 1998

Foster Higgins: National Survey of Employer-Sponsored Health Plans, 11th Edition. New York, Foster Higgins, 1997

Gabbard GO: The big chill: the transition from residency to managed care nightmare. Academic Psychiatry 16:119–126, 1992

Gold MR: Effects of the growth of managed care on academic medical centers and graduate medical education. Academic Medicine 71:828–838, 1996

Grazier KL, Eselius LL, Hu T, et al: Effects of a mental health carve-out on use, costs and payers: a four-year study. J Behav Health Serv Res 26:381–389, 1999

Gresenz CR, Sturm R: Who leaves managed behavioral health care? J Behav Health Serv Res 26:390–400, 1999

Herzlinger R: Market-Driven Health Care. Reading, MA, Addison, 1996

Lazarus A: Afterword: is managed care psychiatry's internecine war? in Controversies in Managed Mental Health Care. Edited by Lazarus A. Washington, DC, American Psychiatric Press, 1996, pp 403–410

Lieberman JA, Rush AJ: Redefining the role of psychiatry in medicine. Am J Psychiatry 153:1388–1397, 1996

Meyer RE: The economics of survival in academic psychiatry. Academic Psychiatry 17:149–160, 1993

Meyer RE, Sotsky SM: Managed care and the role and training of psychiatrists. Health Aff (Millwood) 14:65–77, 1995

Mohl PC: What is a balanced program? Academic Psychiatry 19:94–100, 1995

National Committee for Quality Assurance: Draft Accreditation Standards for Managed Behavioral Healthcare Organizations. Washington, DC, National Committee for Quality Assurance, 1996

OPEN MINDS: Over 72% of insured Americans are enrolled in MBHO. The Behavioral Health and Social Service Industry Analyst 11(4):9, 1999a

OPEN MINDS: States Profiles, 1999, on Public Sector Managed Behavioral Health Care. http://www.openminds.com/IndustryResources/publicsector.htm, 1999b

OPEN MINDS: OPEN MINDS Yearbook of Managed Behavioral Health Market Share in the United States, 2000–2001. Gettysburg, PA, OPEN MINDS, 2000

Residency Review Committee for Psychiatry: Program Requirements for Residency Training in Psychiatry: Effective January 1, 2001. Chicago, IL, Residency Review Committee for Psychiatry, 2000

Riba MB, Carli T: Will academic psychiatry survive managed care? in Controversies in Managed Mental Health Care. Edited by Lazarus A. Washington, DC, American Psychiatric Press, 1996, pp 81–98

Roberts LW, McCarty T, Lyketsos C, et al: What and how psychiatry residents at ten training programs wish to learn about ethics. Academic Psychiatry 20:131–143, 1996

Sabin JE: The moral myopia of academic psychiatry: a response to Glen O. Gabbard's "The Big Chill." Academic Psychiatry 17(3), 1993

Sabin JE, Borus JF: Mental health teaching and research in managed care, in Managed Mental Health Care: Administrative and Clinical Issues. Edited by Feldman JL, Fitzpatrick RJ. Washington, DC, American Psychiatric Press, 1992, pp 185–202

Schnapp WB, Stone S, Van Norman J, et al: Teaching ethics in psychiatry: a problem-based learning approach. Academic Psychiatry 20:144–149, 1996

Senge PM: The Fifth Discipline: The Art and Practice of the Learning Organization. New York, Doubleday, 1990

Sharfstein SS, Schreter R: Psychiatrists in the new medical marketplace. Journal of Practical Psychiatry and Behavioral Health 5:132–141, 1999

Shore JH: Psychiatry at a crossroad: our role in primary care. Am J Psychiatry 153:1398–1403, 1996

Sparer MS: Managing the managed care revolution: states and the new Medicaid, in Competitive Managed Care: The Emerging Health Care System. Edited by Wilkerson JD, Devers KJ, Given RS. San Francisco, CA, Jossey-Bass, 1997, pp 231–258

Sperry L, Grissom G, Brill P, et al: Changing clinicians' practice patterns and managed care culture with outcomes systems. Psychiatric Annals 27:127–132, 1997

Steenbarger BN, Budman SH: Group psychotherapy and managed behavioral healthcare: current trends and future challenges. Int J Group Psychother 46:297–310, 1996

Steenbarger BN, Smith HB, Budman SH: Integrating science and practice in outcomes assessment: a bolder model for a managed era. Psychotherapy 33:246–253, 1996

Sturm R, Wells KB: How can care for depression become more cost-effective? JAMA 273:51–58, 1995

Talbott JA: Future directions, in Textbook of Administrative Psychiatry. Edited by Talbott JA, Hales RE, Keill SL. Washington, DC, American Psychiatric Press, 1992, pp 563–584

Talbott JA, Hales RE, Keill SL (eds): Textbook of Administrative Psychiatry. Washington, DC, American Psychiatric Press, 1992

Tobias S: Behavioral health helps AMCs stave off extinction. Behavioral Healthcare Tomorrow 7(6):17, 1998

Weiner J: Forecasting the effects of health care reform on US physician workforce requirements: evidence from HMO staffing patterns. JAMA 272:222–230, 1994

8

The Medical Director's Role in Organized Care Delivery Systems

David Pollack, M.D.

Kenneth Minkoff, M.D.

It may seem axiomatic to psychiatrists reading this textbook that defined, formal psychiatric leadership (through a designated medical director or similar position) is essential to the functioning of any mental health program. However, this is not often the case. For many years, mental health administrators, beset by funding pressures, have sought to reduce costs by restricting the use of expensive psychiatrists to reimbursable activities, thus narrowing or even eliminating the medical director function (Dewey and Astrachan 1985; Diamond et al. 1985; Knox 1985; Pollack and Cutler 1992). For many such administrators, the value of formal psychiatric leadership has given way to cost considerations.

At the same time, dramatic changes have taken place in both public and private mental health systems. In the public sector, community support system evolution, privatization, competition, and public sector managed care have transformed the traditional system (e.g., community mental health centers [CMHCs] and state public hospitals) into much more complex mental health organizations that manage or participate in elaborate systems of care. Some programs are being taken over by larger healthcare systems, some are merging or developing networks with other similar or complementary organizations, and others are expanding their organizations to include heretofore private sector activities (Broskowski and Eaddy 1994; Cuffel et al. 1994; Hoge et al. 1994; Intergovernmental Health Policy Project 1994; Minkoff 1994; Minkoff and Pollack 1997).

A parallel phenomenon has been occurring on the private side, with previously unaffiliated providers joining larger groups to expand their market share. Many of these private sector organizations have begun to compete for public sector contracts and clients, in some cases leading to mergers, partnerships, or affiliations with community or public provider organizations. In some cases private organizations have assumed the administrative or management aspects of some or all of the contracts for certain public providers. Thus, providers and administrators from the private side have had to become more familiar and competent with the kinds of patients and delivery system issues previously associated primarily with the public sector (Clark et al. 1994; Dorwart 1990; Dorwart and Epstein 1992, 1993;

J. L. Feldman and Fitzpatrick 1992; S. Feldman 1992; S. Feldman, S. Baler, S. Penner: "Roles for Private Managed Care Companies in the Public Sector," unpublished manuscript, 1995; Freeman and Trabin 1994; Patterson 1993; Pomerantz et al. 1994).

In these complex systems, it is increasingly important to clarify the types and amount of psychiatric leadership that is required, as the conflict between the potential clinical and organizational value of competent psychiatric leadership and the pressure for cost containment continues and may even be stimulated.

We believe that the progressive increase in complexity of organized public and private delivery systems, and the expansion of capitated or other prepaid (fixed budget) methods for financing care, support and, in fact, require the increased development of appropriate administrative roles for psychiatrists. We argue for the proper use of psychiatric leadership in such systems and, most important, for the development of these valuable administrative skills in current and potential psychiatric leaders. Such policies and practices can lead to improved clinical outcomes, better quality of service, better use of clinical staff (including the psychiatrists who provide direct clinical services), enhanced teamwork and efficiency, and improved relationships with collaborating providers and agencies. In addition, these factors in the long run will be cost effective, as they contribute to overall quality and efficiency of clinical management, which, itself, is pivotal to the organization's maintaining fiscal solvency.

In this chapter we 1) clarify how the role of psychiatric leadership in organized delivery systems has changed; 2) describe the evolution of guidelines for psychiatric leadership in organized systems, including a sample job description; 3) discuss the skills associated with the recommended functions and duties within this job description; and 4) identify the variety of complex internal and external relationships that must be managed for success as a medical director in an organized mental healthcare setting.

It is important to note that although we describe these functions as residing in a specific individual—the medical director—we really are using the term as a convenient shorthand for the multiple variations on this theme. Some organizations have multiple medical directors, some have a primary medical director and several associate medical directors, some have medical directors for specific programs but not for the agency as a whole, and some staff psychiatrists perform certain administrative functions while mainly providing direct clinical service. Whatever the arrangement, we are convinced of the need to have psychiatric administrators with formal and overt administrative responsibilities.

It is also important to emphasize that the functions of the medical director are distinct from those of the chief executive officer (CEO) of the organization, even if the CEO is a psychiatrist. In complex systems the CEO functions primarily as an administrator and tends to be much more detached from the day-to-day operations. The medical director, by contrast, is more integrated into the service operations and clinical life of the organization and is a vital member of the management team.

The Changing Roles of Psychiatric Leadership in Organized Care Settings

One or two decades ago, the traditional public sector provider—a CMHC, a public hospital, or a substance abuse clinic—was typically a well-defined entity, relying almost exclusively on public funds and serving public patients with fixed budget or cost-reimbursement funding allocations; a defined public mandate to serve a particular patient base in a specified catchment area; a public sector ethos valuing altruism, continuity, collegiality, and opposing competition, rapid change, and profit; and an organizational ethos, often fostered by volunteer citizen boards, valuing a low-key, somewhat cautious and "laid-back" but nurturant management style.

Over the past decade, CMHCs—and other formerly "public mental health" entities—have been steadily transformed by a variety of forces into what Ray et al. (1997) have termed *community behavioral health provider organizations* (CBHPOs), which must be flexible, entrepreneurial, and fiscally accountable, much like private sector businesses. At the same time, private providers also have evolved into behavioral health provider organizations, with many of the characteristics of organized public sector programs. These transformations have been necessary to deal with the following issues:

1. *Transformation of public and private mental health funding:* Privatization initiatives and increasingly competitive public contracting processes have broken down the boundary between traditionally public and private sector organizations. CBHPOs exist now in a competitive marketplace and must

compete with other organizations, both public and private, for healthcare contracts. This involves addressing new populations (e.g., substance abusers) and developing new capabilities (e.g., marketing) and products (e.g., employee assistance programs [EAPs]). Public and private managed care initiatives make these changes even more pressing. A related change is the breakdown of traditional concepts of "community." Catchment areas have been enlarged, and geographical limitations often have disappeared; populations are defined increasingly by source of payment rather than by geography.

2. *Increased accountability:* Funding pressures have caused both public and private payers to make escalating demands for accountability of all providers. This involves a range of issues: productivity, practice guidelines, utilization management, quality management, customer satisfaction, and outcome assessment. These have created culture shock in many public settings.

3. *Horizontal and vertical integration: evolution of systems and networks:* Increasingly, CBHPOs are integrating horizontally into networks and vertically into complex systems to respond to payer demands for broader geographical (regional or statewide) contracting and comprehensive service systems to maximize continuity and utilization efficiency. This has resulted in a dramatic expansion of organizational complexity.

4. *Increased needs for fiscal and technological sophistication:* The emergence of capitation and risk-based contracting and the increasing need for sophisticated clinical and management information systems have completed the metamorphosis of many "sleepy" CMHCs (and, likewise, many solo and group private practitioners) into full-fledged businesses, with much more demanding accountability for managers, including psychiatric managers.

How have these radical changes affected the role of psychiatric leadership? In the 1970s–1980s, it was common for CMHCs, private group practices, public and private hospitals, and other mental health organizations to have psychiatrists in the role of executive director, not simply as medical director (Diamond et al. 1985, 1991; Knox 1985; Langsley and Barter 1983; Thompson and Bass 1984). Administration per se was typically viewed as a simple task, distinctly secondary in value to sophisticated senior clinical or academic leadership in defining the culture and functioning of the organization. Psychiatrists at other levels of the organization who were in medical director or even program director roles had similar expectations of providing clinical leadership, vision, direction, and accountability with a lesser need for specific administrative or management expertise (Pollack and Cutler 1992; Ranz et al. 1997). Being a "good doctor" with collaborative skills and a sense of responsibility was often sufficient.

During the mid-1980s and the 1990s, as these systems underwent change, the role of the executive director enlarged, becoming increasingly important and powerful, and the role of medical (and strictly clinical) leadership became less well defined. Executive directors were required to be managers first, often with postgraduate training in business or public health administration. Clinical background was no longer a necessity for leadership and was seen in some organizations as potentially detrimental to the managerial and business focus. Conflicts emerged in many settings between the executive director and the medical director, each unclear about the other's role definition, programmatic purview, and authority.

Guidelines for Psychiatric Leadership

In response to these issues, within CMHCs in particular, the American Association of Community Psychiatrists (AACP; 1991) developed "Guidelines for Psychiatric Practice in CMHCs," with a sample job description, to clarify the importance of the role of the medical director and the nature of the collaborative relationship between the medical director and the executive director. These guidelines were subsequently adopted by the American Psychiatric Association (APA) as official standards (American Association of Community Psychiatrists 1991). A similar set of guidelines was developed by the APA for psychiatrists working in health maintenance organizations.

The essence of these guidelines is that the medical director must be empowered to have authority over the quality of clinical care but that this authority cannot exist in a vacuum. The medical director's job description includes a requirement for involvement in a wider range of administrative and management duties and investment of nonclinical time in collaboration with other members of the management team. Given that allocation of administrative time to a psychiatrist leader is expensive, the successful medical director must perform as a manager with sufficient energy and skill so that others clearly see that this time is well spent. Psychiatrists who lack the skills to be effective managers or choose not to assume that role still may be valued as clinical leaders in organized care settings. However, they run the risk of being marginalized within the organizational structure and are often treated as staff clinicians without reference to their leadership capabilities.

As CMHCs have evolved into CBHPOs and even larger integrated delivery systems or networks of CBHPOs, and as similar changes have occurred elsewhere, the earlier guidelines for psychiatric leadership have remained relevant, but the specific demands of the leadership role have become increasingly complex. As a consequence, in 1995, the AACP updated the guidelines in a new document, titled "Guidelines for Psychiatric Leadership in Organized Delivery Systems for Treatment of Psychiatric and Substance Disorders," and again incorporated a model job description (American Association of Community Psychiatrists 1995). We participated extensively in this project. This AACP document was, like its predecessor, adopted by the APA and now represents a national standard for psychiatric leadership in public and private delivery systems. The more recent guidelines are reprinted in Table 8–1, and the model job description is shown in Table 8–2.

Critical Administrative Skills

Let us now examine the skills that are necessary for the medical director to succeed within these guidelines and job functions.

Maintaining a Strong Clinical Presence

However skillful the medical director becomes as a manager, he or she must continue to represent the importance of good clinical care as the organization's ultimate mission. This facilitates the ability of the organization as a whole to shift more into a business mind-set without loss of clinical principles or quality of care.

The medical director does this in several ways: providing direct clinical care, providing clinical supervision and teaching, articulating a clinical mission, and continually striving to solve management and fiscal problems in a manner that maintains a focus on clinical values.

Learning to Use Management Tools

Despite the tendency of mental health provider systems, and psychiatrists in general, to be somewhat informal and antibureaucratic, the medical director for any organized care delivery system must become comfortable with management tools. Because psychiatrists are trained as clinicians, not managers, and community clinics are often very process-oriented, there can be significant resistance to developing the kind of internal structures and accountability methods that are necessary today for the mental health program to carry out its organizational mission in the external environment of privatization, competition, prepaid funding, regulation, and managed care.

Medical directors therefore must learn the following skills:

- Understanding the nature of the formal organizational structure and how to work within it (and when it is necessary to work around it); becoming comfortable with the exercise of organizational, as well as clinical, authority
- Developing and using protocols, policies, and procedures to standardize administrative and clinical functioning
- Developing and using job descriptions, productivity standards, and employee evaluation instruments to monitor the performance of clinical staff, which transmit the values of the organization and justify staffing decisions
- Developing basic competency in fiscal, regulatory, and reimbursement issues to be able to address billing and budgetary problems in a helpful way and to integrate clinical sensibility into the solution of fiscal problems

Using Management Tools to Enhance Clinical Quality

Using management tools to enhance clinical quality is the natural outgrowth of the first two skills. The medical director must go beyond viewing quality assurance and utilization management as "necessary evils" and learn to use them in an integrated manner to solve problems, create new interventions, and enhance outcomes.

This involves using continuous quality improvement or total quality management methods to answer real clinical questions: Are our groups effective? Are our consumers satisfied? Are we overlooking substance

TABLE 8–1. American Association of Community Psychiatrists, "Guidelines for Psychiatric Leadership in Organized Delivery Systems for Treatment of Psychiatric and Substance Disorders"

Principles

1. All organized mental health service delivery systems should identify one psychiatrist as the Medical Director and ensure that that individual has adequate salaried time to perform his/her administrative responsibilities. In systems which are so large as to encompass organized subsystems, each such subsystem should have its own Medical Director as defined herein. In addition, in any system which is sufficiently complex, the Medical Director should designate Associate Medical Directors to ensure adequate supervision of psychiatric services in order to maintain high standards of care in all system components.

2. Each program within an organized delivery system must have one individual identified to provide medical/clinical direction for that program, with the amount of time allocated for that function to be commensurate with the size and complexity of clinical need of that program.

3. The Medical Director shall have ultimate clinical authority, but must function primarily as a collaborator and team member, both with the administration and with clinicians of other disciplines, in order to be maximally effective in accomplishing the goals and functions of the position.

4. The Medical Director shall be delegated ultimate authority and responsibility for ensuring psychiatric oversight in each of the following clinical activities:
    a. *Emergency Services:* Review of all dispositions through a defined protocol.
    b. *Acute Care Services:* Admission and discharge decisions, level of care determinations, and direct supervision of care.
    c. *Psychopharmacology:* Direct evaluation of all patients and/or supervision of nurse prescribers through a defined protocol.
    d. *Outpatient:* Participation and leadership in regular interdisciplinary team case reviews, including signing off on diagnoses and treatment plans.
    e. *Long-Term Support/Rehabilitative/Residential Services:* Participation and leadership in interdisciplinary treatment plan reviews.
    f. *Other Medical Care*

5. The Medical Director shall be delegated the ultimate authority and responsibility for ensuring psychiatric involvement and/or oversight in each of the following administrative areas:
    a. Development of job descriptions for system psychiatrists.
    b. Establishment of criteria for adequate psychiatric staffing within the system.
    c. Recruitment and supervision of psychiatrists.
    d. Staff training.
    e. Quality Assurance, CQI, Risk Management, and Outcome Evaluation.
    f. Utilization Review, Level of Care determinations, and appeals to third party payers.
    g. Developing standards of practice for psychiatric services in each program/level of care.
    h. Developing standards for continuity of case management and care as patients move through the system.
    i. Developing policies regarding medical and psychiatric evaluation, laboratory studies, risk assessment, treatment protocols, admission and discharge criteria, administrative discharge criteria.
    j. Medical Records/Documentation standards.
    k. Involvement in program budgeting, program planning, and program development.
    l. Establishment of criteria and processes for ensuring that clinical resources and programs are adequate and appropriate for the population served.

Note. CQI = continuous quality improvement.
Source. Excerpted from American Association of Community Psychiatrists: "Guidelines for Psychiatric Leadership in Organized Delivery Systems for Treatment of Psychiatric and Substance Disorders." *Community Psychiatrist,* Autumn 1995, pp 6–7. Used with permission.

abuse disorders? Are our day treatment patients stagnating? Is our psychopharmacology current? Do our patients function any better than they did before? Are the service use patterns consistent with clinical needs?

Similarly, as external managed care and internal case management gradually come together in capitated systems, the medical director must participate in and even lead efforts to design clear criteria for variations of service intensity (or levels of care) and a utilization management system for staff to make clinically appropriate decisions. This is not only necessary for the clinical relevance of those criteria and instruments but also

TABLE 8–2. Model job description for the system medical director

Responsibilities

Unless the Chief Executive Officer (CEO) is properly trained and qualified to serve this purpose, the Medical Director has ultimate authority and responsibility for the medical/psychiatric services of the System. Specifically, this includes responsibility for:

1. Assuring that all System patients receive appropriate evaluation, diagnoses, treatment, and medical screening, and that medical/psychiatric care is appropriately documented in the medical record.

2. Assuring psychiatric involvement in the development, approval, and review of all Policies, Procedures, and Protocols that govern clinical care.

3. Ensuring the availability of adequate psychiatric staffing to provide clinical, medical, administrative leadership, and clinical care throughout the system.

4. Developing job descriptions for staff psychiatrists that are comprehensive, and permit involvement in therapeutic and program development activities, as well as application of specific medical expertise.

5. Recruiting, evaluating, and supervising physicians (including residents and medical students), and overseeing the peer review process.

6. Assuring that all clinical staff receive appropriate clinical supervision, staff development, and in-service training.

7. Assuring, through an interdisciplinary process, the appropriate credentialing, privileging, and performance review of all clinical staff.

8. Providing direct psychiatric services.

9. Advising the CEO regarding the development and review of the System's programs, positions, and budgets that impact clinical services.

10. Assisting the CEO by participating in a clearly defined and regular relationship with the Board of Directors.

11. Participate with the CEO in making liaisons with private and public payers, in particular with Medical Directors or equivalent clinical leadership in payer organizations.

12. Assuring the quality of treatment and related services provided by the System's professional staff, through participation (directly or by designee) in the System's ongoing quality assurance and audit processes.

13. Providing oversight to ensure appropriate utilization of services throughout the System, by developing an appropriate continuum of programs; identifying level of care criteria, standards of practice, and psychiatric supervision for each program; and creating a system for internal review of level of care determinations and appeal of adverse UR decisions.

14. Participating in the development of a clinically relevant, outcome evaluation process.

15. Providing liaison for the System with community physicians, hospital staff, and other professionals and agencies with regard to psychiatric services.

16. Developing and maintaining, whenever possible, training programs in concert with various medical schools and graduate educational programs.

The Medical Director, by licensure, training, and prior clinical/administrative experience, shall be qualified to carry out these functions, and shall have an approximate minimum of 50% of his/her time allocated to administration. In all but the smallest settings, this position should be no less than 32 hours per week.

Note. UR = utilization review.
Source. Excerpted from American Association of Community Psychiatrists: "Guidelines for Psychiatric Leadership in Organized Delivery Systems for Treatment of Psychiatric and Substance Disorders." *Community Psychiatrist,* Autumn 1995, pp 6–7. Used with permission.

enhances the influence of clinical judgment on the ultimate continuum of services to be provided in organized care delivery systems. AACP is in the process of field testing one such instrument, the Level of Care Utilization System for Psychiatric and Addictions Services (LOCUS) (American Association of Community Psychiatrists 1997).

Keeping Pace With Management Technology

Psychiatric leadership requires increasing familiarity with computer technology, implementation and management of information systems, outcome measurement, and data manipulation (Lyons et al. 1997; Wells et al. 1995). The medical director must develop sufficient computer competence to be conversant with rapidly expanding organizational and data management technology.

Maintaining a Collaborative Presence in the Management Team

Because many psychiatrists, especially those who have worked in community settings, see themselves as inherently collaborative, this skill may seem deceptively simple. It is actually the most difficult. As the demands on organization managers become more complex and fiscally driven, the medical director is likely to identify less and less with administrative concerns and may retreat increasingly into the clinical role. This may set the stage for a deeper rift over values and direction later on. The medical director cannot give up on the management team, however stressful such continuing engagement may be. As the medical representative on the management team, the psychiatric leader must recognize the wide range of internal and external relationships that must be effectively cultivated and maintained. These important management-related liaisons are specific, but not exclusive, to the medical director.

Key Relationships

In addition to the specific roles and responsibilities that the medical director in community and other organized care delivery settings must be able to perform, it is important to identify the key relationships that this person must attend to in order to realize fully the organization's administrative agenda. In this section we use some anecdotal examples to describe these key relationships, with emphasis on the relationship skills as well as the clinical and administrative knowledge needed to develop and maintain appropriate influence in such relationships.

We have grouped these relationships into two relatively distinct types: those that are internal to the organization and those that are external. Among the key internal relationships are those with the CEO, other managers and supervisors, the clinical staff, patients, and the agency's board of advisors or directors. External relationships include consumer and family advocacy organizations, outside clinical liaisons, third-party payers, policymaking and regulating entities, and organizations involved in training, research, and program evaluation.

Chief Executive Officer

It is vital that the medical director and the CEO have a close and compatible relationship. The medical director, who has a biopsychosocial perspective unique to psychiatry and provides appropriate clinical insights about programmatic issues, must serve as a key clinical advisor to the CEO. The advice often will include information about the actual functioning and morale of the clinical staff, information that the medical director often has direct access to because of his or her clinical activities, whereas the CEO may be too far removed from the direct service activities to have an accurate reading of the "pulse" of the organization. Often, the medical director will be the only manager who is aware of clinical or programmatic conflicts, especially those that are related to the interface between separate programs within the agency. An example might be warfare between a case management team and a residential facility that houses many of the patients served by that team. The medical director must have some degree of authority over budget and personnel related to clinical activities, at least those that are directly related to medical services, such as physicians, nurses, laboratory personnel, and pharmacy personnel. The relationship with the CEO can make or break the medical director's opportunity to have this direct budgetary influence. In many ways, this relationship is the most critical, because the CEO's tacit or active support is essential to enable many of the following relationships to work well or to even occur.

Management and Supervisory Staff

The way in which the medical director interacts with other managers and supervisors is important both for its influence on how clinical services will be provided and managed and for its modeling effect on how other medical providers within the organization will be perceived and treated. The emphasis on interdisciplinary respect, and maintaining an atmosphere of mutual learning, applies as much to the general administrative activities that take place on a management team or within the supervision of a clinical program as it does to the interactions with direct clinical staff (described in the following subsection). A willingness to listen to others, to help to facilitate group problem solving, and to apply appropriate psychodynamic understanding and occasional interpretations of the organization's behavior, without insisting on personal credit for agency programs or accomplishments, are some of the skills and characteristics that may allow the medical director to succeed at this level of activity.

Clinical Staff

The medical director must directly influence the process and content of clinical activities, both medical and nonmedical. This means helping to create and guide clinical policies and procedures to ensure that patients' clinical needs predominate. These policies include standards of practice and some of the more bureaucratic aspects of clinical policies, such as documentation standards, rules regarding confidentiality, release of information, and critical incident reports. At the same time, the medical director must serve as a senior clinician, providing regularly scheduled and ad hoc clinical consultation and supervision to all staff. The clinical credibility of the medical director may need to be proven through the participation in the direct care of patients. How well this person performs clinically may be compromised by the extent of the administrative activities he or she may be required to perform, so it is equally important that the medical director be willing to defer to and learn graciously from the clinical expertise of the other expert clinicians in the agency, regardless of whether they are psychiatrists.

Consumers and Patients

The medical director's visibility within the agency makes it especially important for him or her to model the kind of respect for consumers that the consumer empowerment movement and good clinical practice require. Through the kinds of behaviors shown to patients, who are either known or unfamiliar, in direct clinical service activities or just in passing in the hall, the medical director sets the tone for how other clinical staff and how the agency's administration will be perceived and respected. The medical director should be a leader in formulating and implementing policies related to consumer involvement in the agency, ethical practices, and the use of consumers as employees within the organization. This may involve the recruitment and inclusion of consumers on various agency committees or advisory panels. The medical director's attitude toward such issues and individuals can have a great effect on whether patients feel respected and honored for their input.

Agency Board

The CEO must maintain a strong primary relationship with the agency's board of directors, but this relationship can benefit greatly from the use of key management personnel. In particular, the medical director should be directly involved in some board activities, if only on an intermittent basis. The key functions within this relationship involve explaining and translating difficult concepts associated with clinical practices, quality assurance and quality improvement, and risk reduction. The presence of the medical director at board meetings can often increase the credibility of the level of quality and the professional reputation of the agency staff in the eyes of the board.

Consumer and Family Advocacy Organizations

Among the various public relations functions the medical director may perform, none is as critical as maintaining an effective, respectful, and responsive relationship with the key consumer and family advocacy organizations in the community. The same principles of behavior described above, regarding patients within the agency, apply to the way one relates to these groups. Often, they look to the medical director as a representative of the psychiatric establishment and use opportunities such as casual contacts or public speaking engagements to "ask the doctor" questions that are important to their (or their loved one's) care or to their understanding of mental illness. Often, they use these opportunities to ventilate about the egregious ways they have been treated. Or they may seek support for certain policy or funding issues. In any case, the medical director's response and attitude is something about which one cannot be cavalier. Consumers and family members transfer surplus power to such an official and deserve to be heard, respected, and provided honest and direct answers, even if the information is at variance with their expectations.

Outside Clinical Liaisons

The medical director often serves as, or is perceived to be, the primary clinical liaison to other clinical and social service organizations. This is particularly true for primary care providers, health clinics, and medical directors of health plans. With the increasing presence of prepaid health plans, health maintenance organizations, and other organized managed care delivery systems, primary care providers have a growing role in the assessment, treatment, and referral for specialty care of persons with psychiatric disorders. Under these managed care arrangements, it is also important to relate to primary care providers more effectively to facilitate and ensure the provision of quality primary care services, especially for adults with severe and persistent mental disorders and children with serious emotional disorders. The interface with primary care has become one of the most critical areas of focus in mental healthcare delivery (Pincus 1987; Pollack and Goetz 1997; Simon 1995). The medical director must be involved in the development of consultation and linkage models, the negotiation of such arrangements, and the staffing and supervision of whatever liaisons emerge.

Third-Party Payers

Community and other organized care systems have become increasingly involved in developing specific contractual relationships with payers, such as prepaid health plans, including Medicaid managed mental healthcare systems. The successful negotiation and maintenance of such contracts may or may not require the participation of the medical director. However, ensuring quality clinical services in such contracts and maintaining adequate access to services for patients who manifest the greatest need appear to require substantial participation by a medical director. The medical director can provide oversight for the planning process to make sure such quality standards are incorporated without giving in to excessive pressure to cut costs. The medical director's presence also can add credibility to the negotiating team, especially when dealing with representatives from health plans, some of whom may have medical backgrounds.

Policymaking and Regulating Entities

Whether the care delivery organization is involved in predominantly prepaid funding contracts or fee-for-service revenue-generating activities, substantial outside regulations and quality standards are likely to affect the administration of the organization. As stated above, the medical director can provide valuable assistance to the process of adhering to such rules by helping to guide the internal processes associated with quality assurance and standards of care. The medical director also can be critical to the relationship with such external monitors, whether in the communications associated with such monitoring or even in the more important role of participating in the development and implementation of the standards themselves. Many medical directors throughout the United States have expanded their influence by gaining access to regional or statewide mental health authorities or other planning bodies and participating in activities such as the development of clinical record standards, role definitions for specific clinical disciplines, health plan benefit packages, and clinically relevant formulary and laboratory restrictions.

Organizations Involved in Training, Research, and Program Evaluation

Mental health provider organizations often have found it advantageous to establish links with academic institutions, such as professional training programs, to provide training and research opportunities for students and faculty from those organizations. In exchange, they usually have been able to recruit graduates from those programs to join their staff. In addition, the association with academic institutions can lend prestige and credibility to such programs. Similarly, community and other organized care providers may find themselves needing the services of outside organizations that do program evaluations. In all of these relationships, the involvement of the medical director can be useful to clarify expectations, generate ideas, improve the collaboration potential, and maintain the professional connections between the organizations.

Conclusion

In this chapter, we describe the value of and need for psychiatric leadership in organized mental healthcare delivery programs and systems at any level of complexity. We outline specific standards for the responsibilities and authority of the medical director role. Our thesis is that the expense of psychiatric leadership is more than sufficiently justified by its clinical effect and cost effectiveness, especially if psychiatric leaders are allowed and encouraged to develop the administrative, managerial, and collaborative skills that are herein defined and described.

References

American Association of Community Psychiatrists: Guidelines for psychiatric practice in CMHCs. Psychiatric News, April 5, 1991, p 32

American Association of Community Psychiatrists: Guidelines for psychiatric leadership in organized delivery systems for treatment of psychiatric and substance disorders. Community Psychiatrist, Autumn 1995, pp 6–7

American Association of Community Psychiatrists: Level of Care Utilization System for Psychiatric and Addiction Services, Version 1.5. Erie, PA, Deerfield Behavioral Health Network, 1997 (http://www.dbhn.com). See also AACP (http://www.comm.psych.pitt.edu)

Broskowski A, Eaddy M: Community mental health centers in a managed care environment. Adm Policy Ment Health 21:335–352, 1994

Clark RE, Dorwart RA, Epstein SS: Managing competition in public and private mental health agencies: implications for services and policy. Milbank Q 72:653–678, 1994

Cuffel BJ, Snowden L, Masland MC, et al: Managed mental health care in the public sector (Working Paper No. 6-94). Berkeley, CA, Institute for Mental Health Services Research, 1994

Dewey L, Astrachan B: Organizational issues in recruitment and retention of psychiatrists by CMHCs, in Community Mental Health Centers and Psychiatrists. Washington, DC, American Psychiatric Association and National Council of Community Mental Health Centers, 1985

Diamond H, Cutler D, Langsley D, et al: Training, recruitment, and retention of psychiatrists in CMHCs: issues and answers, in Community Mental Health Centers and Psychiatrists. Washington, DC, American Psychiatric Association and National Council of Community Mental Health Centers, 1985, pp 32–50

Diamond R, Stein L, Susser E: Essential and nonessential roles for psychiatrists in community mental health centers. Hosp Community Psychiatry 42:187–189, 1991

Dorwart RA: Managed mental health care: myths and realities in the 1990s. Hosp Community Psychiatry 41:1087–1091, 1990

Dorwart RA, Epstein SS: Economics and managed mental health care: the HMO as a crucible for cost-effective care, in Managed Mental Health Care: Administrative and Clinical Issues. Edited by Feldman SL, Fitzpatrick R. Washington, DC, American Psychiatric Press, 1992, pp 11–27

Dorwart RA, Epstein SS: Privatization and Mental Health Care: A Fragile Balance. Westport, CT, Auburn House, 1993

Feldman JL, Fitzpatrick RJ (eds): Managed Mental Health Care: Administrative and Clinical Issues. Washington, DC, American Psychiatric Press, 1992

Feldman S (ed): Managed Mental Health Services. Springfield, IL, Charles C Thomas, 1992

Freeman MA, Trabin T: Managed Behavioral Healthcare: History, Models, Key Issues, and Future Course. Washington, DC, Center for Mental Health Services, 1994

Hoge MA, Davidson L, Griffith EEH, et al: Defining managed care in public-sector psychiatry. Hosp Community Psychiatry 45:1085–1089, 1994

Intergovernmental Health Policy Project: Medicaid Managed Care and Mental Health: An Overview of Section 1115 Programs. Washington, DC, George Washington University, 1994

Knox M: National register reveals profile of service providers. National Council News, September 1985, p 1

Langsley D, Barter J: Psychiatric roles in the community mental health center. Hosp Community Psychiatry 34:729–733, 1983

Lyons JS, Howard KI, O'Mahoney MT, et al: The Measurement and Management of Clinical Outcomes in Mental Health. New York, John Wiley & Sons, 1997

Minkoff K: Community mental health in the nineties: PSMC. Community Ment Health J 30:317–321, 1994

Minkoff K, Pollack (eds): Managed Mental Health Care in the Public Sector: A Survival Manual. Toronto, Ontario, Harwood Academic, 1997

Patterson DY: Twenty-first century managed mental health: point of service treatment networks. Adm Policy Ment Health 21:27–34, 1993

Pincus H: Patient oriented models for linking primary care and mental health care. Gen Hosp Psychiatry 9:95–101, 1987

Pollack D, Cutler D: Psychiatry in community mental health centers: everyone can win. Community Ment Health J 28:259–267, 1992

Pollack D, Goetz R: Psychiatric interface with primary care, in Managed Mental Health Care in the Public Sector: A Survival Manual. Edited by Minkoff K, Pollack D. Toronto, Ontario, Harwood Academic, 1997, pp 217–232

Pomerantz JM, Liptzin B, Carter AH, et al: The professional affiliation group: a new model for managed mental health care. Hosp Community Psychiatry 45:308–310, 1994

Ranz J, Eilenberg J, Rosenheck S: The psychiatrist's role as medical director: task distributions and job satisfaction. Psychiatr Serv 48:915–920, 1997

Ray C, Oss M, Slayton L: Program management issues: introduction, in Managed Mental Health Care in the Public Sector: A Survival Manual. Edited by Minkoff K, Pollack D. Toronto, Ontario, Harwood Academic, 1997, pp 127–130

Simon G: Mental health and primary care liaison in a staff model HMO. Paper presented at the annual meeting of the American Psychiatric Association, Miami, FL, May 1995

Thompson J, Bass R: Changing staffing patterns in community mental health centers. Hosp Community Psychiatry 35:1107–1114, 1984

Wells KGB, Astrachan BIM, Tischler GL, et al: Issues and approaches in evaluating managed mental health care. Milbank Q 73:57–75, 1995

❖ Section III ❖

New Administrative
Psychiatry Concepts

Robert E. Hales, M.D., M.B.A., Section Editor

Introduction

Robert E. Hales, M.D., M.B.A.

This section is intended to provide the reader with information on new core administrative concepts that have resulted from the managed healthcare revolution sweeping across the United States. In particular, the chapters focus on several issues of importance to psychiatrists who work in managed care organizations or who must interact frequently with such organizations.

In Chapter 9, Yohanna and O'Mahoney provide a comprehensive overview on how to establish a behavioral health network. The authors emphasize that numerous organizational and staffing issues must be considered before such a network is created, especially in capitated environments, in which the behavioral health network is responsible for providing all mental healthcare for a defined population at an agreed-on per-member per-month rate. Psychiatrists must be quite careful in how they design such a system to ensure that mental health services can be provided within the available financial constraints. The chapters that follow in this section develop to a fuller extent many of the important issues raised by Yohanna and O'Mahoney in Chapter 9.

In Chapter 10, Bennett discusses what needs to be done to maintain a behavioral health network after it has been established. Among the points he emphasizes are several needs: to refine and shape activities, to enhance quality management functions, to provide care management activities, to focus on provider relations and education, and to ensure that the administrative support functions are adequate to maintain the system. Bennett eloquently emphasizes throughout his chapter that maintaining a behavioral health network requires a continuous process of differentiation, redefinition, and improvement. Once the behavioral health network has been established and a number of policies and procedures have been implemented and refined, the network must be appropriately staffed.

In Chapter 11, Osher provides a complete overview of staffing the network. He emphasizes how the role of the psychiatrist has been transformed from that of an individual, solo practitioner to one in which the psychiatrist works as a member of a coordinated, multidisciplinary treatment delivery system. In this managed care era, psychiatrists' roles and responsibilities are increasingly dedicated to diagnostic evaluation, medication management, and clinical supervision. The provision of individual psychotherapy, unfortunately, has been reduced. In addition to the normal array of professional staff (psychiatrists, psychologists, social workers, psychiatric nurses, and professional counselors), an important administrative staff of case managers, consumer employees, and management information specialists play key roles in ensuring the successful administrative operation of the behavioral health network. The professional and administrative staff who work in a managed mental healthcare system also must be competent in clinical, cultural, economic, and ethical areas, and training in each of these subjects must be continued. Osher emphasizes the need for continued education and training, not only for mental health staff but also for the community providers who may be providing care to network patients.

In Chapter 12, Simon provides a comprehensive overview on the topic of cost calculation, capitation, and redesigning systems. An important question psychiatrists must ask themselves is whether the amount of capitation funds being offered to them or their group is adequate to provide care for the population to be served. As Simon emphasizes in Chapter 12, many important patient issues affect the intensity and level of mental health services. Such issues include age; employment status; and, if employed, type of industry (blue collar vs. white collar, high technology vs. manufacturing, etc.). Other important issues are the extent of services included within the capitated payment: outpatient, partial hospitalization, inpatient, detoxification, substance abuse treatment programs, and so on. Based on the array and intensity of services included within the capitation rate, systems must be designed to ensure that this care is, in fact, delivered.

An increasingly important issue in managed mental healthcare is determining and measuring outcomes. In Chapter 13, Kramer and Smith provide an excellent overview of this rapidly evolving area. From one perspective, managed mental healthcare has caused providers to be more "customer-oriented," not only toward their patients but also toward their referral sources (primary care physicians, insurance companies, or employers). In determining the quality of services being delivered in a managed behavioral care network, a wide spectrum of potential clinical and administrative outcomes may be measured. Patient satisfaction and employer satisfaction with the quality of services are extremely important. Also, employers want to be assured that their employees in fact do improve with the treatment received from managed mental healthcare providers and that, as a result, these employees take fewer sick days and are more productive at work. Also, managers of behavioral health networks want to evaluate the quality of services delivered by their contracted mental health providers, and, as Kramer and Smith em-

phasize in Chapter 13, managers may use a variety of outcome measures to assess these providers.

The final chapter in this section is Chapter 14, "Health Information and Confidentiality," by Wald. As mental health clinicians know, obtaining authorization for outpatient, inpatient, or partial hospitalization services requires the treating physician to provide sufficient documentation to a utilization review person, who must determine the level of care and number of sessions (or hospital days). Also, when a prescription for a psychotropic medication is written, this information is usually entered into a comprehensive database and is identified with the particular patient being treated. A significant adverse effect of managed care, as implied in these examples, has been a dissemination of confidential information for administrative purposes to many other individuals not involved in the treatment of the patient. For some patients, this system has resulted in their inability to obtain life insurance, disability insurance, or medical insurance. In addition, because the primary care physician acts as a "gatekeeper" in many managed care systems, psychiatrists, psychologists, and social workers frequently need to provide written feedback to the primary care physician about the patient's response to treatment. This process is often essential to obtain additional outpatient visits. Although conveying psychiatric information to the primary care physician is necessary, such information not only will appear in the patient's medical record but also may be widely disseminated to other non–mental health personnel. For all of these reasons, the safeguarding of mental health medical records and of confidentiality between patient and provider is an extremely important issue that must be addressed in the development of any behavioral health network.

In summary, Section III, "New Administrative Psychiatry Concepts," provides the reader with core information that can help individuals seeking to design their own behavioral health network. By studying this section, clinicians and administrators will learn important principles in order to establish and maintain a behavioral health network, to provide appropriate staffing to the network, to calculate a capitated rate that would support the cost of such a network, to design outcome measures that would document the quality and effectiveness of the network, and to develop medical records and documentation procedures for mental health treatment while maintaining confidentiality for patients being served by the network.

9

Behavioral Health Network Establishment

Daniel Yohanna, M.D.
Michael T. O'Mahoney, Ph.D.

As clearly described in Section II, behavioral health delivery and financing systems are changing rapidly. We present one important element of this change process—the establishment of behavioral health networks. This "integration" of behavioral health services is in response to explicit market demands that behavioral health providers reform and improve their services, especially in the broad areas of affordability and accountability.

By the end of 1995, 161 million Americans belonged to some form of managed healthcare plan. This total represents more than 60% of the total insured population (Institute of Medicine 1990). This compares with only 29 million members in 1988 (American Medical Association 1990). As this chapter is being written, this number has continued to grow, although certain types of managed care organizations seem to be increasingly in favor.

Managed care organizations have taken on several forms, including health maintenance organizations (HMOs), point-of-service plans (POS), preferred provider organizations (PPOs), management services organizations (MSOs), and managed behavioral health

care organizations (MBHOs). There are "carve-in" behavioral programs, in which the programs are part of a larger multispecialty network, and "carve-outs," in which the behavioral programs are separate and distinct from the rest of the multispecialty medical group, with their own providers, financial arrangements, and utilization and quality management capabilities. Up to now, the growth of these managed care organizations has been driven mostly by cost containment.

Affordability

In the United States, healthcare system employers, unions, and government agencies are the major purchasers of healthcare. From the time that mental health services began to be reimbursed by health insurance until the late 1970s or early 1980s, behavioral healthcare costs were mostly not an issue; that is, they represented 3% or 4% of the healthcare dollar paid by the employer and did not draw much attention.

Beginning in the early 1980s, the demand for behavioral health services began to increase. The factors that fueled this increase included destigmatization of such services, improved treatments, increased stress on individuals and families, and the increasing availability of service. Costs to employers (especially those related to inpatient psychiatric services for adolescents and for chemical dependence treatment) began to increase at the rate of 30%–40% per year, and the existing review procedures followed by medical-surgical utilization management companies were inadequate to control these increases.

Employers began their attempt to control these cost increases by modifying the designs of the employee health benefit plans. Mental health and chemical dependence treatment costs were controlled by attempting to reduce consumer demand, provider use, or the amounts providers charged. These first-generation strategies typically did not control costs very well and also had the important disadvantage of limiting access to appropriate care for some of those who needed it.

Carve-out managed mental health firms began to emerge in the mid-1980s to deal with the explosion in behavioral healthcare costs being experienced by employers by promising to ensure that benefit dollars would be used to deliver only "medically necessary" behavioral healthcare. These firms used several utilization management strategies to control costs, including

- Requiring referral to specialty care by a gatekeeper—a primary care physician, employee assistance professional, or a centralized referral line staffed by behavioral health professionals
- Requiring precertification for intensive (inpatient and partial hospital) services
- Requiring concurrent utilization review to ensure "medical necessity"
- Developing preferred provider panels of physicians who agreed to reduced fees and practice protocols

Cost containment could be viewed initially as controlling two aspects: the demand side (i.e., through restricting benefits, limiting access to service through precertification or gatekeeper models, and utilization review) and the supply side (i.e., restricting provider networks and risk-sharing arrangements through capitation and other incentive arrangements) (Schwartz 1993).

These carve-out firms provided effective cost management and gradually set the stage for the reform of the behavioral health delivery system. They emphasized easy access to appropriate service, which led to the development by providers of better crisis intervention, "wraparound" alternative services, aggressive case finding, and more comprehensive assessment. These companies also emphasized ensuring that care took place in the most appropriate setting and using established standards of care, leading to the development of a continuum of care, flexible benefits, and clinically reasonable care management criteria.

These emerging managed mental health systems were being built on an integrated platform of clinical services delivered by contracted providers operating in a reimbursement system with appropriate incentives. Patients theoretically entered through a single point of entry and had access to the entire range of treatment modalities, integrated into a comprehensive program that ensured smooth transition between levels and careful linkage.

Solo behavioral health practices began to disappear, and large delivery systems began to emerge. Affordability of behavioral health services became a less pressing problem, at least in the private market. The challenge of administrators for 2001 and beyond is for behavioral health systems to develop self-managing, integrated systems of care to improve efficiency while maintaining cost effectiveness, achieve economies of scale, and develop an enhanced ability to work with smaller financial margins.

The alternative is to focus on cost containment by less thoughtful means. In some areas of the United States, organizations are offering increasingly restrictive networks and benefits. These strategies appear to be failing, as employers are being faced with increased costs in handling employee complaints ("Psychiatric delivery systems are changing for the better" 1993), and the restricted nature of care may cause an increase in morbidity, which will ultimately drive up the overall costs of providing healthcare. Organized psychiatry is quite uncertain about managed care and is increasingly voicing its concerns (Sabin 1995). Recent exposés in the media also have been increasingly critical of behavioral managed care.

Accountability

Another important reason for the rapid growth and success of the managed behavioral health industry was the loss of faith by payers in the ability of providers to be accountable. Payers turned to managed care in search of assurance that they were receiving value for their health insurance dollar. From now on, organized provider systems will need to demonstrate value, clinical excellence, and, increasingly, clinical and cost effectiveness. For the foreseeable future, managed care organizations will most likely continue in their intermediary role as purchasing agent for the payer. Behavioral health networks will need to be able to show the managed care organizations that they can provide appropriate, cost-effective care; improve functional health status; and maintain information-reporting capabilities that will assist the managed care organizations in reporting compliance to standards back to the payers.

Evolution of managed care into this area is evidenced by the rapid growth of protocols, guidelines, and "medical necessity" criteria. Sharfstein et al. (1992) pointed out that models of managing costs through demand-side and supply-side containment, combined with managing care through medical appropriateness criteria, will produce the best value. This will be elaborated further in the system through outcome studies to prove the value of this approach. Behavioral health networks will need to take on this role of demonstrating effectiveness.

Why Should a Network Be Established?

Managed care organizations, without doubt, have lowered healthcare costs. Compared with the older indemnity plans, managed care has lowered the rates of use of inpatient days (Lutz 1991; Perry 1991), lowered the rates of use of expensive tests, and, in some cases, increased the amount of preventive care provided for its members. What has yet to be proven is improved outcomes in terms of health status of its members (Miller and Luft 1994).

As stated earlier in this chapter, the purchasers of healthcare set the rules. They have successfully solved their most pressing cost problems by use of the intermediaries, the managed behavioral health industry. We believe that the managed behavioral health industry *will gradually fade,* to be replaced by more efficient and effective self-managed behavioral health networks. Our basic assumptions are that

- Third-party managed behavioral health is too costly.
- Payers will increasingly contract with organized provider systems with proven effectiveness, on a shared-risk basis.

- Providers will be required to meet established standards for access, appropriateness, and effectiveness.
- Providers will have to improve their ability to understand and control costs.

Provider networks will need to coalesce and develop the internal capabilities that have been served by third-party managed care entities. Their first task will be to prove the independent capability to contain costs. This will be accomplished, at least in the larger markets, almost entirely by the force of the marketplace. Behavioral health networks will arise and compete with one another for market share, at first almost completely on the basis of cost. Quality will be assessed in the areas of access, comprehensiveness, and satisfaction of members and employers. Processes will need to be continually improved to ensure better customer service.

Creating a behavioral health network will allow for pooling of capital and intellectual resources, potentially greater leverage in negotiating and contracting with health plans and employers, and increased opportunity to offer a comprehensive continuum of care. A central infrastructure should be able to support more comprehensive information management capabilities and enhanced ability to meet the more complex information and reporting requirements of the payers. Managed care has already influenced the evolution of financial and operating information systems of organizations (Marino 1996). Accounting systems are going through an evolution as they approach full integration of utilization and clinical information to provide financial and performance measures in a reliable and timely manner (Marino 1996). Economies of scale and sharing of some expenses should allow the system to become more cost effective and competitive (Dewsnup 1995). Administrators will require special skills in tolerating change, remaining flexible, and at the same time providing a focus and vision for the organization (Wampler et al. 1966).

When Should a Network Be Established?

For many proud provider systems, the allure of "first to market" is a siren song. Somebody has to go first, but it should be noted that it requires considerably less effort and fewer resources to enter a market after someone else. Very few markets are left that have not been explored, so many lessons from competitors exist. A related issue is differentiation of a new provider system from competitors in the market. Differences should be limited to those worth achieving, those that add value rather than simply differentiation.

Types of Organizations

Several different types of structures have evolved since the onset of managed care. In Table 9–1, the different types of organizations are outlined.

In an Institute of Medicine publication titled "Managing Managed Care: Quality Improvement in Behavioral Health" (Edmunds et al. 1997), the separate types of managed care organizations are defined from a variety of sources, including the Employee Assistance Professionals Association, the Joint Commission on Accreditation of Healthcare Organizations (JCAHO), the National Committee for Quality Assurance (NCQA), and the United Healthcare Corporation. In another document, these sources defined the HMO as "an organized system of healthcare that provides a comprehensive range of healthcare services to a voluntarily enrolled population in a geographic area on a primarily prepaid and fixed periodic basis" (Substance Abuse and Mental Health Services Administration 1999).

HMOs generally provide each subscriber with a primary care physician who could be an internist, a family practitioner, a pediatrician, and, in some settings, an obstetrician/gynecologist. The role of the primary care physician in the HMO is to serve as the patient's physician and as the "gatekeeper" of access to specialty services. There are reports, however, of some HMOs allowing "open access" to specialists without first getting a referral from the primary care physician (Kreier 1996). The belief is that as specialists learn their responsibility in an HMO to provide cost-effective care, the presence of a gatekeeper is unnecessary.

HMOs break down into essentially four models: the staff model, the group model, the network model, and the individual practice association model.

In the staff model HMO, all of the practitioners are employed on a salaried basis. This model is usually the most tightly managed and restrictive for its insured subscribers. The practitioners are usually responsible for only those patients covered by the plan. This arrangement is most amenable to management, as the practitioners are generally the most consistent and united in their approach to care. Staff models represent about 5% of HMOs.

TABLE 9–1. Types of managed care organizations

Health maintenance organizations
   Staff models
   Group models
   Network models
   Individual practice associations
Preferred provider organization (PPO)
Point of service (POS)
Management services organization (MSO)
Managed behavioral health organization (MBHO)
Business provider organization (BSO)
Employee assistance program (EAP)

In the group model, the practitioners are in a group and are paid by the HMO at a capitated rate. The members of the group then distribute money among the members. They are not employees of the HMO.

In the network model, practitioners work out of their own offices and are contracted with an HMO on a negotiated fee-for-service rate or at a capitated rate.

In the individual practice association model, the individual practitioners continue with their individual or group practice and are compensated by the HMO, generally on a negotiated fee-for-service basis. It is the most common type of HMO, constituting 56% of HMOs (Sharfstein et al. 1992). Incentives are set aside for the individual practice association if it achieves certain goals, such as a decrease in inpatient days or the use of other expensive services. Generally, individual practice associations are the most loosely managed of the managed care organizations, and the practitioners are likely to have patients from many HMOs or other types of organizations or who self-pay.

Individual HMOs may represent a pure form or a mixture of these models.

The PPO is defined as "a network discount, fee for service, provider arrangement with incentives to stay inside the network; [it] allows services outside of the PPO network at an increased co-payment and/or deductible; [and it] has structured quality and utilization management" (Substance Abuse and Mental Health Services Administration 1999).

A POS organization is defined as "an organized system of healthcare provided by an HMO model with the option of the delivery of services outside of the network at a higher co-payment or deductible" (Institute of Medicine 2000, p 94). This co-payment or deductible is often higher than the PPO co-payment or deductible. The incentive for the insurance company or employer of a POS plan is the ability to offer more choices while benefiting from the savings offered by an HMO. It is often used as a transitional arrangement by insurance carriers to move insured groups to an HMO that does not have the option of going out of the network. Employees soon realize the added savings in co-payments and deductibles to make the HMO more attractive.

The MSO is defined as "an organization that provides practice management, administration, and support services to individual physicians or group practices" (Substance Abuse and Mental Health Services Administration 1999).

The MBHO is "an organized system of behavioral healthcare delivery usually to a defined population of members of HMOs, PPOs, and other managed care structures; also known as a carve-out" (Substance Abuse and Mental Health Services Administration 1999).

Some companies use employee assistance programs (EAPs), which are company programs used to assist employees or their covered family members in finding solutions to their workplace or personal problems. EAPs often provide referrals to the managed care network of behavioral service and provide some case management of the care rendered. The integration of EAPs and managed care has achieved additional savings for many employers (Lee 1994).

A new concept, in which employers contract directly with providers to provide healthcare for their employees and covered family members, is being called a business provider organization (BPO). Two examples of BPOs are the Georgia Healthcare Partnership in Savannah and the Unity Health Network in St. Louis, Missouri (Gee 1995).

Investor-owned physician practices, also called physician practice management (PPM), are another relatively new network arrangement being developed by companies such as Coastal Healthcare Group and PhyCor, both publicly traded companies (Christianson et al. 1995). The American Medical Association has even encouraged physicians to compete with managed care companies by establishing a capital fund for physicians called Physicians Capital Source to start networks (Friedman 1995).

Provider-owned HMOs is a concept for immature markets, defined as less than 20% managed care penetration (Krampf 1995). In these markets, providers could team up with insurance companies to start their own HMOs. Immature markets are rapidly in decline, however, as managed care extends throughout the United States.

How Should a Network Be Established?

The first step in establishing a network is to develop a fully articulated shared vision. This vision must be stated in the mission and vision statements of the organization. Network development is a difficult process, with unique problems arising in each different market and within each evolving system. The partners must commit completely and for the long haul and must develop a plan to create a whole that is greater than the sum of the parts. The system must add value to the community as a system rather than be an attempt at defensively protecting historic market positions.

The next step is to do market research. Every market is different. The partners must complete a thorough assessment of the needs and the plans of the payers in their local or regional market. They also must assess the behavioral health resources available in the area. It is an error to construct a delivery system to match the specifications of a theoretical "model" system. It is also important to benchmark the progress and current status of competitors in the local market and to set realistic competitive market share goals. This process will also aid in the identification of target markets and product offerings.

A careful consideration of standards of networks would help guide the development of the network to meet standards. For example, NCQA standards delineate issues of quality, access, patient satisfaction, membership, utilization, and finance. A network would need the appropriate elements to meet these standards.

Several components of care would be required in any system. These different entities, their importance, and their place in the puzzle of delivering behavioral healthcare to a population of patients will be determined by local conditions and healthcare needs. An evaluation of existing services will help determine which components are available or need to be developed.

Components of care would include, at a minimum, hospitals; partial hospital programs; intensive outpatient programs; residential programs; individual or groups of outpatient practitioners that include psychiatrists, psychologists, psychiatric nurses, and social workers; and chemical dependence programs and therapists.

Some other step-down programs have been employed to reduce the dependence on more expensive inpatient or residential programs, such as assertive community treatment, traditional and mobile crisis intervention programs, wraparound services, and home care (Glazer 1993).

Wraparound services are services that are intended to assist the person in accessing mental health or other services (i.e., they "enable" the person to obtain services). Examples include transportation, child care services, employment counseling, legal assistance, domestic violence services, and even cash assistance. These services are most identified with public psychiatry and the treatment of the severely and persistently mentally ill.

Services must be accessed through a system or strategy that ensures that the patient is rapidly evaluated and then referred to the appropriate level of care for the appropriate amount of time. Quality, as defined by the Institute of Medicine, is "the degree to which health services for individuals and populations increase the likelihood of desired health outcomes and are consistent with current professional knowledge" (Institute of Medicine 1990, p 21).

To ensure quality and accessibility, several aspects of network development must be considered. A framework to understand this can be adapted from the work of Avedis Donabedian (1980), who described three criteria by which to understand and measure the quality of an organization: structure, process, and outcomes. These concepts are also described in Chapter 13 of this book.

Structural measures of quality include the types of services available in the network, the qualifications or certification of the individuals or the organizations, staffing issues within a group or organization, and adherence to certain requirements or codes (e.g., public health requirements and building and fire codes).

Certification of each of the different components is necessary to begin to evaluate the quality of an entire organization. Several accreditation and regulatory bodies are involved in this process. Some of the more prominent bodies include the JCAHO, the NCQA, the Accreditation Association for Ambulatory Health Care (AAAHC), the Utilization Review Accreditation Commission (URAC), and the Commission on Accreditation of Rehabilitation Facilities (CARF). A number of federal and state agencies have regulatory authority over healthcare organizations, including licensing agencies, insurance commissions, and departments of mental health, public health, and public aid.

Process measures of quality include evaluating the procedures used in treatment and the course of treatment. This would include statistics on the number of people served (such as penetration rates) and the num-

ber of visits or days of service; the appropriateness of levels of care; the determination of medical necessity; measures of access to services such as time on hold on the telephone, wait time until the first appointment, hours of service, and convenience of locations; and maintenance of quality through practice guidelines, pathways, or continuous quality improvement activities.

Outcome measures include measures of improvement of functional levels, symptoms, subjective well-being, and patient satisfaction.

In addition, independent audits of providers should be conducted to ensure adherence to the contracts.

In the development of a network, the structure of the network is partly determined by the patient population and the financing authority. Privately financed systems may differ significantly from publicly financed systems in the components of care, credentialing bodies, patient population, and aspects of care monitored for outcome.

Initial screening for quality of the structure and process of individual practitioners involves their qualifications as indicated by licensure, board certification, practice setting (e.g., office locations, hours of service, days to first appointment, and after-hours coverage), and practice styles (e.g., orientation of practitioners; use of individual, group, and family treatment; and availability of medication consultation). Licensure and certifying organizations for individual practitioners are listed in Table 9–2.

For facilities and institutions, quality assessment of structure includes the types of service available, number of patients served, location, licensure and accreditation, information system capacity, and how effectively they meet the standards of managed care. This last characteristic is important because facilities and institutions use their own resources to decrease utilization, use less restrictive settings, implement guidelines or pathways, and gather vital information for reporting to the managed care entity.

Several accreditation organizations exist for facilities and institutions. These are listed in Table 9–3.

In mental health treatment, with the diversity of programs and settings, network establishment must provide for a smooth continuum of care between inpatient and outpatient programs.

Information Systems

A crucial element in the development of a behavioral health network is an information system, so it deserves

TABLE 9–2. Professional associations, certifying organizations, and accreditation organizations

Professional associations
American Psychological Association
Employee Assistance Professional Association
American Association for Marriage and Family Therapy (AAMFT)
American Academy of Family Practitioners—offers training in addiction medicine
National Association of Social Workers
National Association of Alcohol and Drug Abuse Counselors

Board certification organizations
American Society of Addiction Medicine
National Board of Medical Examiners
American Board of Psychiatry and Neurology; also added qualifications in addiction psychiatry, geriatric psychiatry, child and
  adolescent psychiatry, and forensic psychiatry

Accreditation organizations
American Nurses Credentialing Center

State licensure organizations
National Council of State Boards of Nursing Licenses RNs and Licensed Practical Nurses (LPNs)
Association of State and Provincial Psychology Boards
American Association of State Social Worker Boards

special mention. The system that is developed or purchased will have a powerful effect on the network's developing efficiency and effectiveness, on its services, and on the quality of care it provides. The administrative streamlining resulting from efficient information management also will be vital to cost containment. Marketplace pressure will require rapid information access, effective and efficient communication, careful cost management, and more concrete proof of value by relating clinical outcome to cost. In addition, network providers will require access to complete and accurate patient information in ways that best support clinical decision making, protocol compliance, and case planning. As the members of a developing network come together, they will usually have varying levels of existing sophistication and effectiveness in information management. Given the central importance of information systems, as well as the substantial costs involved in developing a networkwide system, a stepwise developmental approach is recommended:

1. Invest in professional information system consultation from the onset.
2. Bring all the partners up to the best practice level of the most well-developed aspect of the system.
3. Consider an external MSO partner as a source of information system functionality.
4. See the information system as a crucially important tool of integration but not as the "glue" that magi-

TABLE 9–3. Accreditation organizations for facilities and institutions

National Committee for Quality Assurance (NCQA)
Accreditation Association for Ambulatory Health Care
  (AAAHC)
Utilization Review Accreditation Commission (URAC)
Joint Commission on Accreditation of Healthcare
  Organizations (JCAHO)
Commission on Accreditation of Rehabilitation Facilities
  (CARF)

cally creates a network. Learn as you develop and delay the purchase or licensing of the network-developing software until you have built up sufficient infrastructure and sophistication to make optimal use of it. It is easy to overspend on information systems.

Summary

Behavioral health network development will be an essential part of administration as healthcare continues to evolve. It is the mechanism that will integrate clinical care with the economic reality that demands affordability of the services offered, accountability that the services are needed, and proof that the care is effective in reducing morbidity and mortality. In this chapter we have outlined the different arrangements and issues in establishing a network, with the ultimate prediction that the ways of managed care, in its best forms we hope, will be a part of service organizations in the future.

References

American Medical Association: The Current Managed Care Environment: Trends and AMA Perspectives. Paper presented at meeting of the American Medical Association, October 1990, Chicago, IL

Christianson J, Dowd B, Kralewski J, et al: Managed care in the twin cities: what can we learn? Health Aff (Millwood) 14:114–130, 1995

Dewsnup RK: The once and future health care market. Journal of Pension Planning and Compliance 21(2):44–65, 1995

Donabedian A: Explorations in Quality Assessment and Monitoring, Vol 1: The Definition of Quality and Approaches to Its Assessment. Ann Arbor, MI, Health Administration Press, 1980

Edmunds M, Frank R, Hogan M, et al: Managing managed care: quality improvement in behavioral health, in Committee on Quality Assurance and Accreditation Guidelines for Managed Behavioral Health Care, Institute of Medicine. Washington, DC, National Academy Press, 1997

Frank RG, McQuire TG, Newhouse JP: Risk contracts in managed mental health care. Health Aff (Millwood) 14:50–64, 1995

Friedman AS: AMA to help doctors set up own health care networks. National Underwriter (Life/Health/Financial Services) 99(8):3, 1995

Gee EP: Business-provider organizations reap cost and health dividends. Modern Healthcare 25(7):82, 1995

Glazer WM: Psychiatric treatment programs: the continuous services model. Employee Benefits Journal 18(2):30–36, 1993

Institute of Medicine: Medicare: A Strategy for Quality Assurance, Vol 1. Washington, DC, National Academy Press, 1990

Institute of Medicine: Managed care systems and emerging infections: challenges and opportunities for strengthening surveillance, research, and prevention. Workshop summary, 2000, p 94

Krampf L: Provider-owned HMOs target unsaturated markets. Health Care Strategic Management 13(3):1–24, 1995

Kreier R: HMOs without gatekeepers. American Medical News 39(29):1, 27, 1996

Lee FC: Controlling costs through managed behavioral care. Human Resources Professional 7(6):3–6, 1994

Lutz S: Troubled times for psych hospitals. Modern Healthcare 21(50):26–33, 1991

Marino GV: Medical group practice: enhancing the basis for managed care planning. The CPA Journal 66(1):74–75, 1996

Miller RH, Luft HS: Managed care plan performance since 1980. JAMA 272:1512–1519, 1994

Perry L: Pressure from payers continues to slow growth of psychiatric hospitals: chains report decline. Modern Healthcare 21(20):70–74, 1991

Psychiatric delivery systems are changing for the better. Business and Health, September 1993, pp 15–22

Sabin J: Organized psychiatry and managed care: quality improvement or holy war? Health Aff (Millwood) 14:32–33, 1995

Schwartz MP: Big insurers fine-tune managed care programs. National Underwriter (Life/Health/Financial Services) 97(36):3, 50, 1993

Sharfstein SS, Goldman HH, Arana J: The market for mental health care: new rules of reimbursement and new delivery systems, in Textbook of Administrative Psychiatry. Edited by Talbott JA, Hales RE, Keill SL. Washington, DC, American Psychiatric Press, 1992, pp 91–115

Substance Abuse and Mental Health Administration, Center for Substance Abuse Prevention, Division of Workplace Programs, Workplace Managed Care: Working Glossary of Terms. Presented at 7th WMC Steering Committee Meeting. Version: April 30, 1999

Wampler J, Frank D, Fogel K: Strategic alliances: an integrated health system alternative. Frontiers of Health Services Management 13(1):53–56, 1966

Selected Readings

Abrams HS: Harvard community health plan's mental health design project: a managerial and clinical partnership. Psychiatr Q 64:13–31, 1993

Arons BS, Frank RG, Goldman HH, et al: Mental health and substance abuse coverage under health reform. Health Aff (Millwood) 13:192–205, 1994

Beck DF, Dempsey J: The managed care time clock: what's making it tick? Health Care Supervisor 14(3):1–12, 1996

Bennett MJ: The greening of the HMO: implications for prepaid psychiatry. Am J Psychiatry 145:1544–1549, 1988

Bittker TE: The industrialization of American psychiatry. Am J Psychiatry 142:149–154, 1985

Borok LS: The use of relational databases in health care information systems. J Health Care Finance 21(4):6–12, 1995

Boyle PJ, Callahan D: Managed care in mental health: the ethical issues. Health Aff (Millwood) 14:7–22, 1995

Business and Health Magazine: The State of Health Care in America. Montvale, NJ, Medical Economics Publishing, 1995

Cerne F: Money and management. Hospital and Health Networks 69(1):32–36, 1995

England MJ, Vaccaro VA: New systems to manage mental health care. Health Aff (Millwood) 10:129–137, 1991

Frank RG, McQuire TG, Newhouse JP: Risk contracts in managed mental health care. Health Aff (Millwood) 14:50–64, 1995

Gold MR, Hurley R, Lake T, et al: National survey of the arrangements managed-care plans make with physicians. N Engl J Med 333:1678–1683, 1995

Grates GF: Managed care marketing: the next generation. Broker World 14(11):80–84+, 1994

Hutton DH: Organizing and managing primary care practice networks. Healthcare Executive 10(2):17–21, 1995

Iglehart JK: Health policy report: managed care and mental health. N Engl J Med 334:131–135, 1996

Pyle TO, Connell S, Hurley RE: Seamless; reply. Frontiers of Health Services Management 9(4):42–45, 1993

Ricks CS: Managed care will end era of provider networks. Modern Healthcare 26(13):92, 1996

Sheffert DG: Insurer/network pacts offer affordable care. Best's Review (Life/Health) 95(10):64–68, 1995

Shore MF, Beigel A: The challenges posed by managed behavioral health care. N Engl J Med 339:116–118, 1996

Talbott JF: Managing for change in behavioral health care. Continuum 3:37–43, 1996

❖ 10 ❖

Behavioral Health Network Maintenance

Michael J. Bennett, M.D.

The concept of *maintenance,* which conjures visions of a handyperson with tools strapped to his or her belt, is most unromantic. Alluding to the Hindu *arasmas,* however, Erik Erikson suggested a more lofty vision: that maintenance (householding in the service of "maintenance of the world") is the proper task of adulthood (Erikson 1978, p. 22). In the world of healthcare, as with adulthood, maintenance activities presume that a certain plateau or state of stability (maturity) has been achieved. Because of the dynamic nature of change, however, evolving behavioral health networks (BHNs) never meet such a definition. The first principle, therefore, of maintaining a BHN is that the network is always in a state of becoming.

The BHN may be characterized as an array of services and providers assembled by the manager of a behavioral healthcare organization (MBHO) to provide necessary mental health and substance abuse care to an enrolled population. It is the job of the MBHO to transform a loose assembly of clinical resources into a system that is integrated both vertically and horizontally, so that it operates as though it were a collaborative system without walls. The contemporary BHN is the residue of earlier forms of networks (Bennett 1996), and it is dis-tinguished from preferred provider organizations (PPOs) and independent practice associations (IPAs) by the introduction of managerial techniques at every level of the system. These techniques include selection, credentialing, and ongoing evaluation of providers; oversight of caregiving activities; and monitoring of the quality and cost of services. Contemporary BHNs are the lifeblood of the organizations that form and manage them. The MBHO contracts with various clients (i.e., federal and state governments, HMOs, self-insuring corporations), usually in some form of risk-sharing arrangement. The MBHO manages its risk largely through managing the BHN.

Despite the difficulty of identifying a *maintenance phase,* certain activities are essential to the smooth operation of a BHN (Table 10–1).

The first function, refining and shaping the network, relates largely to growth, turnover, and the demands of new contracts. In addition, the inclusion of clinical resources reflects shifting priorities and norms, as the array of available services evolves in response to the environment and to new knowledge. Such shaping also reflects the requirements of special populations and may include resources lying outside the formal

TABLE 10–1. The six functions of a behavioral health network

Function	Examples of function
Refining and shaping	Growth, subspecialization, new services
Care management	Shaping and monitoring clinical services
Quality management	Monitoring and enhancing quality of care
Risk management	Monitoring and diminishing risk
Provider relations and education	Rapport, support, guidance, appeals
Administrative and support services	Information systems, claims, customer service

healthcare system (e.g., self-help programs, wrap-around services). In addition to micro matters such as staffing and recruitment (i.e., of subspecialists, programs, and services), shaping also involves macro matters: changing configurations of service delivery (i.e., group rather than individual practice) or changing relationships between management and clinical providers (i.e., case rates or subcapitation).

Care management activities are the successor to *benefit management* and *utilization management,* which may be understood as antecedent forms of managed care. Care management requires intermediaries (i.e., care managers, physician advisors) whose job it is to oversee (and, increasingly, to shape) the care provided. Operating at the interface of management and clinical practice, care managers are involved in all six functions. In order to work effectively, they must be supported by information systems that allow efficient communication of clinical material to them and rapid, clear, and timely responses from them to the providers of care. This important support function takes place in an era of rapidly advancing information processing technology. Network growth, in particular, places demands on such technology to link providers with the care managers and with each other. This latter type of linkage transforms the network from solo and group entities in competition with each other (Bennett 1994) into a collaborative enterprise, bringing about the coordination of care necessary in today's highly subspecialized environment. Kane et al. (1995) described the use of a clinical management information system to provide not only the information necessary to monitor care but also the baseline and follow-up data necessary to assess the quality and utility of services provided.

As the healthcare system has adapted to demands for cost containment, the spotlight has fallen increasingly on quality management as the distinguishing feature of organized systems of care. Quality, defined most broadly, refers to the three aspects of healthcare identified by Donabedian: structure, process, and outcome (Donabedian 1969, 1980); therefore, the monitoring and documented systematic enhancement of quality is crucial to the organizations that compete for healthcare business. Concerns about manifest quality enhancement drive the system and are reflected in all six categories of maintenance.

Risk management refers not only to concerns about organizational liability (e.g., meeting contractual obligations and the requirements of law) but also to the identification, monitoring, and reduction of clinical risk (e.g., treatment of the suicidal patient). As an overarching aspect of organizational performance, risk management is closely related to the concept of continuous quality improvement. In considering relevance to network maintenance, this chapter focuses primarily on the management of clinical risk.

The maintenance of a network involves, next, those activities designed to enhance rapport, identify and solve problems, and contribute to the improved performance of the caregivers. These activities include opportunities for exchange and feedback, training, and the development of due process when disagreements lead to denials of authorization or termination of network membership. Ordinarily this function involves a provider relations department and various committees at both central and local levels (e.g., quality improvement committees, provider credentialing and review boards), in which provider participation is increasingly common. In addition, an MBHO may develop other methods to relate to its providers, ranging from booths and other activities at national professional organization conventions to newsletters to Web sites, subserving the functions of both communication and education.

Finally, a variety of support functions must be maintained, expanded, and periodically updated. These functions include processes that allow for credentialing and re-credentialing, timely and appropriate referral to network providers, prompt claims payment, and the expedited processing of appeals. They depend on an intact, effective information system that is capable of expanding to accommodate a continuously changing network.

In considering BHN maintenance, this chapter emphasizes three domains: managing care, managing quality, and managing risk.

Managing Care

The BHN exists for only one reason: to provide services to populations of enrolled members when those members become patients. The structure, process, and outcome of care provided in the healthcare community have for many years been regarded as the sole business of the principals involved: primarily providers of care and their patients. With the growth of managed care in the 1990s, however, payers have increasingly exerted their influence through intermediaries. The contemporary network is created and maintained with an eye toward meeting payer demand for value, that is, the highest quality care at the lowest possible cost. These considerations are operationalized for the individual patient at the care manager–provider interface. Following selection and organization of a network, therefore, it becomes necessary to determine whether the payer is receiving such value and to take steps to enhance value. This assessment falls within the domain of quality management, and enhancement consists of a series of activities designed to make care as efficient and effective as possible.

Although antecedents of the contemporary BHN, the IPA and the PPO, relied on the management of benefits to contain cost (their primary mandate), the additional mandate of enhancing quality requires greater involvement in the process of care. Care managers and psychiatric overseers must be recruited, trained, and supervised for this role. Formal training programs and clear lines of authority, supervision, and communication are essential. Because training is not provided for such roles within professional degree programs, it must be provided by the overseeing organization. The function of care management falls somewhere between peer review and consultation, with considerable variation in mission depending on the relationship between network clinicians and the overseeing behavioral healthcare manager. In risk-sharing arrangements, for example, the manager's involvement in individual cases may be minimal. In fee-for-service arrangements, however, which remain the norm, care managers render authorization decisions that may considerably influence clinical decision making. The instrument used for this purpose is the organization's *care management guidelines*: a set of criteria and indicators that determine the appropriate level and site of care, services, and service personnel based on the concept of *medical necessity*. These guidelines, which are developed collaboratively, are published and shared with clini-

cians. Book et al. (1996) described an example of a process and product common to most of the MBHOs.

Under the influence of monitoring organizations such as the National Committee for Quality Assurance (NCQA), the process by which guidelines used to precertify and review treatment decisions are developed and used is being standardized and the "black box" phenomenon (Pincus et al. 1996) reduced. An MBHO is responsible not only for developing and teaching such guidelines but also for periodically updating and revising them. Because large (especially national) clients, the federal government, and some state governments may require their own guidelines, an MBHO must ensure that care management staff are familiar with all guidelines they may be called on to use. This requirement poses a great educational and supervisory challenge, because language and conceptual differences among guidelines may be significant, though the principles are usually consistent. The sharing of care management guidelines with network providers, once a considerable logistical problem, will be greatly facilitated by the Internet.

Care management guidelines presume that clinicians and overseers of care share basic clinical assumptions. Because networks may be quite large, however, this is often not the case, and efforts must be made to convey a clinical philosophy or, in some cases, specific expectations regarding the evaluation and treatment process. For example, it is commonly assumed that clinicians will routinely screen for the presence of substance use disorders, consider psychopharmacologic evaluation and/or intervention for depressed patients, and employ family treatment methodologies when dealing with children or adolescents. Many clinicians, however, owing either to lack of knowledge or contrasting clinical orientations, may have different views or convictions. Guidelines must, therefore, also convey general expectations regarding accepted community standards. In this regard, an overlap exists between care management guidelines and practice guidelines, and the distinctions between the two are likely to become progressively less distinct as overseers move from monitoring to shaping care. In addition, as BHNs become involved with populations that have more severe and persistent forms of mental disorder, which is the case with the trend toward privatizing programs dealing with such populations, care management will also evolve. In discussing changes in the British National Health Service, Thornicroft et al. (1993) pointed to the need for a more interventionist model of care management when dealing with such patients. Such changes will likely occur in the United States as well. A report written by a consumer provided a poignant account of the value to the patient of such an interventionist role (Ware 1995).

Although communication with network providers may be accomplished through newsletters, direct mailing, or electronic means, education of clinicians and retraining pose greater challenges. Though changes are taking place, the average clinician remains poorly trained to adapt to the demands of contemporary managed care (Bennett 1993a). Most MBHOs attempt to address this need through working with the Institute for Behavioral Healthcare, an educational resource, or other trainers; through sponsorship; or through providing their own seminars and workshops. Finally, the BHN provider must be encouraged to relate effectively to the wider array of other healthcare resources used by his or her patients. Such resources include primary care and other medical clinicians, self-help programs, psychosocial rehabilitation resources, and other mental health providers. Collaboration in caregiving runs counter to the dyadic model that has represented the dominant paradigm of mental healthcare since the 1950s (Bennett 1993b, 1997). The care manager's function extends to supporting, encouraging, and facilitating such interaction and collaboration. These functions may be accomplished both formally (i.e., through educational programs aimed at such constituencies) or through expectations conveyed through the primary network provider in a given case. As with care management guidelines, these functions imply shared clinical values, which may or may not be the case. Once again, an overlap exists between practice guidelines and the overarching domains of quality and risk management.

Managing Quality

With the evolution of networks from loose affiliations to more tightly managed and integrated systems of care, a gradual shift in emphasis has occurred: from cost containment to a more balanced set of objectives that embrace the key parameters of quality. NCQA, whose imprimatur is highly prized by BHOs, requires that quality management be more than a presence; the expectation is that concerns about quality will drive the system. Donabedian's three dimensions of quality—structure, process, and outcome—remain organizing concepts within a framework of continuous improve-

ment (Donabedian 1969, 1980). The cycle of quality improvement requires 1) that methods be in place to identify, measure, and monitor quality indicators, 2) that initiatives be undertaken to improve identified shortcomings, and 3) that progress and change be documented. The network's performance is measured and addressed primarily through this sequence.

In constructing (and continuously reshaping) the network, the evaluation of the individual clinicians, agencies, and facilities that compose it must begin with credentialing. Under the influence of NCQA and client organizations (those that employ the BHO and provide its enrollees or patients), this process has become highly systematized. It involves not only primary source verification with regard to training, licensure, qualifications, ethical and legal status, and, in many instances, indications of readiness to work within a managed system of care, but also (especially with high-volume providers) closer scrutiny through on-site inspection and chart review. This assessment may be performed by the BHO or delegated to organizations that specialize in such services. Questions such as accessibility for both average and disabled patients, adequacy and security of records, and privacy of the setting are evaluated. Periodic re-credentialing involves repeated assessments of these parameters and consideration of performance since the last review. Considerable resources are required to perform these functions in a credible, timely manner. The American Managed Behavioral Healthcare Association, which includes representatives of some of the larger companies, has begun to develop a standardized method for accomplishing the routine tasks involved, with the aim of reducing unnecessary duplication (Gruttardaro 1996).

Performance review has historically focused on three measures: patient satisfaction, utilization patterns, and care manager review. Although these measures remain important, only a broad picture of performance that includes multiple parameters will provide reliable information. BHOs have been slow to develop such capacity. Methods for gauging outcome represent a rapidly growing component of quality improvement programs, and as these are developed they will become an important element in measuring provider performance. For the provider who is known to the system, data are retained on availability (i.e., access for new and returning patients), incident reports (both favorable and adverse), member complaints, and favorable or problematic interactions with the care management system. These elements, in addition to a profile of the individual's (or the group's) pattern of practice, provide a necessary third dimension to the data on utilization. As the professional community debates the matter of what constitutes excellence in clinical practice, the resulting standards will be adopted by BHOs and used in assessing and monitoring performance.

Performance monitoring provides a basis for selective referral or designation of favored (or unfavored) status, which may be based on the specific, demonstrated skills of the provider (i.e., added qualifications in geriatric or substance use disorders) or on an overall assessment of the provider's effectiveness and efficiency. Providers whose patterns fall outside the norm are so informed and offered assistance in making necessary changes. Actions that may be taken range from the provision of specific feedback to various forms of limiting practice or, in extreme instances, termination. As required by NCQA and by many client organizations, methods must be in place to inform clinicians of the reasons for termination, even when a contractual clause allowing "termination without cause" is invoked. Several BHOs have joined a program through the American Psychiatric Association in which delineation of cause for termination is provided in all cases involving psychiatrists. Such "due process" represents both quality and risk management principles.

The assessment and monitoring of quality within organized settings, including BHNs, have become of general interest. The Institute of Medicine evaluated the state of the art of quality assessment in MBHOs and found them varied and wanting (News and Notes 1997b). The Institute recommended broader consumer involvement and federal and state oversight to prevent abuses. A spate of legislation has addressed issues of unwarranted coercion of network providers (i.e., "gag rules"), as network development and maintenance have seriously eroded the autonomy of providers. Druss and Rosenheck (1997), considering the impact of NCQA's use of the Health Plan Employer Data and Information Set (HEDIS), have criticized the limitations of this widely used "report card," which requires only tracking of aftercare appointments for hospital-discharged depressed patients as an indicator of quality of mental health management. Most BHOs have already gone beyond the HEDIS requirements, driven largely by the desire to compete successfully for the business of an informed payer. The extraordinary attention being given to managed behavioral healthcare contrasts with the extraordinary neglect of the quality of mental health services in the United States even as

late as 1990. This attention also indicates the degree to which the expanding presence of managed behavioral healthcare has raised both consciousness and anxiety. The results of such intense scrutiny are likely to be positive for the organizations, for the providers, and, most important, for the patients who increasingly receive care within such systems.

Finally, in considering the matter of quality, the issue of practice guidelines must be taken into account. NCQA has set expectations, as have many client organizations, requiring that BHOs develop and share with their providers expectations about what constitutes good care. Some organizations have developed their own guidelines, and others have relied primarily on guidelines developed by professional organizations (Agency for Health Care Policy and Research 1993; American Psychiatric Association 1993, 1994, 1995a, 1995b; American Society of Addiction Medicine 1996) or by a consensus process (Expert Consensus Panel for Bipolar Disorder 1996; Expert Consensus Panel for Schizophrenia 1996). Most organizations have resisted the notion of practice standards as posing too great a threat of liability and not being consistent with the current state of knowledge in the field.

Merit Behavioral Care Corporation (MBC), one of the largest of the BHOs, has begun to develop guidelines for the treatment of specific clinical quandaries or impasses rather than guidelines based on diagnosis per se, while endorsing selective disorder-based guidelines produced by professional organizations or a consensus process. The assumption underlying this policy is that the credibility of guidelines produced outside the organization will be greater, and the process used to generate credible guidelines exceeds the resources of a single organization. The method used by MBC has been iterative, involving network providers and national experts. Internally produced guidelines (e.g., on the assessment and management of the suicidal patient) have been promulgated through a provider newsletter and distributed free of charge to network members, and providers have been helped to obtain guidelines in the public domain. A report released by the U.S. Office of Technology Assessment (OTA) pointed to the importance of provider participation in guideline development and the wide dissemination of such guidelines (News and Notes 1994).

The major method of implementing guidelines, however they are derived, is through the educated case manager, whose job includes "championing" a knowledge-based approach to care. Although guideline development presents prospects for improvement in practice by reducing unwarranted variability and encouraging knowledge-based clinical decision making, problems remain. A report published by the General Accounting Office commented on the tendency of BHOs to use published guidelines selectively, in order to simplify them or adapt them to perceived needs (News and Notes 1997a). A major concern among such organizations is the overly inclusive nature of guidelines published by professional organizations and their lack of specificity. As the OTA report suggested, however, a potential for bias exists when guidelines are developed locally or when they reflect too narrow a perspective. Ultimately, BHOs must reconcile their interest in shaping provider behavior with the evolving standards in the community. Given the great interest in guidelines among payers, professional organizations, and regulatory bodies, this aspect of network maintenance will become increasingly important in coming years.

Managing Risk

Mental health practice involves risk, and that risk is likely to be shared by both providers and managers of care (Appelbaum 1993; Sederer and Bennett 1996; Soltys 1995). Risk may be a particularly important consideration when network providers are asked to practice in a manner that may deviate from the community norm, for example, when they are asked to treat mental illness in patients who might ordinarily be hospitalized on an ambulatory basis or to discharge patients to lower levels of care before the illness requiring hospitalization is in a state of full remission. Sound risk management must take into account the evolving legal trend to regard both the BHO and the provider as sharing a duty to the patient and therefore as potentially liable in the event of an adverse outcome. This shared duty places considerable pressure on the BHO to obtain risk assessment information from the provider and to ensure that risk is managed properly.

In addition to clinical risk (e.g., with the potentially suicidal or homicidal patient), network managers must take steps to conform to legal and contractual requirements with regard to provider contracting and the discipline and termination of network members. To address these requirements in an atmosphere that is often contentious and in a culture that is often litigious creates the need for integrating clinical and legal functions at all levels of the system.

Both Sederer and Bennett (1996) and Appelbaum (1993) identified the discrepancy that may exist between the BHO and the practitioner with regard to individual patient advocacy and fiduciary responsibility. The network provider is bound by an ethical duty to advocate for the individual patient, whereas the BHO must concern itself with the cost-effective care of populations, which involves duties both to enrollees who are not (yet) patients and to active patients. This distinction may lead to disagreements, and all methods must resolve such disagreements promptly and in a manner that does not have an adverse effect on patient well-being. Mechanisms for appeal, which are part of all contracts, must be combined with effective communication if favorable relationships are to be preserved and adversarial situations avoided.

When adverse incidents do occur, they must be reviewed and their causes addressed, as a matter of avoiding liability and meeting contractual obligations. The adverse incident audit is a powerful tool to identify and rectify systems and clinician issues that may have contributed to a bad outcome. Kinzie et al. (1992) described the value of mortality and morbidity conferences in pointing the way to corrective action in a university hospital. Within a network, a review and often a conference involving the providers and managers of care takes place, for example, following a patient suicide, but under somewhat different circumstances. First, the provider is often wary of the legal risks of review and may be advised by his or her attorney not to participate or, in some cases, not to forward information. Such resistance violates the contractual obligation to participate in quality and risk management activities, which is usually a clear requirement. Second, the provider may be reluctant to participate on a personal basis, following the trauma of such an event. Finally, the provider may not personally know or have reason to trust the reviewer and may demur as a result. The response to such resistance must come from a peer and must be personal: educational, supportive, exhortative, even while indicating that the provider's network status will be enhanced by cooperation and diminished by its absence. Every effort is made in such reviews to reduce the exposure and risk to all parties while providing a useful service.

Risk management strategies include education of care managers, other staff, and providers about key tenets; such education is part of routine training programs. Care management staff must be familiar with the principles of sound documentation, the duty to protect and to warn, and the duty to report and staff must be prepared to advise network providers regarding such matters. The maintenance of good records, by the care manager and the provider, is the best guarantee of legal protection in the event of untoward incidents.

Summary

The contemporary BHN is shaped to deliver effective and efficient care to populations of enrollees. As the healthcare system continues to evolve, managed care continues to be redefined to bring it into alignment with the expectations of increasingly knowledgeable payers and healthcare consumers. For organizations seeking to compete as managers of care, the network is the key to success: the end product, the only product.

This chapter has considered the essential elements of network maintenance: a continuous process of differentiation, redefinition, and improvement. The key elements are the management of the process of care (with an eye toward seeking the best outcomes), the management of quality (and its enhancement), and the management of risk (and its diminution). Continuous improvement is the theme that links these three elements with each other and with three other elements of network maintenance: provider relations, shaping and growth of the network, and provision of services to support these functions.

As Americans have opted for managed systems of healthcare that provide a wide choice of providers, access to specialized services, and services provided close to home, the network has largely displaced the staff model HMO as the dominant model of managed behavioral healthcare. Because providers may be geographically remote from each other and from the BHO, and because they are not employees of the BHO, methods must be found to promote coordinated care of consistently high quality while conserving costs. Such methods require the establishment and maintenance of rapport with practitioners, agencies, and facilities that may be culturally diverse and committed to differing clinical values and perspectives. Shortell (1993) suggested that the breadth, depth, and geographical concentration of resources in a network are the variables that must be addressed and managed if the system is to function effectively. I consider maintenance to be the management of obstacles to integration.

As managed systems become progressively more collaborative, old ideas about control and inspection are replaced by the principles of shared accountability and shared risk. This change is a product of movement toward partnerships and joint ventures involving network participants and BHOs. It calls for a reconsideration of incentives and a replacement of compliance with alliance. Within emerging configurations, maintenance activities must be predicated on commitments to excellence and to continuous improvement in performance. Education, reduction of unwarranted variations in practice, and experimentation with new methods replace investment in the status quo under such circumstances. The organization, or its subunits (increasingly, group practices that mirror the network as a whole), take on the characteristics of what Senge (1990) called the learning organization: one committed to acquiring and utilizing knowledge in the service of new paradigms of health and illness. For the practitioner, this means investment in the promotion of health and wellness and willingness to consider the needs of populations and matters of allocation in the course of making decisions about individual patients.

The paradox, of course, is the seeming contradiction in the use of the term *maintenance* to characterize the activities of an organization that is committed to constant change. Only by taking the long view, perhaps in the manner suggested by Erikson, can the matter be resolved; the maintenance of change and continuous improvement is the ultimate goal.

References

Agency for Health Care Policy and Research: Depression in Primary Care: Vol 2. Treatment of Major Depression. Rockville, MD, U. S. Department of Health and Human Services, Agency for Health Care Policy and Research, 1993

American Psychiatric Association: Practice guidelines for major depressive disorder in adults. Am J Psychiatry 150 (suppl):1–26, 1993

American Psychiatric Association: Practice guidelines for the treatment of patients with bipolar disorder. Am J Psychiatry 151 (suppl):1–36, 1994

American Psychiatric Association: Practice guidelines for psychiatric evaluation of adults. Am J Psychiatry 152 (suppl):63–80, 1995a

American Psychiatric Association: Practice guidelines for the treatment of patients with substance use disorders: alcohol, cocaine, opioids. Am J Psychiatry 152 (suppl):1–59, 1995b

American Society of Addiction Medicine: Patient Placement Criteria for the Treatment of Substance-Related Disorders, 2nd Edition (ASAM PPC-2). Chevy Chase, MD, American Society of Addiction Medicine, 1996

Appelbaum P: Legal liability and managed care. Am Psychol 48:251–257, 1993

Bennett M: The importance in teaching the principles of managed care. Behavioral Healthcare Tomorrow 2:28–32, 1993a

Bennett M: View from the bridge: reflections of a recovering staff model HMO psychiatrist. Psychiatr Q 64:45–75, 1993b

Bennett M: Are competing psychotherapists manageable? Managed Care Quarterly 2:36–42, 1994

Bennett M: Will the transition into integrated networks appear seamless? in Controversies in Managed Mental Health Care. Edited by Lazarus A. Washington, DC, APA Press, 1996, pp 371–382

Bennett M: Focal psychotherapy, in Acute Care Psychiatry: Diagnosis and Treatment. Edited by Sederer L, Rothschild A. Baltimore, MD, Williams & Wilkins, 1997, pp 355–375

Book J, Harbin H, Marques C, et al: Should the ASAM criteria be adopted as a national standard, in Controversies in Managed Mental Health Care. Edited by Lazarus A. Washington, DC, APA Press, 1996, pp 143–158

Donabedian A: A Guide to Medical Care Administration: Medical Care Appraisal. New York, American Public Health Association, 1969

Donabedian A: Exploration in Quality Assessment and Monitoring: The Definition of Quality and Approaches to Its Assessment. Ann Arbor, MI, Health Association Press, 1980

Druss B, Rosenheck R: Evaluation of HEDIS measure of behavioral health care quality. Psychiatr Serv 48:71–76, 1997

Erikson E: Adulthood. New York, WW Norton, 1978

Expert Consensus Panel for Bipolar Disorder: Treatment of bipolar disorder. J Clin Psychiatry 57 (suppl 12a):5–88, 1996

Expert Consensus Panel for Schizophrenia: Treatment of schizophrenia. J Clin Psychiatry 57 (suppl 12b):5–58, 1996

Gruttardaro D: Centralized credential verification for mental health and substance abuse. Behavioral Healthcare Tomorrow 5:41–45, 1996

Kane L, Bartlett J, Potthoff S: Building an empirically based outcomes information system for managed mental health care. Psychiatr Serv 46:459–461, 1995

Kinzie J, Maricle R, Bloom J, et al: Improving quality through psychiatric mortality and morbidity conferences in a university hospital. Hosp Community Psychiatry 43:470–474, 1992

News and Notes: Burgeoning clinical practice guidelines prompt concerns about conflicts, bias and credibility. Psychiatr Serv 45:1244–1245, 1994

News and Notes: Health plans modify practice guidelines to meet local needs. Psychiatr Serv 48:118, 1997a

News and Notes: Report from Institute of Medicine focuses on use of quality measures to improve behavioral health care. Psychiatr Serv 48:118–119, 1997b

Pincus H, Zarin D, West J: Peering into the "black box": measuring outcomes of managed care. Arch Gen Psychiatry 53:870–877, 1996

Sederer L, Bennett M: Managed mental health care in the United States: a status report. Adm Policy Ment Health 23:289–306, 1996

Senge P: The Fifth Discipline: The Art and Practice of the Learning Organization. New York, Doubleday/Currency, 1990.

Shortell S: Creating organized delivery systems: the barriers and facilitators. Hospital Health Services Administration 38:447–466, 1993

Soltys S: Risk management strategies in the provision of mental health services. Psychiatr Serv 46:473–476, 1995

Thornicroft G, Ward P, James S: Care management and mental health. Br Med J 306:768–771, 1993

Ware T: The value of case management for a consumer. Psychiatr Serv 46:1231–1232, 1995

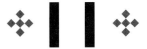

Staffing Behavioral Health Systems

Fred C. Osher, M.D.

Given the increasing demand for cost-effective behavioral health services in the managed care environment, the allocation of human resources within systems of care is one of the most critical issues confronting system designers. Although the preponderance of behavioral health service costs is for personnel, few data are available about what blend of human resources delivering what types of services to which subpopulations of patients results in the best outcomes. Absent these data, systems of care are governed by historic networks of providers, a fledgling effort at the development of clinical guidelines for care, and prevailing market forces. In this chapter I outline considerations for behavioral health systems design related to the appropriate composition, competencies, training, credentialing, and management of our industry's most important asset—human resources. As with previous chapters, an emphasis is placed on the type of work force required to work in managed care environments.

Many forces contribute to the dynamic landscape of human resource management in behavioral health settings. Traditionally, the knowledge base and scientific advances within the mental health field have driven treatment. These advances can have large and unpredictable effects on staffing needs. For example, advances in psychopharmacology and the understanding of

brain-based disorders have vastly changed the practice of psychiatry over the past several decades. The wide variety of medication options, with increasing efficacy, has altered the nature of the doctor-patient relationship toward the identification of diagnosable syndromes constituting "purer" disorders with increasingly specific treatments. As such, medication regimens have gained in simplicity and acceptability to a point at which the largest prescribers of psychotropic medications are not behavioral specialists but primary care physicians. While evidence mounts as to the risks and benefits of mental healthcare being provided by these practitioners (Shore 1996; Sturm and Wells 1995; Wells et al. 1994), no one disputes its impact on the site of care for most mental disorders and the attendant shift in medical work force needs. Psychiatry is now commonly considered a tertiary care specialty, and in many systems its providers play a consultative role to primary care systems. In addition, referrals to specialty mental health services are often made via primary care gatekeeping models.

The emphasis on outcomes has pushed the development of briefer and at times more intensive models of care to achieve similar or better outcomes at lower costs. One has only to look at the evolution of briefer cognitive psychotherapy models and the reduction of insurance-financed insight-oriented psychotherapies to appreciate the shifting training and staffing issues within mental health systems. Short-term, goal-oriented treatment has become the standard; most patients receive a course of treatment in a small number of sessions. Assuming no change in the incidence and prevalence of mental disorders, briefer and more effective treatments should require fewer clinicians.

Instead of the state of science and technology predominantly determining the nature of treatment, our society is now focused on rising healthcare expenditures and is increasingly willing to accept limitations on its application. The era of unlimited resources for both research and clinical services is over, and the management of care is focused on obtaining the biggest bang for the buck. This resource rationing coincides with broad acceptance of the principle of least restrictive alternatives to shape the site, and staffing patterns, of mental health practice. Therefore, the locus of care has increasingly moved from high-cost medical inpatient settings to relatively low-cost community-based systems of care. This has shifted mental health personnel from more medically trained physicians and nurses to community providers with a broad array of biological, psychological, and social skills. Although the policy of deinstitutionalization was borne out of primarily humanitarian concerns for providing care to those with severe mental illnesses in the least restrictive settings, it also served the economic agendas of most states, whose taxpayers poorly accepted burgeoning budgets. One can see the downsizing of the state hospital census, from a high of 585,000 patients in the 1960s to the current level of less than 100,000, juxtaposed with the rapid growth of psychosocial rehabilitation programs over that same period. Since the 1980s, psychosocial rehabilitation services have grown dramatically. Conservative estimates of the psychosocial rehabilitation work force are now 100,000 staff persons working in more than 7,000 agencies (Department of Health and Human Services 1996). Now, as efforts to contain costs mount, and capitation financing strategies grow, the role of psychosocial rehabilitation and ultimately funding support is forcing close monitoring of utilization and outcomes that may shift resources away from these services.

Work Force Assessment

To determine appropriate staffing, a clear articulation of the mission of each provider or service sector is required. The organizational values will have a large effect on the allocation of personnel resources. If training is an important part of the mission, then the need for seasoned personnel with professional backgrounds and supervision experience will be important. If generating knowledge is a central part of the mission, then research backgrounds and the capacity to capture research dollars will be emphasized. Increasingly, the central mission of many agencies, particularly those associated with managed care organizations (MCOs) is to provide effective mental healthcare in the least costly fashion. Market forces create incentives for managers to employ the least costly staff members to deliver any care that the managers have credentialed them for and that the staff members are competent to do. As such, psychiatrists can be seen narrowly as the workers licensed to prescribe medication; the impact of this perception is to reserve physician time for medication evaluations. This role constriction has implications for the recruitment and retention of physician staff. For psychological treatments, including psychotherapy, agencies principally concerned with cost will direct care to lower cost nonphysicians.

With the transformation of healthcare purchasers from patients to benefits managers, the assessment of work force composition has changed dramatically (Table 11–1). In the past, the patient's assessment of his or her mental health needs, and of the provider competencies required to meet those needs, determined the type, length, and, in turn, cost of care. The patients' beliefs, informed or not, that a particular type of provider (often a specialist) was necessary for care was the basis for choosing a provider, making appointments, and ensuring that the bill was paid. Now care managers are assessing need, interpreting medical necessity criteria, monitoring the quality of care, and authorizing continued services. Program administrators must address many questions in determining the appropriate composition of their mental health work force: What services are to be provided, and how will administrators manage the behavioral health benefit? Who will be served, and how will these patients be identified? How will full-time equivalents be defined, and what will the direct care expectancies be? What are consumers' expectations about the professional backgrounds of their providers? What geographic access does any given patient need to the range of mental health professionals in the community?

Hospitals (psychiatric or general), clinics (within mental health settings or outside them), or academic

TABLE 11–1. Factors to consider in work force assessment

What population is targeted for care? How will the population be identified?
What staff competencies are legally required?
What staff competencies are expected by patients/ consumers?
What resources are available for personnel?
What geographic access is required?
Is training central to the agency mission?
Is knowledge generation central to the agency mission?

settings will all have different requirements based both on their missions and on standards set by accrediting agencies. Typically, an MCO contracts with a provider network of clinicians, institutions, group practices, and agencies. In return for being included in the network, the provider agrees to practice within the company guidelines. The provider will be responsible for collecting any co-payments from the patient and will be paid by the MCO on either a capitated or a fee-for-service basis. Providers may receive subcapitation contracts from the MCO and go at-risk for the care provided. In the latter arrangement, the providers control the staffing pattern, but they assume the same cost incentives that govern the MCO.

Few data exist to inform decisions about staffing composition and staffing levels. Standardization and generalization of workloads are impossible because of the number of variables affecting patient need (e.g., patient age, level of disability, interpersonal and case management support). These variables similarly affect assumptions regarding the percentage of direct clinical care or average length of stay. This knowledge gap must be addressed by services research.

Work Force Composition

The growing emphasis on coordinated, multidisciplinary treatment delivery has been associated with improved access and quality of mental healthcare. Depending on the patients' needs, following adequate triage activities, nonphysician mental health practitioners work solely or in collaboration with psychiatrists. The value of diverse clinical and theoretical perspectives has been cited as an important feature in delivering care to persons with complex disorders and multiple problems. A secondary effect of multidisciplinary

service settings has been the continued blurring of mental health professional boundaries. To outsiders, it is often difficult to understand where medical treatment ends and nonmedical services begin. The nature of these role relationships has a large influence on required staffing patterns. Increasingly, the supervisory relationship defines mental health roles (Benarroche and Astrachan 1983). In this model, one professional has clinical responsibility (both legally and ethically) for another professional's or a nonprofessional's work. State regulations or professional organizations may specify the type and intensity of supervision required for licensure. The supervisory model extends the expertise of professional staff to most patients through the work of mental health workers who have less experience or training. Although professionals have historically valued the educational aspects of supervision, they have raised concerns regarding the liability imparted by these administrative relationships. Federal financing agencies are concerned about the quality of supervision, particularly as it relates to the oversight of psychiatric resident education. Recent Medicare guidelines from the Health Care Financing Administration have sought to delineate the nature of clinical supervision with an insistence on direct observation of trainee services. This policy clarification has a significant impact on the staffing patterns within academic settings.

The Mental Health Work Force: Titles and Roles

Professional Staff

The range of human resources available to provide elements of mental healthcare is broad, and providers' skill sets frequently overlap. Core mental health disciplines include psychiatry, psychology, social work, and psychiatric nursing (Table 11–2). In addition, practitioners of occupational therapy, counseling, and marriage and family therapy provide significant amounts of mental health treatment, psychosocial rehabilitation, and school psychology. Not all of these disciplines are recognized in all states, and licensing and credentialing may not be standardized. Nonetheless, the appropriate ratio of these disciplines in mental health settings is the subject of intense debate.

The role of psychiatrists in mental health systems can be either narrowly defined to reduce direct personnel costs or expanded in recognition of their being the

TABLE 11–2. Roles and responsibilities of professional staff

Staff	Roles and responsibilities
Psychiatrists	Diagnostic evaluation Medication management Psychotherapy Clinical supervision
Psychologists	Diagnostic evaluation Psychotherapy Clinical supervision
Social workers	Psychotherapy Accessing entitlements and income supports Care management Environmental interventions
Psychiatric nurses	Diagnostic evaluation Medication administration Psychotherapy
Professional counselors	Guidance and consulting Psychotherapy Crisis intervention Functional assessment

only mental health professionals grounded in biology and psychology with a medical tradition focused on epidemiology, etiology, and differential diagnosis. With more than 29,000 clinically active psychiatrists (Department of Health and Human Services 1996), the United States has the lowest psychiatrist-patient ratio and the highest absolute number of psychiatrists in the world (Weissman 1994). Depending on one's perspective, there are either too many or too few psychiatrists for the country's mental health needs. Psychologists are involved in every type of mental health setting, and the number of licensed psychologists has risen from 20,000 in 1975 to almost 70,000 in 1995 (Department of Health and Human Services 1996). Their roles encompass all aspects of clinical care, and recent demonstrations have explored their capacity to prescribe psychotropic medication (Cullen and Newman 1997). The issue of prescribing privileges for psychologists is likely to bring together the professional psychological associations with MCOs, where the role expansion and cost-cutting agendas are well aligned.

Nursing generalists and advanced practice psychiatric nurses provide a wide range of mental health services. About 35 states have granted nurse practitioners either complementary authority (requiring physician supervision) or substitute authority (not requiring phy-

sician supervision) for prescribing medication. Research is needed to determine the effect of these regulatory approaches on clinical outcomes. Again, MCOs are keenly interested in prescribing roles for nurses.

Social workers have been major providers of mental health services for over a century. Their training emphasizes the blending of individual and environmental interventions. Private group practice and outpatient clinic work are the fastest growing settings for an estimated 180,000 clinically trained social workers in the United States (Department of Health and Human Services 1996). As a group, social workers bring a breadth of skills at a cost typically below other mental health professionals. As such, they are increasingly sought after within behavioral health systems.

Nonprofessional Staff

Increasingly, consumers are being used as staff members in multidisciplinary settings to engage difficult-to-reach patients who have severe mental illnesses. The value of firsthand experience with mental disorders and treatment systems may give an individual the capacity for empathy and improve the development of therapeutic alliances with difficult-to-engage patient populations. The few reported studies suggest that the presence of consumers affords important opportunities yet creates significant challenges related to boundaries and stressors leading to decompensation (Dixon et al. 1994; Mowbray et al. 1996). Self-help groups and consumer-run drop-in centers, while not typically counted in staffing plans, have been cited by some behavioral health organizations as providers of significant adjunctive care. A question arises as to the effectiveness of these nonprofessional services replacing more treatment-oriented programs.

Case management services range from brokered models with primarily a linkage function to integrated treatment teams providing treatment, rehabilitation, and social services. Often nonprofessionally trained case managers provide a critical component of care for patients with severe mental illnesses. These staff members may or may not have bachelor's degrees and spend large portions of their work day in direct clinical contact. They are often the most underpaid and overworked staff members in community mental health systems. Of paramount importance are adequate oversight and supervision of their encounters.

The increased emphasis on utilization review and quality management has created the need for a new cadre of behavioral health staff with primarily nonclinical responsibilities. The need for management information systems capable of generating reports and documentation for multiple applications has increased a reliance on information specialists to help the clinical enterprise. Increasing demands for documentation and review have also shifted staff resources from clinical to administrative activity. This remains a hidden cost of quality management operations and presumably is offset by the cost savings realized from the elimination of so-called unnecessary services. Table 11–3 summarizes the roles and responsibilities of nonprofessional staff.

Specialists Versus Generalists

The tenets of primary care and the need to reduce health expenditures have challenged the healthcare professions to provide gatekeeping and screening functions inherent in managed care approaches. Thus, the generalist brings a breadth and flexibility that are welcome in most settings. Also, the compartmentalization of behavioral disorders has been seen as a mismatch with the complex problems that patients typically bring when seeking care from mental health professionals. Indeed, calls are surfacing for the integration of health services to provide comprehensive, holistic, and effective service. We can see a clear example of this in responding to the needs of persons with comorbid mental and addictive disorders. Epidemiologic data (Kessler et al. 1996) have shown that the prevalence of dual diagnoses is high and that in some settings the modal patient is likely to have dual disorders. Staff members whom we have trained exclusively within the mental health system with few skills in working with addictive disorders often feel uncomfortable and may be ill prepared to effectively address both disorders in an integrated manner. Cross-trained individuals with broad skills enhance both the clinical outcomes and the system efficiency.

Licensing, Credentialing, and Provider Profiling

The Institute of Medicine defines quality of care as "the degree to which health services for individuals and populations increase the likelihood of desired health outcomes and are consistent with current professional knowledge" (Institute of Medicine 1990, p. 21). Yet,

TABLE 11–3. Roles and responsibilities of nonprofessional staff

Staff	Roles and responsibilities
Case managers (bachelor's prepared or less)	Engagement of patient Linkage to essential services and supports Monitoring of social and health status
Consumer employees	Engagement of patients/ consumers Liaison to professional staff Counseling on community integration
Management information specialists	Data collection and analysis Documentation and billing Technology support

how is one to know which blend of staffing will work in which setting? With which population? To achieve what outcomes? Licensing and credentialing of practitioners can be only one dimension of staffing a mental health system, and even in this dimension, a correlation may not exist between desirable outcomes and an individual's training. Nonetheless, licensure of practitioners plays a critical role in consumer protection.

MCOs typically have a system for credentialing professionals as providers. This system generally starts with professional licensing and may include a variety of inclusion criteria (e.g., certification) and exclusion criteria (e.g., history of malpractice litigation). With varying emphases, MCOs may also have a mechanism in which training, licensing, and quality of care are validated.

Missing from this process is an assessment of whether the licensing and credentialing on which staffing decisions are made reflect best practices from the perspective of system planners. Although the methods and emphases in delivering mental healthcare have changed dramatically, the licensing and credentialing criteria have not. Small and isolated efforts have been made to expose trainees to managed care practices and principles, but professional associations and schools have not developed focused agendas in these areas, and state licensing boards tend to follow the lead of these associations.

With the absence of defined practice standards in managed care, an internal system for rating providers has evolved, based on practice patterns and outcomes. Increasingly, attention is being focused on the use of provider profiles in determining the cost and effectiveness of care. Elements of these profiles include the number of visits by provider per episode of treatment, the cost of care by provider per episode of treatment, client satisfaction data, and client outcomes data. These data can be used as corrective feedback to providers within the network and to influence referral patterns. They can also be used to select a network of providers with a demonstrated capacity to manage utilization successfully. This method of provider profiling is often not shared externally and may have a significant impact on referral to providers and the composition of the provider network. Providers who are the subject of frequent consumer complaints or who practice outside of the MCO guidelines may be subject to adverse referral patterns.

Staff Competencies: Training and Retraining

In traditional independent practice, clinicians were free to design interventions with little outside clinical review. The emphasis was frequently on patient insight, and the responsibility for payment was typically the patient's concern. This frequently resulted in long-term open-ended therapies; as such, training was geared toward this approach. With the arrival of managed care, requirements for goal-specific, well-documented interventions have become the norm, and medical necessity criteria govern the length of care. A third party, the managed behavioral healthcare organization, now brokers the decision to begin or end care—previously the province of the clinician and the patient—with an incentive for reducing expenditures. This fundamental shift has brought with it a new list of competencies and skill sets for today's practitioners. They must be familiar with management information systems and quality management criteria and procedures and must have the capacity to juggle quality and cost-of-care issues. Table 11–4 highlights staff competencies relevant to changing behavioral healthcare delivery systems.

TABLE 11–4. Types of staff competencies required in managed care systems

Clinical
Cultural
Economic
Ethical

Clinical Competencies

Much has been written about the clinical competencies required of the mental health work force in the twenty-first century. Increasing emphasis will be placed on the development of problem-oriented, goal-directed treatment; the use of group and alternative low-cost treatments; knowledge of appropriate community alternatives to higher cost inpatient and residential care; and the principles of quality management. Authorization procedures will limit time for extensive evaluations, and treatment plans will likely be less precise. Clinicians will need to be aware of and practice cost-effective treatments supported by services research data.

Cultural Competencies

Racial and ethnic minorities frequently lack access to behavioral healthcare, let alone care that is culturally appropriate. One of the more difficult staffing issues in the development of networks of providers is preservation of the capacity to serve these minority populations. To create smaller and more efficiently staffed organizations, the retention of a culturally diverse staff is critical. Often the excuse for not having a culturally diverse staff is that research has not proven the effectiveness of these culturally defined interventions. This lack of data should not weaken attention to this critical staffing dimension (Institute of Medicine 1997). Related to the issue of cultural diversity is an organization's capacity to serve persons with disabilities such as deafness or blindness. Bringing in the personnel and skill sets necessary to serve these special populations can be labor intensive but is no less important in ensuring access to appropriate care.

Economic Competencies

For managed care principles to be implemented effectively, the organization's staff must be aware of and share the organization's values. The value that all services provided are necessary and medically appropriate is central to the mission and performance of MCOs. It is equally important that the staff share the value that the goal of care is to increase the patient's independence and to reduce reliance on treatment settings and providers. For persons with severe and persistent mental illnesses, this goal becomes the achievement of the highest functional capacity with the lowest utilization of mental health services. These philosophic values are the cornerstones of economic performance and must be embraced by the network of providers in a sharing of the business and clinical objectives of the system of care. Providers must have the capacity to view simultaneously their contributions to both the patients seeking their care and the system they represent.

Ethical Competencies

In staffing a behavioral health system, the clinical and economic incentives must be aligned in a way that does not create clinician discomfort nor violate ethical standards of health care. In past fee-for-service financing arrangements, concerns were primarily related to the overprovision of services and the attendant costs. In today's managed care environments, particularly those using capitated financing, the danger is the underprovision of services as a way of staying within budget or increasing one's profit margin. There should be no prohibition of or contractual limitations on practitioners' discussing clinically appropriate treatment with their patients and families. It is important that staff be aware of strategies for maintaining confidentiality while meeting the needs of practitioners to coordinate care and move patients between levels of care.

It is for these reasons that attention to medical ethics is critical. To help staff negotiate these ethical dilemmas, McFarland et al. (1997) offered two general strategies: 1) the development of clear guidelines to guide service utilization throughout the service continuum, including level-of-care criteria and practice standards, and 2) the training of staff in required utilization management skills in level-of-care determinations, treatment planning, and relating to utilization reviewers.

Conclusion

In these times of accelerated changes within behavioral health services delivery systems, organizational staffing is the most important consideration. The type of personnel employed will determine success in both attaining organizational objectives and remaining cost effective. Achieving a balance between the economic and clinical goals of a system is critical. Since available data to guide personnel decisions are lacking, a clear and pressing need for research exists.

References

Benarroche CL, Astrachan BM: Interprofessional role relationships in psychiatric administration, in Psychiatric Administration: A Comprehensive Text for the Clinician-Executive. Edited by Talbott JA, Kaplan SR. New York, Grune & Stratton, 1983, pp 223–236

Cullen EA, Newman R: In pursuit of prescription privileges. Professional Psychology: Research and Practice 28:101–106, 1997

Department of Health and Human Services, Center for Mental Health Services: Mental Health, United States, 1996. Edited by Manderscheid RW, Sonnenschein MA. Washington, DC, U.S. Government Printing Office, 1996

Dixon L, Krauss N, Lehman A: Consumers as service providers: the promise and the challenge. Community Ment Health J 30:615–625,1994

Institute of Medicine: Medicare: A Strategy for Quality Assurance, Vol 1. Washington, DC, National Academy Press, 1990

Institute of Medicine: Managing Managed Care: Quality Improvement in Behavioral Health. Washington, DC, National Academy Press, 1997

Kessler RC, Nelson CB, McGonagle KA, et al: The epidemiology of co-occurring addictive and mental disorders: implications for prevention and service utilization. Am J Orthopsychiatry 66:17–31, 1996

McFarland B, Minkoff K, Roman B, et al: Utilization Management in Managed Mental Health Care in the Public Sector: A Survival Manual. Edited by Minkoff K, Pollack D. Amsterdam, Harwood Academic Publishers, 1997, pp 151–168

Mowbray CT, Moxley DP, Thrasher S, et al: Consumers as community support providers: issues created by role innovation. Community Ment Health J 32:47–67, 1996

Shore JH: Psychiatry at a crossroad: our role in primary care. Am J Psychiatry 153:1398–1403, 1996

Sturm R, Wells KB: How can care for depression become more cost effective? JAMA 273:51–58, 1995

Weissman S: American psychiatry in the 21st century: the discipline, its practice, and its work force. Bull Menninger Clin 58:502–518, 1994

Wells KB, Katon W, Rogers B, et al: Use of minor tranquilizers and antidepressant medication by depressed outpatients: results from the medical outcomes study. Am J Psychiatry 151:694–700, 1994

❖ 12 ❖

Capitated Financing and Population-Based Care

Gregory E. Simon, M.D., M.P.H.

Capitation: The Motivation for Population-Based Care

Among mental health providers, discussions of capitated financing have focused primarily on potential negative effects. As a larger portion of the population is enrolled in capitated managed care networks, providers fear exclusion based on arbitrary (and often proprietary) practice profiles. For providers participating in capitated plans, financial incentives can create uncomfortable and inappropriate conflicts of interest. In some areas, large health plans competing for market share have triggered a "race to the bottom"—slashing capitation rates to levels inadequate to support even minimally adequate mental healthcare. All too often, the concept of capitation has become synonymous with inadequate levels of service and perverse economic incentives.

Capitated financing has the potential, however, to shift clinical priorities toward areas of greatest need. *Capitation* is a population-based method for financing medical and mental healthcare. Consequently, capitated financing should encourage population-based approaches to organizing and delivering services. These approaches have the potential to significantly improve the quality and effectiveness of mental healthcare across the entire population.

From Patients to Populations

Traditional medical and mental health practice is essentially reactive, responding to the immediate needs of those who present for care. In such a reactive system, care received is determined primarily by patients' perceived need and ability to pay (through insurance coverage or personal resources). Epidemiologic data suggest that this arrangement is far from perfect in matching treatment resources to those with greatest clinical need. Of community residents with psychiatric or substance use disorders, only approximately 15% receive any specialty mental health treatment, and more than 60% receive no professional treatment at all (Regier et al. 1993). Among those with bipolar disorder

Supported by National Institute of Mental Health Grant 51338.

or schizophrenia, the proportion receiving specialty treatment remains only 50%–60%. Use of specialty mental healthcare is strongly influenced by nonclinical factors such as race (Olfson and Klerman 1992; Padgett et al. 1994), insurance coverage (Landerman et al. 1994; Simon et al. 1996a), and level of education (Leaf et al. 1988; Simon et al. 1994).

Financial responsibility for care can be a strong incentive to look beyond the group of patients currently seeking treatment. Capitated financing arrangements assign responsibility to provide all needed health (or mental health) care for a defined population. The responsible healthcare system is liable for all costs of treatment and consequences of nontreatment. If health plans are actually held accountable by patients and purchasers, population-based financing of care will encourage population-based organization of care. Ongoing responsibility for a defined population also creates incentives for health plans and providers to focus on more effective management of chronic or recurrent conditions. Preventing relapse of depression or schizophrenia will probably prove more cost effective in the long run than repeated episodes of acute treatment. However, incentives for better long-term management exist only in health systems with low turnover. A capitated health plan has little incentive to plan for long-term care of members likely to belong to another plan within 2 years.

The General Health Care System

Capitated financing arrangements should help to focus attention on interactions between mental health services and the larger healthcare system. Financial responsibility for all health needs of a defined population allows a view of mental health treatment that is not limited to mental health providers or mental health facilities. A unified financing arrangement can help to unify clinical services across the de facto mental health system: primary care, medical specialists, emergency rooms, and mental health facilities (Regier et al. 1993). The true costs of treating mental disorders can be more readily linked to the effect of untreated mental disorders in the general medical system (Simon et al. 1995a, 1995b). These advantages are realized only when financing and delivery of mental health services are integrated with general medical care. As discussed later in this chapter, subcapitation or carve-out arrangements may perpetuate the compartmentalization of traditional fee-for-service care.

Obligation to Purchasers

Capitation arrangements make explicit providers' obligations to employers and other purchasers of healthcare. Under traditional fee-for-service financing, transactions between providers and payers focus on a unit of clinical service (e.g., visit, procedure, hospital day). In general, purchasers (including employers, government programs, and individual patients) are not fundamentally interested in purchasing health services. They are hoping to "purchase" improved health by purchasing healthcare. Specific health services are important only if they contribute to the ultimate good in this transaction—improved physical or mental health. Capitated financing arrangements more accurately reflect the contributions of both sides to this transaction. Purchasers provide a specified amount to maintain or improve the health of those covered. Providers accept, along with this payment, an obligation to provide services necessary to maintain or improve health. Providers' obligations focus on the outcome (improved health) more than the process (specific units of service).

Is Capitation Only About Cost-Cutting?

The previous subsections focus on the potential for capitated financing arrangements to reorganize care around improving the health of the entire population. Unfortunately, most existing capitated arrangements have realized little of this potential. Costs of care are more immediate and easily measured than improved health or quality of service. Lacking good data on health outcomes and quality, many capitated plans focused strictly on reducing costs. Resulting savings have been diverted from direct treatment and used to either increase profits or reduce premiums in hopes of increasing market share. Few capitated systems have made organized efforts to increase delivery of effective services across the covered population. Several current and future developments should help to shift the balance of health and mental health decision making away from cost alone and back toward quality of care. Practice guidelines for the management of common mental disorders are helping to define appropriate levels of care and establish standards against which health plans can be judged (American Psychiatric Association 1993, 1994; Depression Guideline Panel 1993). Sophisticated purchasers are requiring evidence of appropriate care in the form of report cards (e.g., the set of HEDIS performance indicators) and accreditation processes (e.g., National Committee on Quality Assurance). Routine measurement of treatment outcomes and satisfaction has become more common. Focusing attention on treatment effectiveness should give capitated systems added incentive to concentrate on population-based health improvement. The sections below describe key steps in that process.

Developing a Population-Based Perspective

Designing or redesigning mental health services for an entire population begins with a population-based view of clinical needs and current utilization. This view should incorporate existing data on disease epidemiology, use of services, and costs. Data from the population of interest are invaluable, but extrapolation from external data sources often is necessary. Steps in developing this population-based view are described below.

Disease Epidemiology

A comprehensive view of mental health needs in the population begins with cross-sectional epidemiology: describing the current prevalence of mental disorders. Although community-based epidemiologic surveys are the gold standard for estimating population prevalence, conducting community-based surveys within individual health plans would be expensive and probably unnecessary. Two large United States community surveys (the Epidemiologic Catchment Area Survey [Regier et al. 1988] and the National Comorbidity Survey [Kessler et al. 1994]) provide a reasonable basis for estimating community prevalence. Several surveys of anxiety, depressive, and alcohol use disorders among primary care patients showed general similarity of prevalence estimates across a broad range of patient characteristics and practice settings (Nielsen and Williams 1980; Philbrick et al. 1996; Simon and VonKorff 1995; Spitzer et al. 1994; VonKorff et al. 1987). Estimates from these external sources must be adjusted to reflect sociodemographic characteristics of the covered population of interest. In general, prevalence rates of anxiety and depressive disorders show modest variation by ethnicity (slightly lower among nonwhites) and significant variation by sex (higher among women) and age

(highest in early adulthood and declining after middle age) (Kessler et al. 1994; Regier et al. 1988). More severe disorders show less variability with ethnicity and sex but still decline in prevalence after middle age (Regier et al. 1988). Most disorders appear more prevalent among those of lower socioeconomic status (Kessler et al. 1994; Regier et al. 1988). Consequently, these relevant characteristics of the population of interest must be considered when estimating prevalence and service need. General population estimates will be least applicable in populations that differ markedly in these important characteristics (e.g., Medicare risk contracts, capitated Medicaid contracts, predominantly male military populations).

Static information on disease prevalence must be supplemented by an understanding of illness patterns over time. For example, estimates of the prevalence of current major depressive disorder in the community range from 3% to 7%, whereas lifetime prevalence may be as high as 20% (Angst 1992; Kessler et al. 1994; Regier et al. 1988). Most patients recover from major depression, but most of those who recover experience a recurrence (Angst 1992). A significant minority have a chronic course. This picture contrasts with that for schizophrenia, which typically shows higher rates of chronicity and a higher ratio of current to lifetime prevalence (Regier et al. 1988). These differences in temporal patterns have important implications for the organization of care.

Patterns of Service Use

In the general population, those with psychiatric disorders are distributed across all types and levels of treatment. Sites of care include inpatient, day treatment or partial hospitalization, outpatient specialty treatment, primary care, and the voluntary service sector (e.g., clergy, self-help organizations). The distribution of people with psychiatric illness across these various sectors will vary considerably by diagnosis and healthcare system (Regier et al. 1993). Figure 12–1 illustrates the sites of care for those with depressive illness in a typical health plan population. Rates of service use can be compared with estimated prevalence rates in the covered population. Gross mismatches between estimated prevalence and rates of treatment are the crudest indication of under- or overtreatment. Rough equality of prevalence rates and treatment rates, however, does not necessarily imply appropriate care. For example, although the prevalence of benzodiazepine use may be roughly equivalent to the community prevalence of significant anxiety disorders, most benzodiazepines are prescribed to those without specific psychiatric diagnoses (Simon et al. 1996b). Matching diagnoses with service use data will indicate which categories of patients receive which type of mental healthcare. In general, those with more severe illness will receive higher levels of treatment (Regier et al. 1993), but this pattern has many exceptions. Discovering and understanding these exceptions is a vital step in population-based care planning.

A longitudinal view of service use is necessary to understand need and use in a population. Recurrent brief episodes of care may reflect the underlying clinical course (i.e., recurrent illness with good recovery), but this pattern also may suggest insufficient attention to maintenance treatment and relapse prevention. Some patterns of use (e.g., multiple hospitalizations without associated follow-up care) may indicate important gaps in the current system of care. Patients may use services from multiple sectors (e.g., primary care and outpatient specialty) simultaneously and will move from one sector to another over time. Goldberg used the term *filter* to describe the factors that influence movement from one care sector to another (Goldberg and Huxley 1980).

Burden of Illness

The overall burden of any psychiatric disorder depends on disease prevalence and disease effect. Significant effects of psychiatric disorders include work loss, decreased productivity, increased dependence on social welfare programs, and impaired family roles. Less severe but more prevalent disorders may have a lower effect per affected individual but a greater effect across the population. For example, subthreshold depressive disorders appear to account for as great a burden of lost productivity as major depression (Broadhead et al. 1990). Considering average effect for all those with any diagnosis, however, ignores significant variability among individuals. Impairment typically concentrates in those with the most severe or recurrent illness.

The pattern of healthcare costs for psychiatric disorders also varies considerably across conditions. Depressive and anxiety disorders are associated with significant increases in use of general medical services (Simon et al. 1995a). In the entire population, most patients with depressive and anxiety disorders receive no treatment or are treated exclusively in primary care

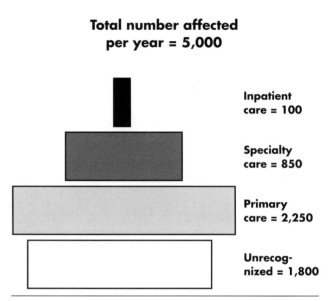

Total number affected per year = 5,000

Inpatient care = 100

Specialty care = 850

Primary care = 2,250

Unrecognized = 1,800

FIGURE 12–1. Sites of care for depression across the entire population (based on covered population of 100,000).

(Regier et al. 1993). Consequently, the excess general healthcare costs attributable to depressive and anxiety disorders in the population are many times the direct costs of specialty mental health treatment (Simon et al. 1995b). The pattern seen for more severe mental disorders is typically quite different. Most patients receive some specialty treatment, and many use inpatient psychiatric services (Regier et al. 1993). Although psychotic disorders also are associated with increased use of medical services, this increase is smaller than that seen for depressive and anxiety disorders (Simon 1992). Severe affective disorders and psychotic disorders have their greatest effect in the mental health specialty sector.

The disability associated with psychiatric disorders may have varying effects on families, employers, and public welfare programs. For example, depressive disorders are most prevalent among women and those in early adulthood and middle age. The functional impairment associated with depression will have the greatest effect on work productivity and care of children. For many employers, depression is one of the leading causes of work loss due to illness (Conti and Burton 1994). In contrast, psychotic disorders are associated with decreased fertility and often preclude gainful employment. The burden on families may be felt more by parents than by spouses and children. The impairment due to psychotic disorders may have a greater effect on disability insurance systems and public welfare programs than on employers.

Redesigning the Population-Based System

Establishing Priority Clinical Areas

The various steps described earlier in this chapter will yield a population-based view of treatment needs and current treatment patterns. This view should include the full range of mental health conditions and mental health services. Redesign efforts, however, must be more focused. Mental health providers and systems have finite quantities of attention, energy, and time available for reorganization. Success depends critically on focus and follow-through. A sequential approach (one priority at a time) has a much greater chance of successful implementation than a more global strategy. Important factors to consider in ranking clinical priorities are described below and summarized in Table 12–1.

Prevalence

Overall prevalence is probably the most important criterion for establishing redesign priorities. This does not imply that rare conditions are not deserving of appropriate, high-quality clinical care. For rare conditions, however, a focus on individuals rather than populations is probably appropriate.

Burden on Patients, Families, and Purchasers

Decisions about organizational priorities must incorporate the priorities of the various customers of mental healthcare. In most cases these groups will agree on priorities for clinical redesign and service improvement. As mentioned above, priorities of purchasers will vary according to characteristics of the population covered. The list of stakeholder interests in Table 12–1 intentionally excludes the priorities of providers. Traditional mental health practice has allowed providers to focus on particular clinical areas or treatment modalities because of personal interest or ideology. Population-based planning gives providers' preferences much less weight than those of patients, families, and purchasers.

Current Resource Use

Health services costs for a particular condition indicate both the current resources devoted to treatment and the potential resources available in redesigned programs. In most cases, priorities based on current treatment costs will agree closely with those based on prevalence and disease burden.

TABLE 12–1. Setting priorities for population-based system redesign

Prevalence in the population
Burden on affected patients
Burden on family members
Burden on employers/purchasers
Current resource use
Availability of effective treatment

Availability of Effective Treatment

Although disease prevalence, burden, and cost are central to establishing priorities, reorganizing care will produce little benefit if effective treatments are not available. Consequently, evidence of treatment efficacy (and actual effectiveness) must influence priority-setting. Redesign efforts could focus on reducing use of ineffective treatments, but programs with positive messages should probably take priority. In many health systems, capitation and redesign programs have focused almost exclusively on reducing costs and restricting access to care. Understandably, providers have objected to efforts that appear to place cost savings before clinical needs. Redesign programs that focus on expanding and guaranteeing the delivery of effective treatments are more likely to gain providers' trust and cooperation than programs focused on restricting less effective treatments.

Identifying Key Areas for Redesign

Understanding the flow of patients through the complete healthcare system is necessary to identify key transition points in the process of care. Service use data can be organized to describe a typical episode of care for a given condition. Figure 12–2 illustrates the beginning of an episode of care for major depression. The picture of an episode of care should include all common points of first contact with the treatment system, including contacts with general medical providers. In the early stages of an episode of depression treatment, key steps include the initial diagnostic assessment (major depression vs. dysthymia vs. other depressive disorder) and the choice of first-line treatment (psychotherapy vs. pharmacotherapy). These transition points have major implications for subsequent clinical management and resource use. The picture of an episode of care should include common treatment paths and clinical outcomes, as well as uncommon but important events (because of morbidity, mortality, or treatment costs). If

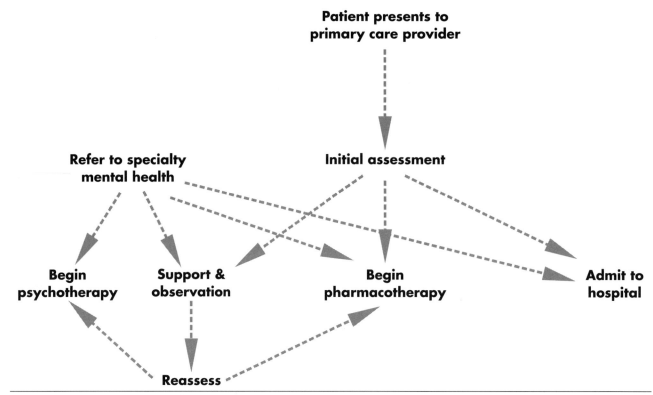

FIGURE 12–2. Flow diagram of initial process of care for depressive illness after presentation in primary care.

possible, estimates of the proportion of patients following different paths should be based on actual data. These estimates are too often based on the expert opinion of specialists—opinions that are unduly influenced by the most severely ill or intensively treated patients.

Comparison of current care processes with ideal patterns will identify important gaps in the current organization and delivery of care. Ideal care patterns can be constructed from outcomes research, treatment guidelines (American Psychiatric Association 1993, 1994; Depression Guideline Panel 1993), and local expert opinion. For the example shown in Figure 12–2, we can identify specific steps that should be part of the initial evaluation of a patient presenting with symptoms of depression. Table 12–2 lists desired steps in the initial clinical examination, which should be completed regardless of the location (e.g., mental health clinic, primary care clinic, emergency room) or type of provider. Appropriate care requires completion and documentation of each of these steps. Data to compare current practice with ideal processes can come from a variety of sources: administrative databases, medical records, and patient or provider surveys. These data sources can help to identify gaps in current treatment and to evaluate the effect of redesign efforts.

TABLE 12–2. Key steps in initial evaluation of depressive symptoms

Assess alcohol use/abuse/dependence
Formally assess for major depressive episode with DSM-IV criteria
Assess suicide risk
Assess history of mania or hypomania
Inquire about current psychotic symptoms
Collect details of prior treatment (pharmacotherapy and psychotherapy)
Inquire about patient's treatment preferences

Considering the Full Range of Options for Improving Care

A population-based approach to redesigning clinical programs should consider the widest range of options, including options not usually considered clinical. Efforts to close gaps in current care processes will sometimes involve typical clinical interventions within the mental health specialty service (e.g., staffing changes, provider training, new clinical programs). Population-based approaches often will involve the larger health-care system and may involve new roles for mental healthcare providers as educators and consultants. In some cases, population-based redesign may call for interventions drawn from public health programs rather than clinical practice. For example, a significant minority of patients with depressive disorders currently receive no treatment from either primary care providers or medical specialists. Clinically oriented strategies to increase the availability of treatment include provider training to improve recognition and routine screening of primary care patients. An alternative nonclinical strategy would include direct education of health plan members through the health plan's monthly newsletter (or the health plan's Internet home page). The latter strategy would be much less expensive than routine screening and might be more effective than screening for reaching patients with covert depression. Other examples of nonclinical interventions or programs include self-care programs, alliances with community groups or advocacy organizations, and cooperative health promotion efforts with employers.

Monitoring Process and Outcomes

Monitoring of process and outcomes across the entire population is essential to the success of redesign efforts. The same sources of data used to identify gaps in practice can be used to determine how well those gaps have been closed. Unfortunately, many administrative data systems can yield only aggregate data on groups of patients treated weeks or months ago. Research on improving practice through feedback suggests that improvement is greatest with feedback that is current and patient-specific (Litzelman et al. 1993; McDonald et al. 1996). Ideally, feedback to providers should identify specific patients for whom care is not up to standards and recommend patient-specific plans for improvement.

Integrating Cost Effectiveness Information Into Clinical Planning

Choices among competing priorities must be guided by data on expected cost and effectiveness. Unfortunately, claims regarding cost effectiveness have too often been invoked to justify denial of care or attempts to reduce cost. In fact, few treatments or programs can be judged "not cost effective" in absolute terms. Most decisions involve treatments or programs that yield clinical benefits but carry additional costs. Any clinical program can only be judged cost effective or ineffective compared with some other potential use of the same resources. For example, research suggests several options to improve the quality of acute-phase pharmacotherapy for depression: increasing the proportion of patients treated by psychiatrists (Sturm and Wells 1995), increasing the use of psychiatric consultation services in primary care (Katon et al. 1995), or promoting the use of newer (and more expensive) antidepressants (Simon et al. 1996c). Each of these choices is likely to increase the proportion of patients receiving recommended levels of treatment and may increase the likelihood of good clinical outcome. Distributing resources available for quality improvement among these options depends on the ratio of improved outcome and increased cost for each choice.

Estimates of treatment effectiveness and cost must be translated from controlled research to real-world practice. Unfortunately, most predictions of cost and effectiveness involve considerable extrapolation. Treatment effectiveness data are often drawn from controlled clinical trials. The patients, providers, and treatment protocols in such studies often differ dramatically from real-world practice. Positive outcomes seen under controlled conditions are often difficult to achieve in practice. Real-world decision makers must consider differences in patients and providers when attempting to generalize from published cost effectiveness data. The slippage from research to practice is greatest with more complex or intensive treatments. Predictions of treatment or program cost often depend on expert opinion or resources used in clinical trials. Specialist experts, accustomed to the most difficult and treatment-resistant patients, often overestimate resources used in primary care and community practice. As with effectiveness data, utilization data from research patients treated under research protocols may generalize poorly to actual practice. Cost or utilization data from the actual population of interest may be more useful than published estimates. If possible, key parameters in published cost effectiveness studies (e.g., hospitalization rates, treatment adherence rates, outpatient visit frequency) should be compared with any available local data.

Differences in cost effectiveness of alternative treatment strategies must be weighed against differences in patients' preferences. When choosing among treatments or programs with similar clinical benefits, potential small differences in cost may not justify large differences in patient satisfaction. For example, pharmacotherapy and specific psychotherapies appear equally effective for acute-phase treatment of most cases of major depression. Depending on assumptions about frequency of contact and nature of continuation/maintenance treatment, either choice may appear slightly less expensive. Many patients, however, strongly prefer psychotherapy or pharmacotherapy (Schulberg et al. 1995). Attempts to direct patients away from a preferred treatment are likely to produce decreased satisfaction and decreased effectiveness. Strong preferences are more important than small savings.

Establishing Capitation Arrangements

Questions to Ask

Providers or group practices planning to enter new capitation arrangements must predict need for various components of mental healthcare. Historical data on utilization may be the best guide. Without such data, planners should consider various characteristics of the population and insurance system likely to influence service use. Major factors to consider are listed in Table 12–3.

Setting Capitation Rates

In most cases, capitation rates will be determined more by market forces than by epidemiologic data. For example, typical capitation rates for carve-out mental health services in employed populations range from as low as $2 per person per month to as high as $8. These variations appear determined more by local or regional variations in employer demands and practice patterns than by differences in prevalence or severity of illness. Monthly per-person costs for Medicare and Medicaid populations also vary widely, reflecting the heterogeneity of these programs. For example, aged Medicare beneficiaries typically have lower mental health claims than do young adults, but costs for disabled Medicare beneficiaries are typically several times those for employed populations. Similarly, enrollees in Medicaid Aid to Families with Dependent Children (AFDC) typically have mental health claims similar to or somewhat higher than other insured samples, whereas Medicaid "General Assistance" or "General Relief" enrollees have much higher utilization.

TABLE 12–3. Factors to consider when predicting service use

Historical utilization data

Population demographics
  Age (mental health use is highest in young adulthood and middle age)
  Sex (mental health use is lower in males)
  Ethnicity (mental health use is typically lower in nonwhite populations)

Local practice patterns
  Inpatient use patterns (prevailing hospitalization rates and lengths of stay)
  Penetration rate (proportion of population receiving any mental health specialty care)

Insurance coverage
  Degree of cost-sharing (co-payments or co-insurance)
  Inclusion of patients disabled by mental disorders

Variations on the Theme of Capitation

The discussion above reviews issues common to most capitated mental health systems. Various permutations of capitated financing raise several specific concerns and potential problems. Several of these are discussed below.

Cream-Skimming, Adverse Selection, and Risk Adjustment

Fair competition among health plans or provider groups requires that competing plans be responsible for similar groups of patients—similar prevalence and severity of illness and similar expected treatment costs. A plan that manages to attract a healthier, less expensive population (cream-skimming) will clearly gain an unfair advantage. Although few health plans openly practice cream-skimming, many engage in marketing targeted toward healthier potential members. Conversely, a plan that attracts a sicker or more expensive population (adverse selection) will have a significant disadvantage. Fear of adverse selection often is cited by health plans as a reason for not providing more generous mental health benefit plans than the competition. Clearly, these incentives to seek out healthier members or avoid sicker ones divert attention and resources away from providing better health services. Risk adjustment methods use measurable characteristics of enrolled populations to adjust capitation payments and restore fair competition. At present, risk adjustment is practically limited to member characteristics available from administrative data systems. Candidates for mental health risk adjustment include the same measures described earlier as indicators of a population's need for mental health treatment: age, sex, socioeconomic status (or some proxy measure), and treatment history. Fair competition among health plans and more comprehensive insurance coverage of mental health treatment will probably depend on the development of accurate and efficient methods for risk adjustment.

Varying Provider Incentives

Although capitated financing arrangements are often similar at the health plan level (a fixed monthly rate or premium for each person covered), financial arrangements with individual providers vary widely. Providers may still be reimbursed on a fee-for-service basis, may be capitated at the provider level, may receive a fixed salary, or may have some hybrid arrangement between salary and capitation (e.g., salary with bonuses or holdbacks according to use or costs). These various provider financial incentives can have both positive and negative effects on overall quality of care. Fixed salaries create no financial incentives for over- or undertreatment or for increased clinical productivity. Fee-for-service reimbursement creates clear incentives for increased clinician productivity but can also encourage overtreatment. When providers are responsible for a fixed panel of patients, fee-for-service reimbursement can encourage churning (more frequent visits than necessary, substitution of reimbursed visits for unreimbursed telephone calls). Capitated reimbursement of providers (or small groups) can create incentives for undertreatment. These incentives are strongest when outpatient providers are also at risk for potentially large inpatient expenses. The potential negative incentives of provider capitation on quality of care can be mitigated if patients are allowed to transfer easily among providers or groups. Providers will have greater incentives to improve quality and patient satisfaction if patients are encouraged to vote with their feet (and their premiums).

Subcapitation and Carve-Outs

Separation of mental health and general medical health capitation rates can create a different (and often undesirable) set of incentives for providers and administrators. Separate capitation rates will reduce attention to both the costs of mental disorders in the general medical system and the potential cost savings from improved mental health treatment. Both medical and mental health providers may respond to new incentives for patient dumping (shifting of responsibility and cost onto a different budget). Separate budgeting processes also make integrated planning and redesign difficult. Complete carve-out of mental health services by a separate organization represents the most extreme form of this separation. Under carve-out arrangements, medical and mental health systems have separate budgets, separate cultures, separate planning, and sometimes separate stockholders.

Distinct financing for various components of mental health treatment also can create complex incentives. Separate capitation rates for inpatient and outpatient services create no financial incentive for outpatient providers to control inpatient expenditures. In fact, such arrangements can encourage outpatient providers to hospitalize sicker patients more often to avoid intensive and expensive outpatient treatment. Integrated financing of inpatient and outpatient care encourages use of intensive outpatient services and other alternatives to hospitalization. Resources can be directed to the most cost-effective program of treatment. As discussed earlier, however, placing individuals or small groups of providers at risk for inpatient expenditures can create inappropriately strong financial incentives to deny inpatient care.

Point-of-Service Plans

Point-of-service coverage arrangements allow patients to choose between in-plan and out-of-plan providers for any episode of care. Visits to out-of-plan providers typically require higher co-payments or co-insurance. In most such plans, the internal mental health system is at risk for out-of-plan use either through direct responsibility for payment or loss of capitation funding for members choosing external providers. These hybrid insurance arrangements have grown rapidly in recent years because of purchaser demands and (in some cases) regulatory requirements.

Insurance plans with point-of-service options create a different set of incentives and challenges. Under such an arrangement, internal and external providers compete for the same population of patients (and the same premiums). If this competition is a fair one, patients are likely to benefit. Providers will then compete by providing more effective, convenient, and satisfying care. Without a locked-in base of members, internal providers and administrators must become more responsive to patients' needs and requests. Such arrangements, however, are prone to the same distortions as competition among health plans—cream-skimming to attract the healthiest patients and adverse selection, which punishes those who perform well treating sicker patients.

Capitation for the More Severely Ill

Various economic forces will probably increase the portion of patients with severe mental illness treated in capitated systems. State and federal policies are encouraging those covered by Medicare and Medicaid to enroll in managed care plans. Health plans in competitive markets actively seek Medicare and Medicaid enrollees.

Capitated systems serving the severely mentally ill may need specific mechanisms to ensure that the most vulnerable receive appropriate treatment. Almost all capitated systems attempt to limit the supply of mental health services, but few make organized efforts to ensure that limited resources are directed to those with the greatest need. Access to outpatient services is too often controlled by cost-sharing (co-payments and co-insurance) and queuing (limited appointment availability and long wait times). In such a system, those with the greatest need will be significantly disadvantaged. Patients with severe mental illness are typically less able to afford co-payments or co-insurance and often lack the motivation or organization necessary to deal with wait times and crowded provider schedules. Early experience with capitated care for public sector patients gives credence to some of these fears: the more severely ill may experience poorer functional outcomes (Lurie et al. 1992). Separate programs or pathways for patients with severe disorders may be necessary to ensure appropriate access to treatment.

Summary

Capitated financing arrangements have the potential to improve the delivery of mental health services to all those in need of care. Population-based financing of care should encourage population-based planning and organization of services. Capitated financing also can encourage a more integrated view of all aspects of mental healthcare (e.g., outpatient, day treatment, inpatient) and a more integrated view of mental disorders and mental health treatment within the healthcare system. Breaking the link between reimbursement and specific units of service allows administrators and clinicians to focus on the ultimate goal of care—improved mental health—rather than on intermediate steps such as numbers of visits or hospital days.

A transition to capitated financing also brings potential risks. Although capitation can eliminate some of the undesirable financial incentives of fee-for-service financing, it can create undesirable incentives of its own. Dissolving all links between service and reimbursement can also eliminate incentives for clinician productivity and high service quality. Placing individual physicians or small groups at risk for all aspects of care can create powerful incentives to withhold expensive treatments. Without accurate methods for risk assessment and risk adjustment, health plans or medical groups may be encouraged to compete by seeking healthy members and excluding the sick.

Population-based organization and delivery of care will certainly require major shifts in orientation for administrators and providers. The focus of planning and redesign efforts must broaden from patients currently seeking treatment to the entire covered population, including those treated by medical providers and those not receiving any treatment. Quality improvement must consider each step in an episode of care to identify critical gaps in current processes. In some cases, the most effective intervention for closing these gaps will be a nonclinical one (e.g., community outreach, public education, self-care programs).

Since the mid-1980s, capitated financing of mental healthcare has developed an unfortunate reputation among providers and patients. Capitation has too often been linked with efforts to reduce costs and deny service. The promise of population-based care has remained only a promise. In fact, capitated financing is not a mechanism for reducing the resources devoted to mental healthcare. Overall spending on mental health is determined by the value patients, purchasers, and governmental agencies place on mental health treatment. Capitated financing is one tool for reorganizing the delivery of general medical and mental healthcare. When used in combination with the other tools (population-based planning and redesign), capitation can help to ensure that resources available for mental health treatment are used in the way that most improves the population's health.

References

American Psychiatric Association: Practice guideline for major depressive disorder in adults. Am J Psychiatry 150:S1–S26, 1993

American Psychiatric Association: Practice guideline for the treatment of patients with bipolar disorder. Am J Psychiatry 151:S1–S36, 1994

Angst J: Epidemiology of depression. Psychopharmacology 106 (suppl):S71–S74, 1992

Broadhead WE, Blazer DG, George LK, et al: Depression, disability days and days lost from work in a prospective epidemiologic survey. JAMA 264:2524–2528, 1990

Conti DJ, Burton WN: The economic burden of depression in a workplace. J Occup Med 36:983–988, 1994

Depression Guideline Panel: Depression in Primary Care: Clinical Practice Guideline. Rockville, MD, U.S. Department of Health and Human Services, Public Health Service, Agency for Health Care Policy and Research, 1993

Goldberg DP, Huxley P: Mental Illness in the Community: The Pathways to Psychiatric Care. New York, Tavistock, 1980

Katon W, VonKorff M, Lin E, et al: Collaborative management to achieve treatment guidelines: impact on depression in primary care. JAMA 273:1026–1031, 1995

Kessler RC, McGonagle KA, Zhao S, et al: Lifetime and 12-month prevalence of DSM-III-R psychiatric disorders in the United States. Arch Gen Psychiatry 51:8–19, 1994

Landerman LR, Burns BJ, Swartz MS, et al: The relationship between insurance coverage and psychiatric disorder in predicting use of mental health services. Am J Psychiatry 151:1785–1790, 1994

Leaf PF, Bruce ML, Tischler GL, et al: Factors affecting the utilization of specialty and general medical mental health services. Med Care 26:9–26, 1988

Litzelman DK, Dittus RS, Miller ME, et al: Requiring physicians to respond to computerized reminders improves their compliance with preventive care protocols. J Gen Intern Med 8:311–317, 1993

Lurie N, Moscovice IS, Finch M, et al: Does capitation affect the health of the chronically mentally ill? Results from a randomized trial. JAMA 267:3300–3304, 1992

McDonald CJ, Overhage JM, Tierney WM, et al: The promise of computerized feedback systems for diabetes care. Ann Intern Med 124:170–174, 1996

Nielsen AC, Williams TA: Depression in ambulatory medical patients: prevalence by self-report questionnaire and recognition by nonpsychiatric physicians. Arch Gen Psychiatry 37:999–1004, 1980

Olfson M, Klerman GL: Depressive symptoms and mental health service utilization in a community sample. Soc Psychiatry Psychiatr Epidemiol 27:161–167, 1992

Padgett DK, Patrick C, Burns BJ, et al: Ethnicity and the use of outpatient mental health services in a national insured population. Am J Public Health 84:222–226, 1994

Philbrick JT, Connelly JE, Wofford AB: The prevalence of mental disorders in rural office practice. J Gen Intern Med 11:9–15, 1996

Regier DA, Boyd JH, Burke JD, et al: One-month prevalence of mental disorders in the United States. Arch Gen Psychiatry 45:977–986, 1988

Regier DA, Narrow WE, Rae DS, et al: The de facto US mental and addictive disorders service system: Epidemiologic Catchment Area prospective 1-year prevalence rates of disorders and services. Arch Gen Psychiatry 50:85–94, 1993

Schulberg HC, Block MR, Madonia MJ, et al: Applicability of clinical pharmacotherapy guidelines for major depression in primary care settings. Arch Fam Med 4:106–112, 1995

Simon GE: Psychiatric disorder and functional somatic symptoms as predictors of health care use. Psychiatr Med 10:49–60, 1992

Simon G, VonKorff M: Results from the Seattle Centre, in Mental Illness in General Health Care. Edited by Ustun TB, Sartorius N. New York, Wiley, 1995, 265–284

Simon GE, VonKorff M, Durham ML: Predictors of outpatient mental health utilization in an HMO primary care sample. Am J Psychiatry 151:908–913, 1994

Simon GE, Ormel J, VonKorff M, et al: Health care costs associated with depressive and anxiety disorders in primary care. Am J Psychiatry 152:352–357, 1995a

Simon GE, VonKorff M, Barlow W: Health care costs of primary care patients with recognized depression. Arch Gen Psychiatry 52:850–856, 1995b

Simon GE, Grothaus L, Durham ML, et al: Impact of visit co-payments on outpatient mental health utilization by members of a health maintenance organization. Am J Psychiatry 153:331–338, 1996a

Simon GE, VonKorff M, Barlow W, et al: Predictors of chronic benzodiazepine use in a health maintenance organization sample. J Clin Epidemiol 49:1067–1073, 1996b

Simon GE, VonKorff M, Heiligenstein JH, et al: Initial antidepressant selection in primary care: effectiveness and cost of fluoxetine vs. tricyclic antidepressants. JAMA 275:1897–1902, 1996c

Spitzer RL, Williams JBW, Kroenke K, et al: Utility of a new procedure for diagnosing mental disorders in primary care: the PRIME-MD 1000 study. JAMA 272:1749–1756, 1994

Sturm R, Wells KB: How can care for depression become more cost-effective? JAMA 273:51–58, 1995

VonKorff M, Shapiro S, Burke JD, et al: Anxiety and depression in a primary care clinic: comparison of Diagnostic Interview Schedule, General Health Questionnaire, and practitioner assessments. Arch Gen Psychiatry 44:152–156, 1987

❖ 13 ❖

Behavioral Health Outcomes

Patient and System

Teresa L. Kramer, Ph.D.

G. Richard Smith, M.D.

At least 40 years have been devoted to determining the efficacy of mental health treatment. Despite the initial and yet controversial findings of Eysenck (1952) that psychotherapy is ineffective, numerous studies have been published documenting the benefits of both psychotherapy (cf. Bergin and Garfield 1994; Garfield and Bergin 1986) and pharmacologic treatments (Klein et al. 1980). Since then, psychotherapy research has moved in focus from showing that psychotherapy is generally helpful to questioning which interventions are efficacious for specific clinical problems. A similar shift in research emphasis has occurred in psychopharmacy studies. Further refinement of these types of studies has led to research known as clinical trials, which typically consist of highly detailed therapy and treatment manuals that clinicians follow for specific diagnostic conditions (Goldfried and Wolfe 1996). Although these studies have been crucial in the development of our knowledge about the curative potential of mental health treatment, they use rigorous research conditions that may limit their generalizability to "real-world" settings.

As a result, we know little about the effectiveness of various routine mental health interventions. Much of the literature to date has shown that specific treatments work under specific "conditions"—that is, when patients meet certain diagnostic criteria, when comorbidity is limited, and when clinical interventions are carefully outlined and monitored. What is not so apparent is how deviations from the clinical trials research model influence outcomes; in other words, how effective is treatment when patients present with multiple problems and diagnoses in variable clinical settings and receive an array of treatments by different types of providers?

Changing trends in the delivery, financing, and management of healthcare have created a need to better understand the components and complexities of care to improve the overall effectiveness of treatment. New developments in the administration and financing of healthcare have undoubtedly influenced the accessibility and quality of care in recent years. In addition, market demand, competition, and increased pressure to meet accreditation guidelines and report card standards have forced various delivery systems to alter the way in which services are provided over time and accessed by patients. In addition, multiple stakeholders, including payers, insurers, and consumers, also are advocating for more data that can determine whether limited costs compromise the accessibility to and/or outcome of treatment and, eventually, the health of larger populations. These combined forces have prompted individual providers, as well as systems of care, to evaluate the cost effectiveness of various treatments and to determine whether patients are improving and are satisfied with the services they receive. Consequently, patient outcomes are as popular today as personality testing and psychotherapy process research were in the 1970s and 1980s. (See, for example, recent issues of *Psychiatric Annals* [February 1997] and *American Psychologist* [October 1996], which are devoted almost exclusively to the various economic, ethical, methodological, and policy questions that confront evaluators of patient outcomes.)

Understanding the widespread effect of healthcare policies and reform is an even more difficult and complex undertaking than assessment of individual patients or patient groups but one that deserves considerable attention as more and more organizations move into new healthcare paradigms. These issues are beyond the scope of this chapter, but they are important to consider in the context of outcomes assessment and subsequent initiatives to improve the quality of care within various delivery systems.

Given the increased need for information pertaining to outcomes of patient care, in this chapter we explore relevant issues to consider in establishing state-of-the-art outcomes programs that will permit reliable and valid evaluation of patients and patient care systems. The following topics are reviewed in this chapter:

- Elements of care to assess
- Definition of outcomes management systems
- Patient outcomes (generic vs. diagnostic-specific assessments; domains of health to be assessed; use of a tracer condition; sampling vs. population data)
- Organizational or systemic outcomes
- Implementation of outcomes systems (needs assessment, selection of instruments, methodological issues, data analysis, and costs)
- Integration into the quality improvement process

Elements of Care

The elements of medical care have been described by Donabedian (1980) as consisting of structure, process, and outcome (see Figure 13–1). *Structure* refers to the resources used in the provision of care and the more stable arrangements under which care is provided (e.g., budgeting, staffing, management style and organization, and information systems). *Process* refers to the activities that constitute care (e.g., practice guidelines, length of care, level of care, accessibility, and use of high-risk procedures). *Outcome* refers to the consequences to health on an individual and social level (e.g., psychological and physical symptomatology, critical events, quality of life, and legal and social consequences).

Any and all of these components may be evaluated as part of an overall evaluation plan, depending on the needs of the provider and/or organization. Changes in one component (e.g., the location of the facility) may affect another (e.g., patient access and outcome). However, process and outcome of care will be the two components focused on in this chapter because they are most frequently the targets of quality improvement activities and, therefore, the objects of ongoing evaluations.

Definition of an Outcomes Management System

The goal of an outcomes management system is to assess patient characteristics, processes of treatment, and outcomes of routine care in order to monitor and/or improve mental health and substance abuse treatment and outcomes. In line with this goal, outcomes management systems may be designed to accomplish a number of objectives, which may improve value, quality, decision making, effectiveness, accountability, and marketing efforts (see Figure 13–2).

The critical components of such a system include the following:

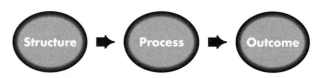

FIGURE 13–1. Elements of medical care.

Value:	To determine benefit for outcome dollar
Quality:	To improve behavioral health outcomes
Decision making:	To inform clinicians and managers
Effectiveness:	To determine what works
Accountability:	To provide evidence of patient outcomes
Coercion:	To relieve pressure
Marketing:	To maintain or increase market share

FIGURE 13–2. Goals of outcome assessment.

- Ability to verify that patients evaluated in the system meet diagnostic criteria for the condition(s) under study
- Ability to provide valid and reliable data about salient patient outcomes
- Ability to measure prognostic variables to permit comparisons across groups
- Ability to assess the type and extent of treatment the patient received for the target condition(s) across various healthcare delivery settings

Outcomes systems or programs are often used to describe new approaches to obtaining clinical data at the patient and organizational level. Such systems contain the mechanisms to obtain patient-level data pertaining to several domains, some of which are relevant across all areas of health—functioning, disability, quality of life, patient satisfaction, general health status, and mental health status (Smith 1996). Others are more pertinent to mental health and include disease or disorder status, disease or disorder severity, and disease- or disorder-specific functioning (Smith et al. 1997b). Prognostic variables, also known as case-mix variables, also should be included to aid in predicting treatment outcome. To be effective, outcomes systems often obtain data pertaining to the process of care, including treatment modality, duration and intensity, type of provider, and use of other medical services and/or therapeutic interventions; this enables the evaluator to begin developing hypotheses about what patient outcomes are associated with particular treatment processes.

Outcomes systems, designed to obtain clinical information about patients, are different from other forms of clinical research in a number of ways. First, the objectives of outcomes systems are to monitor or enhance patient care and the quality of services, as opposed to confirming research hypotheses. Although hypotheses may be generated from the outcomes system, the lack of experimental conditions (e.g., randomization, inclusion of comparison groups) limits the scientific conclusions that can be drawn from the data.

Second, technological advances in the last few decades have improved the ability to create and use large databases and elaborate information systems relevant for assessing outcomes. For example, outcomes systems can be designed to include data on claims, authorizations for treatment, appointment scheduling, pharmacy use, and other healthcare services received during the course of treatment. These revolutionary technological changes and sophisticated data systems now allow providers and organizational leaders to easily assess the costs of multiple treatment interventions on large groups of patients rather than just examining small groups who theoretically receive only one type of treatment intervention by a clinician trained in that method.

Outcomes systems also are designed to assess what occurs "naturally" in a clinical setting. First, ethical considerations prohibit providers from establishing waiting lists or placebo conditions to assess treatment without informed consent and important research safeguards. Second, adherence to established practice guidelines may limit the treatment plan developed by a provider. In addition, experimental treatments are not reimbursed, which also may influence decision making on the part of the provider. Finally, other external constraints, such as utilization review under a managed care environment, are other factors to consider in development of an outcomes system. These types of limitations usually do not affect traditional clinical research efforts.

Unlike efficacy or clinical trials research, outcomes systems are designed to inform key decision makers about focus areas for the quality improvement process. This represents an application of the data to the actual setting in which outcomes assessment occurs, which will have an immediate effect on the care provided to the patient. By comparison, efficacy studies may be conducted in clinical settings but often have little relevance to the specific quality improvement plan of an organization.

Finally, multiple treatment sites have become the focus of outcomes assessment. In traditional clinical research, efficacy is assessed primarily in a mental health setting in which trained mental health clinicians provide the treatment. Now, with so many family practitioners, primary care physicians, and other generalists providing psychosocial interventions, it becomes imperative to evaluate patient outcomes in the context of multidisciplinary, multisite interactions.

Patient Outcomes

To conduct comprehensive and informative outcomes assessment at the patient level, measures of functioning and symptomatology should be taken at baseline, periodically throughout treatment, and at follow-up intervals. As a result, changes over time can be calculated and analyzed in conjunction with appropriate case-mix data, such as initial symptoms, demographic variables, and compliance with treatment. An estimate of treatment effect can then be calculated (Bartlett 1997).

Generic Versus Disease-Specific Assessments

One of the primary questions in developing an outcomes system is whether to include generic or disease-specific assessments. Generic systems assess global symptomatology and/or functioning; the use of similar instruments across disorders provides extensive information on a wide array of symptoms across patient groups. On the other hand, disease- or disorder-specific systems assess patient diagnosis and diagnostic severity, which provides very specific information about a patient's condition.

Both types of outcomes systems are associated with certain advantages and disadvantages. Generic assessment is simpler to design and implement. One or two instruments that contain multiple symptom domains can be selected and easily administered for an entire patient population. Unfortunately, generic assessments do not show how a particular disease entity responds to specific treatment interventions.

In comparison, disease-specific systems lead to specific knowledge of a patient's disorder, which may respond differentially to various treatment approaches. By establishing a relatively homogeneous group of patients who can be treated in a consistent manner, providers and provider organizations can more realistically assess the effectiveness of care. For example, diagnostic entities such as major depression, schizophrenia, alcohol abuse, panic disorder, or eating disorders respond to different medications and therapeutic modalities, which are easier to measure with uniform measurement tools.

Use of a Tracer Condition

The use of a tracer condition, a single condition that is followed within an organization, rather than assessing patients with any disorder facilitates the evaluation of a particular disorder or disease over time (Kessner et al. 1973; Wells 1985). Also, because fewer patients are monitored, the selection of a tracer condition reduces the burden of assessment to the system. In choosing a tracer condition, it is important to determine that valid and reliable assessment tools are available to measure that condition and that an adequate number of patients in the organization present with that condition to ensure that meaningful data will be obtained (Smith et al. 1997a). In addition, the following selection criteria should be considered:

1. *The condition is common in the clinical setting.* If it takes 6 months to collect data on only a few patients, the information obtained will not be meaningful to the system and will discourage provider participation.
2. *Clinical change is expected, and effective treatment(s) exist.* Certain conditions, such as conduct disorder in adolescents or Axis II diagnoses in adults, are generally not amenable to change within most measurement time frames, whereas other conditions, such as depression, respond more rapidly to certain types of treatment.
3. *Providers agree that outcomes information pertaining to this condition is relevant and important to the quality of care.* Because provider participation is such a significant factor in the success of outcomes assessment, it is important that the data obtained have clinical relevance to all parties involved and that providers, in particular, believe that the effort is worth the results.

Interestingly, a combination approach of generic and diagnostic-specific assessments may well serve providers and organizations interested in both types of outcomes (Smith 1996). For example, a generic assessment at baseline coupled with a disorder- or disease-specific assessment at follow-up may prove to yield the desired information in a timely and inexpensive manner. An initial generic assessment of the patient population also may generate further clinical questions, which could form the basis for smaller, more disease-focused studies of selected groups of patients.

Sampling Versus Entire Population Data

Experts in the area of quality improvement argue in favor of collecting data by sampling as opposed to universal inspection (Deming 1986; Juran 1988). Certainly, sampling is a much less expensive way of monitoring health outcomes, if care is taken to ensure that the sample is truly representative of the population at large. On the other hand, measuring everyone is far more meaningful to the individual clinician and easier to implement systemwide than is assessing every "nth" person.

Organizational or Systemic Outcomes

Market demands have increased the need for systems-level outcomes data, sometimes referred to as *performance* or *process information*. Systems-level data may be aggregate patient data, aggregate provider data, or organizational data. Aggregate patient-level data, as discussed earlier in this chapter, provide some estimation of treatment effectiveness. At this level, much-needed information relevant to the organization's ability to provide quality care is available. Practice patterns can be analyzed to determine whether patients' conditions are being diagnosed accurately and treated appropriately. Other questions may be answered through aggregate data, such as whether specific patient characteristics predict response to medication or whether certain treatment programs are more effective in reducing patient distress.

Aggregate provider data, which may include information on outcomes, costs, and patient satisfaction, can be used to distinguish provider practices and competencies. For example, a particular provider may consistently fail to detect the presence of a depressive disorder in his patients, resulting in an inadequate treatment plan and poorer outcomes. Also referred to as *provider profiling*, this type of measurement has raised considerable concerns among providers who resent the close scrutiny of their clinical practices; however, if used in conjunction with education and consultation, this type of assessment can lead to improved care.

Systems-level data may be used to evaluate the effectiveness of programs or organizations, in general. Currently, several groups are developing and implementing report cards, which provide information on quality of care within managed care organizations, delivery systems, provider networks, and specific facilities. These groups include the National Committee for Quality Assurance (NCQA); the Joint Commission on Accreditation of Healthcare Organizations (JCAHO) and its new ORYX initiative, the American Managed Behavioral Healthcare Association (AMBHA); and the

Center for Mental Health Services (CMHS) within the Substance Abuse and Mental Health Services Administration of the federal government. As a result, some performance indicators have been targeted by the industry as markers of quality care. These indicators will set the standards for care in several domains, including accessibility, quality, clinical appropriateness, outcomes, patient satisfaction, and prevention.

Outcomes systems also can provide patient satisfaction data to be used in a marketing plan, to document the effects of changes in practice procedures on patient health, to supplement clinical information and assist in treatment planning and review, and to track patients longitudinally to determine changes in patient care and health status. As an organization undertakes new contracts or business, develops new programs, increases or reduces personnel, or changes other procedures, assessment of the associated clinical effects is helpful. As systems data are collected over time, it will become important for providers and organizations to monitor trends in patient care, particularly as the structure and process of services shift.

Implementation of Outcomes Systems

The key to a successful outcomes system is careful planning, selection of instruments, systematic implementation, and routine feedback to correct any problems that become apparent as clinicians and patients use the system. Six aspects of the implementation process are described: needs assessment; selection of instruments; methodology, including staff preparation and patient involvement; data analysis; costs; and integration into the organization's quality improvement plan (see Figure 13–3).

Needs Assessment

Implementation of an outcomes system requires significant commitment on the part of upper management from initial planning stages to final analysis of results (which will ultimately inform decision-making processes and potentially change organizational practices) (Smith et al. 1997a). Therefore, the leaders of an organization must become knowledgeable about the intricate details involved in establishing an outcomes system and learn basics aspects of research design, statistical

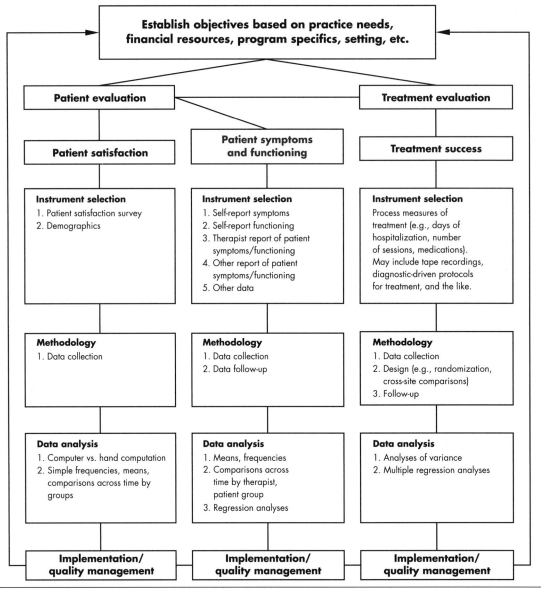

FIGURE 13–3. Decision tree for developing outcomes management systems.

analyses, and methodological issues. Upper management also must assume that such an endeavor will cost substantially in terms of human resources and financial expenditures but that undertaking this type of work can be seen as a capital investment in the future of the organization.

By establishing objectives at the outset, developers of an outcomes system can determine which variables to monitor as well as the frequency, duration, and method of measurement. The overall goal is to develop a cohesive and systematic program of measurement that will ultimately improve the quality of care provided and ensure that an organization remains competitive in the mental health industry.

Selection of Instruments

An important consideration in the development of an outcomes system is the selection of the specific measures to assess the patient's mental health status and functioning. The instruments must provide valid and reliable data, reflect the patient's and provider's perspectives, adapt to changes in clinical knowledge and practice, and be standardized to allow for comparisons across groups (Smith et al. 1997b). Unfortunately, few assessment tools (generic or diagnostic-specific) meet these standards, resulting in considerable controversy in the field about what specific aspects of the patient's mental health should be assessed and the best approach to measuring them.

In mental health outcomes assessment, several patient variables may be evaluated, including primary symptoms, comorbid symptoms, functioning levels, and demographics. As a result, outcomes assessment usually consists of more than one assessment tool, assembled into a battery of measures, and administered directly to the patient and/or completed by the primary caregiver or clinician.

Global, self-report instruments that are currently popular for the generic assessment of patient status include the Brief Symptom Inventory (BSI; Derogatis 1985), the Behavior and Symptom Identification Scale (BASIS-32; Eisen et al. 1994), the SF-36 (Ware and Sherbourne 1991), and the Outcome Questionnaire (OQ-45; Lambert et al. 1994). Use of these instruments allows for a general profile of the patient's functioning and symptom status, which can be easily monitored over time.

In comparison, outcomes tools that assess disease- or condition-specific symptoms allow for clustering of relatively homogeneous patients and assessment of specific treatment applications. Examples of diagnostic-specific outcomes assessment tools include modules assessing major depression, alcohol abuse/dependence, panic disorder, and substance abuse/dependence developed by the Centers for Mental Healthcare Research at the University of Arkansas for Medical Sciences. Each module contains items pertaining to disease-specific symptoms and functioning, sociodemographics, prognostic/case-mix variables, treatment use, outcomes of care, and general health.

Treatment or process variables, including treatment modality, duration and intensity, type of provider, and use of other medical services and/or therapeutic interventions, are also helpful additions to an outcomes evaluation. This information, when analyzed in conjunction with symptom change, provides important data for assessing the effectiveness of care and, when appropriate, the comparability of various treatment approaches.

Whenever possible, normative data should be solicited from the authors of the instruments selected or from other groups conducting similar outcomes systems to permit comparisons across sites. Benchmarking such as this allows organizations to search for and apply significantly better practices that result in quality care and improved health. Furthermore, by sharing outcomes data in pursuit of best practice methods and procedures, organizations can contribute significantly to the development of new technology, more effective treatments, and enhanced delivery of services (Camp and Tweet 1994).

Methodological Issues

In collecting data, organizations must decide whether all or a sample of patients will be assessed, depending on the results of the needs assessment, the size of the population to be monitored, and the importance of individual patient data versus systemwide information (Smith et al. 1997b). One important issue to consider in assessing only a select group of patients is how those patients will be screened for participation in the outcomes system. The number of patients assessed should be large enough to allow for even distribution of demographic variables, provider types, severity of symptoms, and treatment conditions. This may not be difficult to achieve at the outset of the assessment, but follow-up of patients who are representative of the larger group seems to be one of the most critical barriers to completion of successful outcomes systems.

Timing of administration of the measures is important from the patient's standpoint in order to avoid paperwork that, because of its burden, interferes with clinical interventions and services. For this reason, patients should be informed at the scheduling of their first appointment that important clinical data will be requested from them, with accommodations made for early arrival. The important issue here is that patients understand that the clinical data obtained will be used to develop an appropriate treatment plan rather than tossed aside with no clinical review. If patients understand the benefits of complying with the assessment protocol, they are more likely to participate in its completion.

Other methods have been documented to facilitate patient participation in outcomes assessment, including therapist involvement, distribution of surveys in the office (as opposed to home mailings), follow-up postcards and/or telephone calls to remind patients to complete the measures, and various incentives such as small payments and entry into lottery systems. Although these have all been effective in improving response rates, most outcomes studies in clinical settings attain maximum follow-up rates of 30%–60%. Generally, follow-up rates of 70%–80% are desired to ensure that the treatment population is adequately represented. Another option is to conduct telephone follow-up queries, although this can be extremely time-consuming and expensive. It is important to keep in mind that outcomes assessments that are well defined, limited, and targeted to a smaller population are more likely to result in higher response rates because more resources can be allocated toward closely tracking and contacting patients.

Regardless of the response rates obtained, care should be taken to understand how and to what extent patients who complete measures at follow-up intervals differ from those who do not (i.e., are they more seriously ill; do they belong to a particular minority, age, or socioeconomic group; or are they generally less satisfied?). Sometimes focus studies targeted at noncompliant patients can provide additional information about these issues.

It probably seems quite obvious at this point that without appropriate staff orientation and training, outcomes studies will fail in an organization. Just as it is imperative that top management be invested in the project, clinicians and support staff should be involved in initial decision making, planning, and implementation. Most important, clinicians need to believe that the information obtained will be clinically relevant to their individual patients and that aggregate data will result in meaningful organizational changes. Support staff, who may be responsible for distributing the outcomes measures to patients or who may be asked questions by patients completing measures in the waiting room, should be equally well informed.

Many outcomes systems have failed because clinicians and support staff were not well prepared or because front-line personnel did not have the resources to follow through on the project as originally planned. Orientation or training sessions should include an overview and purpose of the outcomes system, dissemination and review of the measures (staff members may appreciate time allotted for them to complete the measures), distribution of a manual that explains in detail the methodology of the system (e.g., who is responsible for various phases of the project, what exactly to communicate to the patient, copies of letters or consent forms the patients may receive), and an in-depth discussion of possible barriers or difficulties that may be encountered. The more attention devoted to including and motivating clinicians and staff, the easier the outcomes system will be to implement.

In addition, the perspectives of the patient or patient's family are critical to the entire outcomes process and can be included through self-report; development of consumer focus groups; involvement in the assessment process, including the feedback phase; and acknowledgment of the various socioeconomic and cultural factors that may influence symptomatology, functioning, and use of services. These considerations, consistent with the principles of continuous quality improvement (CQI) to be discussed below, may uncover problems and conflicting values in the outcomes system and organization of care.

Data Analysis

Information systems have evolved into complex networks of data, which may include claims requests and payments, medical and mental health use, pharmaceutical orders, appointment scheduling, and personal information such as diagnoses, demographics, and medical record contents. The dilemma confronting developers of outcomes systems is no longer whether to integrate outcomes data into the larger information systems, but to what extent and how. The more systemic information required, the more likely the outcomes program will be linked with other databases, thus allowing for a more comprehensive analysis of the organization's responsiveness to patients and overall quality of care provided.

Individual patient data should be analyzed in as timely a manner as possible to provide immediate feedback to the clinician and patient. Although the outcomes project may last 12 months or longer, interim analyses also should be conducted on aggregate data to ensure that reliable information is obtained, software equipment is operable, errors in data entry are deleted, programming is accurate (accounting for missing variables), and clinically relevant and meaningful findings are produced. Constant vigilance is required to safeguard the integrity of the data.

Final data analyses should be conducted in accordance with the goals established at the outset of the project and in a format that is easily read and understood. Graphs and other figures facilitate comprehension and can be converted efficiently into overheads and slides for presentations to staff, management, payers, and other stakeholders.

Costs

Costs for implementation can range anywhere from several hundred to thousands of dollars, depending on the nature, extent, and complexity of the outcomes system. Whether these investments actually result in eventual cost savings because of improved efficiency in services and/or healthier patients remains to be determined through empirical research. Nonetheless, a budget should be developed that includes expenses for the

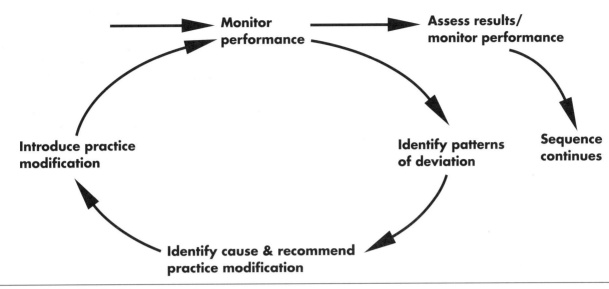

FIGURE 13–4. Feedback loop for quality improvement.
Source. Modified from Donabedian 1990.

various system elements, such as measures (costs will differ depending on whether the measures are proprietary), postage (initial and return), supplies (particularly software and computers), and copying (for letters, consent forms, and preparation of reports). The highest costs will be for outcomes systems personnel, such as a project coordinator, data analyst, and consultant, if desired.

Integration Into the Quality Improvement Process

Total quality management is a term derived from the quality movement in manufacturing and service industries, which emphasizes integration of all organizational activities to achieve the goal of servicing customers (Cortada and Woods 1995). *CQI* is the term applied in the healthcare sector to the use of total quality management (Chowanec 1994). Both ideas provide the philosophy, techniques, and experience to improve competitiveness and cost effectiveness by creating a quality mind-set throughout the organization. As the behavioral healthcare industry incorporates quality concepts and processes into the evaluation and ongoing management of clinical delivery systems, there has been increased pressure to scrutinize specific aspects of delivery systems, including clinical documentation and authorization for services, credentialing of providers, complaint procedures, utilization review, accessibility, and outcomes. In addition, benchmarking efforts are under way to measure best practice indicators, which

will ultimately lead to organizations modifying their standards of care to improve overall performance (Watson 1993).

CQI can be applied in healthcare delivery systems to improve outcomes (Chowanec 1994); however, outcomes measurement must be a critical component of this effort. Patient, provider, and systems assessment can identify patterns of deviation or success. This information, when communicated to providers, organizational leaders, and payers, can result in new ideas for practice management, processes of care, and treatment programs. To accomplish this cycle of feedback (see Figure 13–4), reports pertaining to outcomes data should be discussed with all persons in the organization. Providers should be informed about their individual performance, and, in the case of satisfaction surveys, comments made by patients about providers should be addressed. Aggregate data should be reviewed periodically by management and included in the agenda of annual meetings and reports, with specific recommendations accompanying the findings. Information relevant to support staff should be discussed with them and action plans developed for improving service. Subsequently, the outcomes system should be revised as services are changed or new programs are developed, in conjunction with the establishment of CQI goals, objectives, and annual plans. In essence, outcomes systems should trigger programming modifications, educational and training sessions, team development, guideline implementation, and other organizational programs to maximize patient care.

Summary

Outcomes systems are targeted toward specific groups of patients, consist of reliable and valid measures, have programmatic questions that can be answered with actionable results, and encompass different variables, including patient and system characteristics and costs. Outcomes systems also must be integrated into the goals of the organization and be continually redesigned to accommodate the changing visions and programs of the organization.

Escalating expenses for behavioral health treatment, coupled with external pressure from employers, payers, government agencies, consumers, and other stakeholder groups, have forced clinicians and delivery systems to develop more cost-effective services, while verifying that the services they provide result in positive outcomes for patients. This trend has resulted in an increased emphasis on outcomes systems that are often adopted into the overall quality improvement goals, objectives, and plans of the organization. By better understanding the process, structure, *and* outcomes of care, providers and organizations can more carefully develop and execute treatment interventions that will maximize accessibility, improve care, and ultimately result in healthier populations.

References

Bartlett J: Treatment outcomes: the psychiatrist's and health care executive's perspectives. Psychiatric Annals 27:100–103, 1997

Bergin AE, Garfield SL (eds): Handbook of Psychotherapy and Behavioral Change, 4th Edition. New York, Wiley, 1994

Camp RC, Tweet HG: Benchmarking applied to healthcare. Journal on Quality Improvement 20(5):229–238, 1994

Chowanec GD: Continuous quality improvement: conceptual foundations and application to mental health care. Hosp Community Psychiatry 45:789–793, 1994

Cortada JW, Woods JA: The McGraw-Hill Encyclopedia of Quality Terms and Concepts. New York, McGraw-Hill, 1995

Deming WE: Out of the Crisis. Cambridge, MA, MIT Center for Advanced Engineering Study, 1986

Derogatis L: Brief Symptom Inventory. Minneapolis, MN, National Computer Systems, 1985

Donabedian A: Explorations in Quality Assessment and Monitoring, Vol 1: The Definition of Quality and Approaches to Its Assessment. Ann Arbor, MI, Health Administrative Press, 1980

Donabedian A: Specialization in clinical performance monitoring. Quality Assurance and Utilization Review 5(4):114–120, 1990

Eisen SV, Dill DL, Grob MC: Reliability and validity of a brief patient-report instrument for psychiatric outcome evaluation. Hosp Community Psychiatry 45:242–247, 1994

Eysenck HJ: The effects of psychotherapy: an evaluation. J Consult Clin Psychol 16:391–324, 1952

Garfield SL, Bergin AE (eds): Handbook of Psychotherapy and Behavioral Change. New York, Wiley, 1986

Goldfried MR, Wolfe BE: Psychotherapy practice and research: repairing a strained alliance. Am Psychol 51:1007–1016, 1996

Juran JM: Juran on Planning for Quality. New York, Free Press, 1988

Kessner DM, Kalk CE, Singer J: Assessing health quality—the case for tracers. N Engl J Med 288:189–194, 1973

Klein DR, Gittelman R, Quitkin F, et al: Diagnosis and Drug Treatment of Psychiatric Disorders: Adults and Children, 2nd Edition. Baltimore, MD, Williams & Wilkins, 1980

Lambert MJ, Lunnen K, Umphress V, et al: Administration and Scoring Manual for the Outcomes Questionnaire (OQ-45. 1). Salt Lake City, UT, IHC Center for Behavioral Healthcare Efficacy, 1994

Smith GR: State of the science of mental health and substance abuse patient outcomes assessment. New Dir Ment Health Serv 71:59–67, 1996

Smith GR, Fischer EP, Nordquist CR, et al: Implementing outcomes management systems in mental health settings. Psychiatr Serv 48:364–368, 1997a

Smith GR, Rost K, Fischer EP, et al: Assessing the effectiveness of mental health care in routine clinical practice: characteristics, development, and uses of patient outcomes modules. Evaluation and the Health Professions 20:65–80, 1997b

Ware JE, Sherbourne CD: The SF-36 Short Form Health Status Survey I: Conceptual Framework and Item Selection. Boston, MA, New England Medical Centers Hospital, International Resource Center for Health Care Assessment, 1991

Watson GH: Strategic Benchmarking. New York, Wiley, 1993

Wells KB: Depression as a Tracer Condition for the National Study of Medical Care Outcomes—Background Review. Santa Monica, CA, RAND, 1985

❖ 14 ❖

Health Information and Confidentiality

Jonathan S. Wald, M.D., M.P.H.

The topics of security and confidentiality in healthcare are important because inappropriate use of patient information is possible in connection with almost every activity within a healthcare setting, as well as wherever identifiable health information is used beyond it. Changes in healthcare delivery in the United States, including increasing management of care by third parties, collaborative care teams within and across healthcare systems, and consolidation among physicians and hospitals (Deloitte and Touche 1996), have resulted in more information about patients flowing to greater numbers of individuals inside and outside the clinical setting. The proliferation of databases containing person-identifiable health and demographic information outside of the healthcare system further increases the potential exposure of personal information beyond its intended audience, especially when links between health data and other personal information are forged in unanticipated ways.

In this chapter, I define the challenges facing patients, providers, and society as a whole in maintaining confidentiality; identify many of the important threats to confidentiality; and address the organizational strategies needed to manage those threats. The development of effective protective strategies requires examination of root processes and assumptions concerning information sharing in healthcare.

The Oath of Hippocrates addressed the importance of confidentiality (Bartlett 1968, p. 88):

> Whatsoever things I see or hear concerning the life of men, in my attendance on the sick or even apart therefrom, which ought not be noised abroad, I will keep silence thereon, counting such things to be as sacred secrets.

The topic of confidentiality in medical care has received much attention within psychiatry because of the damage that can befall the patient whose personal information is divulged inappropriately. Furthermore, the basic history-taking and therapeutic activities essential to careful evaluation and treatment often require self-disclosure by the patient, which is impossible without a high degree of confidence in the therapist. Stigmatization of those with mental illness has further intensified concerns about psychiatric information.

But the behavioral health record represents only a portion of mental health information available to potential users; the general medical record, with its gynecological, infectious disease, oncological, and psycho-social documentation, is very detailed and revealing as well. Outside of the health record, a high volume of health information is found in public and private databases with their own access rules. The challenge of protecting patient information has never been more difficult.

Traditionally, the discussion of confidentiality in the medical record focused on laws, regulations, and formal procedures for storing and releasing charted information. This chapter places the subject in the broader context of health information privacy, recognizing that there is widespread, unregulated use of information beyond the understood use when it was shared.

Health Information, Confidentiality, Privacy, and Security

Health information, in this discussion, broadly refers to any information obtained in the course of providing care or delivering care services that identifies or can be readily associated with a person.

Confidentiality, privacy, and security are each important in discussing threats to health information and countermeasures to protect it. The *Comprehensive Textbook of Psychiatry* (Kaplan and Sadock 1989, p. 2118) defines *confidentiality* as "the obligation of the professional to keep in confidence whatever information is shared by the patient, absent specific permission." Thus, confidentiality requires a shared understanding of the professional's and the patient's expectations, an appreciation of the context in which information was divulged, and consideration of other requirements (e.g., insurance reimbursement, legal) that may require information disclosure.

Privacy is the ability of an individual to keep information that is not intended to be shared out of public view. Privacy and confidentiality are often used interchangeably by patients and providers. Erosion of privacy has been particularly severe in recent years as 1) individuals sometimes unwittingly reveal personal preferences and behavior through credit card purchases, grocery purchases, and release of their Social Security number, and 2) companies building large databases aggregating personal information from public sources provide information services to the marketplace of individuals and

organizations that wish to purchase such information (Bernstein 1997).

Security encompasses the administrative and technical methods for keeping data available, reliable, and safe from destruction, modification, or tampering (Bakker 1994). A significant challenge is to control data flow. Weaknesses in security, such as unlocked doors and file cabinets, poor surveillance of restricted work areas, and release of the health record without explicit identification of the requester, can compromise confidentiality. As the technology for storing and sharing health information advances from paper to electronic patient records, new threats such as disk failures, power failures, network failures, and software failures are added to the more traditional threats inherent in managing paper. No record systems are secure against all risks and threats. Explicit choices about which security methods to support (plan, implement, and maintain) must reflect the effects and costs of such protection.

Care and Confidentiality Risks

Managing information flow within a healthcare organization to support quality care and to maintain effective confidentiality at the same time creates a fundamental tension. There is an irreconcilable conflict between the "risk of compromised care" and the "risk of inappropriate disclosure" when health information is withheld or shared among workers in a healthcare organization (Figure 14–1). Discussions that focus on obtaining and sharing clinical information for patient care reasons but that do not consider confidentiality issues are unbalanced. Similarly, efforts to address confidentiality concerns that ignore the care risks that increase when certain patient-specific data are unavailable or missing ignore the mandate to provide quality care. The two are linked because resources expended on maintaining security are not available for patient care and vice versa. As long as our society continues to value both high-quality care and patient confidentiality, we must be careful to address both priorities.

Risk of Compromised Care

Substantial evidence in areas of behavioral health and medical care indicates that the level of care and the level of health services delivery vary over geography, over time, and among individual providers and recipients of

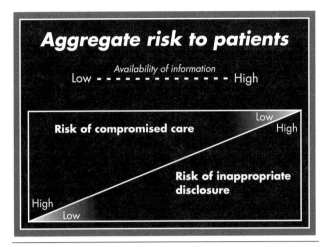

FIGURE 14–1. Irreconcilable conflict between the risk of compromised care and the risk of inappropriate disclosure of information.

care. The effect of inadequate information on patient care has increasingly been documented with clinical metrics such as adverse drug events (Bates et al. 1995), unnecessary laboratory tests (Schoenenberger et al. 1995), unnecessary immunizations in children (Murphy et al. 1997), and costs of care associated with those outcomes (Bates et al. 1995; Murphy et al. 1997; Pestotnik et al. 1990; Schoenenberger et al. 1995).

For example, in acute care medical settings, an estimated 30% of all adverse drug events are preventable, and almost 80% of *those* adverse drug events could be prevented if relevant clinical information were available at the right time to the right person in the right context (Bates et al. 1995). This would amount to hundreds of preventable adverse drug events per year in a large hospital facility, saving millions of dollars in recurrent avoided costs and generating large annual reductions in length of stay. Another study found that the availability of timely test results reduced laboratory test ordering 13% compared with physicians without ready access to test results (Tierney et al. 1987).

Large epidemiologic studies show that depression, anxiety disorders, and other psychiatric conditions in primary care populations go undetected or are detected after much delay (Department of Health and Human Services 1993). This problem is intensified by the disparate collection and storage of health information in multiple locations without a system for linking and integrating it over time for an individual. Poor communication of information also creates clinical and economic costs. Studies of cross-coverage in teaching hospitals identified a sixfold increase in the risk of an

adverse drug event when a patient was cared for by a "covering" physician than when cared for by the "primary" physician (Petersen et al. 1994). The serious effect of lost information and the lack of continuity when a patient transfers care from one therapist or therapy setting to another is well known by all who practice and receive healthcare.

Risk of Inappropriate Disclosure

Tremendous variation is seen both in the practice of healthcare and in the methods used by healthcare organizations to protect confidentiality. To preserve the confidentiality of patients, an organization must successfully 1) guide individual employee behavior, 2) understand how the organization's administrative practices raise or lower confidentiality risks, 3) adopt policies and procedures that are protective of patients, 4) establish a high-level commitment to confidentiality, and 5) allocate funds for security/confidentiality projects. Vulnerabilities to intentional or unintentional breaches are numerous, and every organization can identify areas needing improvement after even brief self-assessment. For example, inadequate shredding of paper or uncontrolled access to sensitive data is commonly found, and patient information is often overheard in the hospital elevator from physicians ("Study finds disregard for patient confidentiality," 1995). Stories abound in which the white-jacketed "doctor" who reviews the patient record is in fact a newspaper spy. In Massachusetts a former hospital employee's password was used to obtain telephone and demographic information from confidential files, which was then used to make obscene telephone calls to patients and their families (Brelis 1995).

A New England health maintenance organization in 1995 made front-page news when the organization failed to adjust its clinical note-taking practices while making the transition to a new centralized record and computerized notes system (Bass 1995). Some patients carrying their own charts from one appointment to another noticed detailed psychiatric notes included in the same folder with progress notes from medical visits. Mental health workers had not considered altering their detailed "process" notes when the psychiatric and medical records were combined.

Systemic Risk From Information Flow

Controlling the flow of patient-identifiable clinical information within and outside of a healthcare organization is difficult because our healthcare "system" was never designed to do this in a coordinated fashion. Information recorded for one purpose is used for another. Most patients (and providers, for that matter) are poorly informed about the extent to which information is copied and stored beyond the clinic or hospital. For example, clinical information typically recorded in the course of a medical or psychiatric visit is frequently released to insurers to verify that services have been performed. From there, it may be re-released to the Medical Information Bureau, a nonprofit trade association that again re-releases it to other insurers and member organizations who seek to reduce the likelihood of fraudulent claims.

Another example involves prescriptions. Retail pharmacies use diagnostic and treatment information to support their claims to pharmacy benefits managers, who in turn use the information to perform utilization review and to suggest generic substitutions to the patient's physician. State groups, including the health department, the bureau of vital statistics, and the agency collecting hospital discharge data, also store copies of patient information to fulfill their various objectives. Groups such as the Joint Commission on Accreditation of Healthcare Organizations (JCAHO) and the National Committee for Quality Assurance (NCQA) obtain and store clinical information for regulatory reasons.

It is ironic that videotape rental lists receive far more protection by federal legislation than health information does. Lack of policy leads to inadvertent and deliberate sharing of data. One company that buys and sells patient drug information for the pharmaceutical industry (Kolata 1995) said that the data sold to the company often included patient names and Social Security numbers because the sellers of the data were not sophisticated enough to remove them. Calls by consumer advocates to strictly limit the flow of identifiable information within the healthcare industry, and to intensify efforts to obtain informed consent, have been met with support from a number of groups (Woodward 1995). But simple steps to improve the situation have been difficult, in part because there is no singular view on which uses of medical information are reasonable and which are not. A comprehensive National Research Council report on confidentiality in healthcare (Clayton et al. 1997, pp. 3–19) points out that

> systemic risks arise from deep differences among stakeholders as to what constitutes fair information

practice. Every stakeholder that receives data about a patient has an argument to support its claims about a bona fide need for patient information. No consensus exists across society regarding the legitimacy of these needs and against which they can be independently assessed. Nor does consensus exist regarding the uses made of such information.

The report differentiates the challenge in healthcare from other industries:

> [T]his lack of consensus differentiates the security problem in the health care field from that of the military or financial communities, for example, where a general consensus on information policy exists. As a consequence, security technology and practices from these other communities should be adopted only with great care.

Distinct from the "systemic risk" problem, it is the "insider threat" that has been an immediate concern for security experts in healthcare organizations.

Risk From the Insider Threat

Within an organization, it is inevitable that some with access to patient information may look at it without an appropriate reason. This is especially easy with the paper record (Wald 1996), which offers clinical, scheduling, billing, demographic, and other kinds of information to each staff member. Access controls are limited; self-control is the main strategy for protecting information from inappropriate viewing. There is little or no tracking of the use of paper-based information. Records spend uncharted time on desks, in automobiles, and in unlocked file drawers while awaiting "processing." They are copied and faxed for a variety of reasons. Security experts agree that for a few hundred dollars almost any experienced investigator can obtain health information about an individual.

The increasing use of computers to store and retrieve health information permits the introduction of tighter controls over who has access to what information. This in itself can help to clearly identify the number and type of individuals with authorized access to health information, but security strategies with information systems are often not addressed adequately. Furthermore, the features of simultaneous access and availability over a wide geographical area offered by computers offset the diminished risk from blocking access to unauthorized users.

Laws and Regulations Affecting Privacy

Despite a strong culture of privacy felt by many in the United States, nowhere in the Constitution is there an explicit statement of a right to privacy. Privacy practices in general are based on federal statutes and state laws. Privacy in healthcare is also influenced by recent legislation called the Health Insurance Portability and Accountability Act (HIPAA) of 1996. The overall effect of federal and state regulations is a thin patchwork that allows needed flexibility in the management of health information in most settings but provides inadequate guidance to many organizations in the healthcare industry (Clayton et al. 1997).

Federal and State Laws

The Privacy Act of 1974 established protections for personal information in record-keeping systems operated by, or subcontracted to, federal agencies. It provides that individuals have the right to know about their personal information being stored in a governmental system, have the right to access and retain a copy of that information, and have the right to prevent disclosure without explicit consent (for uses beyond the original consent and certain "routine" uses). It also provides a mechanism for allowing individuals to request amendments to their record in the case of inaccurate, incomplete, irrelevant, or untimely information. Organizations such as the Indian Health Service, the Department of Veterans Affairs, the Department of Defense, the Health Care Financing Administration (HCFA) for Medicare beneficiaries, and other federally funded registries must adhere to these protections.

Federal statutes covering federally funded drug or alcohol abuse treatment facilities restrict release of information pertaining to the diagnosis, treatment, or identity of persons cared for at those facilities. These supersede state laws on confidentiality. The Americans With Disabilities Act (ADA) has no provisions to cover health information but has deterred employers in some instances from collecting and maintaining information that would subject the employer to litigation under the ADA (Clayton et al. 1997, pp. 2–3). The Medicare rules for participation by hospitals in Medicare programs require confidentiality procedures such as release of information only with consent and protections against unauthorized access.

The HIPAA established federal standards for the availability and portability of group and individual health insurance coverage, helping individuals who change jobs, lose jobs, or otherwise lose their health insurance to maintain coverage. It also limits the "pre-existing condition" exclusions commonly used by insurers to deny coverage. In this context, it seeks to promote electronic exchange of administrative and financial data to improve appropriate information sharing, while taking steps to protect the confidentiality and security of transmitted health information. As described in the National Research Council report (Clayton et al. 1997, pp. 2–12),

> The Secretary [of Health and Human Services is] required to adopt security standards that take into account (1) the technical capabilities of record systems used to maintain health information; (2) the costs of security measures; (3) the need for training persons who have access to health information; (4) the value of audit trails in computerized record systems; and (5) the needs and capabilities of small health care providers and rural health care providers. [HIPAA] requires that each person who maintains or transmits health information shall maintain reasonable and appropriate administrative, technical, and physical safeguards to ensure the integrity and confidentiality of the information; to protect against any reasonably anticipated (1) threats or hazards to the security or integrity of the information and (2) unauthorized uses or disclosures of the information; and to ensure that a health care clearinghouse, if it is part of a larger organization, has policies and security procedures that isolate its activities with respect to processing information in a manner that prevents unauthorized access to such information.

The implementation and enforcement of HIPAA will unfold in the near future. Its effect on the vulnerability of patient information to confidentiality threats remains to be seen.

Nonuniform state statutes and regulations provide for the use and dissemination of health information, the right of patients to review their medical records, and special protections of certain types of health data such as HIV status, substance abuse, and mental health information. Many states lack these provisions. Even when present, these regulations are weakened by a lack of penalties for violating them and by little or no attention to limiting information redisclosure (Gostin et al. 1996; Institute of Medicine 1994). There is much room for individual interpretation within the loose framework of state and federal laws.

Industry Regulation

Triennial evaluations of healthcare organizations by the JCAHO include surveys of confidentiality policies and practices. JCAHO defines an effective process as one that addresses 1) access permission (who gains access to what information); 2) release permission (when information may be released and when information may be deleted from the record); 3) countermeasures to intrusion, corruption, or damage; 4) the user's commitment to confidentiality; and 5) actions taken when a breach is detected (Joint Commission on Accreditation of Healthcare Organizations 1997). However, little detailed examination takes place during site visits. Organizations usually only need to show that policies and procedures are in place rather than how well (or poorly) they are working.

Exceptions to Confidentiality Protections

To protect an individual's care, and the public health interest, most jurisdictions allow that information may be released without the usual consents for reasons of patient incompetence, for involuntary commitment, for duties to inform third parties, and for reportable conditions such as certain communicable diseases and child abuse (Kaplan and Sadock 1989).

Organizational Strategies to Protect Confidentiality

A series of well-planned, iterative steps are helpful in developing and maintaining effective confidentiality strategies within an organization, whether large or small. Assessment of current strengths and weaknesses, clear articulation of policies and procedures, and implementation of action plans that reflect principles, common sense, and balance between competing priorities have the greatest cumulative effect in reducing unnecessary patient risks.

Establish a Confidentiality Mandate

A crucial first step is the consensus building and critical buy-in by top executives and the board of directors (or similar authority) that a mandate for confidentiality protections for patients exists and that it will be supported by the organization. The task of writing or updating a policy can help create clarity among key members of an organi-

zation. Some large organizations create a security officer role, typically reporting to the head of quality assurance or risk management (or heading either department). Some organizations have adopted a "Patient/Client Bill of Rights," which can be an effective vehicle for communicating internally and a teaching tool for the patient.

The confidentiality mission is directly driven by principles. It is also motivated by the assumption that confidentiality breaches occur both unintentionally and, at times, deliberately in every health organization. The Pentagon predicted 500,000 attacks on its information systems in 1996, based on collected data (General Accounting Office 1996). Just as incident reports in acute care settings are now recognized to be insensitive in estimating the rates of adverse drug events (Cullen et al. 1995) (much less monitoring and correcting them), executives who are reassured by few or no reports of confidentiality problems need to perform more systematic study; typically, this will reveal multiple areas of concern.

Establish Policies and Procedures

The organizational mandate is then translated into specific policies and resultant activities addressing areas such as 1) informed consent; 2) information collection, storage, retrieval, and release; 3) information flow within the office/clinic/hospital/organizational setting; 4) education and awareness training for all employees; and 5) careful credentialing of workers and coordination of privileges with human resources. As pointed out in the National Research Council report, systemic flow of information is a large source of risk that must be understood and communicated with patients. Education and awareness training are large, recurring expenses that must be budgeted and carried out for any overall approach to succeed. Credentialing is important because patients rely heavily on professional codes of conduct in the use of their information to protect them from inappropriate disclosure. Coordination with human resources is more important with the widening use of information systems: timely creation, deletion, and modification of passwords permitting a user access to patient data are paramount. All five of these areas are scrutinized carefully during the investigation of an alleged breach and may affect an eventual settlement.

It is common for information requirements and information flow to vary between different clinical settings, such as acute care versus outpatient care versus emergency care areas. Security procedures must be tailored to each setting. Furthermore, information practices evolve over time. When insurance reporting requirements change, or two clinics become one, or new information systems are designed and deployed, the rationale and effectiveness of current security and confidentiality strategies must be reevaluated in the new context. Information system changes are increasingly common and have particular importance in security and confidentiality because of their effect on information flow and information use.

Role of Information Systems

The use of computers to assist in medical and psychiatric care has grown substantially in the past decade and will continue to expand rapidly in the near future. Historically, most early systems used in healthcare were for billing and administrative purposes, but early adopters of clinical systems (1970s and 1980s) have shown that substantial improvements in care and control of costs can be achieved through the use of well-planned and carefully implemented projects. Interest in automation has intensified with the rise of managed care and pressures to contain healthcare costs. Many believe that electronic patient record systems are essential despite their cost and complexity because they 1) track patient information over time, 2) perform outcomes measurement, 3) proactively guide care delivery from the acute care to the outpatient to the home-based setting, and 4) provide detailed analyses of costs, quality, and efficiency of health services delivery.

The confidentiality-related capabilities of automated systems include the ability to block access to a record or parts of the record to selected users, to prompt users to declare their role with a patient before looking at the chart, to selectively display information to a particular user, and to inform the patient (or others) who has looked at his or her record and why (Wald 1996). These functions are systematically performed with paper-based systems. Of particular use in one mental health setting are "monitored notes" (Wald et al. 1994), which allow the author of a note containing particularly sensitive information to change its status to "monitored." This change does not restrict access to the note but causes a text message to be presented to the user who opens the note, requesting a detailed reason for why the note is about to be accessed. This permits the user to pause and consider whether it is important to view that particular note. If the note is read, an e-mail is automatically generated to the note's author with the date, time, user, and reason for lookup.

Automated systems also lead to new vulnerabilities. As the old norm of lost records and incomplete records gives way to "just in time" records that are up-to-date, viewed wherever and whenever is convenient, and filtered logically to show just the relevant information to each care team member, the potential number of users, and their ease of access to information, increases. Security for information systems can be violated intentionally or accidentally and may lead to serious leaks of information unless strong countermeasures are employed physically (e.g., locked doors), technically, and administratively. Comprehensive reviews of security and confidentiality in healthcare information systems are available. An unintended benefit of introducing information technology in healthcare has been the stimulation of vigorous discussion and debate about the development of more effective privacy and confidentiality strategies in healthcare.

Accountability and Access Control Strategies

Confidentiality strategies essentially fall into two broad categories—they either guide appropriate use of information by heightening accountability or control access to information. Accountability strategies such as 1) a signed employee agreement to protect patient information, 2) an acknowledgment that disciplinary action up to and including termination is taken as a result of misuse of information, 3) a unique password to authenticate the user to the information system, 4) reminders in public areas and on the computer screen to control discussion and sharing of information beyond its intended uses, and 5) monitored notes are examples of techniques that increase an individual's sense of responsibility and motivation to conform to established policies and practices in an organization (to "do the right thing"). Accountability strategies form the foundation of all confidentiality strategies.

Access restriction strategies limit a user's ability to view patient information. Examples include physical security procedures such as locked doors, surveillance of work areas for unauthorized individuals, and software locks (passwords). Ultimately, each access restriction strategy requires strong authentication (positive identification) of individuals in order to work. This is well served by identification badges and information system passwords. Authentication via the telephone and fax is also important. Weakened access restrictions are problematic. Passwords that are inappropriately shared, are easily guessed or obtained (e.g., from the sticker on the keyboard), or persist for terminated employees can compromise the patient. Special access controls for health information that is considered "sensitive" have helped patients by protecting their mental health records, for example. But maintaining special protections in healthcare, characterized more by loose management of information than by consistent controls, is insufficient to protect patients.

Overcoming Confidentiality Barriers

Acceptable levels of protection for health information are possible with a systematic approach to confidentiality, provided that several barriers are overcome. First, there has been a lack of awareness within organizations, between organizations, and in the public. This situation is changing rapidly, but continual emphasis and effort regarding confidentiality are needed. Second, there has been no coordinated public (and private) demand for benchmarking and monitoring confidentiality of health information. Third, there are few economic incentives for spending the time, effort, and money on revamping information management within organizations. Avoidance of lawsuits can generate some budgetary justification, but the sustained commitment to improving policies, procedures, and technology has not easily been justified by healthcare executives without near-catastrophic incidents ("Computers, confidentiality, and health care," 1995). Fourth, consolidation and increased competition in healthcare have diverted attention from security to dozens of other urgent priorities of organizations, many of which have more tangible benefits (or avoided costs). Fifth, simple solutions do not exist.

Risk cannot be eliminated. Strategies that are developed one year must be reevaluated in subsequent years and as the organization and its technology change. Focus on access control alone is insufficient. Arbitrary decisions about which information will be considered (and tagged) "very sensitive" or "sensitive" (all clinical information) have some effect but still miss the mark. Systemic flow of information throughout the healthcare industry is not centrally regulated or controlled. Individuals will always behave imperfectly. Access controls alone are insufficient because it is impossible to accurately predict what information will be needed by what user at what time for what purpose.

Optimizing confidentiality requires the reexamination of information-sharing practices within and out-

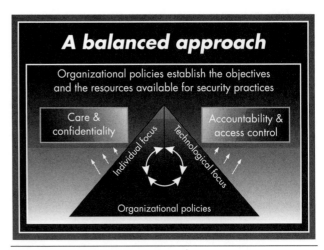

FIGURE 14–2. Key balances in confidentiality strategies within an organization.

side an organization. Improved accountability methods for both paper-based and electronic information are important. A proactive systems approach that assumes that breaches will occur, and takes countermeasures to safeguard against them, is critical.

Conclusion

The challenge of maintaining confidentiality in healthcare has become more difficult and must be addressed from a variety of perspectives (Affiliated Health Information Networks of New England Patient Confidentiality and Privacy Work Group 1996; Bunschoten 1996; Computerized Patient Record Institute; Donaldson and Lohr 1994; Lawrence 1994; Tomes 1994). Information collected for one purpose is frequently used for another. Health care organizations often have inadequate policies and partially effective strategies for improving confidentiality and security yet are growing more reliant on health data to improve quality and lower costs of care. Consumers, increasingly worried by the threat of a deliberate or unintentional breach of confidentiality involving a healthcare organization, are also worried about the growing disclosure risks as a result of systemic sharing and aggregation of information.

The fundamental tension between care and confidentiality will persist. Balanced efforts toward clear policies, individual behavior shaped by ongoing training and awareness, and careful use of technology can lead to sustained risk reductions for the patient through access control strategies and accountability strategies (Figure 14–2). Protecting confidentiality as information flows beyond the individual organization will require coordinated efforts and regulations that do not exist today. As healthcare matures as a "knowledge industry," it will become more important for control of person-identifiable information transactions to be in some way "brokered" by the patient or an authorized representative.

Consistency among policies, practices, and procedures, including strong authentication steps, careful access controls, and detailed logging of when, how, and why information is used, will go a long way toward protecting the patient. Changes in healthcare organizations, in the alignment of clinical and economic incentives, in the form and use of the health record, and in the technologies for both sharing and protecting information will challenge users of health information to maintain consistency and prioritize the protection of the individual.

References

Affiliated Health Information Networks of New England Patient Confidentiality and Privacy Work Group: Confidentiality of health data—an exploration of principles, policies and practices. Proceedings of a public meeting to announce interim standards, March 28, 1996. Boston, Massachusetts Health Data Consortium, 1996

Bakker AR: Security in medical information systems, in Yearbook of Medical Informatics 1993. Edited by Bemmel van JH, McCray AT. Schattauer Verlag, Stuttgart, Germany, 1994, pp 52–60

Bartlett J: Bartlett's Quotations. Little, Brown, 1968, p 88

Bass A: HMO puts confidential records on-line. Boston Globe, March 7, 1995, p 1

Bates DW, Cullen DJ, Laird N, et al: Incidence of adverse drug events and potential adverse drug events: implications for prevention: ADE Prevention Study Group. JAMA 274:29–34, 1995

Bernstein N: Lives on File: The erosion of privacy—a special report: personal files via computer offer money and pose threat. New York Times, June 12, 1997, p 1

Brelis M: Patients' files allegedly used for obscene calls. Boston Globe, March 11, 1995, p 1

Bunschoten B: Striking a Balance Between Access and Security. Health Data Management, May 1996, pp 69–72

Clayton PD, Boebert EW, DeFriese GH, et al: For the Record: Protecting Electronic Health Information: A Report of the National Research Council. Washington, DC, National Academy Press, 1997

Computerized Patient Record Institute (CPRI); http://www.cpri.org; 1000 East Woodfield Road, Suite 102, Schaumburg, IL 60173; (708) 706-6746; FAX (708) 706-6747

Computers, confidentiality, and health care (advertisement). Boston Globe, March 17, 1995, p 17

Cullen DJ, Bates DW. Small SD, et al: The incident reporting system does not detect adverse drug events: a problem for quality improvement. Jt Comm J Qual Improv 21(10):541–548, 1995

Deloitte and Touche: U.S. Hospitals and the Future of Health Care. Philadelphia, PA, DeLoitte and Touche, 1996

Department of Health and Human Services, Public Health Service, Agency for Health Care Policy and Research: Depression in primary care: detection, diagnosis, and treatment. J Psychosoc Nurs Ment Health Serv 31(6):19–28, 1993

General Accounting Office: Information Security: Computer Attacks at Department of Defense Pose Increasing Risks. Washington, DC, General Accounting Office, May 1996

Gostin LO, Lazzarini Z, Neslund VS, et al: The public health information infrastructure: a national review of the law on health information privacy. JAMA 275:1921–1927, 1996

Institute of Medicine, Committee on Regional Health Data Networks: Health Data in the Information Age: Use, Disclosure, and Privacy. Edited by Donaldson MS, Lohr KN. Washington, DC, National Academy Press, 1994

Joint Commission on Accreditation of Healthcare Organizations: Comprehensive Accreditation Manual for Hospitals—The Official Handbook. Oakbrook Terrace, IL, Joint Commission on Accreditation of Healthcare Organizations, 1997

Kaplan SI, Sadock BJ: Comprehensive Textbook of Psychiatry, 5th Edition. Baltimore, MD, Williams & Wilkins, 1989

Kolata G: When patients' records are commodities for sale. New York Times, November 15, 1995, p 1

Lawrence LM: Safeguarding the confidentiality of automated medical information. Journal on Quality Improvement 20(11):639–646, 1994

Murphy TV, Pastor P, Medley F: Factors associated with unnecessary immunization given to children. Pediatr Infect Dis J 16:47–52, 1997

Pestotnik SL, Evans RS, Burke JP, et al: Therapeutic antibiotic monitoring: surveillance using a computerised expert system. Am J Med 88:43–48, 1990

Petersen LA, Brennan TA, O'Neil AC, et al: Does housestaff discontinuity of care increase the risk for preventable adverse events? Ann Intern Med 121:866–872, 1994

Schoenenberger RA, Tanasijevic MJ, Jha A, et al: Appropriateness of antiepileptic drug level monitoring. JAMA 274:1622–1626, 1995

Study finds disregard for patient confidentiality. San Francisco Chronicle, July 4, 1995, p A8

Tierney WM, McDonald CJ, Martin DK, et al: Computerized display of past test results: effect on outpatient testing. Ann Intern Med 107:569–574, 1987

Tomes JP: Healthcare Privacy & Confidentiality: The Complete Legal Guide. Chicago, IL, Probus Publishing, 1994

Wald JS: Dialogue privacy protection: paper or computer records? Best strategies for clinical delivery systems. Behavioral Healthcare Tomorrow 5(1):39, 42, 44, 1996

Wald JS: Optimizing patient confidentiality through the use of health care information systems, in Proceedings of the Annual HIMSS Conference 3:61–70, 1997

Wald JS, Rind D, Safran C: Protecting confidentiality in an electronic medical record: feedback to the author when someone reads a clinical note. American Medical Informatics Association Spring Proceedings, 1994, p 42

Woodward B: The computer-based patient record and confidentiality. N Engl J Med 333:1419–1422, 1995

❖ Section IV ❖

New Concepts for a Changing Behavioral Health System

Judith H. Browne, R.N., M.S.N., Section Editor

Introduction

Judith H. Browne, R.N., M.S.N.

We in healthcare are now in a stage like chrysalis. In the world of moths and butterflies, chrysalis is that stage during metamorphosis when the insect is in tumultuous change but still wrapped in its cocoon, and anything seems possible. At this point in the development of healthcare, it is difficult to imagine how we might emerge. The increasing need to control costs has set in motion a metamorphosis that calls into question our most basic underlying principles about healthcare. Healthcare costs have been on the rise for some time; it is not a new problem. In 1974, Lewis Thomas, who was then president of the Memorial Sloan-Kettering Cancer Center in New York, addressed the issue of skyrocketing healthcare costs:

> Whatever sum we spent last year was only discovered after we'd spent it, and nobody can be sure what next year's bill will be. The social scientists, attracted by problems of this magnitude, are beginning to swarm in from all quarters to take a closer look, and the economists are all over the place, pursing their lips and shaking their heads....(Thomas 1974/1995)

Social scientists and economists are not the only ones who have an interest in the problem of escalating healthcare costs. As government leaders move toward managed care to control those costs, others have come forward to voice their opinions and stake their claims. Any taxpayer or citizen, in fact, has a significant stake in the outcome of this debate. We are all, in a very real sense, stakeholders in the process.

Each day we hear or see a different view of the matter. Whenever such a flurry of activity occurs, with so many stakeholders involved, it is difficult to discern the "true" picture. Those of us in the profession, especially, must keep our perspective. That may prove especially troublesome as we try to balance our personal economic needs and our professional commitments to those in our care.

As we discuss new roles for behavioral health players, we learn from Sabin and Borus, in Chapter 15, how the science and economics of behavioral healthcare, not new knowledge, are shaping that change. The emerging domain of primary behavioral healthcare will provide opportunities for strong alliances between specialty behavioral healthcare clinicians and primary care physicians and their allied nurse practitioners. Sabin and Borus discuss the reconfiguration of the boundaries between primary medical care and behavioral healthcare, offering examples of models for implementing the new concepts. Klamen, Flaherty, and Astrachan discuss in Chapter 16 the implications of these developments for psychiatrists, and I examine in Chapter 17 the implications for other healthcare professionals. Multiple avenues of service delivery have spawned diverse career pathways, and new and dynamic careers in medicine will surely surface. A move away from individual craftsmanship and a "duty to the patient" toward a situation in which accountability is shifting to a broader responsibility to society and the payers is significantly changing the roles that physicians play. This is resulting in an increasing role as a collaborator with primary care physicians and emerging opportunities in the growth of specialty areas such as geropsychiatry, neuropsychiatry, and women's mental health. Lazarus notes in Chapter 18 that one-third of the physicians already in practice change careers. This is even more likely in administrative roles. Lazarus addresses careers that are likely to emerge in greater demand such as "physician executives" and "entrepreneurs" and those that cater to behavioral problems of a chronic nature.

We are not the only ones who will play a part. As we learn from Mowbray, Moxley, and Van Tosh, in Chapter 19, and from Lefley, in Chapter 20, we will be working collaboratively and side by side with primary consumers and their families, who are taking increasingly more active roles in the design and delivery of care. The move away from the focus on pathogenesis, in which families were viewed as contributing to the cause of the problem, has led to a growing appreciation that families can play a vital role in the recovery and rehabilitative process. Consumers and their supporting families have much to teach us.

We who specialize in behavioral healthcare have learned the importance of treating the mind and the body in an integrated fashion. Many caregivers take an even more holistic approach, knowing that it is important to deal with human beings in all their aspects: physical, mental, emotional, cultural, and spiritual. Consumers and their families are often the ones who guide us to this vision.

Developments in managed care and partnerships in the public and private sectors have shown government policymakers that specialized program management can preserve quality behavioral healthcare and expand access while responding to mounting budget pressures. Partnerships that include managed care organizations, providers, consumers, and their families can create innovative programs that expand access to behavioral healthcare, integrate primary and behavioral healthcare, reduce costs, and increase consumer satisfaction. The fiscal realities have provided increased pressure for caregivers to document the value of care from a clinical outcome, member satisfaction, and cost perspective. Although this approach is generating useful data that validate the effectiveness of behavioral care, legitimate concerns exist about how to ensure appropriate decision making that provides the best long-term outcomes. Sabin reminds us that the leaders in the field need to ensure that practice changes driven by economic incentives are supported by a strong knowledge base built on decades of research.

What is certain is that everyone has an opinion about the matter, and the debate continues. Whatever the outcome, we encourage the debate and hope that what takes wing will provide long-term improvements in service and behavioral care outcomes.

References

Thomas L: The Lives of a Cell: Notes of a Biology Watcher. 1974. Reprinted, New York, Viking Penguin, 1995

❖ 15 ❖

Changing Roles in Primary Behavioral Healthcare

James E. Sabin, M.D.

Jonathan F. Borus, M.D.

Clinical, administrative, and financial relationships between the specialty mental health sector and primary care medicine are changing rapidly. This process of change will continue with even more speed, flux, and potential for both benefit and harm in the near future. If research and widely available publications had the power to drive practice change, more change would have occurred well before now. The fact that primary care clinicians provide treatment to the majority of patients with mental disorders has been abundantly clear since the mid-1980s (Regier et al. 1978), and the fact that as many as half of the patients seen in primary care do not have any definable medical disorder has been well known even longer (Stoeckle et al. 1964). Health system inertia, vested professional interests, and paradigms that sharply separate mind from body (Beitman et al. 1982) have perpetuated relatively rigid barriers between mental and physical healthcare. The changes we are now witnessing are driven by the economics of the managed care revolution, not new knowledge. It is up to leaders in the field to ensure that practice changes that ensue from the new economic incentives of managed care build on the strong knowledge base provided by more than three decades of research and clinical experimentation.

This chapter takes as its title the recent term for the new relationships emerging between specialty mental health services and primary care. In the complex contemporary environment, *primary behavioral healthcare* refers to at least three related but distinct activities: 1) behavioral healthcare delivered by primary care clinicians, 2) specialty behavioral healthcare delivered in the primary care setting, and 3) innovative programs that integrate elements of primary care and specialty behavioral healthcare into new formats. Each of these enterprises reflects an aspect of primary behavioral healthcare; none encompasses the full scope or future of the field.

We define primary behavioral healthcare as the clinical domain concerned with effectiveness (enhancing clinical outcomes) and efficiency (obtaining maximum value per unit of expenditure) at the interface of specialty behavioral healthcare and primary care. Because the clinical techniques and program formats that make up primary behavioral healthcare are still very much in flux, we have organized this chapter around a series of concepts and strategic considerations that leaders and front-line clinicians will need to understand in order to influence development in the field. We first address the reconfiguration of boundaries between primary medical care and specialty behavioral healthcare. We then consider behavioral healthcare approaches to three clinical populations—patients with what have traditionally been conceptualized as medical disorders; patients with traditional psychiatric disorders; and patients with somatization, who are sometimes dismissed as the "worried well." Although in clinical circumstances these groups often overlap, we believe it is heuristically useful to examine them separately. Because our objective is to provide practical administrative guidance we present a series of program examples (introduced by bullets) to illustrate major models for implementing primary behavioral healthcare concepts. Finally, we speculate about strategies to further develop this area in the coming years.

The Emerging Primacy of Primary Care

From an international perspective, the U.S. healthcare system has been unusual in the degree to which it has been dominated by the medical specialties—including the mental health specialties—in terms of leadership, funding, status, and clinician numbers (Block et al. 1996). In other countries, virtually all efforts to improve access, public health, and what the British call "value for money" depend on robust primary care leadership of the health system. The managed care revolution appears to be redressing the imbalance between primary care and the specialties in the United States by making primary care clinicians captains of the referral process and, frequently, financial gatekeepers as well.

Primary care physicians and their allied nurse practitioners (which we henceforth refer to collectively as PCPs) have the incentive under capitation and other fixed reimbursement systems to avoid excessive referrals to specialists and to provide as much of the care themselves as possible. They must do so under increasingly tight time restrictions and clinical productivity requirements. The high prevalence of behavioral disorders seen in primary medical care settings has raised a number of issues concerning the boundaries, communications, and collaboration between PCPs and behavioral healthcare clinicians. Issues currently being addressed include 1) how much of the treatment for behavioral disorders PCPs can, want to, and are prepared to provide within the restrictions of their practice settings, 2) what PCPs want from behavioral healthcare clinicians in terms of teaching, consultation, and communication to coordinate care, and 3) what administrative guidelines and mechanisms are needed to optimize the efficiency of the PCP–behavioral healthcare interface.

Within the specialty behavioral healthcare sector itself, managed care has fostered adoption of a primary care model for psychotherapeutic practice (Cummings and VandenBos 1979). Primary care clinicians organize treatment around the chief complaint and anticipate a continuing relationship in which the patient may return to deal with other issues. Using a primary care approach allows behavioral healthcare clinicians to focus on the current symptoms or developmental impasse without taking a superficial or reductionistic view of the patient, combining empathy with efficiency (Sabin 1995).

In addition to the many clinical, epidemiologic, and conceptual reasons for specialty behavioral healthcare clinicians to adopt a primary care model and work closely with PCPs, the fact that power and financial control increasingly reside within the primary care sector makes seeking close collaboration a practical necessity (Wulsin 1996). In the years to come, PCPs will become progressively more influential in determining how much money is allocated to behavioral healthcare and which clinicians and groups become part of care networks. Prudent psychiatric administrators will treat their increasingly powerful primary care colleagues as both crucial customers and vital potential allies. The fact that behavioral interventions have the potential to improve patient satisfaction, clinician satisfaction, and medical outcomes while reducing overall healthcare costs will be the most important leverage for developing these alliances.

Using Behavioral Healthcare Expertise to Improve Care for Patients With Medical Disorders

Psychosocial factors and coexisting psychiatric conditions can make many of the cardiovascular, gastrointestinal, respiratory, and other medical disorders treated in primary care more severe or refractory to treatment. Multiple studies amply demonstrate that psychiatric and substance abuse comorbidities increase the impact and costs of medical conditions. In the Medical Outcomes Study, patients with coronary artery disease and depressive symptoms lost twice as much social functioning as patients with coronary artery disease alone (Wells et al. 1989). Patients with diabetes or hypertension who had comorbid anxiety disorder had substantially worse mental and physical function than did similar patients without anxiety disorder (Sherbourne et al. 1996). In a study of patients undergoing ambulatory electrocardiographic monitoring, feelings of tension, frustration, and sadness doubled the risk of myocardial ischemia during the subsequent hour (Gullette et al. 1997). Depression, cognitive impairment, high interpersonal sensitivity, and hostility all predicted increased medical hospital utilization over a 4-year period (Saravay et al. 1996). Finally, comorbid depressive or anxiety disorders led to persistent, substantial increases in medical costs above and beyond the costs associated with the psychiatric condition itself (Simon et al. 1995a, 1995b), and comorbid substance abuse leads to substantial increases in utilization and medical costs not only for the designated patient but also for family members (Holder 1987).

Behavioral interventions can often improve clinical status and reduce overall costs for patients whose medical conditions are complicated by dysfunctional behavioral and cognitive patterns and by psychiatric comorbidities. With the aging of the general population and increasing prevalence of chronic medical conditions, behavioral interventions for patients with medical disorders will be increasingly important. The following four examples illustrate the kinds of behavioral healthcare interventions that have been effective for patients with medical disorders:

- Between 1905 and 1923, Joseph Hersey Pratt treated tuberculosis in poor urban patients, using what he called the class method, in weekly sessions that met in the basement of a Boston church (Sabin 1990). Pratt initially designed the class as an efficiency measure but soon recognized that the group format improved morale, enhanced adherence to the demanding medical regimen of enforced rest on tenement rooftops, and allowed his patients to achieve outcomes at least as good as those achieved by the well-to-do at the best tuberculosis sanitoria.

- In the 1970s, Spiegel developed a group program for women with metastatic breast cancer on the hypothesis—confirmed by the study—that the group experience would improve the women's mood and coping with their malignancy (Spiegel et al. 1981). At the 10-year follow-up, Spiegel made a serendipitous discovery—the patients receiving treatment in his groups survived longer (Spiegel et al. 1989). This important finding appears to have been replicated with patients whose malignant melanoma had a good prognosis. In a controlled study, patients who participated in a 6-week group program that focused on stress management, coping skills, education, and support had better mood and function, enhanced immune system performance, and—6 years later—a trend toward better survival (Fawzy et al. 1993).

- The Colorado Permanente Medical Care Program developed and studied a group program similar to the one developed by Pratt, except that the Permanente program is addressed to elderly patients (with ages, on average, in the 70s) with at least one chronic medical condition (Beck et al. 1997). The remarkably simple format, replicated at Vanguard Medical Associates and elsewhere, has PCPs meeting monthly with groups of elderly patients for 90–120 minutes. Meetings include education about topics as diverse as medication management, emergency care, arthritis, depression, advance directives, and addictions, and the meetings include time for questions, socialization, and group involvement in planning for future meetings. Patients in the Colorado study reported increased satisfaction with their medical care, increased rates of immunizations for pneumonia and influenza and completion of advance directives, decreased emergency room visits, and decreased hospital readmissions. The PCPs reported increased satisfaction in their care of older patients. Taking into account the full cost of the intervention, the Colorado group found that it produced a 5% decrease in overall medical costs.

- The Arthritis Self-Management Program (ASMP) developed at Stanford University represents an innovative collaboration between clinician-researchers and the voluntary sector. The intervention consists of a 12-hour program taught in six 2-hour-long weekly sessions, generally led by trained lay leaders, many of whom themselves have arthritis (Lorig and Holman 1993). The curriculum, which is designed to increase the patients' ability to cope with the impact of arthritis, leads to a prolonged reduction in pain, depression, and medical visits despite continued progression of the underlying condition (Lorig et al. 1993). To date, more than 100,000 arthritis patients have participated in the ASMP.

Given the increasing burden of chronic illness in an aging population, combined with an increasing pressure for productivity in primary care practice that leads to brief, symptom-focused visits, group or class-based interventions provide the same promise of efficiency and clinical effectiveness that Pratt identified in the early 1900s. The evidence suggests that patients value these interventions, and many studies report some combination of improved clinical status, reduced cost, and, almost invariably, clinician satisfaction. Lorig (1995) argued persuasively that a validated educational intervention such as ASMP should be regarded as a medically necessary component of treatment, not an optional frill. By the late 1990s, continuing care group programs for patients with chronic psychiatric disorders (Sabin 1978) were well recognized and widely applied. The next decades will almost certainly see development and dissemination of similar behavioral healthcare approaches to a widening range of chronic medical illnesses as part of the overall treatment of these conditions in managed healthcare systems (Wagner et al. 1996).

Treating Psychiatric Disorders in Primary Care

The best-conceptualized model for treating psychiatric disorders in primary care comes from the United Kingdom, which has provided universal access to PCPs under the National Health Service (NHS) since 1948. In the early 1980s, Goldberg (1991) found that of the 250–315 per 1,000 people in the British population who had a mental disorder, 230 saw their PCP, 100 were given the correct diagnosis, and 20 (less than 10%) were referred to behavioral healthcare specialists. Jenkins (1992), then principal medical officer for mental health in the NHS, argued that because each PCP had on average 300–600 patients with depression and anxiety, and 7 patients with severe and persisting mental illness, the most efficient NHS approach to caring for patients with psychiatric disorders was to expect PCPs to provide treatment to the large majority of them; to support the PCPs with education, guidelines for treating

the common forms of depression and anxiety, and practice-based master's-level counselors; and to reserve use of psychiatrists for consultation to PCPs and direct treatment of the most severe and most complex cases.

Although the United States has relatively more behavioral healthcare specialists and fewer PCPs than the United Kingdom, data from the Epidemiologic Catchment Area Survey in the early 1980s showed that even prior to the growth of managed care, PCPs in the United States provided care for a larger segment (43%) of people with mental and addiction disorders than did behavioral specialists (40%) (Regier et al. 1993). In the foreseeable future, diagnosis and treatment of psychiatric disorders will depend even more on the primary care sector, as managed care organizations require PCP approval for specialty referrals and put PCPs at financial risk for the costs of specialty care.

Depression, as a common psychiatric disorder in primary care practice and cause of substantial morbidity and mortality, is the best studied psychiatric condition in primary care. In the Medical Outcomes Study, although depressive symptoms were more common in primary care practice than were arthritis, diabetes, heart disease, or lung disease, only half of the depressed patients had their condition detected, with lower rates of detection in prepaid compared with fee-for-service settings (Wells et al. 1996). Comparably depressed patients are more than twice as likely to receive appropriate antidepressant treatment and counseling from psychiatrists than from PCPs. The following examples illustrate two approaches to improving outcomes for patients with psychiatric disorders in the primary care setting:

• In a remarkable series of epidemiologic and outcome studies of the clinical manifestations, costs, and treatment of depression in the primary care setting, researchers at the Group Health Cooperative of Puget Sound (GHCPS) demonstrated that a carefully managed multipronged intervention that includes patient education, systematic follow-up, education of primary care physicians, and integration of behavioral healthcare specialists into the primary care setting led to significant improvements in patient adherence to adequate antidepressant medication, satisfaction with care, and self-reported symptomatology (Katon et al. 1995). In one iteration of the authors' model a psychologist trained in a manual-guided form of cognitive-behavioral treatment provided four to six weekly appointments (2.5–3.5

contact hours) in the primary care clinic, reviewed the patient's status with a consulting psychiatrist, and brought clinical management recommendations to the PCP, who handled the medication (Katon et al. 1996). The GHCPS approach is currently being implemented and evaluated throughout the Kaiser Permanente system.

- Another innovative program that uses new communication technologies is the Massachusetts General Hospital's Psychiatric TeleConsultation Unit (PTCU), which uses integrated computer and telephonic technology to provide immediate psychiatric consultation availability to PCPs 40 hours per week. Consultation-liaison psychiatrists are available to answer PCPs' diagnostic and treatment questions about their patients. Consultation about psychopharmacologic alternatives, doses and side effects, additional behavioral interventions that might help the patient, and rapid referrals for specialist care when appropriate can all be accomplished via telephone, often while the patient is still in the PCP's office. This service has been very well received by the PCPs and demonstrates psychiatry's desire to work collaboratively in serving the behavioral healthcare needs of primary care patients.

Substantial knowledge is available about accurate diagnosis and effective treatment of depression. The most promising way to improve the overall cost effectiveness of care for depression is to increase the reliability with which depressed patients are recognized, given correct diagnoses, and provided with well-established psychotherapeutic and psychopharmacologic treatments in primary care (Sturm and Wells 1995). The GHCPS demonstrated that a practical program requiring relatively modest resource investment could accomplish this goal. Although treatments and programs will continue to evolve, this is an area where psychiatric administrators can know the right thing to do.

Using Behavioral Healthcare Expertise to Improve Care for Patients Who Somatize

Lipowski (1988) provided a useful and widely accepted definition of *somatization* as "a tendency to experience and communicate somatic distress and symptoms unaccounted for by pathological findings, to attribute them to physical illness, and to seek medical help for them" (p. 1359). In one study of 500 consecutive outpatients, 80% reported at least one, and two-thirds reported multiple, symptoms, among which fatigue, back pain, dyspnea, headache, and indigestion were the most common. The majority of these symptoms were medically unexplained, and only 50% of the patients experienced benefit from the recommended medical treatment (Kroenke et al. 1990). Although symptoms are the leading reason patients visit clinicians, they "at the same time are among the last things a [clinician] wants to see" (Kroenke 1992, p. 3S). Patients with somatization experience substantial distress, seek care frequently, rarely benefit from conventional medical interventions, and create significant costs, leading to intense frustration for both patients and clinicians (Barsky and Borus 1995).

In the current environment of increased accountability for clinical and financial outcomes, patients who generate substantial costs without reaping significant benefit or experiencing satisfaction with their care represent a catastrophic healthcare system failure. Forward thinking behavioral healthcare leaders will make helping PCPs achieve better results with this large group of patients a high priority. The following three examples illustrate the kinds of programs that have been effective:

- A simple but carefully planned educative consultation, in which PCPs in Arkansas received a consultation letter with extremely practical advice about how to provide treatment to specific somatizing patients who had been identified by screening, showed that a limited but timely and precisely targeted intervention could lead to improved physical functioning and a 30% reduction in medical care costs (Rost et al. 1994; Smith et al. 1995). This educational intervention, like the PTCU program at the Massachusetts General Hospital, fits the industrial model of a just-in-time supply function, as the PCPs were given directed advice about specific patients they were currently seeing, as opposed to being encouraged to attend a grand rounds or continuing medical education program on somatization, interventions less likely to have tangible impact on clinical outcomes. The fact that the consultation was delivered by letter has extremely important practical implications, because it suggests the possibility that behavioral healthcare programs will be able to exploit electronic linkages to provide outpatient consultation services to geographically dispersed PCPs for patients with somatization and other disorders. This potential joining together of traditional consultation-liaison concepts with new communication technologies will almost certainly be an area of significant future program development.

- In a Dutch study, 6–16 hours of individual cognitive-behavioral treatment, delivered in a medical clinic by behavioral healthcare specialists focused on dysfunctional health-related cognitive patterns, has been demonstrated to decrease symptoms, improve sleep, and improve overall function (Speckens et al. 1995). Because third-party payers are unlikely to support such a resource-intensive treatment, Barsky demonstrated that a similar cognitive-behavioral intervention for somatizing high utilizers can be delivered efficiently in a group setting (Barsky 1996). A long-standing program at Vanguard Medical Associates has applied this kind of group-based approach to patients with somatization in a six-session class called the Personal Health Improvement Program, in which 5–20 patients use workbooks, structured class exercises, and homework to learn and practice new self-observational and self-management skills. A standardized leader-training program has been developed, and the intervention appears to be reproducible at other sites, conducted by leaders from a wide range of disciplines, including PCPs. Participation in the program leads to increased patient satisfaction, improved physical and emotional function, and reduced medical utilization (McLeod and Budd 1997).
- Americans invest substantial personal resources in what the American biomedical establishment calls alternative medicine. One form of primary behavioral healthcare seeks to re-engineer alternative approaches to connect them to the medical mainstream. Meditation, introduced by the Buddha 2,500 years ago, is perhaps the most widely practiced of these alternative approaches and is readily adaptable to the primary care setting, as exemplified by a program at the University of Massachusetts Medical Center involving a meditation-based stress clinic to which PCPs may easily refer distressed patients (Kabat-Zinn 1990).

These and other successful behavioral approaches to the treatment of somatization disorders share four core ingredients. First, they make the often-stigmatized somatizing patients feel welcome by taking their distress seriously and not blaming them for their condition. Second, they teach the patients practical cognitive reframing of expectations and behavioral self-management skills that can immediately be practiced and applied and that are potentially useful whether or not a diagnosable medical illness is present. Third, unlike earlier approaches to somatization, these programs do not assume that somatizing patients are "neurotics" who refuse to acknowledge underlying psychiatric disorders—an assumption that appears to have been false (Simon and VonKorff 1991) as well as offensive to the patients. Finally, and as important as the content of the programs, they apply just-in-time consultation methods, systematic leader training, and enough managerial sophistication and perseverance to overcome the usual barriers to the use of behavioral approaches with medical patients.

Future-Oriented Administrative Strategies

Medical school deans, observers and critics of the healthcare system, patient advocates, and many others recurrently lament the dehumanization of healthcare and relative neglect of integrative biopsychosocial approaches. Given that the biopsychosocial model is not difficult to understand and has great face validity and that integrative approaches of the sort described in this chapter are neither rocket science nor very costly (compared with many technological interventions), why should this much lamented separation of mind and body be such a tenacious element of healthcare in the United States?

We do not believe the problem is one of deficient evidence, concepts, pilot studies, or demonstration projects. Although studies of the effectiveness of behavioral interventions can and should be held to the highest standards of methodology and analysis, biotechnical interventions that have no better or even less research support, and that cost significantly more, are routinely implemented without controversy. To use a clinical concept, the problem appears to be one of resistance.

An adequate analysis of the barriers to implementing primary behavioral healthcare strategies would require a chapter of its own. However, the current economic pressures on healthcare, which in the United States play out through use of competitive market forces as the engine of healthcare system change, may provide the crucial kinetic energy that will allow administrators to implement long-resisted changes and disseminate new interventions. Managed care is intrinsically atheoretical, which means that the legacy of mind-body dualism has no intrinsic managerial appeal. And because management is a results-oriented process, resistances based on the vested interests of the health professions and the inertia of existing program formats do not carry significant weight. Thus, it is not unreasonable to hope that the managed care revolution can have positive implications for dissemination and implementation of valuable forms of behavioral healthcare.

Current experience suggests that many different ways of relating medical and behavioral expertise in primary care can be effective if there is close collaboration and ongoing communication among the providers to coordinate their care. Good collaboration between physically separate clinicians may be sufficient to treat uncomplicated comorbidities (e.g., lupus and depression), but some more difficult and complex biopsychosocial situations (e.g., hospice care) will require a highly integrated system with co-location and/or close in-person coordination of caregivers (Doherty et al. 1996). Although telephone, video, and electronic mail communication certainly facilitate integration of medical and behavioral components of care, physical proximity and budgetary integration are probably necessary to provide a high level of medical-behavioral integration on a sustained basis (Paulsen 1996).

Although the U.S. healthcare system has traditionally separated specialty behavioral healthcare from primary and specialty medical care, the population takes a much less specialized approach to psychosocial distress. The majority of patients with addictive and mental disorders receive treatment within the medical sector, and a substantial portion are seen in the alternative medicine, nonmedical human services, and nonprofessional voluntary sectors (Regier et al. 1993). Contemporary models of primary care practice, which describe the PCP-patient dialogue as potentially "meander[ing] seamlessly and meaningfully into conversations about work, friendships, hopes, worldviews, and faith" (Inui 1996, p. 171), offer a strong foundation for a central PCP role in delivering behavioral healthcare. However, this kind of care takes time, and many reimbursement schemes punish PCPs who want to provide it in their practices (Eisenberg 1992). Innovative re-engineering of the care process, such as locating behavioral specialists in the primary care setting, using new technologies to facilitate just-in-time brief consultation, and developing innovative class and group formats for delivering behavioral healthcare may increase efficiency, but structuring incentives to allow the provision of care by PCPs that will not fit into a 7- or 10-minute primary care appointment will also be necessary.

As mentioned earlier in this chapter, many clinical issues at the primary care–behavioral healthcare interface require further study to determine the most effective and efficient ways to provide care. In addition, administrators must also determine how to optimally align the financial incentives to stimulate integrated primary and behavioral healthcare. In a single general health and behavioral health capitation model, in which specialist care is paid out of a budget controlled by PCPs, PCPs have incentives to minimize use of specialist care. Such incentives can delay needed mental health treatment and promote excessive, and at times inappropriate, use of psychoactive medications. For example, consider that the greatest proportion of prescriptions for selective serotonin reuptake inhibitors are written by PCPs, not psychiatrists. In a carve-out or subcapitation model, with a preset, fixed payment for behavioral healthcare, PCPs have incentives to refer all patients with emotional distress to behavioral healthcare specialists. Both single capitation and subcapitation models provide mixed incentives to behavioral healthcare specialists for working closely with PCPs to help the latter treat behavioral disorders in their patients. Such collaboration is likely to increase the number of patients receiving treatment solely from PCPs but will also increase PCPs' recognition of mental disorders and direct their referrals to the behavioral healthcare specialists with whom they work closely. (Administrators must also determine how to allocate the expense of time and personnel for intensive behavioral healthcare specialists' work with PCPs—is this a medical or a behavioral healthcare expense if it decreases total healthcare utilization?) Last, further experience is needed to determine the most efficient ways to provide utilization management and quality monitoring for patients with behavioral disorders. Most PCPs lack sufficient time or expertise to manage and monitor their patients' specialty behavioral healthcare, and these important functions are probably best shared by closely communicating primary and behavioral healthcare providers and administrators.

In years to come, skillful administrators will have substantial opportunities to improve care and ultimately contain or reduce costs by integrating primary medical care and behavioral healthcare within well-managed systems of care. Although we will certainly see new biopsychosocial conceptualizations and clinical breakthroughs, progress in primary behavioral healthcare will in large degree consist of doing well what we already know how to do but previously have not had the will to implement widely.

References

Barsky AJ: Hypochondriasis: medical management and psychiatric treatment. Psychosomatics 37:48–56, 1996

Barsky AJ, Borus JF: Somatization and medicalization in the era of managed care. JAMA 274:1931–1934, 1995

Beck A, Scott J, Williams P, et al: A randomized trial of group outpatient visits for chronically ill older HMO members: the cooperative health care clinic. Journal of the American Geriatric Society 45:543–549, 1997

Beitman BD, Williamson P, Featherstone H, et al: Resistance to physician use of the biopsychosocial model. Gen Hosp Psychiatry 4:81–83, 1982

Block SD, Clark-Chiarelli N, Peters AS, et al: Academia's chilly climate for primary care. JAMA 276:677–682, 1996

Cummings NA, VandenBos G: The general practice of psychology. Professional Psychology: Research and Practice 10:430–440, 1979

Doherty WJ, McDaniel SH, Baird MA: Five levels of primary care/behavioral healthcare collaboration. Behavioral Healthcare Tomorrow 5:25–27, 1996

Eisenberg L: Treating depression and anxiety in primary care. N Engl J Med 326:1080–1084, 1992

Fawzy FI, Fawzy NW, Hyun CS, et al: Malignant melanoma: effects of an early structured psychiatric intervention, coping, and affective state on recurrence and survival 6 years later. Arch Gen Psychiatry 50:681–689, 1993

Goldberg D: Filters to care-a model, in Indicators for Mental Health in the Population. Edited by Jenkins R, Griffiths S. London, HMSO, 1991, pp 30–37

Gullette ECD, Blumenthal JA, Babyak M, et al: Effects of mental stress on myocardial ischemia during daily life. JAMA 277:1521–1526, 1997

Holder HD: Alcoholism treatment and potential health care cost savings. Med Care 25:52–71, 1987

Inui TS: What are the sciences of relationship-centered primary care? J Fam Pract 42:171–178, 1996

Jenkins R: Developments in the primary care of mental illness-a forward look. International Review of Psychiatry 4:237–242, 1992

Kabat-Zinn J: Full Catastrophe Living: Using the Wisdom of Your Body and Mind to Face Stress, Pain, and Illness. New York, Dell, 1990

Katon W, VonKorff M, Lin E, et al: Collaborative management to achieve treatment guidelines: impact on depression in primary care. JAMA 273:1026–1031, 1995

Katon W, Robinson P, Von Korff M, et al: A multifaceted intervention to improve treatment of depression in primary care. Arch Gen Psychiatry 53:924–932, 1996

Kroenke K: Symptoms and medical patients: an untended field. Am J Med 92 (suppl 1A):3S–6S, 1992

Kroenke K, Arrington ME, Mangelsdorff AD: The prevalence of symptoms in medical outpatients and the adequacy of therapy. Arch Int Med 150:1685–1689, 1990

Lipowski ZJ: Somatization: the concept and its clinical application. Am J Psychiatry 145:1358–1368, 1988

Lorig KR: Patient education: treatment or nice extra? Br J Rheumatol 34:703–704, 1995

Lorig KR, Holman HR: Arthritis self-management studies: a twelve-year review. Health Educ Q 20:17–28, 1993

Lorig KR, Mazonson PD, Holman HR: Evidence suggesting that health education for self-management in patients with chronic arthritis has sustained health benefits while reducing health care costs. Arthritis Rheum 36:439–446, 1993

McLeod CC, Budd MA: Treatment of somatization in primary care: evaluation of the personal health improvement program. HMO Practice 11:88–94, 1997

Paulsen RH: Psychiatry and primary care as neighbors: from the Promethean primary care physician to multidisciplinary clinic. Int J Psychiatry Med 26:113–125, 1996

Regier DA, Goldberg JD, Taube CA: The de facto U.S. mental health services system: a public health perspective. Arch Gen Psychiatry 35:685–693, 1978

Regier DA, Narrow WE, Rae DS, et al: The de facto U.S. mental and addictive disorders service system: Epidemiologic Catchment Area prospective 1 year prevalence rate of disorders and services. Arch Gen Psychiatry 50: 85–94, 1993

Rost K, Kashner TM, Smith GR: Effectiveness of psychiatric intervention with somatization disorder patients: improved outcomes at reduced costs. Gen Hosp Psychiatry 16:381–387, 1994

Sabin JE: Research findings on chronic mental illness: a model for continuing care in the health maintenance organization. Compr Psychiatry 19:83–95, 1978

Sabin JE: Joseph Hersey Pratt's cost-effective class method and its contemporary application: some problems in biopsychosocial innovation. Psychiatry 53:169–184, 1990

Sabin JE: Time-efficient long-term psychotherapy in managed care. Harv Rev Psychiatry 3:163–165, 1995

Saravay SM, Pollack S, Steinberg MD, et al: Four year followup of the influence of psychological comorbidity on medical rehospitalization. Am J Psychiatry 153:397–403, 1996

Sherbourne CD, Wells KB, Meredith LS, et al: Comorbid anxiety disorder and the functioning and well-being of chronically ill patients of general medical providers. Arch Gen Psychiatry 53:889–895, 1996

Simon GE, VonKorff M: Somatization and psychiatric disorder in the NIMH Epidemiologic Catchment Area Study. Am J Psychiatry 148:1494–1500, 1991

Simon GE, Ormel J, VonKorff, et al: Health care costs associated with depressive and anxiety disorders in primary care. Am J Psychiatry 152:353–357, 1995a

Simon GE, VonKorff M, Barlow W: Health care costs of primary care patients with recognized depression. Arch Gen Psychiatry 52:850–856, 1995b

Smith GR, Rost K, Kashner M: A trial of the effect of a standardized psychiatric consultation on health outcomes and costs in somatizing patients. Arch Gen Psychiatry 52:238–243, 1995

Speckens AEM, van Hemert AM, Spinhoven P, et al: Cognitive behavioral therapy for medically unexplained physical symptoms: a randomized clinical trial. BMJ 311:1328–1332, 1995

Spiegel D, Bloom JR, Yalom I: Group support for patients with metastatic cancer: a randomized prospective outcome study. Arch Gen Psychiatry 38:527–533, 1981

Spiegel D, Bloom JR, Kraemer HC, et al: Effect of psychosocial treatment on survival of patients with metastatic breast cancer. Lancet 2: 888–891, 1989

Stoeckle JD, Zola IK, Davidson G: The quantity and significance of psychological distress in medical patients. Journal of Chronic Diseases 17:959–970, 1964

Sturm R, Wells KB: How can care for depression become more cost-effective? JAMA 273:51–58, 1995

Wagner EH, Austin BT, Von Korff M: Organizing care for patients with chronic illness. Milbank Q 74:445–467, 1996

Wells KB, Stewart A, Hays RD, et al: The functioning and well-being of depressed patients: results from the Medical Outcomes Study. JAMA 262:914–919, 1989

Wells KB, Sturm R, Sherbourne CD, et al: Caring for Depression. Cambridge, Harvard University Press, 1996

Wulsin LR: An agenda for primary care psychiatry. Psychosomatics 37:93–99, 1996

❖ 16 ❖

Changing Roles for Psychiatrists

Debra L. Klamen, M.D.
Joseph A. Flaherty, M.D.
Boris M. Astrachan, M.D.

The Psychiatrist and the Profession of Medicine

Sociologists have considered for many years the issue of what *profession* means (Carr-Saunders and Wilson 1933; Freidson 1970; Greenwood 1965; Parsons 1954). From the writings of sociologists come two critical elements that define a profession. First, a profession must possess a body of specialized knowledge. This requirement has several implications, including the necessity of a long apprenticeship to acquire the necessary knowledge, the control of entry into the profession through examinations of the knowledge acquired, and thus, the control of the number of professionals. Because those holding the specialized knowledge required of the profession will argue that no other is competent to determine whether good practice is being followed, the power to self-regulate also belongs to a professional group.

The second critical element that defines a profession such as medicine is that of objective, emotionally detached service to clients. Clients must trust the professional and share intimate worries and problems. To be of service, the professional must remain detached,

see the client as a case, and not become emotionally involved to the extent that he or she loses objectivity. A set of professional ethics and etiquette helps to maintain this delicate balance, and members of the profession are expected to share in these common values and uphold them (Ben-David 1964).

Professions such as medicine also serve to stabilize society. By dealing with personal problems in a detached, objective manner, the idiosyncratic expression of distress is minimized (Parsons 1951). In addition, professionals define and limit the ways in which they define and deal with deviancy from societal norms (Freidson 1970). In exchange for this stability, and the professional's commitment to serve, society bestows protection and rewards in the form of autonomy, power, and social and economic status. Medicine as a profession thus serves individual patients, society at large, and its practitioners.

Professions have no clear organizational structure and no evident central or leading part. Their boundaries are maintained by multiple enterprises that are often unconnected, and at times in conflict, with one another. A profession cannot be understood as a single enterprise. The environment in which the profession exists is at the very least a national environment with complex expectations and demands. In a complex society, professions must accomplish multiple tasks.

The physician's role as a medical professional includes that of Aesculapian Authority—the granting to the healer of the right to probe human minds and bodies in ways permitted by no one else. As a healer, the physician must sit with the suffering of another. It is the physician's role to explain and clarify, to determine what is sickness and what is not. Once this has been determined, it is the physician's role to offer relief from suffering using the skills and science of the profession, whether in the form of emotional support and hope, biological intervention, or both. The role of the physician is carried out within the framework of the doctor-patient relationship, a dyadic relationship exemplified by the confidentiality of the patient's communication with the doctor.

Astrachan, Adler, Levinson, and others have defined four major tasks of psychiatry and identified the perspectives required of each task (Adler et al. 1981; Astrachan et al. 1976; Benarroche and Astrachan 1982; Sledge et al. 1995):

1. Diagnosing, curing, and limiting illness—*the medical perspective*. The work of this area is to evaluate and diagnose the patient's illness and provide appropriate treatment.

2. Reducing defect and enabling those with defect to live more normal lives—*the rehabilitative perspective*. The work of this area is to treat residual defects following acute medical treatment in order to prevent further deterioration, restore functioning, and improve the level of adaptation.

3. Controlling socially deviant behavior—*the societal-legal perspective*. Psychiatrists are often called upon by the legal-correctional system in its efforts to control forms of social deviance considered to be the result of mental illness or impairment. The social control task of psychiatry involves providing treatment to any individual who is committed or diverted to psychiatric care by the legal system.

4. Fostering growth and competence—*the educational-developmental perspective*. The primary task in this area is not to treat an illness but rather to enhance the individual's potential for development, an exploration of impeded growth.

Though interconnected, these tasks are distinct and separable. They are all within the legitimate domain of psychiatric practice.

The nature of the physician's role, including that of the psychiatrist, is changing rapidly in today's healthcare system, mirroring the changes occurring in the world of work at large. The manner in which care is delivered, the structure of institutions providing care, the financing of care, and the ability of medicine to continue its sole control over practice are all being reshaped. Healthcare is being increasingly constrained by the growing emphasis on increased efficiency, decreased cost, and front-line accountability. Medical corporations are moving toward team production and away from individual craftsmanship. The physician is seen increasingly as an employee. These changes have resulted in alterations in how psychiatrists practice.

The substitution of less powerful (and usually less extensively trained) groups of health professionals for tasks previously undertaken by those in more powerful (and usually more expensive) positions is one change that has resulted in the new healthcare climate. The emphasis on care delivered in the most cost-effective manner possible has been a catalyst for this change. "What matters is the outcome of the intervention, not the status of the person who intervenes" (Hopkins et al. 1996). As long as there are no legal obstacles, and patients are happy, care given by a less trained and lower-paid person is being substituted. Indeed, the acceptability of the substituted healthcare professional, in many cases, has been shown to be equal to that of the traditional healthcare provider (Carzoli et al. 1994; David et al. 1982; Dowling et al. 1995; Hill et al. 1994; Holmes 1994; Maule 1994; Royal College of Surgeons of England and the Society of Cardiothoracic Surgeons 1994; Spitzer et al. 1974a, 1974b; van der Horst 1992). This has become possible secondary to the routinization of technical skills and the development of a multiplicity of new professions ready to take over tasks previously performed by physicians.

In organized treatment structures, physicians, including psychiatrists, work within hierarchical role relationships, unlike the peer systems in which they previously functioned. The restructuring of the marketplace from solo or small group providers to multi-institutional, investor-owned healthcare corporations increasingly requires physicians to rely on complex organizational and financial arrangements to carry out their work (Light and Levine 1988). Hierarchical structures, including management, give structure to work, ensure quality, and secure resources required for the work (Astrachan et al. 1997). Efficiency is maximized through the concentration of expertise, skill, and authority in the hands of senior managers. Managers rather than peers define the scope of the work. By its very nature, such settings limit autonomy and collegiality.

The movement into hierarchical systems has meant the diminution of physician autonomy and the interpolation of third parties into the doctor-patient relationship. The increasingly technical and organizational complexities of modern medicine, the rise of investor-owned healthcare corporations, and the current attempts to control healthcare costs are all eroding professional control. To this end, physicians are being subjected to forms of corporate control such as incentive pay structures and restrictions on practice patterns. It may feel as if there are now three people in the psychiatrist's office: the psychiatrist, the patient, and the third-party payer, raising questions of intrusion on the tradition of doctor-patient confidentiality. In an ever more competitive healthcare environment, institutions vigorously manage their resources and their practitioners, emphasizing bottom-line decision making, through mechanisms such as defining or limiting practice privileges, by identifying who shall have access to care, by monitoring use of service, and by limiting economic risks and emphasizing economic returns (Relman 1980). Physicians are continually required to justify inpatient stay recommendations and outpatient treatment plans to insurers or to managed care companies. They are asked to justify the prescription of various classes of medications; their peer groups and often the managed care industry establish standards for review of their practices and procedures. Hospitals discourage the admission and treatment of patients whose care is supported by certain payers and encourage the treatment of others. The physician's behavior is frequently constrained by organizational policy and practice.

There has been a shift in accountability mechanisms in all of medical care. We have moved from a paradigm in which the practitioner primarily owed a duty to the patient and secondarily owed a duty to the profession to one in which third parties are increasingly and apparently legitimately involved in the clinical relationship. Government now insists on its right to be in the middle of the doctor-patient relationship. Payers and their agents are involved, and families and advocates also insist on a voice. Accountability mechanisms seem to proliferate. They are structured both within and external to organizations. Management of care occurs not only through external agencies as an imposition on physician and hospital practice but increasingly also within hospitals and other healthcare settings.

The values of the marketplace and the world of commerce became the catalysts for these sweeping changes. Starr (1982) described the corporatization of healthcare in the early 1980s. Since then, corporations have dramatically and powerfully entered into the world of healthcare. They have reshaped the healthcare environment. Corporate policy now dominates where public policy once ruled. Practice increasingly is organized into systems of care. The for-profit sector saw opportunity in the healthcare arena as the capacity of medicine to generate profit increased. Companies that could oversee complex financial empires seemed ideally suited for administering hospitals, nursing homes, or managed care firms. As the corporatization of healthcare and the commercialization of medicine became dominating principles, entities once regarded as services having economic components came to be seen primarily as businesses (Tischler and Astrachan 1996). The control of care has moved from the owner of the office (the physician) to the owners of the institutions (financiers, banks, insurance companies, and the public and private capital markets). Rather than cooperation and care, these new owners have primary goals of competition; cash flow; and low-cost, high-margin service delivery.

A shift from the biopsychosocial model to a more biological emphasis on practice has also contributed to the changes seen in today's healthcare system. Although the academic enterprise historically has paid lip service to a biopsychosocial model, research increasingly emphasizes biological understanding of mechanisms of disease and disorder. Research support and the major journals now emphasize neurobiology. The 1980s and beyond have been witness to explosive growth in the neurosciences. Powerful new biological techniques are changing the way in which the brain is understood. The field of psychopharmacology has dramatically altered the practice of psychiatry. Treatment responsivity has helped modify nosological categories. Changes in nosology have fueled a revolution in epidemiologic research. Diagnostic imaging technologies have become increasingly sophisticated and, with increasing precision, reflect the nature of underlying biological processes.

The use of information technology, a rapidly expanding arena, serves the goals of corporatization and allows for its exponential growth by enhancing productivity, fostering greater accountability, and facilitating control by management. Computers can establish algorithms for types of care with standard defaults as well as red flags alerting the physician or case manager of potential danger in the history, physical examination, or treatment. Computers allow for substitution of professionals by less well-trained individuals supported by a sophisticated ability to access and use information. They can support examination of drug interactions, medication side effects, patient education, and cost profiling. Such methods inform both the physician and the providers and allow for more rational decision making. In addition, information is now available about practice variation, from a wide range of sources, allowing comparisons of hospital with hospital and practitioner with practitioner.

The rise of consumerism and advocacy has accounted for some of the role changes. In the midst of the more organized care systems, patients, families, and their advocates insist on some measure of accountability. Patient or family organizations provide a voice for many people who too often were not heard. They generally insist on an emphasis on humane medical care supported by psychosocial and other rehabilitative programs. Many of those served are dissatisfied with care and with many caregivers and have definite views about how they should be treated. In addition, there is much greater emphasis on providing sufficient information to patients and to their relatives so that they can make informed choices.

New roles are being formed and reformed for psychiatrists almost as quickly as healthcare itself changes. Managed care has created or altered the roles of psychiatrists in relating to case managers, other mental health professionals (i.e., in split care), medical directors, and peer reviewers. The rapidly changing nature of the work of primary care physicians has opened up new opportunities for collaboration with psychiatrists. Doctor-organized group practices or limited liability corporations are also being formed in response to the changing healthcare environment.

Case management has considerable potential as a means of organizing and delivering mental health services in a cost-effective manner (Sledge et al. 1995). Case management reflects two basic but apparently contradictory underlying processes: increasing access to services and limiting costs. In addition, case management functions have a role in all of the task areas of psychiatry—medical, rehabilitation (psychological, social, and vocational), social control, and growth and development (Astrachan et al. 1976). A clinically oriented coordinating, linking, and integrating function is needed, not only for cost-control efforts but also to ensure

quality of services, particularly for patients with persistent illnesses that wax and wane and are likely to require different levels of intensity of care and different kinds of services at different times. Psychiatrists must understand the role of case management in the provision of psychiatric services. The tension between limiting and enhancing access to care, on the one hand, and setting priorities across task areas, on the other, is always present.

Extraordinary variation exists in the nature of the split care of a patient between psychiatrists and other mental health professionals. Clinical staff generally expect that the psychiatrist will participate in the assessment and treatment of patients' medical problems (or will arrange for appropriate referral) and will be responsible for the evaluation and monitoring of psychopharmacologic therapies. But the medical backup role often expands into a variety of other activities. These activities include organizationally required societal-legal tasks such as assessments for involuntary commitments, evaluations to help determine eligibility for public aid or rehabilitation services, preparation of psychiatric reports for third-party payers, and forensic assessment; management tasks such as assessment of and arrangement for the physical containment or isolation of violent or self-injurious patients; and other technical services such as the provision of a second opinion to other mental health workers for diagnostic or treatment purposes.

When a psychiatrist serves as a medical backup, the goal of the interprofessional association is good patient care. To assume that responsibility, the physician has to identify 1) the framework in which care will be delivered, from a medical or rehabilitative perspective (within each perspective varying degrees of autonomy are possible for other professionals; consequently, the nature of the appropriate interprofessional relationship may also vary), 2) the training, clinical experience, and credentials of the associated professionals, 3) the patient's characteristics, 4) the organizational structure of the institution in which care is being delivered (including specifics about lines of accountability for treatment integration and monitoring), and 5) the legal and clinical requirements for the psychiatrist's presence as mandated by healthcare legislation or contractual requirements. Medical backup thus implies a flexible role that has to be adapted to specific circumstances, to the nature and membership of therapeutic teams, and to the demands of the organizational setting. Depending on these variables, the psychiatric backup may be involved in prescriptive, collaborative, consultative, or supervisory relationships (Benarroche and Astrachan 1982). Administrators must insist that the role of medical backup be defined in ways that protect patient care, identify accountability relationships, allow for the legitimate discharge of medical responsibility, and permit the appropriate level of autonomous or supervised practice of the other professional.

The Psychiatrist and Managed Care

Psychiatrists find themselves relating to or working within managed care organizations in a number of ways. Many psychiatrists relate to managed care organizations as a condition of payment for providing treatment. The managed care company approves the patient's entry into treatment and certifies sessions of outpatient care or days of inpatient care. In most cases, managed care serves to control costs and, far more rarely, to manage care. In some programs, intensive (focused) case management programs may be available to provide enhancements to traditional services but usually only if the patient selects services within a particular clinical network. In these situations, both care and costs may be managed.

Decisions about level and intensity of care generally are driven by considerations of medical necessity and risk. The definition of care is usually framed within the medical task area as previously identified; and issues of diagnosis, acute resolution of symptoms, and follow-up for monitoring and medical management predominate.

Some managed care companies tend to split care, with social workers or psychologists providing psychotherapeutic services and psychiatrists providing psychopharmacologic treatment. Other managed care organizations have concluded, at least in the treatment of moderate to severe depression, that the provision of all care by a psychiatrist is most cost effective. In split therapy, practitioners must be clear about the relationship to the nonmedical collaborator and have clear models in mind for resolution of problems should they arise.

In dealing with managed care companies, practitioners must understand that the case managers with whom they interact are often well-trained clinicians. They have an organized approach to care that emphasizes clear goals for treatment, time-focused treatment, elaboration of a clear treatment plan, attention to risk factors, concern with complicating substance abuse or medical problems, and explicit discharge planning. Responding to case managers courteously within a focused treatment framework often allows for comfortable interaction and approval of care.

Because the field is maturing, risk protocols and protocols that define indications for treatment by level of care are usually available from the managed care company. The practitioner needs to be clear about the explicit or implicit model of care and whether he or she wants to be bound by such a model. In general, flat-out denial of payment usually requires peer-to-peer interaction. Thus, in such cases practitioners have the opportunity to deal directly with clinical peers to discuss clinical concerns. Although medical necessity may slide into a rehabilitative framework with the expectation that rehabilitation today will lead to less cost tomorrow, it rarely slides over into the educational-developmental task area (i.e., improving quality of life, enhancing relationships). When there are disagreements about care, appeals processes may be sought, and in some cases appeals processes may even extend to the corporation that contracts with and uses the managed care firm as its vendor for services. Concerns that reach the employees' company (particularly if the company is a substantial contractor for care) often draw explicit attention to problem areas.

IBM developed a mental health advisory board that reviews quality concerns in the program its vendor provides (Astrachan et al. 1995). Other companies have developed user groups to jointly monitor quality-of-care issues. Quality is often more difficult to address when mental health services are subcontracted from a health maintenance organization (HMO) to a managed care vendor, as overall dollars allocated to care are fewer, and patient and practitioner are several layers removed from the corporation that is purchasing services.

The Psychiatrist in the Managed Care Company

The role of psychiatrists in HMOs varies from working in organized mental health units (e.g., Kaiser-Permanente, Harvard Community Health, Humana) to monitoring carve-out services in other HMOs. Several large HMOs have developed extensive mental health services. In these programs, psychiatrists often are involved in medication management, in consultation to other mental health practitioners, and in supervision of time-limited focused psychotherapy. Research generally identifies

HMO practitioners as less likely to identify certain mental disorders; yet, in HMOs at least, as many individuals receive mental healthcare as in the private sector. Generally in the HMO, the modal mental health practitioner is a nurse or social worker, and length of treatment is less than in the specialty treatment sector (Wells et al. 1989a, 1989b, 1995). Psychiatrists are expected to collaborate in care, to educate colleagues, and to treat the most severe illnesses. (See section "The Psychiatrist and Primary Care Practice.")

In managed care companies, roles for psychiatrists are growing. Such companies need medical directors (large accounts may have an account medical director). Medical directors supervise the group of practitioners who review care. If focused on a specific account, they will interact with the medical office of the company (occupational health program) and the corporate human resources department. They will be charged with helping to develop clinical guidelines, with reviewing criteria for network membership, with oversight of exceptions to policy regarding network membership (e.g., review of malpractice history and decision to allow into network), and with the development of new programs (mobile crisis teams).

The Psychiatrist and Primary Care Practice

Over half of all patients with behavioral problems are seen in the primary care sector. These patients tend to be less severely disturbed than patients seen in the specialty sector, but substantial overlap exists. Primary care physicians (PCPs) have been learning more about diagnosis and about psychopharmacology than in the past. Some PCPs also are becoming involved in developing addiction programs. Yet, in general, most PCPs willingly collaborate with mental health specialists in cases with moderate to severe levels of psychopathology and in settings in which psychiatric physicians have demonstrated their interest in developing programs that serve the needs of PCPs and their patients (Astrachan et al. 1997).

Effective collaboration requires that psychiatrists rapidly respond to requests for consultation, increasing service with no additional cost. Emergency requests must receive high priority, and if at all possible, patients must be seen within a few hours of the request (within one day, at maximum). Psychiatrists or psychiatric practices need to be available during some evening hours and on some weekend days.

Psychiatrists need to treat their PCP colleagues as real colleagues and as customers, to determine if they wish to continue following the patient for the emotional problem and, if so, arranging for further consultation, as needed. If care is to be moved to the specialty sector, the psychiatrist has a responsibility to provide such information as may be useful to the PCP in practice. Psychiatrists need to respond rapidly and fully to colleagues' requests for information and must be prepared to pick up the most troublesome patients. Psychiatrists, in order to be credible to PCPs, need to behave like caring specialists and to be available round the clock. They cannot treat PCP colleagues as less than intelligent individuals who ought not be trusted to work with ill patients. They must be willing to teach and to refer their patients to PCPs. In this manner, psychiatrists add value to the PCP beyond patient care, strengthening the relationship with the PCP and encouraging future referrals in a cost-effective manner. Educating practitioners in order to identify patients who need psychiatric care and systematizing procedures for accessing care further reduce clinical barriers and costs and improve practice competitiveness. In addition, psychiatrists who wish to collaborate with PCPs need to know how to work with addicted patients, must know the effects of addiction on physical health, and must be able to arrange for the continuing care of such patients.

Managed care offers interesting opportunities and challenges to traditional patient-centered consultation and referral practices. The opportunity to add quality improvement into the triad of efficiency, accountability, and decreased cost is available. For example, when psychiatry and primary care share capitation and risk (through either carve-out or subcapitation), the importance of joint preventive activities is clear. For various high-risk groups, joint psychiatry–primary care prevention programs can have real payoffs from both economic and quality perspectives. Prepartum screening for depression and substance abuse can reduce maternal and infant morbidity. Valid and reliable screening instruments have been developed for anxiety disorders and depression. Linking the use of such instruments to clinical algorithms might permit PCPs to attend to mild and moderate cases with rapid referral to a psychiatrist for more severe cases. Developing group programs for individuals undergoing the trauma of divorce may limit later medical care.

An active psychiatry group with appropriately trained professional staff located in a primary care practice can establish group programs that combine psychoeducation and therapy—for example, support groups directed at patients with pain, sickle cell anemia, or cancer. Vigorous psychosocial programs can be useful in enhancing quality of care and in limiting costs. Psychiatrists need not be primary care physicians, but they must understand the constraints on primary care practice and how to work within those constraints.

The Psychiatrist in Public-Community Psychiatry

We anticipate rapid change and opportunity for careers in the public-community psychiatry sector and in this section describe the current opportunities and how these opportunities may change in the near future.

Traditional Public-Community Careers

Although most of the opportunities for careers in the public-community psychiatry sector are still available, changes are taking place within each area.

Community Mental Health Centers

Community mental health centers (CMHCs) are increasingly competing for behavioral healthcare opportunities. They are diversifying services, expanding their funding bases, and increasingly becoming part of integrated networks. Many states are recognizing the shortcomings of a rapid move to the privatization of Medicaid and the treatment of severe mental illness by managed care companies with little experience or modeling in the care of patients with chronic illness. To the extent that CMHCs have been successful in using continuum-of-care models and implementing outreach programs and assertive community training projects that allow the severely mentally ill population to function in the community, they are likely to be asked to participate in these newly forming public managed care consortia. In such settings, the CMHC psychiatrist will continue to function in roles varying from direct patient care to team leader to liaison and arbitrator of larger systems of care.

Work Within State Code Agencies

The extent of privatization, which will have marked regional variation, will be a determining factor for opportunities within state code agencies. For example, some states will close a proportion of their state hospitals and privatize the care of most of the severely mentally ill population; this will leave two special populations remaining within state hospital systems: severely mentally ill and demented patients and the criminally insane. Similarly, regional variations will exist in the extent to which states privatize care of patients in the prison system, although opportunities with this population will likely increase as the population grows and the public calls for treatment intervention, particularly for those incarcerated for substance abuse–related problems. Psychiatrists who have received training in mental health administration, including business and legal expertise, will be in high demand to direct the clinical operations in state code agencies, regardless of the degree of privatization.

Veterans Administration

Although the Veterans Administration (VA) will likely remain open to psychiatry, particularly for psychiatrists with subspecialty training in geriatrics and addictions, the VA's move to consolidation of regions and other changes will also require psychiatrists to have some training and familiarity with networking and community services. As the VA serves an increasingly elderly population, a decreasing patient base will limit new opportunities in this area.

Public Health Psychiatry

Public health psychiatry is largely supported by the federal government. Decisions about the federal government's role in providing healthcare are obviously affected by political decisions and are consequently difficult to predict. Areas in which opportunities have existed (e.g., underserved populations, homeless populations) may receive private services as the marketplace recognizes need. Programs with the Bureau of Indian Affairs will likely continue to employ psychiatrists for the Native American population.

Potential New Public–Community Sector Roles

We envision that what we know of as the public sector will privatize much psychiatric care in the first decade of the twenty-first century and that therefore direct patient care work with traditional public sector populations will not be significantly different from that in the private sector. However, state agencies are unlikely to relinquish their responsibility to their clients through a wholesale conversion to managed care. Rather, they are likely to form partnerships with managed care companies, provider networks, and universities as well as better links or umbrella structures for dealing with one another (e.g., child welfare, mental health, substance abuse, corrections). In this new scenario psychiatrists can develop new provider roles. They will need special training with particular populations and methods of community psychiatry; however, they may now become employees of a larger provider organization rather than the state. In addition, and importantly, as state agencies enter into complex relationships with managed care entities, they will also need psychiatrists with specific interests and skills. These skills include monitoring performance and checking boundaries among the many entities providing and managing mental healthcare, credentialing and profiling providers, and identifying best practices. These psychiatrists will need competence in utilization review, computerized information retrieval, data analyses, and quality management. They will likely also find it useful or even necessary to take courses and obtain certificates from private organizations that credential such skills in healthcare professionals.

Although a great deal of psychiatric training and practice, like the rest of medicine, will emphasize the generalist orientation, academic and practice opportunities will continue to be available in subspecialty areas. One provision, however, that will be different from the emerging specialties of the 1980s and 1990s will be a concentration on patients with major and severe mental illness. This emphasis is the result of the intersection of three vectors all pushing psychiatry to concentrate, if not limit, itself to individuals with major psychiatric disorders: 1) the rise in the organization and power of consumer mental health organizations driven largely by parents and siblings of patients with schizophrenia and bipolar disorder, 2) the recognition by industry and payers that effective treatment of the major disorders can be reflected in genuine cost savings, and 3) the incorporation of the National Institute of Mental Health into the National Institutes of Health and the subsequent pressures to have that institute become more biological and disease focused. A related factor in subspecialization predictions is that subspecializations will move from the historical emphasis on modes of delivery (e.g., consultation-liaison, psychotherapy, community) to a disease model such as in the medical subspecialties and to divisions reflecting demographic boundaries (e.g., children, geriatrics, women). To a great extent, as subspecialty training moves back into the medical school setting, the need for psychiatric departments to tie subspecialty training to their research

strengths may reemerge. Given these provisions and assumptions, the likely subspecialty opportunities in the twenty-first century can be delineated.

Neuropsychiatry

Several factors are driving the development of neuropsychiatry: the rapid development of imaging technologies along with rapid translational research that finds practical clinical applications for these new technologies; increased interest and capacity to measure potential efficacy of pharmacologic agents by examining brain activity before and during drug treatment; the closer linkage of psychiatry to both the clinical and basic neurosciences; the corporatization of medicine that has led to the recognition that the term "neuropsychiatry" has less stigma and more market value than just psychiatry alone; and the relative failure of our colleagues in neurology and rehabilitation medicine to recognize their potential to compete with psychiatry in the treatment and rehabilitation of patients following stroke, brain surgery, brain trauma, and seizure disorders. To a great extent the basic training of psychiatrists that allows them to sit and communicate with psychotic patients will also serve them well in this subspecialty and will guarantee that psychiatrists will be the providers of this care. Thus far, neuropsychiatry, like its cousin, geropsychiatry, has been largely a diagnostic branch of the profession. This situation is likely to change in the direction of embracing treatment. Neuropsychiatric treatments, while benefiting from technology and development of novel pharmacologic agents, have been slow to link strongly to rehabilitative professionals. To a large extent, neuropsychiatrists have represented what was not long ago referred to as "white coat" psychiatrists because of their similarity to other medical practitioners. This difference will become less striking as the tasks of the rest of psychiatry become more aligned with them. They will still serve as a major force between general psychiatry and the rest of medicine. As such, they will also continually range between the two professional domains, at times becoming temporarily captive by medicine. Their tasks will require more extensive training in neurology and the neurosciences as well as detailed knowledge acquisition and training in neuroradiology and imaging techniques.

Geropsychiatry

The two central driving forces behind the continued development of geropsychiatry are the graying of the population as baby boomers enter retirement and the cumulative body of specialized knowledge and skills necessary to effectively work with this population group. There will continue to be overlap between geropsychiatry and neuropsychiatry, particularly in the area of delirium and dementias secondary to stroke, multiple and single cerebrovascular accidents, vitamin deficiencies, viral and postviral encephalopathies, cancer, drug interactions, and newly discovered treatable and untreatable causes of brain syndromes. Like neuropsychiatry, geropsychiatry has been a subspecialty that has concentrated on diagnostic rigor. However, geropsychiatry will differentiate itself in several ways in the area of treatment. As the population ages, the average life expectancy will continue to rise, although it will likely plateau in the upper 80s without major investment in genetic engineering and organ transplantation. Although we anticipate new drug therapies for dementia, geropsychiatrists will also have a central concern with the treatment of basic psychiatric disorders in the elderly, such as anxiety disorders, depression, transient psychotic disorders, and chronic or remitting illnesses such as schizophrenia and bipolar disorder. In addition, more attention will be paid to quality of life and social functioning related to adjustment disorders secondary to medical illness and impairment; to addictions from prescription drugs, illegal drugs, and alcohol; and to the range of mourning and grief reactions, both normal and pathological, so common in the elderly. Geropsychiatry practitioners will need to become familiar with the rapidly growing knowledge base in geriatric psychiatry and gerontology (both biological and psychosocial), which includes pharmacokinetic and pharmacodynamic age-related changes; the changing metabolism; perceptual and cognitive changes in aging; and the development of assessment methods, both through interview and technology, for use in the elderly. Although geropsychiatrists will need neurological training, they will also need to benefit from geriatric medicine, psychology, and sociology. We also anticipate the development of newer psychotherapies, not only age-adjustment to brief psychotherapy and grief work but also sociotherapeutic interventions in the areas of home and respite care, group homes, establishment of foster families, and new social networks—efforts intended to reduce the current trend toward nursing home placement and to enable the elderly to finish their lives with greater dignity and sense of personal accomplishment.

Women's Mental Health

Subspecialty areas such as women's mental health beg the question of whether psychiatry continues to sprawl wildly in all directions and respond to social calls for fads and political correctness. The early developments in women's mental health also led to the mistaken assumption that it was predominantly about psychotherapy and feminist theory and might not be applicable to all women or be significantly related to the practice of general psychiatry. Based on our definition of a profession, we feel confident that this emerging subspecialty is a substantive professional subdomain. The reasoning is clear: Women's mental health has a growing base of specialized knowledge and treatments. These knowledge areas include psychopharmacologic issues during pregnancy and postpartum (e.g., pharmacokinetics, pharmacodynamics, and teratogenicity), disorders that are unique to women (related to pregnancy, estrous cycles, and menopause), disorders that disproportionately affect women (e.g., depression, non-war-related posttraumatic stress disorder, panic disorder), and the different presentations of other disorders in women compared with men. In addition, women's mental health as a subspecialty will continue to utilize the growing knowledge base on gender differences, both psychosocial and biological, and studies of the psychology of women and of families. The natural medical ally for this group of practitioners will be obstetrics and gynecology; a great deal of the subspecialty's success will depend on how well it can be of service to obstetrics and gynecology in areas such as pregnancy counseling, peripartum disorders, depression related to fertility and miscarriage, and adjustments to the effects of cancer surgery and reconstruction on women. In this area, very much like in geriatrics, the practitioner will need to recognize the tremendous variance in psychology, biology, and attitudes toward health among women so as to avoid the trap of generalizing and thereby stereotyping.

Addictions

Addiction has already emerged as a distinct and useful subspecialty. Although key professional issues exist— for example, whether the field can be open to subspecialty training from a primary care basic residency base as well from psychiatry—the subspecialty will continue to be defined by its knowledge and skills. In this regard, addiction psychiatry appears to be on the verge of new knowledge acquisition and ready to move beyond the standard treatment modules that were strongly developed through the treatment of married, employed, middle-aged, middle-class, Christian men. Although the 12-step philosophy has considerable merit and a good track record, and although Alcoholics Anonymous is still the most successful program for abstinence with common addictions, the demographics of addictions are changing. Women, immigrants, and the elderly are increasingly becoming addicted. Also changing are the types of drugs of addiction and abuse, for example, crack cocaine, designer stimulants, inhalants, novel psychedelics, and prescription drugs, including methadone. In addition, breakthroughs in neuroscience and imaging technology are beginning to have a positive influence on the field of addiction and will likely lead to new methods of prevention, early recognition, and treatment. The modern addiction specialist will need to become conversant with these new findings and be well grounded in basic internal medicine and epidemiology.

Conclusions

In developing a framework for understanding practice, Astrachan et al. (1976) described a number of task areas, noting that no one task area encompassed all of practice, nor was any area inherently more valuable than any other. They also noted that at various times public definition may emphasize one area over another. Today, medical tasks have assumed primacy in psychiatric practice, and new role opportunities reflect this shift in value.

Managed care, primary care relationships, new public psychiatry roles, and new areas of subspecialty practice all largely emphasize medical tasks, with psychosocial and rehabilitative emphases assuming somewhat diminished importance. Practicing primarily in a medical framework does not mean forsaking one's emphasis on the psychosocial but rather understanding that today the medical task area drives the engine of practice and that psychosocial practice relates to this emphasis and will continue to do so—at least for the next several years.

References

Adler D, Astrachan B, Levinson D: A framework for the analysis of theoretical and therapeutic approaches to schizophrenia. Psychiatry 44:1–12, 1981

Astrachan B, Levinson D, Adler D: The impact of national health insurance on psychiatric tasks and practice. Arch Gen Psychiatry 33:785–794, 1976

Astrachan BM, Essock S, Kahn R, et al: The role of a payor advisory board in managed mental healthcare: the IBM approach to quality mental health care. Adm Policy Ment Health 22:581–595, 1995

Astrachan BM, Flaherty JA, Astrachan J: Psychiatry, primary care and managed care: an executive perspective. Psychiatr Ann 27(6):440–443, 1997

Benarroche CL, Astrachan BM: Interprofessional role relationships, in Psychiatric Administration. Edited by Talbott JA, Kaplan SR. New York, Grune & Stratton, 1982, pp 223–236

Ben-David J: Professions in the class system of present-day societies. Current Sociology 13:247–330, 1964

Carr-Saunders AM, Wilson PA: The Professions. Oxford, Clarendon, 1933

Carzoli RP, Martinez-Cruz M, Cuevas LL, et al: Comparison of neonatal nurse practitioners, physician assistants, and residents in the neonatal intensive care unit. Arch Pediatr Adolesc Med 148:1271–1276, 1994

David R, Enderby P, Bainton D: Treatment of acquired aphasia: speech therapists and volunteers compared. J Neurol Neurosurg Psychiatry 45:957–961, 1982

Dowling S, Barrett S, West R: With nurse practitioners, who needs house officers? BMJ 31:309–313, 1995

Freidson E: Profession of Medicine—A Study of the Sociology of Applied Knowledge. New York, Dodd, Mead, 1970

Greenwood E: Attributes of a profession, in Social Welfare Institutions—A Sociological Reader. Edited by Zald MN. New York, Wiley, 1965, pp 509–523

Hill J, Harmer R, Wright V, et al: An evaluation of the effectiveness, safety and acceptability of a nurse practitioner in a rheumatology outpatient clinic. Br J Rheumatol 33:283–288, 1994

Holmes S: Development of the cardiac surgeon assistant. British Journal of Nursing 3:204–210, 1994

Hopkins A, Solomon J, Abelson J: Shifting boundaries in professional care. J R Soc Med 89:364–371, 1996

Light D, Levine S: The changing character of the medical profession: a theoretical overview. Milbank Q 66 (suppl 2):10–32, 1988

Maule WF: Screening for colorectal cancer by nurse endoscopists. N Engl J Med 330:183–187, 1994

Parsons T: The Social System. Glencoe, IL, Free Press, 1951

Parsons T: Essays in Sociological Theory, Revised Edition. Glencoe, IL, Free Press, 1954

Relman AS: The new medical-industrial complex. N Engl J Med 303:963–970, 1980

Royal College of Surgeons of England and the Society of Cardiothoracic Surgeons: Cardiac Surgeons' Assistants: Guidelines for Heads of Departments. London, Royal College, 1994

Sledge WH, Astrachan BM, Thompson K, et al: Case management in psychiatry: an analysis of tasks. Am J Psychiatry 152:1259–1265, 1995

Spitzer WO, Sackett DL, Sibley JC, et al: The Burlington randomized trial of the nurse practitioner: health outcomes of patients. Ann Intern Med 80:137–142, 1974a

Spitzer WO, Sackett DL, Sibley JC, et al: The Burlington randomized trial of the nurse practitioner. N Engl J Med 290:251–256, 1974b

Starr P: The Social Transformation of American Medicine. New York, Basic Books, 1982

Tischler GL, Astrachan BM: A funny thing happened on the way to reform. Arch Gen Psychiatry 53:959–963, 1996

van der Horst M: Canada's health care system provides lessons for NPs. Nurse Practitioner 8:44–57, 1992

Wells KB, Hays RD, Burnham MA, et al: Detection of depressive disorder for patients receiving prepaid or fee-for-service care: results from the Medical Outcomes Study. JAMA 262:3298–3302, 1989a

Wells KB, Stewart A, Hays R, et al: The functioning and well-being of depressed patients: results from the Medical Outcomes Study. JAMA 262:914–919, 1989b

Wells KB, Astrachan BM, Tischler GL, et al: Issues and approaches in evaluating managed mental health care. Milbank Q 73:57–75, 1995

❖ 17 ❖

Changing Roles of Mental Health Professionals

Judith H. Browne, R.N., M.S.N.

In this chapter I cover briefly the pivotal events that influenced the growth and development of professional roles for those in behavioral health who are not physicians. A look back at the early roles of key behavioral professionals such as social workers, nurses, and psychologists provides the perspective needed to appreciate the current changing environment. The most significant development in recent years is the advent of managed healthcare, affecting not only how care is delivered but also those who deliver it. Managed care has altered roles for various professionals in the field of behavioral healthcare, and new professional responsibilities—and job opportunities—continue to evolve.

Brief History

Psychiatric Movement

Psychiatry and behavioral health practice as we know it are, in the grand scheme of things, very new. Only in the late 1800s did the German physician Emil Kraepelin first classify mental health as a separate medical model. Because of his efforts, others soon recognized mental health as a separate, legitimate field of medi-

cine, but they still misunderstood treatment and ostracized psychiatrists and their patients (Richardson 1993).

Before Kraepelin, many people misunderstood the symptoms of mental illness and called them invasions by evil spirits. Priests usually attempted exorcism, and if that failed, the afflicted found themselves in asylums, often in chains and restraints (Menninger 1997). No one consulted physicians because the symptoms were commonly believed to have a supernatural cause rather than a physical or mental one.

Societies created asylums to protect themselves from the insane and other so-called social misfits, but none provided any treatment. Not until the eighteenth century did Phillippe Pinel in France introduce the idea of mental illness and apply scientific theories to the disease (Richardson 1993).

Benjamin Rush, considered the father of modern American psychiatry, continued Pinel's work with hospital reform in the nineteenth century (Richardson 1993). As a senior physician at Pennsylvania Hospital, Rush began his work with the mentally ill, shunning the cruel practices that had been routine for hundreds of years. With cautious clinical observation, he developed a more compassionate and curative procedure for treating mental illness, and in 1812, he published the first American textbook on psychiatry, *Medical Inquiries and Observations Upon the Diseases of the Mind* (Leitch 1978).

More than 100 years later, psychiatry continued to be misunderstood; psychiatrists were viewed as "alienists" who still practiced in asylums far removed from cities and towns. This separatist attitude by physicians prompted some necessary changes. In 1925 Karl Menninger converted a farmhouse into the Menninger Sanitarium because local hospitals refused to see his patients, but even sanitariums like Menninger's remained in rural, out-of-the-way places far from the general populace and city hospitals (Menninger 1994).

State mental hospitals evolved from sanitariums and were never well funded, resulting in poor care and overcrowded conditions. This state of affairs, coupled with the lack of effective treatments for psychiatric illness—in medicine, success is demonstrated by a cure—fueled negative public opinion about the mentally ill and those caring for them (Eisdorfer and Cohen 1997).

The real growth of the psychiatric movement came during World War II with the recognition that 20% of war casualties were related to psychiatric illness (Menninger 1994). Psychiatrists on the front lines helped soldiers stay on active duty and worked to rehabilitate those with posttraumatic stress and other emotional disorders related to the war. After the war many young physicians sought psychiatric training, dramatically expanding the number of psychiatric residents and sparking public interest in new methods of care.

In the 1950s the discovery of the world's first effective neuroleptic drug, chlorpromazine, began a new era in psychiatric care. Originally tested as an experimental antihistamine on emotionally ill patients in France, chlorpromazine was the first of many successful medications used to treat severe mental illness, finally offering a glimmer of hope to patients and their families. Because of such pharmaceutical advancements, psychiatry broadened its scope to include not just psychotherapy but also biology. This broader view dramatically changed the roles of psychiatrists and supporting nonprofessionals (Menninger 1994). This shift in focus and change in roles also opened the door to an enormous reduction in hospitalizations and the development of alternative levels of care including partial hospitalization and outpatient treatments for conditions traditionally considered untreatable. By 1954 there were 1,234 outpatient clinics, an increase of almost 70% from pre–World War II numbers (Richardson

1993). This type of shift would be repeated with the advent of managed care, again making a significant change in the modalities of treatment and the roles of behavioral healthcare professionals.

Congress passed the Mental Health Study Act in 1955, establishing a 3-year study searching for recommendations on a nationwide system to treat mental illness (Menninger 1994). The results of the study brought about the Action for Mental Health, laying the groundwork for the Mental Retardation Facilities and Community Mental Health Centers Construction Act of 1964. This movement established a fund for community mental health centers (CMHCs) constructed to provide emergency care, inpatient, outpatient, day treatment, consultation, and education services to individuals regardless of their ability to pay (Richardson 1993).

National Institute of Mental Health Training Funds

During the same time period that Congress enacted its laws, research and training dollars from the National Institute of Mental Health provided more opportunities for many physicians and other professionals such as nurses, psychologists, and social workers (Eisdorfer and Cohen 1997). This funding during the 1950s and 1960s covered training costs and provided living stipends in exchange for graduates practicing for a period of time in the public sector. As this funding declined, parallel decreases in enrollment followed for nonphysician providers such as nurses (Krauss 1993).

Community Mental Health Center Legislation

During the Carter Administration, legislation established CMHCs, creating a public sector mental health delivery system directed toward community systems of care. This care provided needed assistance to individuals navigating the complex mental health system and ensured adequate services for the sickest of the sick. The move to CMHCs created jobs for many nonpsychiatric professionals who would otherwise not have been employed outside the hospital delivery system. This movement also fueled the need for nonphysician professionals in the care delivery system.

The public sector and the community mental health system emerge again in the current managed care debate. The states embrace privatization and managed care as a means to meet demand for services while controlling rising public expenditures. Public-private partnerships between CMHCs and managed care organizations (MCOs) have become a growing force in the competition to win state Medicaid contracts worth millions of dollars. So heated is the competition that a contract award winner is often challenged by the losers. For example, a partnership between an MCO (OPTIONS Health Care, Inc.) and a consortium of CMHCs (Florida Behavioral Health) had its status as a bidder challenged before any contract was awarded. That challenge to one of the first public sector behavioral healthcare carve-outs in 1995 delayed the contract award by almost a year.

Managed Care

Managed care is often thought of as a new event resulting from the need to reduce costs, but it has been around for quite some time. By design, early health maintenance organizations (HMOs) provided comprehensive healthcare to those who might not otherwise receive it. In the 1930s, Kaiser Permanente, one of the largest HMOs, began providing services to shipworkers building vessels for World War II (May et al. 1996). Over time, the plans grew, and the government recognized prepaid healthcare as a cost-effective alternative to traditional fee-for-service indemnity plans. The advent of Medicaid and Medicare and the resulting dramatic increase in healthcare costs led to support for managed care and the passing of the Health Maintenance Organization Act of 1973. The act removed legal impediments to growth and propelled HMO development. Medicaid and Medicare, servicing the poor and the elderly, created a need for coordination of the many aspects of care these populations required. The coordination of care and other less medically oriented care management needs created opportunities for non-physician behavioral healthcare specialists.

Practitioner Roles

Social Workers

Managed care has had a positive impact on social workers and their roles as behavioral healthcare practitioners. In the early 1900s, social workers typically began their practices in charity hospitals and settlement houses in poor neighborhoods. Unlike nurses who practiced almost exclusively in hospitals and psychologists who practiced in offices and schools, social workers assisted individuals and families in their homes and neighborhoods. As mental health services grew after the war, social workers joined the "team" providing key services in inpatient settings under the direction of the psychiatrist. Freedom of Choice legislation in 1977 paved the way for social workers to practice psychotherapy independently by requiring insurers to offer the services of social workers and other licensed therapists (Baker 1994).

The National Association of Social Workers provides the Academy of Certified Social Workers (ACSW) credential. To receive the ACSW credential, social workers must have certain degrees, meet practice requirements, and pass a standard examination. The ACSW credential is the one most often embraced by managed behavioral healthcare organizations (MBHOs) in their network criteria.

Professional Nurses

When nurses first began to receive training around the time of the Civil War, they often served as apprentices. During this apprenticeship and later in practice, nurses invariably ministered their care in a hospital setting under the direction of a doctor. Some 20 years later, when nurses first received training to care for the mentally ill, the focus was much the same. Psychiatrists provided treatment, and nurses generally provided custodial care, concerned primarily with their patients' physical needs. World War II proved to be a catalyst for nurses just as it had been for psychiatrists and psychologists. Nurses became increasingly more involved in group psychotherapy, and after the war, the federal government appropriated a dedicated fund to be used specifically for nurses' training (Richardson 1993). Nursing education today is much more rigorous academically and professionally. Graduate nurses often go on to receive advanced degrees and train side by side with psychiatrists, psychologists, and social workers. Nurses can receive degrees at all levels: 2-year associate's degrees, 4-year bachelor's degrees, and advanced master's and doctoral degrees. Those with associate's degrees usually provide direct care service, whereas those with bachelor's and master's degrees are usually supervisors or teachers. Nurses with doctoral degrees usually teach rather than provide clinical care (Richardson 1993).

Psychologists

In an effort to establish a professional niche, early twentieth-century psychologists stressed their role as scientists—researchers who most often worked in academic settings (Richardson 1993). In early treatment settings, psychiatrists provided treatment using psychotherapy and psychologists did the testing (Baker 1994). As mentioned earlier, World War II sparked real growth and public interest in the field of psychiatry. The war also prompted many prominent European psychoanalysts to leave Europe. Many were psychologists who opened the doors for nonphysicians to practice psychotherapy in the United States (Baker 1994). Because of the influx of European psychologists and the efforts to provide psychotherapy for battle-fatigued troops on the front lines, psychologists saw their clinical practices increase. When the Veterans Administration (VA) expanded its mental health services in VA hospitals, clinical training for psychologists began in earnest. The VA Psychology Training Program began in 1946, and many psychologists continue to receive training there for counseling and clinical practice. All states and the District of Columbia require licensure or certification for psychologists. Most require a doctoral degree when they certify or award a license; however, a few grant a limited license to those who have master's degrees. Psychologists who do not have a license usually practice in schools or CMHCs.

Impact of Managed Care

A Swift and Dramatic Change

Even as Congress struggles to reform the U.S. healthcare delivery system—with the role of managed care as the focus of debate—managed care moves ahead, the driving force changing the practice and reimbursement of healthcare, behavioral healthcare included. The change has been dramatic and swift. In 1980, 9.1 million people were enrolled in HMOs. By 1994, the number had risen to more than 42 million. By 1995, more than 140 million people (95% of the employee population) were in managed care plans (National Association of Social Workers 1995).

Though embraced by employers and federal and state governments, managed care has not generated the same enthusiasm in professional circles nor among the general public. The leadership of the American Psychological Association is adamantly opposed to managed care as applied to the mentally ill. The American Psychiatric Association has vigorously opposed managed care.

In an unlikely alliance, the American Psychiatric Association and the American Psychological Association cooperated to release a Mental Health Bill of Rights aimed at protecting patients by moving control and accountability back to the independent practitioner. This Bill of Rights precludes the use of networks and limits access to information required to evaluate the quality of care. The bill was supported by the major associations for nurses, social workers, counselors, and family therapists; the broad scope of support indicated the degree of impact that managed care has had on professional practice. Over time the Bill of Rights became focused on protecting patients' rights to access selected practitioners and services and to appeal managed care decisions. The bill was a key issue in the platforms of both presidential candidates in the presidential election of 2000. As of early 2001, several versions of the bill were still under revision.

A Radical Impact on the Referral Process

The managed care environment radically alters the essential relationship between the professional and the patient. Historically, consumers chose their provider (usually a psychiatrist or psychologist), who determined an appropriate treatment regimen. It was a direct relationship unhampered by any intrusions. The bills went to an unseen third party (an insurer) who paid them without question.

The nature of managed care usually requires participation in a network and most often requires the consumer or provider to discuss any referral with a behavioral healthcare manager who must authorize the referral for payment. The care manager—often referred to as the gatekeeper—is usually a nurse or mental health professional. The care manager guides the referral and the ensuing care plan and, depending on the plan or the manager, exercises varying control over treatment decisions. That balance is delicate because even though the ultimate treatment decision is always the responsibility of provider and patient, the amount of money available through third-party payment may be critical in influencing the outcome of the decision.

This alteration of the direct relationship between consumer and provider has created a dependent relationship between providers and payers for their supply of patients. Because inclusion in a network and authorization for care are necessary for reimbursement, few members go outside the managed care system for care. This change has had a dramatic impact on practitioner roles.

Managed care networks use volume referrals to negotiate discounts in provider fees. The result is smaller networks and, for those providers not included, limited access to patients. Consequently, competition for network slots has forced practitioners to provide more focused, efficient treatment and to provide practice outcome statistics to demonstrate their value to the managed care companies that control access to the networks. Others have joined single-specialty or multispecialty groups to gain access to a broader base of networks (patients) and to decrease overhead costs to enable them to offer more competitive fees.

Many professional guild associations have spent tremendous amounts of time and money to support legislation to prevent managed care companies from limiting the number of network providers. Twenty-eight states now have "Any Willing Provider" legislation ensuring that all who meet network criteria gain access to the network. In many cases this has not been the benefit providers had hoped for because the large network limits the volume of referrals possible while the discount in fees remains. (Increases in the number of people in managed care plans have provided even more impetus to their efforts.) As of 1996, 74% of employees in firms with more than 200 employees were in HMO plans; an increase of almost 300% in 8 years (Fubini and Antonelli 1997). This trend is a compelling reason for providers to develop alliances with managed care plans in order to have access to patients through their networks.

Group Practices Flourish

The solo nature of the professional practice environment is undergoing significant change. Practicing physicians are moving from solo to group practice, and many are entering practice as employees in preference to independent practice. Data from the American Medical Association indicate that the percentage of patient-care physicians practicing as employees rose from 24.2% in 1983 to 42.3% in 1994. In this same time period, the proportion of self-employed physicians in solo practice fell from 40.5% to 29.3% (Fubini and Antonelli 1997). Most of the changes occurred during the latter half of the 12-year time period, signaling an accelerating trend that was especially pronounced among young physicians and primary care specialists.

Physicians in general are resisting multispecialty practices in favor of joining colleagues with the same specialty. Nearly 70% of physician practice groups are single specialty (Fubini and Antonelli 1997). Similarly, during this period, behavioral healthcare practitioners were leaving solo practices to join group practices. Most often these group practices were also single specialty (behavioral health) but took a multidisciplinary form with the inclusion of behavioral healthcare practitioners of varied disciplines. This move is fueled by behavioral managed care entities seeking to gain efficiencies through the use of single contracting of large provider practices. These large group practices are able to function more autonomously through self-management and have the ability to effectively assume risk under capitated payments. This allows managed care entities—HMOs and behavioral health organizations—to offset some of their financial risk. In fee-for-service arrangements, a gain in market share comes at the expense of discounted fees. That payoff pales in comparison with the assumption of risk and its inherent potential for profit and autonomy. Viewed in this light, it becomes clear that group practices not only offer efficiencies related to the spread of overhead costs but also offer capabilities to assume new financial arrangements with significantly higher profit potential. These group practices are the most valued by managed care companies and consequently will provide the richest referral base.

The advent of group practices assuming risk through capitated payments alters the nature of the competitive roles among various disciplines. Physicians no longer compete with their nonphysician colleagues. Turning over a patient to another who provides care at a lower cost does not mean the loss of a patient (revenue) but rather offers the possibility of increased profit (decreased cost). This trend is evident in primary care and obstetrics where group practices now embrace the very nurse practitioners they once vigorously opposed. It is present also in psychiatry, where social workers and nurses in group practices provide care at the lowest cost. All are mutually dependent on one another for financial success. This change increases the opportunities for nonphysician professionals to enter group practices that once were open only to physicians. It also offers myriad roles in management and care management coordination as the large groups develop functions that mirror those in managed care companies (e.g., medical directors, case managers, appeals coordinators). Group practices operate as businesses and require all the skills necessary to manage the market forces of supply, demand, and finance.

Managed Care Regulating Agencies

The Utilization Review Accreditation Commission (URAC) accredits MCOs. The focus is on the structure and credentials of the organization providing utilization management. Most important for URAC are the qualifications of those directly involved in the review of care. Members of the care review staff and their supervisors must be clinical peers. Consequently, the clinical staff employed in MCOs mirror professionals in independent practice. Because physicians make up the smallest percentage of network providers, there is a significant demand for nonphysician behavioral healthcare professionals in the managed care industry. The peer reviewers must be clinically supported by a physician, also creating roles for psychiatrists as clinical supervisors and psychiatrist peers.

The credentialing process of the National Committee for Quality Assurance (NCQA) will likely be the one that affects practitioners most. By developing an accreditation process and database of comparative information on the quality of managed care plans, the NCQA already has changed the practice environment. The NCQA will have a significant impact because of its rigorous credentialing standards, particularly those applied to MBHOs. HMOs have embraced the NCQA and have consequently changed the standards of criteria for inclusion in the network. NCQA credentialing criteria include several stringent quality initiatives:

- Quality improvement and information
- Primary source credentialing
- Provider site visits
- Utilization management
- Member rights and responsibilities
- Preventive health services
- Medical records

The rigor of this process, particularly primary source credentialing and the requirement of site visits to the provider's office, has added significant financial burdens to all parties. In some cases the provider bears the cost; in others the MCO bears the cost. In either case, the result is more money spent on administration and a shrinking amount of money available to provide needed care. For all the focus on quality, purchasing decisions for healthcare—as for any other service—are driven primarily by price (Fubini and Antonelli 1997). The added costs related to credentialing are not likely to be continually assumed by the managed care entities; rather, they are likely to be passed on to practitioners. Some managed care companies already charge a fee to belong to the network or pass along these and other costs. These costs are increasingly being borne by providers and represent an added burden for solo practitioners who cannot afford the additional overhead and will feel more pressure to join a group practice.

Risks or Fee-for-Service Financing

One of the most significant factors that has altered professional roles is the way behavioral healthcare is financed. Capitation has helped corporate and government purchasers reduce costs while offsetting cost pressures to providers (Fubini and Antonelli 1997). In 1990, healthcare costs were rising at the rate of 9.1% per year. Although still on the rise, the rates of increase in 1994 and 1995 were only one-half the 1990 rate (Fubini and Antonelli 1997).

Historically, the most popular form of financing was payment on a fee-for-service basis. This method of financing inadvertently created incentives for practitioners to provide the most care at the most intensive levels. Because providers received payment for the amount of care (the number of days or sessions) and the level of care (inpatient versus outpatient), and there were relatively few limits (particularly on inpatient care), there was no reason for the providers to seek alternatives to inpatient care. The accepted notion was that more care was better. It is not surprising that some practitioners provided unnecessary treatment and that healthcare costs escalated. To create incentives to use more efficient and less intensive levels of care, managed care entities use capitated payments. The idea is to shift the financial risk and reward to providers, allowing them to share in the profits if they create efficiencies in the system.

In a capitated environment, the incentives are designed to provide care more efficiently. Providers are reimbursed on a per-member per-month basis. In most cases this is a rate per covered person; that is, it is based on the population to be covered regardless of whether or not they use care. The capitation covers every aspect of providing treatment and any required reporting. It is expected that whoever needs care will get it and that all care covered by the benefit will be provided if needed. Any money left over after paying the costs for care and administration is available for profit. Because it is expected that anyone within the covered population will receive the necessary care, it is possible that the amount of money provided may not adequately cover all the needed care. In that case, the provider or the managed care entity is expected to provide the care and absorb the loss. Hence, capitation carries a risk for the provider or the managed care company. Needless to say, the ability to accurately predict utilization and costs is essential for success under this form of reimbursement. With this form of payment the concern is not that overtreatment will occur but rather that people will be denied care in order to promote higher profits. This concern is often addressed by measurable quality objectives designed to ensure that people are not denied care and that the treatment results in positive clinical outcomes.

Managed care companies often assume capitated reimbursement and then subcapitate to providers who assume various levels of this risk. One popular modification of this plan is the case rate, the payment provided per patient for a program of care. In this plan, the provider is paid for every person who receives care, and the rate covers the entire episode of treatment. The goal using any capitated payment plan is to align the incentives for providers and payers by having them share the risk. Providers are free to make decisions about patient care, and analysis of quality of care data helps ensure accountability (Shaffer 1997).

How Roles Are Affected by Managed Care

The knowledge and skills required of practicing professionals are changing dramatically. Today, all professionals need more than the clinical skills and referral sources that worked so well in the past. The single most important predictor of practice success today may be access to the right networks and the best financing arrangements. Practitioners need extensive knowledge of contracting and the ability to assess various group opportunities and financing arrangements, to manage capitation, to evaluate and use computer technology, and to generate reports. To ensure success, providers will need to add business (contracts, cash flow, and margins) and management skills (executive, operational, and clinical) to their repertoire. The managed care environment continues to drive many of these changes.

Primary Care Physicians

The role of the primary care physician (PCP) has flourished as a result of the managed care model. Under managed care, a consumer is assigned a PCP (usually an internist or pediatrician) who assumes overall responsibility for the coordination of care. The PCP in most cases must provide advance authorization for access to specialists of any kind. In many cases, the PCP is responsible not only for care coordination and authorization but also for financing the care. In many models, the PCP receives a pool of money (a per-member per-month capitation). Any authorized care is deducted from the PCP pool. Consequently, the financial incentive is to monitor the use of specialists carefully.

The advent of the PCP, a role similar to the family doctor of days past, has affected the roles of all behavioral healthcare practitioners. Because the PCP must have full knowledge of the whole medical services environment, collaboration and communication links are essential. In addition, the interface has stimulated discussion and debate about the appropriate role of PCPs in the delivery of mental health services. New roles have evolved for mental health practitioners as consultants or colleagues to PCPs, and many primary care practices have established ongoing relationships with mental health professionals to help the practices screen, evaluate, and manage mental healthcare. In many cases, the PCP chooses to manage the patient's medications and to establish relationships with nonphysician professionals.

Psychiatrists

Managed care has had a significant impact on the practice of psychiatry. Historically, psychiatrists provided most of the psychotherapy services. Now that managed care companies have control over access to patients, they usually direct referrals to the most efficient and least costly professional. Consequently, psychiatrists, who are the most highly paid, are called on less often to provide psychotherapy and more often to evaluate medical and biological services. The trend is for psychiatrists to work with patients who have more severe, more complex disorders. As psychiatrists' roles in therapy have diminished, other medical professionals—social workers, nurses, and psychologists—have moved in to fill the gap. Psychiatrists are moving more into executive management roles in the new provider practice organizations.

Professional Nurses

The increased care delivery at the outpatient level and the need to coordinate care and to ensure basic healthcare, especially for vulnerable populations, have had a significant impact on the roles of mental health practitioners in general and nurses in particular.

In fact, among those in the behavioral health field, nurses have experienced the most dramatic changes in professional roles. Unlike social workers, nurses developed their profession in hospital settings. As hospitals downsize and close, nurses are drawn into roles far from their roots. As late as 1988, fewer than 10% of more than 10,000 psychiatric nurses with master's degrees worked in individual or group private practices (Krauss 1993). A large proportion of the nation's nurses receive their training in 2-year associate's degree programs, an education that prepares them primarily for hospital-based roles. Although nurses with bachelor's and master's degrees are well educated and able to perform myriad roles in the out-of-hospital environment, their lack of ties to the managed care networks currently in development makes their move to community-based treatment more difficult (Buerhaus and Staiger 1996). Among psychiatric nurses with master's degrees, 45% still work primarily in hospitals (Krauss 1993).

Two developments enhanced the expansion of nurses' roles in the area of mental health practice: advanced nurses' training provided at the master's and doctorate levels and the advent of the American Nurses Association (ANA) certification programs. These programs began to certify generalist psychiatric nurses and specialist psychiatric nurses with master's and more advanced degrees in adult and child/adolescent psychiatric management. The registered nurse license and certification at the master's degree level not only provide professional credentials but also bestow credibility for nurses who provide independent psychotherapy services. Most MBHOs embrace generalist psychiatric nurses as case managers but require specialist credentials from those who will be included as independent practitioners in their network.

In general medical settings, nurses are the primary care managers. Nurses fill 90% of the roles in rehabilitation, indemnity plans, HMOs, and preferred provider organizations (May et al. 1996). The ANA defines case management as a major career opportunity for nurses and as having "at heart a systematic approach to care" (May et al. 1996). The ANA describes the goals of case management "as providing quality healthcare along a continuum, decreasing fragmentation of care across many settings, enhancing the client's quality of life, and cost containment" (May et al. 1996). The disproportionately high number of nurses serving as case managers provides validation for the acceptance of nurses in this role.

Psychologists

Psychologists, like psychiatrists, have challenged managed care at every turn, but like nurses and social workers, psychologists are changing their practices to meet the needs of the managed care environment. They are certainly not shrinking from the challenge. The number of psychologists in practice (in contrast to the number in scientific roles) is growing rather than shrinking.

Among those psychologists who practice, increasing numbers are in group settings, allowing them to gain access to patients and to offer a wider range of specialized services designed specifically for adolescents, families, or geriatric patients. Many psychologists are joining or starting interdisciplinary practice groups and forming partnerships with PCPs, oncologists, cardiologists, and others to provide direct services through an interdisciplinary team. Some are embracing concepts such as marketing, once unheard of in the field. Others are pursuing privileges for prescriptions. To gain support for these new responsibilities, they are developing educational programs and disseminating model legislation.

Licensed Marriage, Family, and Child Counselors

California, a leader in the development of managed care, passed legislation in the 1980s to license nonphysician behavioral healthcare practitioners across disciplines. This legislation created an overarching independent practitioner role for nonphysician providers in delivering services.

The legislation created licensed marriage, family, and child counselors (LMFCCs) and legitimized independent practice for practitioners with master's or doctorate degrees obtained from an accredited institution. In addition to the educational requirements, LMFCCs need 2 years of supervised experience and must pass an entry examination.

Managed care companies embraced this concept, and when they accepted the LMFCC credential for entry into their networks, the growth of nonphysician practitioners increased dramatically. LMFCCs, regardless of their discipline of origin, practice in the myriad roles available for nonphysician practitioners.

Examples of Managed Care Roles for Mental Health Professionals

Managed care has not only changed the roles that practitioners play in their practice environments but also created numerous roles within the MCOs themselves. One of the most prominent is that of the care manager. Care managers are responsible for intensive case management for clients meeting defined clinical and administrative criteria. They also serve as the primary clinical liaison with providers to ensure that clients receive services in accordance with established guidelines. They ensure coordination of community resources for cases assigned to specialized case management. A sample job description (Figure 17–1) provides the typical responsibilities for case managers.

Network management is also a role most often filled by nonphysician behavioral healthcare professionals. Network managers are usually responsible for the overall day-to-day management of the national organizational networks. This includes development of policies and procedures, management and creation of budgets, management of the department's human and technological resources, interface with other departmental units as part of the management team, interface with other internal and external entities to enhance functioning, support of sales and external efforts, and management of the department's efforts to achieve NCQA standards.

Primary care managers are professionals assigned to primary care practices. They may work directly for the group or as part of the MCO. They interact with primary care practitioners, members, and providers on a daily basis to facilitate the assessment and referral of members seeking access to mental health, substance abuse, or employee assistance program services for outpatient, intensive outpatient, partial hospitalization, or inpatient treatment or crisis intervention.

Quality improvement roles are also predominately filled by nonphysician clinical professionals. They work with the MCO staff and the provider network to analyze service and outcome data and to institute corrective action plans when services in the MCO or in the network do not meet quality benchmarks for best practices.

Innovative methods of delivering healthcare services offer even more opportunities for career development in the future. New roles for various professionals will surely surface, not only providing fresh challenges and responsibilities but also requiring that job descriptions be rewritten.

References

Baker B: The changing face of social work. Common Boundary 12:33–34, 1994

Buerhaus P, Staiger D: Managed care and the nurse workforce. JAMA 276:1487–1493, 1996

Eisdorfer C, Cohen S: How bright is the future for academic psychiatry? The Leifer Health Care Report, Special Report: The State of the Art in Psychiatry, 1997, pp 23–25

Fubini S, Antonelli V (eds): 1997 Health Care Industry Outlook: Healthcare Trends Report. Bethesda, MD, Health Trends, 1997

Krauss J: Health Care Reform: Essential Mental Health Services. Washington, DC, American Nurses Publishing, 1993

Leitch A: A Princeton Companion. Princeton, Princeton University Press, 1978

May C, Schraeder C, Britt T: Managed Care and Case Management: Roles for Professional Nursing. Washington, DC, American Nurses Publishing, 1996, pp 2–19

Menninger W: The future of psychiatry and implications for recruitment. Bull Menninger Clin 58:519–526, 1994

Menninger W: De-stigmatizing psychiatry. The Leifer Health Care Report, Special Report: The State of the Art in Psychiatry, 1997, p 42

National Association of Social Workers: A Brief Look at Managed Mental Health Care. Washington, DC, National Association of Social Workers Press, 1995

Richardson M: Mental health services, in Introduction to Heath Services, 4th Edition. Edited by Williams S, Torrens P. Albany, NY, Delmar, 1993, pp 220–235

Shaffer I: Rewriting the rules of reimbursement. The Leifer Health Care Report, Special Report: The State of the Art in Psychiatry, 1997, pp 6–8

OPTIONS Health Care, Inc.

POSITION DESCRIPTION

JOB TITLE: DIRECT LINE CASE MANAGER

DEPARTMENT: Clinical Operations

SUPERVISOR: Direct Line Team Leader

POSITION CONTROL:

JOB SUMMARY: Interacts with members and providers on a daily basis to facilitate the assessment and referral of members seeking access to their mental health, substance abuse, or EAP services for outpatient, intensive outpatient, partial hospitalization, inpatient treatment, and crisis intervention. Telephonic counseling services for First Call.

PRIMARY RESPONSIBILITIES:

1. Receives, evaluates, refers, and authorizes requests for care from members utilizing client-specific mental health, substance abuse, and EAP criteria.
2. Receives, evaluates, and authorizes care when providers call regarding client-specific mental health, substance abuse, and EAP services.
3. Responsible for triage and management of emergency calls.
4. Responsible for facilitating provider phone assessments.
5. Responsible for data entry and integrity of clinical information reflected by the MHS system.
6. Responsible for member/provider authorization letter generation.
7. Requests and negotiates single case agreements when clinically indicated; follows these requests.
8. Maintains logs and records as required by the team leader or department head.
9. Attends all mandatory staff meetings and assists with mentoring new employees as assigned.
10. Data entry, word processing while working on phone.
11. All other duties as assigned.

SECONDARY RESPONSIBILITIES:

1. Interfaces with Member/Provider Services Department on member/provider concerns or requests for information and assistance.
2. Participates as assigned in Utilization/Peer Review process.
3. Adheres to OPTIONS' and Clinical Management policies and procedures.
4. Participates in clinical and administrative supervision on regular basis.
5. Attends in-service training and meetings as scheduled.
6. Assists in orienting new staff as requested.
7. Provides input/feedback on department's clinical and administrative procedures and concerns.
8. Maintains and demonstrates positive attitude towards work.
9. Maintains clean and safe work area.

FIGURE 17–1. Sample job description for a case manager.

JOB SPECIFICATIONS:

Education: Requires current license in the work state as R.N., L.C.S.W., L.P.C., Ph.D., Clinical Psychologist.

Experience: Three years work experience in a mental health treatment setting.

Knowledge: Knowledge of evaluation and treatment of mental disorders. Understanding of the basic concepts of managed health care. Excellent communication skills—verbal and written. Demonstrated ability to relate effectively to beneficiaries, treatment providers, facility staff, and other professionals.

Supervision Exercised: None.

Supervision Received: Direct Line Team Leader.

Line of Promotion: As qualified.

Physical Requirements: Sits for long periods of time working on a CRT. Near visual acuity essential for preparing and interpreting reports. Finger/hand/arm dexterity required for repetitive motions needed in manipulating keyboards and operating other types of office equipment. Effective oral communication ability essential for managing staff and working with customers telephonically and in person. May be required to lift up to 50 pounds and bend and stoop occasionally while maneuvering and positioning office equipment.

Classification: Non-exempt position

This job description in no way states or implies that these are the only duties to be performed by this employee. The Direct Line Case Manager will be required to follow any other instructions and perform any other duties requested by the Team Leader.

FIGURE 17–1. Sample job description for a case manager. *(continued)*

Source. Published with permission of OPTIONS Healthcare, Inc. May not be reproduced or distributed without the express permission of OPTIONS Healthcare, Inc.

❖ 18 ❖

Changing Careers

Arthur Lazarus, M.D., M.B.A.

I find the great thing in this world, is not so much where we stand, as in what direction we are moving. To reach the port of heaven, we must sail sometimes with the wind, and sometimes against it—but we must sail, and not drift, nor lie at anchor.

"Counsel for the Journey," Oliver Wendell Holmes

The practice of medicine has been dubbed the noblest profession. No other profession endeavors directly to preserve or enhance human life. Pioneering heart surgeon Michael DeBakey (1987) commented, "Medicine is an absorbing, even possessive profession, but the intellectual rewards, humanitarian service, and fulfillment are unsurpassed" (p. 23). DeBakey's words still ring true, even though recent changes in the structure and delivery of medicine may have made the medical profession less appealing and created employment difficulties for newly graduated physicians.

In fact, the shift toward more corporate arrangements for the delivery of healthcare has changed the demand for physicians and the composition of the physician work force (Weiner 1994). It has become necessary for physicians to reevaluate their professional standing in light of these changes. The importance of work cannot be overstated. Freud observed many years ago that a gratifying job is one of the basic requirements of human existence. Rahe (1995) and colleagues, in their classic studies on stress and life-change events, found that business readjustments, employment terminations, and changing responsibilities at work or changing jobs to a different line of work ranked among the most stressful experiences in life. Consequently, physicians in the process of making a career transition need timely and accurate information to help them evaluate alternatives and make informed decisions. In reality, however, career transitions in medicine—and in psychiatry in particular—have rarely been discussed openly. In this chapter I attempt to remove the shroud of mystery surrounding medical career changes.

Research Findings

Many researchers have studied medical career changes following medical school graduation. Generally three questions arise when medical career changes are examined:

1. At what stage are physicians likely to change careers?
2. Are certain physicians more likely to change careers than others?
3. What factors prompt physicians to make a change?

Not all studies define "career change" in the same way. Physicians who have changed careers outside of medicine have been excluded from some studies, thus limiting the cohort to physicians in active practice. Obviously, a different picture emerges when nonpracticing physicians are excluded from the analysis.

Jennett et al. (1990) surveyed 603 medical school graduates of the University of Calgary, Alberta, Canada, who graduated in 1973 to 1985. One hundred and sixty (27%) reported a major medical career change after receiving their M.D. degrees. Compared with family physicians (18%), nearly twice as many specialists (35%) made major changes. Career changes occurred primarily during the first year of residency (42%) but also later in residency (21%) and after entering practice (29%). Common reasons for making a career change were dissatisfaction with the initial choice of a specialty (47%); lifestyle incompatibility (24%); and role model, training, or experience influences (19%). The fact that nearly one-third of physicians changed their careers while in an established practice indicates that "extended exposure to a medical field, the nature of the physicians' clientele, and the envisioned challenges and scopes of a particular discipline no doubt generate new opinions for many doctors regarding their chosen medical careers" (Jennett et al. 1990, p. 49). Women were just as likely as men to change careers.

Kindig et al. (1991) surveyed 867 physicians in administration. These physicians tended to be highly mobile. Senior-level physicians had held four or more positions in a single type of healthcare organization or two positions in different types of organizations. Career advancement required willingness to move between organizations and across organizational types—hospitals, academic medical centers, government agencies, insurance companies, and private industry. Administrative physicians tended to be relatively older, spent little time with patients, and were responsible for activities that spanned the boundary between medicine and management.

Olfson et al. (1993, 1994) conducted research specific to the careers of psychiatrists. They examined professional practice patterns of U.S. psychiatrists and the roles of psychiatrists in organized outpatient mental health settings. Only about 10% of clinical psychiatrists were engaged exclusively in office-based private practice. The majority of psychiatrists worked in multiple settings, served a broad range of patients, and provided a variety of treatments. Increasingly, psychiatrists share the management of severely ill patients with nonmedical mental health professionals.

These findings contrast with statements such as "Career paths for doctors do not exist" (Gumbiner 1994, p. 332) and "By the time a man reaches his psychiatric residency he has already made his basic occupational choices—to enter medicine and to go into the specialty of psychiatry" (Pearlin and Klerman 1966, p. 56). Apparently, one-track careers were typical in the past, but today multiple avenues of service delivery have spawned diverse career pathways.

Trends in Medical Practice

Previous authors have described factors that influence medical student specialty choice (Kassebaum and Szenas 1993; Lee et al. 1995; Rosenthal et al. 1994). Determinants include income potential, indebtedness, the environment and culture of academic medical centers, clinical experience in medical school, lifestyle, professional status, opportunities for research and other intellectual endeavors, and the availability of suitable employment. Although indebtedness may influence the choice of a specialty, income potential is probably less of a driving force than it was in the 1980s (Goldberg 1995). Data from the National Resident Matching Program (1991–1996) suggest that medical students are responding to shifting employment opportunities for generalists relative to specialists, thereby incorporating market conditions into their choice of specialty.

Students who choose psychiatry over other specialties have unique characteristics and values (Lee et al. 1995). Students seeking a career in psychiatry want to understand both body and mind, and positive experiences during the clerkship are critical to the selection of a career in psychiatry. Managed care, the medicalization of psychiatry, and the emphasis on primary care could all negatively influence the choice of psychiatry and recruitment into the field. Indeed, the decrease in the number of U.S. medical students choosing psychiatry as a specialty has been a cause of great concern and alarm (Sierles and Taylor 1995).

A study by the American Medical Association Council on Long Range Planning and Development (1994) identified 33 potential trends likely to occur by 2005. These trends will affect the patient-doctor relationship and the provision of medical care to all segments of society. Moreover, trends in medical practice are likely to shape medical careers in the future. Table 18–1 identifies these trends, many of which can be subsumed under the general heading of managed care.

The drive toward managed care will alter the number and specialty mix of physicians for years to come. Opportunities to specialize, however, will remain for qualified medical students and residents, just as they have for talented trainees in other disciplines. Goodman (1997) commented, "The challenge of managed care to academic medicine is to provide leadership in a competitive marketplace by maintaining high-quality educational standards, funding research, and preparing students for managed care opportunities.... The trend toward managed care indicates that those students knowledgeable of managed care practices will enter the market better prepared for potential job opportunities" (p. 72).

In the future, more physicians will be working in integrated multidisciplinary group practices. Treatment will often be provided by physician assistants. Fewer jobs will be available in hospitals, but more jobs will be available in ambulatory settings. The number of physicians working as salaried employees will increase, and along with this increase will be a need for physicians to develop skills in professional negotiation. Physician autonomy will likely decrease as physicians assume employee status and federal and state governments increase their oversight of care.

TABLE 18–1. Trends in medical practice

Trends in the market for health care
Integrated delivery systems will grow and become more competitive, and some will fail.
Working relationships between physicians and managed care systems will evolve.
Health insurance coverage will expand, community rating will return, and copayments will rise.

Trends in the market for physician services
Medical group practices will incorporate more physicians, and competition for physician services will increase.
Primary care physicians will be in greater demand.
More physicians will work as employees, and the demand for professional negotiations will grow.
Pressure on physician incomes will increase.

Evolving roles of health care players
Physicians will assume more supervisory roles as the range of services provided by nonmedical personnel expands.
Hospitals will be incorporated into large, vertically integrated health delivery systems as business issues assume center stage.
State and federal governments will become more active in health care.

Trends in medical technology
Computers and the Internet will be used more.
Cost-saving technologies will proliferate (e.g., videoconferencing and wireless devices).
Healthy lifestyles and public health issues will be emphasized.

Trends in medical ethics, quality assessment, and standard setting
Outcomes measurements will improve the quality of health care.
Ethical dilemmas will mount as limits on care evolve.
Confidentiality concerns will grow.
Some medical standards will be legislated.

Trends in medical education
Residency training programs will downsize.
Medical schools will recruit more minority students.
A primary care curriculum will be emphasized.

Trends in the market for medical association services
Physician diversity will increase, increasing the need for personal services.

Source.   Adapted from American Medical Association Council on Long Range Planning and Development 1994.

Career changes will also stem from the increasing use of computers and other technology in medical practice. Video conferencing, telemedicine, and computerized lifetime clinical records will enhance information sharing. Technology alone, however, will not ameliorate rural work force shortages. The emphasis on healthy lifestyles will favor medical careers geared toward prevention and wellness, primary intervention, and possibly alternative treatments. However, because the great majority of illnesses are chronic, careers that cater to public health issues, quality improvement, and outcomes measurement will be in demand.

Regardless of career choice, ethical dilemmas will mount, confidentiality concerns will grow, and limits on care will evolve. Medical schools will be pressured to reduce class sizes and residency positions, recruit more minority students, and increase training opportunities in ambulatory and community settings.

Despite downsizing, it is unlikely that even under conditions of a severe physician surplus a large number of physicians will be unemployed, according to health economist Uwe Reinhardt (1997). Reinhardt predicted that even with the impending physician surplus more people with M.D. degrees will be employed in the upper echelons of healthcare administration or other sectors in the economy. Many of these physicians will be entrepreneurs within the health sector itself or in other areas. Reinhardt concluded, "In short, the choice is not 'medical practice' or 'death.' The choice is 'medical practice' or 'any number of exciting and challenging pursuits'" (p. 69).

Career Pathways

Today's healthcare systems and the educational process that produces physicians are not the systems of 15 years ago, nor are they likely to be the systems that predominate in 10 or 15 years. Given the heterogeneity of the medical profession and the ever-changing political and socioeconomic climate, new and dynamic careers in medicine will surely emerge.

Information about career pathways in medicine is based largely on information from interviews of physicians and their autobiographic accounts (Curry 1988; Laster 1996; Lazarus 1996, 1998; Nash 1993; Silberman 1995). Some information, however, has been derived systematically through research (Mogul and Dickstein 1995; Walsh 1987).

Based on interviews with 32 physicians, many of whom are world renowned, Laster (1996) categorized the medical profession into five distinct career pathways (Table 18–2). Each of these pathways can be further subdivided. For example, Lazarus (1996) found that within the field of psychiatry, there were at least 16 distinct career tracks. Some, like private practice and psychoanalysis, are very traditional and deeply ingrained in the profession. Others, such as mental health administration, occupational psychiatry, and health maintenance organization (HMO) practice, are less traditional but can be just as rewarding. Still other career tracks in psychiatry, such as forensic practice, work in the pharmaceutical industry, and participation in organized medicine, may seem unconventional yet usually prove to be highly satisfying.

Silberman (1995) observed that despite rapid changes in the conditions of practice, psychiatrists continue to thrive in diverse settings. Psychiatrists differ by specialty (child and adolescent versus adult), location of practice (urban versus small-city versus rural), nature of practice (multidisciplinary group versus staff model HMO versus hospital), type of practice (psychoanalytic versus psychopharmacologic versus consultation-liaison), and primary area of interest (addiction psychiatry versus geriatric psychiatry versus forensic psychiatric practice). Silberman (1995) noted that successful psychiatrists are competent, energetic, and flexible.

The viability of one career over another may not be related to the content of the field as much as it is to the characteristics and qualifications of the individual physician. Physicians who choose a career in medical management, for example, portray a sense of excitement about their field. They are open to change and tend to be people oriented (Curry 1988). When physicians fail as managers, failure results from personal shortcomings—inadequate management talent or training, failure to lead, inability to fulfill multiple roles, poor interpersonal skills, and so forth (Peters 1994). Both success and failure hinge on personal attributes more than they do on institutional goals and organizational factors.

The Physician Executive

Managed care has created numerous opportunities for physicians interested in careers in administration and management (Lazarus 1994). Many physicians—so-called physician executives—have reached positions of top governance and leadership, such as president and CEO. However, most physician executives make their mark as senior managers, often with titles such as

TABLE 18–2.   The fivefold medical pathway

Internal medicine (e.g., internist, family practitioner, or pediatrician)

Surgery (e.g., general and/or specialized surgeon, obstetrician and gynecologist, otolaryngologist)

Psychiatry

Disciplines removed from ongoing patient care (e.g., anesthesiologist, pathologist, radiologist, nuclear medicine specialist)

Pursuits not related to the practice of medicine (e.g., writer, journalist, broadcaster, musician, executive, entrepreneur, or politician)

Source.   Adapted from Laster 1996.

vice president of medical affairs, chief medical officer, and department or division chair or chief. The key steps in the making of a physician executive, according to Linney (1996), are becoming board certified and practicing at least 3 years, obtaining management experience, furthering one's education, and finding a mentor (Shlian 1995).

As stated earlier, many medical managers have either stopped practicing or reduced their time seeing patients. It's not that practicing and managing are incompatible; it's just that the demand of each makes it very difficult to do both. Medical management will continue to become more specialized (the field may one day be recognized as a board-certifiable specialty by the American Board of Medical Specialties, and it has been recognized as a board-certifiable specialty by the Certifying Commission in Medical Management of the American College of Physician Executives). As this specialization grows, the time and energy required to be a competent and successful administrator will likely compete with time allotted for direct patient care, creating numerous conflicts.

The duties of a high-ranking medical administrator are not always well defined. Most physician executives must coordinate medical staff activities, accreditation surveys, governance issues, credentialing, utilization review, and performance improvement. Those responsibilities have broadened to include product and service line development, strategic planning, financial management, marketing, and physician recruitment and retention. Accordingly, the physician executive's skill set is expanding. More physicians are obtaining master's degrees in business administration and related fields than ever before. In 1994, 9.4% of physicians in management had M.B.A. degrees and another 38% were working on an M.B.A. or planning to pursue one (Anders 1994). For many physicians eager to enter the field of medical management, additional education is becoming a prerequisite.

Skepticism awaits many physicians who assume leadership responsibility. In fact, the term "physician executive" has long been considered an oxymoron. Previously, a physician was selected for a management position because his or her clinical and leadership roles were valued by other physicians, not necessarily by nonphysician managers. However, physicians who have made the successful transition to management have demonstrated an ability to be system thinkers and to understand organizational structure and function. Hospitals and health systems are benefiting from this new generation of physicians because they are more willing and able to join the ranks of senior management. Physician executives are expected to compete on the same turf as their nonmedical counterparts. At the same time, by retaining their white coats, they are expected to relate equally well to other physicians.

Ironically, an assessment of the value of physician executives to organizational effectiveness and performance indicated that in every case where a significant difference existed between physician executives and their nonmedical colleagues, the nonmedical executives always rated the value of physician executives as more important to organizational performance than did the physician executives themselves (Dunham et al. 1994). Physician executives should be reassured to know that they are highly valued by other managers in their organizations.

The Career Change Process

Physician recruiters and career counselors have been besieged by distressed physicians longing to try new fields. However, these same counselors also warn that many physicians who dream of quitting their jobs just want to escape harsh realities—managed care, office politics, a boss they do not like, and so forth. Physicians contemplating a career change often rely on disparate sources of information for advice, from newspaper columnists to self-help books to popular magazines. Seeking a practice solution is not easy because most physicians are particular about location, practice arrangement, and financial compensation. Physicians interested in nonclinical careers may need special guidance to determine which nonclinical options are appropriate for them. The remainder of this chapter outlines an effective decision-making process that physicians can use to determine whether they want to change careers, leave clinical practice, or leave medicine altogether:

1. Do a self-assessment. Examine your priorities and assess your skills. What skills do you now possess that you enjoy using most? Rank your priorities in terms of geography and location, lifestyle, financial needs, and so forth. What trade-offs are you willing to accept? Be flexible in what you consider, and do not eliminate options simply because you fear change. Resistance to change is universal.

2. Seek guidance and personal consulting. Career counseling and vocational tests such as the Strong Interest Inventory and the Myers-Briggs Type Indicator can guide you through the maze of careers and help you focus on what options will work best for you. Counselors and recruiters who have worked with a number of physicians will be particularly tuned in to the job marketplace. Talk to peers, colleagues, or associates who have recently undertaken job searches. Your goal in these conversations is to gain as much knowledge as possible and learn from other people's experiences.

3. Write a powerful resume or, for academically oriented positions, prepare a curriculum vitae. Succinctly outline your education, training, experience, certifications, accomplishments, and publications (if applicable). Make sure the document looks professional. Remember, your resume or curriculum vitae may be the only opportunity you have to present your qualifications to a prospective employer. At this stage, also decide on several references that can be used to assess your strengths (and weaknesses) objectively. References should include physicians as well as teachers, supervisors, and other healthcare professionals.

4. Use different job search methods. The typical methods used to perform a comprehensive job search are personal networking, medical societies and associations, advertisements, the Internet, and physician search firms. Multiple search methods are necessary because the best opportunities are often the most difficult to locate. Keep your curriculum vitae and reference list up-to-date, and take courses, if necessary, that will prepare you for a career change.

5. Learn how to negotiate change. Changing careers creates conflict, and resolving conflict requires negotiation. Developing negotiation skills can help you deal with change and make your present job more palatable.

6. Rely on your instincts. Your subjective feelings and those of your family must be factored into any decision to change careers. Family and relatives may identify issues of which you are not aware. If your career change entails relocating, make sure you have the support of your family. Evaluate housing conditions, the education system, the cultural milieu where you plan to live, and relocation benefits.

Changing careers is easiest if you manage it in an organized and efficient manner. The rewards of your new position will come not only from mastering change but also from being successful in changing times.

References

American Medical Association Council on Long Range Planning and Development: The Future of Medical Practice. Chicago, American Medical Association, 1994

Anders G: A new breed of M.D.s add M.B.A. to vitae. The Wall Street Journal, September 27, 1994, pp B1, B10

Curry W (ed): Roads to Medical Management: Physician Executives' Career Decisions. Tampa, FL, American College of Physician Executives, 1988

DeBakey M: Personal essay, in Medicine: Preserving the Passion. New York, Springer-Verlag, 1987, p 23

Dunham NC, Kindig DA, Schulz R: The value of the physician executive role to organizational effectiveness and performance. Health Care Manage Rev 19:56–63,1994

Goldberg JH: Doctors struggle to keep their earnings up. Medical Economics 72(17):184–202, 1995

Goodman L: Managed care's role in shaping the physician job market. JAMA 277:72, 1997

Gumbiner R: Perspectives of an HMO leader. Inquiry 31:330–333, 1994

Jennett PA, Kishinevsky M, Bryant H, et al: Major changes in medical careers following medical school graduation: when, how often, and why. Acad Med 65:48–49, 1990

Kassebaum DG, Szenas PL: Relationship between indebtedness and the specialty choices of graduating medical students: 1993 update. Acad Med 68:934–937, 1993

Kindig DA, Dunham NC, Chun LM: Career paths of physician executives. Health Care Manage Rev 16:11–20, 1991

Laster L: Life After Medical School. New York, WW Norton, 1996

Lazarus A: Opportunities for psychiatrists in managed care organizations. Psychiatr Serv 45:1206–1210, 1994

Lazarus A (ed): Career Pathways in Psychiatry: Transition in Changing Times. Hillsdale, NJ, Analytic Press, 1996

Lazarus A (ed): M.D./M.B.A.: Physicians on the New Frontier of Medical Management. Tampa, FL, American College of Physician Executives, 1998

Lee EK, Kaltreider N, Crouch J: Pilot study of current factors influencing the choice of psychiatry as a specialty. Am J Psychiatry 152:1066–1069, 1995

Linney BJ: Hope for the Future: A Career Development Guide for Physician Executives. Tampa, FL, American College of Physician Executives, 1996

Mogul KM, Dickstein LJ (eds): Career Planning for Psychiatrists. Washington, DC, American Psychiatric Press, 1995

Nash DB (ed): Future Practice Alternatives in Medicine, 2nd Edition. New York, Igaku-Shoin, 1993

National Resident Matching Program: NRMP Data. Washington, DC, Association of American Medical Colleges, 1991–1996

Olfson M, Klerman GL, Pincus HA: The roles of psychiatrists in organized outpatient mental health settings. Am J Psychiatry 150:625–631, 1993

Olfson M, Pincus HA, Dial TH: Professional practice patterns of U.S. psychiatrists. Am J Psychiatry 151:89–95, 1994

Pearlin LI, Klerman GS: Career preferences of psychiatric residents. Psychiatry 29:56–66, 1966

Peters RM: When Physicians Fail as Managers: An Exploratory Analysis of Career Change Problems. Tampa, FL, American College of Physician Executives, 1994

Rahe RH: Stress and psychiatry, in Comprehensive Textbook of Psychiatry/VI. Edited by Kaplan HI, Saddock BJ. Baltimore, MD, Williams & Wilkins, 1995, pp 1545–1559

Reinhardt U: The impending physician surplus: is it time to quit? JAMA 277:69, 1997

Rosenthal MP, Diamond JJ, Rabinowitz HK, et al: Influence of income, hours worked, and loan repayment on medical students' decision to pursue a primary care career. JAMA 271:914–917, 1994

Shlian DM (ed): Women in Medicine and Management: A Mentoring Guide. Tampa, FL, American College of Physician Executives, 1995

Sierles FS, Taylor MA: Decline of U.S. medical student career choice of psychiatry and what to do about it. Am J Psychiatry 152:1416–1426, 1995

Silberman EK (ed): Successful Psychiatric Practice: Current Dilemmas, Choices, and Solutions. Washington, DC, American Psychiatric Press, 1995

Walsh DC: Corporate Physicians: Between Medicine and Management. New Haven, Yale University Press, 1987

Weiner JP: Forecasting the effects of health reform on U.S. physician workforce requirement: evidence from HMO staffing patterns. 272:222–230, 1994

❖ 19 ❖

Changing Roles for Primary Consumers in Community Psychiatry

Carol T. Mowbray, Ph.D.
David P. Moxley, Ph.D.
Laura Van Tosh

Consumerism continues to grow and diversify as people with serious mental illness involve themselves in the direct provision of supportive and rehabilitative services and in the development, governance, administration, and evaluation of mental health programs (Moxley and Mowbray 1997). The concept of consumers in this chapter refers to those individuals who cope with serious mental illness; those whose functioning is obviated by medical, social, and personal complications; and those who are working toward recovery.[1] "Consumers as providers" means that these individuals can effectively serve other consumers within the context of alternative and established mental health programs and systems. The involvement of consumers in these changing roles has been driven not only by consumer dissat-isfaction with traditional mental health services (L. Van Tosh, unpublished manuscript, 1993) but also by the contribution consumers have made to the formation and perpetuation of innovative types of programs and supports (Mowbray et al. 1997).

In this chapter we examine the changing roles of primary consumers and the challenges psychiatric administrators must address in integrating consumers as providers into service delivery. To achieve this, we offer background on consumer role innovations as well as a framework for understanding consumer service provision. We then identify the administrative issues these role innovations suggest and conclude with the kinds of solutions administrators of psychiatric services should contemplate in addressing the issues proactively.

Development of this chapter was supported in part by a grant to the Ohio Department of Mental Health from the Center for Mental Health Services/Substance Abuse Mental Health Services Administration.

[1] The authors recognize and respect various terms individuals use to describe themselves, for example, consumers, recipients, survivors, ex-patients, or clients. For brevity, *consumer* is used in this chapter.

Background

There is a long history of consumer involvement in provider roles in human services—starting with mental health in the 1940s to 1950s and then substance abuse, aging, and poverty in the 1960s (Moxley and Mowbray 1997). Such innovations are more common in periods of social activism—products of social movements that seek to empower people marginalized by society and to increase the control they have over their own lives (Aronowitz 1992).

Consumers as providers also coincides with a larger consumer movement. Beginning with the efforts of Ralph Nader and the formation of public interest law in the United States, advocates sought to make producers of goods and services more directly accountable to consumers and their representatives (Nader et al. 1976). Reinforced by President Kennedy's consumer bill of rights, the status of the consumer as someone who was to be informed and protected was dramatically strengthened from the 1960s to the early 1980s. Although legal remedies and other protections have since been weakened, contemporary expressions of consumerism can still be found in the total quality improvement movement, which incorporates expectations of consumers as critical indicators of product performance.

New definitions of consumer status introduced by social action movements took root and flourished both within and outside human services. Social movements in the greater society—such as the civil rights (Blumberg 1984), feminist (Feree and Hess 1985), and gay and lesbian movements (Adam 1987)—innovated a range of empowerment practices and principles and translated these into concrete social action. People experiencing discrimination assumed an expectation if not a right to speak out about oppression and inequalities created by social structure. Within the human services arena, antipsychiatry (Chamberlin 1978) and disability rights movements (Shapiro 1993) established new frameworks of service delivery and invested new rights and claims by consumers. These efforts were reinforced by the documentation of institutional abuse produced by social scientists from the 1950s to the 1970s. Often adopting (and adapting) the strategies and tactics of larger social movements, social activists sought to underscore the experience of oppression, the negative effects of labeling, and the disenfranchisement created by service systems (Chu and Trotter 1974). These experiences were translated into a justification for the creation of new roles for consumers.

One of the first examples of consumer involvement in direct mental health services is the founding, in the late 1940s, of Fountain House by a group of ex-patients who called themselves "We Are Not Alone," thus inaugurating the fledgling clubhouse movement (Beard 1976). Here consumers came together to create and operate their own support system in order to fill gaps in services, to develop pragmatic community support systems, and to establish opportunities for affiliation and social interaction. The Joint Commission on Mental Illness and Health, whose report framed the structure of the community mental health model, identified Fountain House and a number of other patient-run alternatives as promising exemplars of how consumers themselves could enhance mental health treatment through their own informal and formal initiatives, supports, and services (Joint Commission on Mental Illness and Health 1961). The commission, however, took a somewhat pessimistic position on these alternatives, noting that they probably could not survive or operate well without the oversight of enlightened mental health professionals.

Although the Joint Commission anticipated consumer role innovation, it did not anticipate the direction and the assertive posture consumers would take. The emergence of the antipsychiatry movement certainly fueled innovation and development of consumers as providers, with the 1970s witnessing the emergence of consumer-run alternatives to mental health services. Based on a social critique of psychiatry, and using constructs of stigma, discrimination, and oppression, members of the ex-patient movement demonstrated the value of alternative support systems and the importance of consumer control (Chamberlin 1978).

These perspectives and resulting organizational and programmatic forms were not readily embraced by established psychiatric and mental health systems. However, emerging community support programs from the late 1970s into the 1980s began to recognize the important if not critical role these alternatives could serve in rehabilitation and recovery. New programmatic structures incorporating consumers as providers became salient within progressive service systems.

This programmatic change was in anticipation of a range of benefits that consumers as providers could create for service recipients and for consumer providers. There were also potential benefits for existing systems of service: opportunities to expand support options in a cost-effective manner and possibly to co-opt consumers who could otherwise create considerable conflict, disruption, or even competitive service alternatives (Moxley and Mowbray 1997). Consumers as providers introduced an element of pragmatism often lacking in psychiatric and clinical services, offering ways of helping people address isolation, crisis, social involvement, and access to community resources.

A Framework for Understanding Consumer-Provider Roles

Although consumer service provision has a long history and substantial current interest as an innovation, the published literature on this topic is diffuse and has not permitted shared learning (L. Van Tosh, unpublished manuscript, 1993). To increase knowledge application, we have proposed a framework and related typology to permit more systematic understanding of variations in consumer roles and the issues involved (Mowbray et al. 1997). As presented in Figure 19–1, the framework uses two organizing dimensions. First, whether or not the alternative is consumer controlled, in recognition of the reality that when disenfranchised groups are merely involved rather than in control, they may have little real impact (Chamberlin 1978). The second dimension, the aim of the alternative—formal service provision versus mutual support—subsumes differences in regulatory requirements, funding bases, legal status, management activities, and the like. The framework produces four types of consumer-service involvement: consumer-controlled alternatives, consumers as employees, self-help, and consumer initiatives.

		Control of alternative	
		Consumer	**Nonconsumer**
Aim of the alternative	**Service provision**	Consumer-run services	Consumers as employees
	Mutual support	Self-help	Consumer initiatives

FIGURE 19–1. A framework for understanding consumer-provider roles.

Consumer-Controlled Alternatives

In consumer-controlled alternatives, formal services are provided through an organization that is governed, administered, and operated exclusively (or nearly so) by consumers. Usually this is a freestanding legal entity with a formal budget, financed through a combination of self-sustaining activities and fee-for-service and/or contracts (e.g., from state government or a local community mental health board). The benefits to consumers include individual and group empowerment from ownership of the service, plus the tangible benefits of employment. Typical models of consumer-controlled alternatives are drop-in centers; others include consumer-run businesses, companion services, case management, and housing assistance. An example of a model consumer-controlled alternative is the program called "on our own," located in Charlottesville, Virginia. This program was started by a group of consumers who were ineligible for or dissatisfied with the limited rehabilitation options available to them. After receiving state funding for a day shelter, they incorporated as a private, nonprofit organization and developed their own policies, rules, and decision-making structures. The philosophy of "on our own" formally endorses the value of choice, using natural support systems, providing comprehensive services, organizing services around people, not places, and emphasizing self-reliance as a goal (Silverman 1997).

Consumers as Employees

In the consumers as employees type of involvement, consumers are hired as staff through a formal organization, usually a community mental health or psychiatric rehabilitation program, which they do not run or control. This organization has its own (nonconsumer) formal governance structure, budget, and organizational and management activities. It purposefully hires consumers in service positions—either through affirmative employment practices or, more commonly, by designating certain positions exclusively for consumers. Typically these consumers are hired to provide support services or to extend the services provided by a nonconsumer professional (i.e., finding jobs or housing, respite work, skill practice in activities of daily living). Increasingly, consumers are also working in credentialed positions. The rationale behind hiring consumers is that they bring to these roles a motivation, sensitivity, and understanding that workers with only professional training cannot. Furthermore, they provide role models for rehabilitation and recovery (Besio and Mahler 1993). Service recipients benefit through services that are more appropriate and useful, consumer providers benefit by having jobs, and the system benefits by having improved services.

An example of a model program that hires consumers is the peer counseling program at Manhattan Psychiatric Center (Oursler 1997). Funded through a grant from the state office of mental health, the program employs four consumers to provide services to other consumers. Peer counselors are supervised by nonconsumer psychiatric center staff and have all the rights, responsibilities, and benefits accorded to other employees. They work in inpatient and day treatment programs with dually diagnosed individuals who have had extended hospitalizations or dependent care experiences to promote rehabilitation readiness. The peer counselors conduct or co-lead (with a professional) consumer groups on topics such as coping with housing crises or planning for the future, accompany consumers to appointments in the community, assume a major role in planning consumer-led programs, and participate in recreational activities with consumers and in treatment team meetings with staff.

Self-Help

In self-help, individuals with a common experience come together voluntarily, operating informal support groups or other programs outside formal systems of care. In contrast to the more differentiated administrative structures found in formal organizations, self-help groups offer little distinction between those who provide help and support and those who receive it. Furthermore, usually there are no formal resources to support operations, nor are there necessarily external funding sources, formal settings for services, or needs to meet external accountability demands and regulations. The rationale behind self-help alternatives is that peer support increases problem-solving capabilities by offering realistic solutions based on others' experiences and enhances the use of social resources by decreasing isolation and allowing opportunities to discuss issues about the self that would be off limits with professionals (Gartner and Riessman 1984). One consumer relates, "There were many times that I needed someone to talk to about feelings of suicide, fear, self-destruction, my hopes and dreams—who I was as a person, not just a mental health client" (Scott 1997). Self-help can fulfill this need. Self-help is provided through local affiliates of national organizations like Recovery, Inc.; Schizophrenics Anonymous; the National Depressive and Manic-Depressive Association; GROW, Inc.; or local grassroots groups started independently by consumers or sometimes professionals.

Consumer Initiatives

Consumer initiatives are probably least represented in the literature but may be the most widespread, with groups of consumers independently initiating activities within mental health or rehabilitation agencies. Although these settings have budgets and formal organizational structures, roles, and procedures, the consumer initiatives within them operate more informally and for mutual support purposes. Resource allocations are usually minimal or nonexistent. The rationale behind this type of alternative is that consumers' experiences can translate into service and support innovations by consumers themselves, within existing programs, uniquely meeting needs that may otherwise be ignored by formal organizations. As in self-help, all consumers can be helpers and help recipients, but with consumer initiatives, there is a stronger rehabilitative focus, with consumers supplying resource information, providing role models, and facilitating empowerment through shared knowledge. These initiatives perhaps best demonstrate the natural leadership potential of psychiatric consumers.

An example of a model consumer initiative is a work and school support group in a community support program, developed and completely facilitated by consumers (Hanna 1997). The consumer-developer of the group was herself a university student and served as a role model as well as a resource person to other group members. Group members gathered strength by supporting each other and by acquiring knowledge about others' successful solutions to problems, their rights under the Americans with Disabilities Act (ADA), and the like.

Administrative Questions and Issues

As the preceding brief descriptions indicate, consumer service provision offers great potential to improve mental health services to individuals with long-term, severe mental illnesses. In fact, these services have usually developed in response to dissatisfactions with the mental health system. The benefits frequently mentioned include increased social support and nurturance, in contrast to formal mental health services that are perceived as not available, accessible, flexible, or individually tailored. Service provision by one's peers produces greater rapport and empathy and consequently a greater willingness to openly disclose problems. The responses of someone "who has been there" can provide greater assurance, more helpful problem-solving assistance, more opportunities for decision making, and greater choice and independence (L. Van Tosh, unpublished manuscript, 1993). Peers may also have more time available for hands-on assistance. Thus, consumer providers are uniquely able to serve as role models. As such, they offer continued hope for the recipient's own rehabilitation and recovery. This, indeed, may be their greatest contribution.

As much as these benefits should be appreciated, administrators also need to grasp the complexity and far-reaching implications that consumer service provision entails. Consumers in provider roles represent a radical change in perceptions of individuals with psychiatric disabilities and a paradigm shift in professional mental health practice. An understanding of the depth and extent of the issues is necessary for determining how and when consumer service provision can best fit within the mental health system and what changes are needed to maximize its utility. Administrators need to address a number of questions in considering this innovation.

What Types of Roles Can Consumers Play?

Consumer service roles most frequently involve peer counseling, working as case manager aides, or leading consumer-based activities. Consumers' functions include advocacy, resource acquisition on behalf of clients, training in community living, socialization, group work, and information dissemination. Consumers have also served as respite workers, educational mentors, housing resident managers, hospital patient advocates, mobile crisis team workers, and so on. Following the onset of a psychiatric illness, individuals report experiences of resuming or assuming professional roles as social worker, psychiatrist, psychologist, professor, administrator, or rehabilitation counselor. Thus, the roles and functions occupied by consumer service providers are extensive and divergent (Mowbray et al. 1997).

How Does Consumer Service Provision Fit In With Existing Mental Health Services?

The extent to which consumer service provision is integrated within mental health systems varies widely. Some consumer-controlled alternatives and self-help groups receive substantial support from established programs, including donated resources such as supplies and equipment or administrative assistance. These programs enjoy referral arrangements wherein consumer services offer an adjunct or alternative. In other locations, mental health programs are distant from or even adversarial to consumer service provision. What accounts for these variations is only open to speculation, possibly including attitudes of mental health administrators or consumer leaders, long-standing tensions, organizational orientations toward empowerment, or overall ideologies about diversity.

For consumer service provision inside mental health agencies, some settings (e.g., inpatient programs that often use more rigid role structures) seem to be more problematic than others. Davidson et al. (1997) described the problems encountered in a traditional day hospital by a peer support group that focused on advocacy, open membership, and confidentiality among the members. When a consumer employee led the group, these values conflicted with the expectations of colleagues and with the way the day program operated.

Another barrier frequently confronted in consumer service provision is the behavior of nonconsumer staff, especially when differential standards are applied to consumer providers. Sometimes nonconsumer staff will lower their performance expectations, based on beneficence or sympathy toward individuals they still view as clients. More frequently, nonconsumer staff find it threatening to view consumers as providers: based on bias, stigma, fears about their own job security, assaults on the boundaries between professional and client status, risks to established professional norms of hierarchical and distanced relationships, or role strains from realignment of attitudes. These reactions are heightened in organizations that foster hierarchies among staff or between staff and clients and in situations in which staff have fewer professional credentials or less status (Jonikas et al. 1997). Such reactions can obviously detract from the success of consumer-provided services by erecting barriers to consumers' abilities to do their jobs, interact with service recipients, or have access to necessary resources.

Are Consumers Available to Fill These Roles on an Ongoing Basis?

Published reports document the large number and wide array of roles consumers have played in direct services. However, there are some noteworthy issues of concern. First, as in many volunteer organizations, psychiatric self-help initiatives may experience high rates of turnover and difficulties in getting peers to assume leadership roles. This can produce burnout in those remaining to carry the load. Second, consumers may experience stress from witnessing a mental health system failing their peers, as it may have failed them. Stress can also result from consumers not feeling secure in their own worth, from lost opportunities or years of disempowering experiences. Third, in the process of serving as role models and providing problem-solving assistance to others, consumer providers may be reminded of their own personal experiences, which could create distress. The similarity between consumer providers and their peers, which produces benefits, can also be a cost, in that boundary issues are more likely to arise for them than for nonconsumer staff. These issues include overidentification with service recipients, disappointment when clients fail to follow through, or an inability to separate one's own issues and anger from those of the service recipients. Nevertheless, as their successes indicate, consumer service providers have by and large been able to overcome these problems and obtain benefits for themselves and their peers.

Some of the ill effects on consumer service providers are directly attributable to biased and discriminatory treatment from nonconsumer staff who see the consumer in a "make-work" position and not really able to contribute meaningfully. Also frequently mentioned are staff assumptions that consumer role performance problems reflect heightened symptomatology when a simpler explanation is warranted, such as the role confusion of a new employee. Furthermore, consumer roles set up by professionals rather than by consumers themselves often lack role clarity and contain unclear performance expectations (Hildebrand et al. 1997).

What Types of Accommodations and Special Arrangements May Be Necessary?

Many program reports indicate that consumers need special training and higher levels of supervision than nonconsumer staff (Weklar and Parker 1997). It is unclear whether these are valid comparisons because most consumers come to paid positions with little or no human services training. Mowbray et al. (1996) found that the supervision needed for peer support specialists decreased over time. Although program administrators are often concerned about consumers maintaining confidentiality, this appears not to be an issue, according to published reports (Mowbray et al. 1997). Administrative costs associated with meeting accommodation needs due to psychiatric disabilities most often involve requests for flexible hours, leave time, sometimes private work space free from distraction, and coverage for absences during hospitalizations (Carling 1993; Mancuso 1997)—none of which appear to be of great magnitude.

An issue that appears to have significant ramifications is failure to involve consumers in planning for consumer service involvement (L. Van Tosh, unpublished manuscript, 1993). Hildebrand et al. (1997) described the problems that resulted when professionals developed a program to hire consumers as life-skills consultants with no input from consumers themselves. Failure to adequately define roles and differentiate peer-based or self-help support from professional mental health treatment is another problem area, often creating confusion and frustration for consumer providers and resentment from nonconsumer staff. Problems can also arise in interpersonal relationships between service recipients and consumer providers in paid roles when principles and rules have not been adequately developed regarding prior relationships, the forming of friendships, or advocacy activities. Many programs fail to address possible conflicts in advance and wind up with situations that are problematic for all parties.

How Should These Innovations Be Structured?

Equitable pay rates, stable hours, and fringe benefits are necessities for consumers in any paid employment situation, particularly because permanent loss of disability benefits can result. Consumer advocates have expressed concern that agencies may be willing to hire consumers, but only into the lowest level positions, without adequate pay or appropriate levels of authority or responsibility (Allen 1997).

A more complex issue is whether service delivery by consumers should be done through designated positions (e.g., peer counselors) or contracts with consumer-controlled alternatives instead of through affirmative employment practices (e.g., actively recruiting and hiring consumers for any staff vacancy). Consumer-designated positions have the advantage of protected work situations that may have more flexibility, support, and safety than those in the competitive market. In contrast, these types of positions almost require self-disclosure as a norm of practice, significantly increasing the stress in a role that already constitutes difficult emotional labor. Furthermore, negative expectations and stigma from supervisors and other staff may degrade consumer performance and negate benefits.

Summary

Although consumer service provision has many reported benefits, its development and implementation are associated with substantial and complex issues (Lehman as cited in L. Van Tosh, unpublished manuscript, 1993). If these issues are not addressed adequately, benefits may indeed be short lived or may occur at an unacceptable cost to the consumer providers.

Administrative Processes to Support Consumer Role Innovation

To facilitate consumer role innovation and make it a viable part of the contemporary provision of community psychiatric service, administrative actions are necessary—particularly concerning consumer employment by agencies. Changes are needed in organizational climate, human resource development, provisions for support needs, and career mobility for consumer providers.

Organizational Climate

Organizational climate forms a critical context within which consumer role innovation will succeed or fail. Attitudes and their expression at all levels must be considered in making consumer role innovation work well and effectively (Bevilacqua et al. 1997). An administrator's support is necessary but not sufficient. Crafting a conducive organizational climate requires a whole system response articulating the value and importance of this innovation from the board down to direct service delivery personnel.

The community board must endorse consumer role innovation to establish a supportive context (D. P. Moxley, "Foundations of Board Performance in Psychosocial Rehabilitation," unpublished manuscript, 1996).

This means surveying prevailing policies and developing an agenda for adopting proactive ones. Policies on credentialing, accommodations, staff development, medical and mental healthcare, and interprofessional communication and confidentiality must incorporate and uphold consumer service provision. A board that is insulated from consumerism or lacking consumer membership may defeat consumer role innovation, equating quality care only with professional credentials. Consciousness raising may be necessary with board education focused on the rationale for consumerism, successful approaches, and information on best practices. Inviting consumers to serve on subcommittees and recruiting consumer members to the board can give this kind of innovation legitimacy and a personalized face and thus serve as critical ways of empowering consumer involvement (D. P. Moxley, "Foundations of Board Development: Building Governance in Community and Social Services," unpublished book manuscript, 1997).

Executive directors, upper echelon division directors, and direct service supervisors must also present a frame of reference and attitudinal set that promotes consumer involvement (Bevilacqua et al. 1997). They should be knowledgeable about requirements under the ADA and other relevant laws. These actors are instrumental in translating organizational policy into direct action and in identifying and resolving barriers to policy implementation. Without this leadership, the intended innovation may not occur.

Direct service providers are also instrumental to successful consumer role innovation. However, they must see it as organizationally sanctioned and emanating out of organizational policy (Zipple et al. 1997). They must have an opportunity to identify issues that can be resolved through education, training, and technical assistance events intentionally undertaken to undergird consumerism. Proactive agency leadership can help staff to make sense of these innovations and to establish consumer roles in service provision as a standard of excellence.

Human Resource Development

These organizational climate initiatives must coincide with responsive human resource development efforts. For employment, the organization must practice affirmative recruitment practices (Zipple et al. 1997). Consumer candidates for paid positions can be identified both within and outside the agency. Good recruitment methods may include advertising in consumer newsletters, forming linkages with consumer groups, conducting recruitment campaigns within programs, and undertaking targeted outreach to particular consumers.

Organizational climate goes hand in hand with human resource development and both join in producing affirmative employment. Whether the agency establishes positions specifically identified for consumers or opens up all positions to consumer hiring is a tactical choice. Movement into consumer role innovation will, however, require the agency to identify affirmative employment as a principal organizational value and to operationalize this value in policies and procedures that support proactive recruitment, innovation in credentialing, and diversification of personnel within the agency (Zipple et al. 1997).

Provisions for Support Needs

Belief in affirmative employment and valuing of diversity (Granger 1997) are not all that are needed. Merely recruiting a fixed number of consumers into service delivery positions does not constitute success; rather it is just the beginning of innovation. Human resource development must also expand into meeting the support needs of consumers employed in service provider roles. Discussions are needed concerning credentialing and salary based on skills, knowledge, and performance rather than education (Griffin-Francell 1997), although many consumers have requisite educational backgrounds. Organizations need to ensure that they do not reinforce marginalization, discrimination, and reduced expectations. Continuing education, mentoring, new systems of credentialing, and pay-for-performance are some of the supports that an affirmative system of employment will offer consumers taking on provider roles (Mowbray et al. 1996). When articulated for all employees, such supports make for an affirmative organization.

Organizational climate, a proactive human resource development system, and specific employment supports will begin to set in motion a successful program of consumer role innovation. However, basic questions face many consumers: Are there long-term benefits? Do these benefits justify commitment to an entry-level role, the redefinition of self based on this role, and acceptance of a minimum wage job? Can the agency compensate for possible relinquishment of disability income and medical benefits (Mowbray et al. 1996)?

Career Mobility for Consumer Providers

Too many consumers report that after they have entered staff positions, they have not moved on as expectations about their possibilities and performance have expanded (Allen 1997). Consumers want to be on career ladders or have salary trajectories like other employees. Serious consumer role innovation means not just crafting new positions but articulating career ladders and a commitment to organizational mobility. These are true tests of an effective program.

Conclusion

What does this mean in practice? Consumers as paid providers should start at a level based on their education or experience; then, based on the acquisition of skill and competencies, they should move into senior positions—perhaps as supervisors, program leaders, directors, or executives. The employing organization takes great care in helping people achieve a sense of competence in their current positions, but it also establishes an expectation that people can advance; the purpose of human resource development is to make this advancement possible if it is desired.

The affirmative agency also recognizes that even its own good intentions may be overwhelmed by structural barriers that surface in the form of discrimination, segregation, and neglect of employees. Supportive alternatives such as mentoring systems, support groups, internal advocacy, and specialized advancement programs can be established to enable sincere and motivated employees to overcome these barriers (Kerouac 1997). More important, successful execution of these initiatives can teach the agency how to overcome barriers and develop effective strategies and tactics to assist all people who might ordinarily be held back.

Whenever organizations undertake significant changes, short-term conflicts are likely to occur. Within the culture of human services, in which assumptions of normality and educational credentials are essential to professional recognition, consumers as providers may be discounted or assigned marginal status. Conflicts that surface at the interface of roles are understandable. For example, consumers receiving services from their peers may expect to interact with them as friends and compatriots, whereas the agency expects consumer providers to perform like other professionals (Allen 1997). Family members may see these changes as compromising the quality of traditional services. Nonconsumer providers may question the competence of their new colleagues or feel resentment because they perceive a double standard. Supervisors may lack knowledge of the ADA or an understanding of how to craft meaningful accommodations.

Such conflicts can be worked out when people come together. They also underscore the importance of proactive preparation. Certainly a supportive organizational climate will help, as will planned supports legitimized by a human resource development framework of affirmative employment. But organizational members must constantly monitor how consumer role innovation may break down at points of interaction between people of different status. Organizational redefinition of alternative credentials; the establishment of quality standards based on best practices; and the use of these standards in training, supervision, and performance evaluation can serve as overarching tactics in reinforcing the idea that people of all types can bring different talents and resources to the work setting (Zipple et al. 1997).

These areas taken together can assist human services organizations in establishing strategies that support consumer role innovation. Simply to implement this innovation without a whole system strategy will not facilitate change and success. Administrators of psychiatric services must recognize that they are reshaping organizational culture when they develop new roles within the agency. Establishing a supportive organizational climate, proactive human resource development policies and practices, specific supports for organizational mobility, and effective interactions across role interfaces are essential features of successful consumer role innovation.

References

Adam BD: The Rise of a Gay and Lesbian Movement. Boston, Twayne, 1987

Allen CR: Project WINS: a consumer's perspective, in Consumers as Providers in Psychiatric Rehabilitation. Edited by Mowbray CT, Moxley, DP, Jasper CA, et al. Columbia, MD, International Association of Psychosocial Rehabilitation Services, 1997, pp 238–242

Aronowitz S: The Politics of Identity. London, Routledge, 1992

Beard J: Psychiatric rehabilitation at Fountain House, in Rehabilitation Medicine and Psychiatry. Edited by Meislin J. Springfield, IL, Charles C. Thomas, 1976

Besio S, Mahler J: Benefits and challenges of using consumer staff in supported housing services. Hospital and Community Psychiatry 44:490–491, 1993

Bevilacqua J, Gads D, Cousins V: Mental health systems development: benefits created by consumer engagement, in Consumers as Providers in Psychiatric Rehabilitation. Edited by Mowbray CT, Moxley, DP, Jasper CA, et al. Columbia, MD, International Association of Psychosocial Rehabilitation Services, 1997, pp 460–470

Blumberg R: Civil Rights: The 1960s Struggle. Boston, Twayne, 1984

Carling PJ: Reasonable accommodations in the work place for individuals with psychiatric disabilities, in Implications of the Americans with Disabilities Act for Psychology. Edited by O'Keefe JE, Bruyere SM. New York, Springer, 1993, pp 103–135

Chamberlin J: On Our Own: Patient-Controlled Alternatives to the Mental Health System. New York, McGraw-Hill, 1978

Chu F, Trotter S: The Madness Establishment: Ralph Nader's Study Group Report on the National Institute of Mental Health. New York, Grossman, 1974

Davidson L, Weingarten R, Steiner J, et al: Integrating prosumers into clinical settings, in Consumers as Providers in Psychiatric Rehabilitation. Edited by Mowbray CT, Moxley, DP, Jasper CA, et al. Columbia, MD, International Association of Psychosocial Rehabilitation Services, 1997, pp 437–457

Feree M, Hess B: Controversy and Coalition: The New Feminist Movement. Boston, Twayne, 1985

Gartner A, Riessman F: The Self-Help Revolution. New York, Human Services Press, 1984

Granger D: Thinking about diversity, in Consumers as Providers in Psychiatric Rehabilitation. Edited by Mowbray CT, Moxley, DP, Jasper CA, et al. Columbia, MD, International Association of Psychosocial Rehabilitation Services, 1997, pp 478–487

Griffin-Francell C: Consumers as providers of psychiatric rehabilitation: reflections by a family member, in Consumers as Providers in Psychiatric Rehabilitation. Edited by Mowbray CT, Moxley, DP, Jasper CA, et al. Columbia, MD, International Association of Psychosocial Rehabilitation Services, 1997, pp 471–477

Hanna B: A consumer as a provider in a work-school support group, in Consumers as Providers in Psychiatric Rehabilitation. Edited by Mowbray CT, Moxley, DP, Jasper CA, et al. Columbia, MD, International Association of Psychosocial Rehabilitation Services, 1997, pp 184–187

Hildebrand K, Jardine L, McVay P, et al: Try another way: transitioning peer support specialists to roles as social and recreational support providers, in Consumers as Providers in Psychiatric Rehabilitation. Edited by Mowbray CT, Moxley, DP, Jasper CA, et al. Columbia, MD, International Association of Psychosocial Rehabilitation Services, 1997, pp 325–333

Joint Commission on Mental Illness and Health: Action for Mental Health. New York, Basic Books, 1961

Jonikas JA, Solomon MD, Cook JA: An inclusion framework: preparing psychosocial rehabilitation programs for the consumer hiring initiative, in Consumers as Providers in Psychiatric Rehabilitation. Edited by Mowbray CT, Moxley, DP, Jasper CA, et al. Columbia, MD, International Association of Psychosocial Rehabilitation Services, 1997, pp 419–436

Kerouac JW: Developing a support group for staff with mental illness, in Consumers as Providers in Psychiatric Rehabilitation. Edited by Mowbray CT, Moxley, DP, Jasper CA, et al. Columbia, MD, International Association of Psychosocial Rehabilitation Services, 1997, pp 397–405

Mancuso LL: Case Studies on Reasonable Accommodations for Workers with Psychiatric Disabilities. Sacramento, CA, California Department of Mental Health, 1997

Mowbray CT, Moxley DP, Thrasher S, et al: Consumers as community support providers: issues created by role innovation. Community Ment Health J 32:47–67, 1996

Mowbray CT, Moxley DP, Jasper CA, et al. (eds): Consumers as Providers in Psychiatric Rehabilitation. Columbia, MD, International Association of Psychosocial Rehabilitation Services, 1997

Moxley DP, Mowbray CT: Consumers as providers: forces and factors legitimizing role innovation in psychiatric rehabilitation, in Consumers as Providers in Psychiatric Rehabilitation. Edited by Mowbray CT, Moxley, DP, Jasper CA, et al. Columbia, MD, International Association of Psychosocial Rehabilitation Services, 1997, pp 2–34

Nader R, Green M, Seligman J: Taming the Giant Corporation. New York, Times Books, 1976

Oursler J: Consumers as providers: a peer counseling program, in Consumers as Providers in Psychiatric Rehabilitation. Edited by Mowbray CT, Moxley, DP, Jasper CA, et al. Columbia, MD, International Association of Psychosocial Rehabilitation Services, 1997, pp 224–237

Scott J: The P.S. Project: together we are living the miracle, in Consumers as Providers in Psychiatric Rehabilitation. Edited by Mowbray CT, Moxley, DP, Jasper CA, et al. Columbia, MD, International Association of Psychosocial Rehabilitation Services, 1997, pp 69–76

Shapiro JP: No Pity: People With Disabilities Forging a New Civil Rights Movement. New York, Times Brooks, 1993

Silverman S: Recovery through partnership: on our own, Charlottesville, Virginia, in Consumers as Providers in Psychiatric Rehabilitation. Edited by Mowbray CT, Moxley DP, Jasper CA, et al. Columbia, MD, International Association of Psychosocial Rehabilitation Services, 1997, pp 126–141

Weklar E, Parker KW: Supporting a consumer employee inside the agency, in Consumers as Providers in Psychiatric Rehabilitation. Edited by Mowbray CT, Moxley, DP, Jasper CA, et al. Columbia, MD, International Association of Psychosocial Rehabilitation Services, 1997, pp 387–396

Zipple AM, Drouin M, Armstrong M, et al: Consumers as colleagues: moving beyond ADA compliance, in Consumers as Providers in Psychiatric Rehabilitation. Edited by Mowbray CT, Moxley, DP, Jasper CA, et al. Columbia, MD, International Association of Psychosocial Rehabilitation Services, 1997, pp 406–418

❖ 20 ❖

Changing Family Roles

Harriet P. Lefley, Ph.D.

Psychiatric care is administered to a wide range of patients in behavioral healthcare systems, and family roles and relationships may vary as a function of the patient's age or functional level, the diagnosis, or the therapeutic modality used. This chapter focuses on families of adults with severe and persistent mental illness. These patients have periodic needs for crisis stabilization and hospitalization and ongoing needs for medication management, community supports, and rehabilitation.

Since the 1970s, marked changes have occurred in families' roles in the service delivery system and in families' relationships with mental health professionals. These changes have paralleled trends in contemporary psychiatric history. They are related to deinstitutionalization and to the waning influence of psychodynamic and family systems theories and their correlative therapies when applied to the major Axis I disorders such as schizophrenia or affective disorders. A proliferation of biological and genetic research findings have counteracted the notion of family interactions as primary etiological factors. Research evidence of biological substrates, as well as family burden research, have tended to alter clinical training and modify sometimes negative attitudes toward families. According to Marsh (1992), models of family pathogenesis have been superseded by models of coping and adaptation (Hatfield and Lefley 1987) and by a paradigm of family competence. In order to enhance families' competencies, pathology-based therapeutic approaches have been replaced by educational approaches responsive to families' expressed needs for information and practical assistance.

In addition to changes in theory, pragmatic needs for family collaboration in caregiving and advocacy began to emerge during deinstitutionalization. The current era of managed care brings similar needs for supportive resources for patients and political allies for providers. The growth of the family movement, the National Alliance for the Mentally Ill (NAMI), has created a major constituency for patients and a powerful political influence to increase funding for research, services, and equitable benefits. The movement has generated alliances with the American Psychiatric Association (APA) and other professional organizations and created new roles for patients' relatives in mental health systems for planning, monitoring, governance, and advisory board membership.

This chapter begins with an assessment of the extent of family involvement with patients who have severe and persistent psychiatric disorders and follows with a brief illustration of the human and practical needs of families coping with mental illness. The discussion traces changing trends in psychiatric history that affect the relations of families and professionals. A collaborative model is proposed in which families, consumers, professionals, and provider institutions can work together for improved care and resource development. This last area deals with administrative policies that offer practical help to families, contributions that families can make to the clinicians who work with their loved ones, managed care, and alliances that affect future directions of mental health services.

The Extent of Family Involvement

An overview of current family studies in the United States suggests that at least 40% of adults with severe and persistent mental illnesses are living with family members, with considerably higher percentages in minority groups (Lefley 1996b). In the most recent national survey of the predominantly white and middle class families of NAMI, 42% were living with the patient (Skinner et al. 1992). Ongoing contact and involvement was maintained with mentally ill family members not living at home. Other research shows that families tend to expend significant time and money on relatives with severe mental illness regardless of living arrangements (Clark and Drake 1994).

Although some studies have reported gratification in the help and companionship accorded by the mentally ill adult, particularly to elderly parents (Greenberg et al. 1994), significant data exist on paranoid abuse and violence (Estroff et al. 1994; Straznickas et al. 1993). In many situations, family members have endured the life strains from 10 to 40 years of illness punctuated by multiple crisis situations and hospitalizations. They have endured this strain during a historical epoch characterized by theories that typically denied any diagnostic or treatment information to the patient's relatives. Adverse experiences with the system are still embedded in the consciousness of many families, and it is important to acknowledge their effects.

Basic Needs of Families

Families of patients want communication, respect as persons, recognition and acknowledgment of the legitimacy of their needs, and some control of the events that affect their lives. These are not abstractions; they are very real, concrete needs, and they are instrumental to successfully fulfilling the long-term role of caregiver or support system for the patient.

In addition to needing understanding and support, family members have practical needs for basic information about psychotic disorders; knowledge of expected effects and side effects of medications; techniques for managing crises and aversive behaviors; and education that will enable them to have appropriate expectations and balance responsibilities toward the patient, other family members, and themselves. In order to help patients and their families, clinicians must have adequate state-of-the-art clinical knowledge, a compassionate awareness of families' experiences with severe mental illness, some training in psychoeducation and behavior management, an understanding of supportive psychotherapy, and a conception of treating chronic mental illness that encompasses a broad, metaclinical view of the service delivery system. Psychiatrists must know the resources needed for community survival and how their availability affects the course of illness and patient care. They also should have some awareness of the impact of psychiatric theories and practices on patients' major support systems—their families.

Historical Family-Professional Relationships

Until fairly recently in psychiatric history, theories of family pathogenesis, related confidentiality issues, and perhaps an uncertain state of knowledge erected communication barriers between clinicians and families. The self-report literature indicates the stark contrast of families' experiences in the medical sector (where family education was standard) and the psychiatric sector. Families' questions about what was wrong with their relative, that is, their natural wish to understand their relative's incomprehensible behavior, were deflected or answered evasively. Inquiries about diagnosis, treatment, and prognosis were not only ignored but also often treated as intrusive and self-serving. In many of the written recollections, families in acute distress felt that clinical staff seemed to perceive them as toxins rather than as suffering human beings. They felt their anguish was often interpreted as contributory psychopathology. Even when staff were sympathetic, confidentiality was an effective barrier to substantive communication (Backlar 1994; Deveson 1991; Group for the Advancement of Psychiatry 1986; Hatfield 1987; Wasow 1995).

Parallel research literature showed significant family burdens as a result of the disruptions and demands of living with a person with mental illness (for overviews see Greenley 1995; Lefley 1996b; Maurin and Boyd 1990). These burdens were not alleviated and sometimes were exacerbated by interactions with practitioners. Although psychodynamic theories tended to exclude families whereas family systems theories insisted on family involvement, the informational barriers persisted. Originating with families of patients with schizophrenia, early systemic theories viewed the patients' symptoms as functional, maintaining a maladaptive homeostasis in a dysfunctional family system. Some families have reported bitterness that although their questions were ignored, they were forced into family therapy against their will. They reported feeling held hostage by the knowledge that hospital policy required this modality and that their relatives would not be served without their reluctant participation (McElroy and McElroy 1994). Many family therapists have acknowledged that these family interaction models were not notably successful in treating the major psychotic disorders and also transmitted a message of familial culpability (Anderson et al. 1986; Marsh 1992; McFarlane and Lukens 1994; Terkelson 1990). The pain of family blaming has been ruefully recalled in interviews with families who felt guilty, bewildered, and frustrated by a lack of information (Backlar 1994; Hatfield 1987; Lefley and Johnson 1990; Wasow 1995).

Although various models of family therapy ultimately became valuable treatment modalities for other conditions, the failure of attempts to eliminate psychosis through family systems approaches generally led to an abandonment of schizophrenia as the focus of interest. Family therapy is still offered by some schools for early-onset schizophrenia (Selvini 1992) but without rigorous empirical support. Proof of effectiveness has come from a totally different paradigm—family psychoeducation (Dixon and Lehman 1996).

Psychoeducational Interventions and Family Education

Family therapists developed psychoeducational models, but they were conceptually differentiated from systemic family therapies and carefully researched (Anderson et al. 1986; Falloon et al. 1984; Goldstein1981; Liberman et al. 1987; McFarlane et al. 1995). The family therapists based their work on a stress-vulnerability model of schizophrenia with no presumption of family pathology.

Despite some variability in the various models developed, all have core elements. These include support for families and acknowledgment of their distress, education about the illness, problem-solving strategies, communication training, and behavior management techniques. The disorder is presented as a biologically based, stress-related illness that leads to multiple problems in living. Education includes information on medications and their side effects, adverse effects of street drugs, stress identification and control, expected rates of improvement, and prodromal signs of decompensation. Communication training enables families to deal with cognitive impairments and to recognize attentional and information-processing deficits as biologically based conditions rather than purposive distancing mechanisms.

Current consensus recommendations for psychosocial treatment for schizophrenia indicate the practice guidelines for family and patient psychoeducation and other family interventions. During hospitalization these include psychoeducation on the nature and treatment of schizophrenia, telephone contact with the family during the first working day, and face-to-face contact within the first three working days. During maintenance outpatient treatment the guidelines stress "Psychoeducation that emphasizes medication compliance, avoidance of stress and identification of prodromal signs." It includes teaching family coping skills aimed at reducing the burden of caring for a mentally ill relative, arranging multifamily groups to decrease isolation among families, and presenting the illness as a "no fault brain disease" (Frances et al. 1996, p. 12). The updated expert consensus guidelines include a guide for patients and families (Weiden et al. 1999).

Outcome data consistently have demonstrated that family psychoeducation reduces the rate of patient relapse (Dixon and Lehman 1996). Among the various models, the least costly approaches seem equally or more beneficial than the more intensive ones. Schooler and Keith (1993) found no significant differences between an intensive in-home behavioral family management intervention combined with a monthly patient-family group (applied family management) when compared with a monthly patient-family group alone (supportive family management). McFarlane et al. (1995) found that psychoeducational multiple-family groups resulted in a significantly longer time to first relapse than did single-family treatment.

The benefits of family psychoeducation are not limited to treatment of schizophrenia. Research evidence suggests that psychoeducation is beneficial for families of persons with bipolar disorder (Goldstein and Miklowitz 1994) and major depression (Holder and Anderson 1990). Nevertheless, these models have not been widely applied. Conceptually, psychoeducation has not been attractive to some NAMI professionals because of its association with a therapeutic rather than an educational paradigm (Hatfield 1994). Solomon (1996) has explored psychoeducational and educational approaches, noting that family education models are aimed not toward deterring patients' relapse but toward improving families' quality of life by reducing stress and burden. The focus is on the family as a whole rather than solely on the relative with mental illness. This is an important consideration for behavioral healthcare specialists whose mission increasingly requires the help of allies in addressing the needs of long-term patient care and in conducting political advocacy for resources.

A Collaborative Model for Families, Patients, and Clinicians

Family members have different roles contingent on their involvement with a single relative or with the universe of mentally ill persons. The family's role must be considered from two vantage points: the individual case-centered level and the societal level. The first vantage point involves an active collaborative relationship with service providers in developing a comprehensive long-range treatment plan for the family's loved one. The second vantage point encompasses a much broader domain, although it may be relevant to resource development for the individual treatment plan.

Practical Help for Families

Families can be helped with direct service provision, information and referrals, service linkages with family groups, and involvement of families in treatment and service delivery planning. Changing the climate in agencies to encourage greater involvement of and collaboration with families may mean training to change staff attitudes. It may involve outreach to families disheartened by their prior experiences with the system. Some families may be on the verge of abandoning the patient because of burnout but would eagerly remain supportive with proper professional help.

Basic Education on Major Mental Illnesses

Regulatory and accreditation bodies, including the Joint Commission on Accreditation of Health Organizations, and APA practice guidelines are beginning to suggest family involvement in treatment or discharge planning. Most families, however, continue to have little knowledge and many unanswered questions.

Information on major mental illnesses, symptoms, medications, research findings, and the like continue to be universal needs of families of patients with chronic illness. This information may be presented in a number of formats. The various psychoeducational models have structured educational modules that may be tailored to an individual agency's needs (e.g., Anderson et al. 1986; Falloon et al. 1984; Liberman et al. 1987). Books developed by NAMI educators are invaluable sources for professionals who wish to address generic and specific family needs (Hatfield 1990). Agencies and institutions may offer a series of public lectures or seminars on special topics of concern to families. In these settings, psychiatrists have a critically important role because they are the experts on psychopharmacology and the biological parameters of behavior.

Psychoeducational Behavior Management Training

The techniques developed in the psychoeducational models have been demonstrably successful in training families to deal with difficult behaviors, recognize prodromals, and avert relapse in many patients. Communication skills, problem-solving methods, and modes of coping with symptomatic behaviors are components of a package of skills that all family members, including the patient, can learn. Psychoeducational interventions were developed as prolonged research projects and may require adaptation to serve the needs of particular agencies and institutions. However, the basic elements may be taught to clinical trainers and families through handouts, videotapes, and other visual aids.

Psychotherapy

Individual therapy with persons who have a mentally ill family member may be beneficial in dealing with guilt, rage, stigmatization, and fantasies of altered life scenarios. Systems-oriented family therapy models have changed considerably since they were first applied in work with families of persons with schizophrenia. New approaches being developed for families of patients with Alzheimer's disease or those with physical disabilities may be relevant to families of persons with mental illness (Rolland 1994). In some cases, therapists may want to use psychodynamic or structural techniques with specific families or indeed focus on breaking a cycle of maladaptive behaviors. The theoretical framework, if any, should focus on a coping rather than a deficit model of functioning (Hatfield and Lefley 1987; Marsh 1992).

Provision of Resources and Training for Community Groups

Contracts between state program offices and mental health agencies have helped the development of local family and consumer groups over the years, spurred by targeted grants from the Community Support Program at the Substance Abuse Mental Health Services Agency. Institutional aid typically involves provision of space and ancillary services (e.g., clerical support, food) for meetings of self-help groups. Other hospitals and behavioral health vendors have offered rooms for meetings as a community service. Many agencies and hospitals are now discovering the virtues of offering family lectures and support groups, not only because of the demonstrated efficacy of psychoeducational interventions but also because in some agencies they may be a reimbursable service. Institutions may also offer professional services such as staff help in training lay facilitators or professionally facilitated support groups. Boundary issues exist that must be resolved in these arrangements. Also, studies have indicated that self-help groups tend to function best on their own without professional leadership (Lefley 1996a).

Referrals to Local NAMI Affiliates and Other Mental Health Organizations

All clinical facilities, particularly those unable to offer the range of family support services suggested in this chapter, should make it a practice to refer family members and patients to the lay support and educational groups available in their localities. For families these groups include the local affiliates of NAMI and may also include the Mental Health Association, Depressive and Manic Depressive Association, and similar organizations (Lefley 1996a).

Benefits of Family Organizations

Education on Illnesses and Resources

Weekly or monthly NAMI meetings are invaluable for educating families about the local service delivery system. Many families learn for the first time in NAMI meetings about the range of mental health facilities in their area, eligibility and admission criteria, the array of services, discharge and referral policies, and the like. Information on entitlement benefits, insurance, housing resources, and case management services is freely offered. NAMI affiliates sponsor many courses for the public on understanding mental illness. The Family-to-Family program, a 12-session family education course developed by a NAMI clinical psychologist (Burland 1992), is now used in multiple sites in almost all states under NAMI sponsorship. The method of training family trainers spreads state-of-the-art knowledge and techniques throughout the 150,000-family NAMI network.

In addition to offering education about mental illnesses and local resources, consumer and family organizations such as the AMI groups increasingly provide the buffers and supports so desperately needed by patients and families in distress. These groups tend to fulfill functions of extended kinship networks, offering psychological support, social and recreational outlets for the previously isolated, and often finding housing and occupations for some of their disabled members.

Family Support Groups

Family support groups are a major forum for families to share their pain and elicit understanding from others who have lived through similar trials. They are sources of comfort and knowledge, providing cathartic ventilation and concrete aid in dealing with crises and other problems. Joining a family support group is an extremely valuable coping mechanism for isolated caregivers. Long-standing members often develop a social support system that offers both companionship and active help in crisis situations. McFarlane et al. (1995) demonstrated the superiority of multiple-family psychoeducational groups to individual family psychoeducation. The findings suggested that supportive elements of the group experience (i.e., the sharing of experiences and development of friendships) may be similar to those found in the informal self-help groups. In research on relatives of persons with severe mental illness, Solomon and Draine (1995) found that more adaptive coping capabilities were associated with membership in an AMI or other family support group.

Political Advocacy

All AMI groups have legislative affairs committees and offer valuable training in political advocacy. For many years, NAMI has held special national leadership conferences to train members in organizational development and for roles as informed advocates and lobbyists. Current regional conferences focus on issues such as state parity legislation, restructuring the healthcare system, and advocating for adoption of well-researched model programs (e.g., Assertive Community Treatment) throughout state systems.

Other Contributions Families Can Make to Clinicians

Case Management Information

With increasing education in the AMI groups, families are becoming valuable sources of information for individual case management. Psychiatrists' interactions with their patients rarely exceed an hour per week and typically far less. Relatives are able to observe diurnal rhythms, mood swings, responses to stress, stimuli that seem to precipitate reactions in patients, areas of fear and anxiety, prodromals of decompensation, and the like. Observations on medication effects and extrapyramidal symptoms are similarly valuable for medication management and patient compliance. This kind of information can maximize professionals' expertise in dealing with patients.

Confidentiality

The boundaries of confidentiality are already stretching thin with managed care and disclosures to third-party payers (Sabin 1997). With families, however, many clinical facilities have maintained a tradition of automatically withholding information. As clinicians increasingly are mandated to involve families in treatment and discharge planning, the need to ask patients for their consent to share information with caregivers puts ownership of confidentiality back into the patient's hands; this conveys respect and may itself have therapeutic value. There are many ways of asking patients, conferring with them about the boundaries of information, and honoring their wishes in ways that will be acceptable to them and to the family. If patients say they do not want involvement of an obviously concerned family, the issues should be explored. Families have long maintained that they do not want to know the patient's private thoughts; they only want information essential for illness management. Working out the parameters and boundaries of disclosure in ways that are responsive to everyone's wishes can be a highly therapeutic intervention.

The new demands for family involvement may finally initiate a situation in which all family members can be brought together in a parity situation to discuss practical issues of aftercare, long-term housing, financial support, medication management, and the like. Working for satisfactory solutions is similar to the problem-solving strategies developed in psychoeducational interventions. The issue of confidentiality has often erected barriers between patients and families. Family involvement becomes a way of bonding and reintegrating the patient with his or her support system.

Information and Referral Benefits to Practitioners

AMI members often receive requests for information on ancillary services, such as psychosocial clubs or housing, from private practitioners working with chronically ill patients. Among families there is an exchange of information and referrals on preferred psychiatrists—those who are perceived as helping their family members, who are both knowledgeable and open to communication. At each annual convention, NAMI hosts an Exemplary Psychiatrist awards ceremony for a large number of psychiatrists throughout the country based on local nominations of favored candidates.

Another reciprocal benefit is the education provided to psychiatric residents who attend meetings. In a public psychiatry module developed at the University of Miami School of Medicine, second-year PGY2 residents have rotated attendance at a local AMI support group. The residents functioned as resource persons for family members wanting information about medications and other issues in illness management. In turn, the residents learned a tremendous amount about the day-to-day lives of their patients, the impact of mental illness on family processes, the operations of the mental health service delivery system, and the interrelation of patients' quality of life with their therapeutic progress (Brauzer et al. 1996; Lefley 1988).

Collaborative Relationships at the Societal Level

Advocacy and resource development have often involved joint efforts of families, professionals, and consumers. Families have collaborated with consumers in joint advocacy for services, for protection against abuse and neglect, and for public education efforts such as the annual Mental Illness Awareness Week. Families have helped consumers develop drop-in centers and have provided support for grant-writing efforts. NAMI has a substantial consumer council operating independently within the organization with representation on the board of directors. The major issue that has divided the two constituencies has been the "rights versus needs" debate, with families supporting, and some consumers opposing, involuntary treatment. However, this debate has not seemed to affect relationships of the major stakeholder groups. Family members and consumers serve as peers and colleagues, mostly with a shared agenda, on mental health planning councils and other advisory and policy-making bodies.

Families have long been involved in joint advocacy efforts and resource development with a range of mental health professionals. Resources developed by families have included housing programs, psychosocial rehabilitation centers, sheltered workshops, vocational training, and other efforts to plug gaps in the service delivery system. The political advocacy efforts of the AMI groups generally target increased funding for services, resources, and research initiatives as well as proper zoning and other legislative changes in mental health law. These efforts include the following:

- Mechanisms to ensure continuing and expanding aid for community support programs, treatment facilities, and residential resources for persons with long-term psychiatric disability
- State and federal policies that will provide incentives for developing guardianship and trust programs

without jeopardizing financial entitlements of persons with psychiatric disabilities
- Incentives for clinical training programs to encourage professionals to work with patients with more severe disorders
- Public and private initiatives for large-scale funding of research on major mental illnesses

NAMI has always had a close association with the APA, including joint advocacy efforts and reciprocal advisory roles. APA officials have been heavily involved in annual NAMI conferences, and psychiatrists have always been involved with NAMI as educators, research advisors, grant reviewers, and political allies. Joint efforts with psychiatrists and other mental health professionals in recent years have focused on funding levels, insurance parity issues, and managed care.

Families and Managed Care

Families have long been concerned about changes in behavioral healthcare. There are obvious benefits in the development of a more capably managed system and in the integration of health and mental health services. Nevertheless, anxieties remain about the possible erosion of public sector services and the breakup of a system that admittedly is defective and inadequate but nevertheless is all we have. Many of the major issues for families are similar to those of psychiatrists and other mental health professionals. Families have the following major concerns:

- The growing threat that financial considerations will supersede quality treatment decisions.
- The needs of chronically ill patients will be ignored in an acute care medical model.
- Under capitated arrangements, health maintenance organizations will shift mental health patients with long-term needs to the public system. Meanwhile, public system resources will be depleted by state contracts with managed care providers.

Other specific concerns are as follows:

- Limited hospitalization and premature discharge of patients with psychotic conditions.
- Emphasis on short-term therapy and denial of long-term supportive psychotherapy in conjunction with medication management.

- Greater emphasis on brief psychotherapy for the "worried well" (i.e., patients with problems in living) who are a more attractive clientele because they require a shorter investment of time and yield a larger payoff in terms of recovery potential and personal reward to therapists.
- Use of lower-cost substitute medications (i.e., substituting older psychotropics for the more expensive atypical neuroleptics).
- Exclusion of nonmedical services, case management needs, and wraparound services needed for survival, leading to erosion of the community support system concept.
- Greater problems in obtaining involuntary interventions and denial of reimbursement for involuntary treatment. The question of whether capitated managed care will pay for involuntary civil commitment is an emerging legal issue (Petrila 1995). Medicaid, too, may make its own determinations and deny reimbursement for court-ordered civil commitment. In either case, the patient may be legally liable for fees for forced hospitalization. Families fear also that such monetary considerations may divert patients needing treatment into the criminal justice system.
- Likelihood that managed behavioral healthcare will not offer family education as part of the treatment package unless framed as a therapeutic modality.
- Unlikely reimbursement for consumer-operated services. Although research suggests that peer counseling and consumer case management may be therapeutic and deter relapse (Nikkel et al. 1992), families fear that patients will be denied this resource because of a lack of credentialing of consumer counselors.

NAMI has developed a publication titled *State Requirements for Managed Behavioral Health Care Carveouts and What They Mean for People with Severe Mental Illness* to educate local affiliates in the monitoring process. The Bazelon Center for Mental Health Law has been encouraging the organization of managed care coalitions in various states to ensure appropriate services and an effective grievance procedure for Medicaid patients.

Conclusions

The roles of patients, families, practitioners, and psychiatric administrators are intermeshed in the process of developing optimal service delivery systems for persons with acute care needs and long-term psychiatric disorders. Collaboration is important both at the individual case-centered level and at the societal level. Pragmatically, the case-centered collaborative model encourages competency building of caregivers and maintenance of patients' major support systems. Collaboration at the societal level is essential for ensuring quality services and research and maintaining professional standards and authority.

Psychiatric practice and mental health systems are presently in flux, and there are threats as well as opportunities in the crafting of new systems. Family members have long been involved in local and national governance and advisory boards and in mental health systems planning. In accordance with federal regulations, many state mental health planning councils now have at least 50% family member and consumer representation. These boards have the responsibility of reviewing and approving the state mental health block grant plan and have a role in shaping the state's contracting with managed care systems.

At both state and national levels, family advocates have an important role in resource development and in initiating and supporting legislation for mental health services and research. Two NAMI family members, Senator Pete Domenici of New Mexico (R) and Senator Paul Wellstone of Minnesota (D), were the recognized bipartisan spearheads behind the insurance parity bill signed by President Clinton in September 1996. The law finally specified that insurers must offer the same monetary benefits for mental illness as for physical illness.

At a meeting of the National Association of Psychiatric Health Systems, Paul Fink, former APA president, stated that "'nobody in their right mind' would make major policy decisions or testify before governmental bodies without including patients or their advocates in the process" (Alliances 1994). The family and consumer constituencies have become a marked political asset, with their advocacy mitigating the perceived vested interests of professional organizations. Families have vested interests of their own, because their quality of life and basic happiness are often contingent on the patient's clinical progress. Administrators and clinicians should always be aware that a patient's potential for rehabilitation and recovery, as well as avoidance of relapse, depends on human supports other than their own.

References

Alliances with advocacy groups urged as psychiatrists try to shape health care reform. Psychiatric News 29(5):8, 1994

Anderson CM, Reiss DJ, Hogarty GE: Schizophrenia and the Family. New York, Guilford, 1986

Backlar P: The Family Face of Schizophrenia. New York, Tarcher/Putnam, 1994

Brauzer B, Lefley HP, Steinbook R: A module for training residents in public mental health systems and community resources. Psychiatr Serv 47:192–194, 1996

Burland J: The Journey of Hope Family Education Course. Baton Rouge, LA, Louisiana Alliance for the Mentally Ill, 1992

Clark RE, Drake RE: Expenditures of time and money of families of people with severe mental illness and substance abuse disorders. Community Ment Health J 30:145–163, 1994

Deveson A: Tell Me I'm Here. New York, Penguin, 1991

Dixon LB, Lehman AF: Family interventions in schizophrenia. Schizophr Bull 21:631–643, 1996

Estroff SE, Zimmer C, Lachicotte WS, et al: The influence of social networks and social support on violence by persons with serious mental illness. Hospital and Psychiatry 45:669–679, 1994

Falloon IRH, Boyd JL, McGill CW: Family Care of Schizophrenia. New York, Guilford, 1984

Frances A, Docherty JP, Kahn DA: The Expert Consensus Guideline Series: treatment of schizophrenia. J Clin Psychiatry 57 (suppl 12B), 1996

Goldstein MJ (ed): New Developments in Interventions With Families of Schizophrenics. New Directions in Mental Health Services, No 12. San Francisco, Jossey-Bass, 1981

Goldstein MJ, Miklowitz DJ: Family interventions for persons with bipolar disorder, in Family Interventions in Mental Illness. Edited by Hatfield AB. New Directions in Mental Health Services, No 62. San Francisco, Jossey-Bass, 1994, pp 23–35

Greenberg JS, Greenley JR, Benedict P: Contributions of persons with serious mental illness to their families. Hosp Community Psychiatry 45:475–480, 1994

Greenley JR (ed): The Family and Mental Illness. Research in Community and Mental Health, Vol 8. Greenwich, CT, JAI Press, 1995

Group for the Advancement of Psychiatry: A Family Affair: Helping Families Cope With Mental Illness. New York, Brunner/Mazel, 1986

Hatfield AB: Families as caregivers: a historical perspective, in Families of the Mentally Ill: Coping and Adaptation. Edited by Hatfield AB, Lefley HP. New York, Guilford, 1987, pp 3–29

Hatfield AB: Family Education in Mental Illness. New York, Guilford, 1990

Hatfield AB: Family education: theory and practice, in Family Interventions in Mental Illness. Edited by Hatfield AB. New Directions for Mental Health Services, No 62. San Francisco, Jossey-Bass, 1994, pp 3–11

Hatfield AB, Lefley, HP (eds): Families of the Mentally Ill: Coping and Adaptation. New York, Guilford, 1987

Holder D, Anderson CM: Psychoeducational family interventions for depressed patients and their families, in Depression and Families: Impact and Treatment. Edited by Keitner GI. Washington, DC, American Psychiatric Press, 1990, pp 157–184

Lefley HP: Training professionals to work with families of chronic patients. Community Ment Health J 24:338–357, 1988

Lefley HP: Advocacy, self-help, and consumer-run services, in Psychiatry. Edited by Tasman A, Kay J, Lieberman JE. Philadelphia, WB Saunders, 1996a, pp 1770–1780

Lefley HP: Family Caregiving in Mental Illness. Thousand Oaks, CA, Sage, 1996b

Lefley HP, Johnson DL (eds): Families as Allies in Treatment of the Mentally Ill: New Directions for Mental Health Professionals. Washington, DC, American Psychiatric Press, 1990

Liberman R, Cardin V, McGill C, et al: Behavioral family management of schizophrenia: clinical outcome and costs. Psychiatr Ann 17:610–619, 1987

Marsh DT: Families and Mental Illness: New Directions in Professional Practice. New York, Praeger, 1992

Maurin J, Boyd C: Burden of mental illness on the family: a critical review. Arch Psychiatr Nurs 4:99–107, 1990

McElroy EM, McElroy PD: Family concerns about confidentiality and the seriously mentally ill: ethical implications, in Helping Families Cope With Mental Illness. Edited by Lefley HP, Wasow M. Newark, NJ, Harwood Academic, 1994, pp 243–257

McFarlane WR, Lukens E: Systems theory revisited: research on family expressed emotion and communication deviance, in Helping Families Cope With Mental Illness. Edited by Lefley HP, Wasow M. Newark, NJ, Harwood Academic, 1994, pp 79–103

McFarlane WR, Lukens E, Link B, et al: Multiple-family groups and psychoeducation in the treatment of schizophrenia. Arch Gen Psychiatry 52:679–687, 1995

Nikkel RE, Smith G, Edwards D: A consumer-operated case management project. Hosp Community Psychiatry 43:577–579, 1992

Petrila J: Who will pay for involuntary civil commitment under capitated managed care? An emerging dilemma. Psychiatr Serv 46:1045–1048, 1995

Rolland JS: Families, Illness, and Disability. New York, Basic Books, 1994

Sabin JE: What confidentiality standards should we advocate for in mental health care, and how should we do it? Psychiatr Serv 48:35–41, 1997

Schooler NR, Keith SJ: The clinical research base for the treatment of schizophrenia. Psychopharmacol Bull 29: 431–446, 1993

Selvini M: Schizophrenia as a family game: posing a challenge to biological psychiatry. Family Therapy Networker 16(3): 81–86, 1992

Skinner EA, Steinwachs DM, Kasper JD: Family perspectives on the service needs of people with serious and persistent mental illness. Innovations and Research 1(3):23–30, 1992

Solomon P: Moving from psychoeducation to family education for families of adults with serious mental illness. Psychiatr Serv 47:1364–1379, 1996

Solomon P, Draine J: Adaptive coping among family members of persons with serious mental illness. Psychiatr Serv 46: 1156–1160, 1995

Straznickas KA, McNiel DE, Binder RL: Violence toward family caregivers by mentally ill relatives. Hosp Community Psychiatry 44:385–387, 1993

Terkelson KG: A historical perspective on family-provider relationships, in Families as Allies in Treatment of the Mentally Ill: New Directions for Mental Health Professionals. Edited by Lefley HP, Johnson DL. Washington, DC, American Psychiatric Press, 1990, pp 3–21

Wasow M: The Skipping Stone: Ripple Effects of Mental Illness on the Family. Palo Alto, CA, Science and Behavior Books, 1995

Weiden PJ, Scheifler PL, McEvoy JP, et al: Expert Consensus Treatment Guidelines for schizophrenia: a guide for patients and families. J Clin Psychiatry 60(suppl 11):73–80, 1999

❖ Section V ❖

How Selected Behavioral Health Systems Are Changing

Toward Integrated Systems

Jose M. Santiago, M.D., Section Editor

Introduction

Jose M. Santiago, M.D.

To remain current and relevant in the behavioral health market, providers have developed three strategies: 1) obtain contracts from employers, payers, or health plans, 2) form alliances and partnerships, and 3) restructure the delivery of services (re-engineering). These approaches demand a pragmatic frame of mind that sets aside ideological considerations, at least to a sufficient degree to allow a strong presence in the market, until a more propitious time when economic survival is no longer as uncertain. Competition continues to be based on cost, not clinical outcomes or functional levels. Efforts by agencies such as the Joint Commission on Accreditation of Healthcare Organizations and the National Committee on Quality Assurance notwithstanding, the focus on quality remains marginal in the United States, except in a few isolated areas of the country.

According to the first strategy, behavioral health providers must obtain contracts as a matter of priority, and the contracts must be based on the most competitive price possible and acceptable. Without these contracts, it is foolish to hope that demand will be sufficient to prevent patients from being channeled to competing providers. In areas of high managed care penetration, health plan enrollees are becoming increasingly dissatisfied with choice restrictions. As a result, point-of-service plans, in which enrollees can receive services from a provider of their choice in exchange for a higher out-of-pocket cost, are in higher demand than traditional health maintenance organizations (HMOs) or even preferred provider organizations.

It remains to be demonstrated that providers can effectively market themselves without engaging in contracts that bring predictable volumes of patients and a foreseeable demand for services. Without contracts, debates over partnerships and restructuring of care are academic. Debates over ideological and ethical issues and even about clinical outcomes are even more remotely connected to survival.

According to the second strategy, in order to effectively fulfill these contracts, behavioral health providers—individual practitioners, corporations, hospitals, and organizations—must link with one another to achieve more effectiveness, efficiency, and profitability. This second strategy has dominated the scene in recent years. In healthcare in general, and in behavioral health in particular, organizations have devoted considerable resources and energy to create structures that are thought to bring added value to the consumers and purchasers of health services. Without these partnerships, organizations have felt vulnerable to buyers of services looking for greater economic efficiency, ease of access, and greater accountability from large conglomerates.

Finally, according to the third strategy, behavioral health processes must be reorganized in order to increase quality, outcomes, and satisfaction, while decreasing costs. This approach, called re-engineering, has challenged traditional modes of thinking and behavior (Hammer and Champy 1993). The "where," "when," and "how" of service delivery have changed profoundly, as illustrated by the dramatic decrease in lengths of stay and the subsequent drop in demand for psychiatric hospital beds.

This section examines closely the second strategy, the formation of alliances and partnerships. Across the United States, the ability to attract contracts has required financial risk assumption strategies. In order to develop successful risk strategies, integrated delivery systems are being created. In this section, several integration tactics are analyzed and the value they provide to patients and payers is examined.

Integrated delivery systems or networks combine several providers into a single organizational structure aimed at the following results (Coddington et al. 1996):

- Improving the quality of care by facilitating the strategy of re-engineering.
- Emphasizing the quality of service as distinct from the quality of the product (e.g., improving hours of service, increasing convenience, and shortening wait times).
- Improving accessibility, a subset of the quality of service.
- Reducing unit costs by requiring higher productivity, economies of scales in joint purchasing, and other methods to decrease the hospital or the patient unit cost. (This approach yields a lower cost that is a direct competitive advantage in today's market.)
- Improving operating efficiency by restructuring the care to yield greater utilization efficiency and reduced cost, substituting cost-effective modalities for expensive ones, and eliminating waste and duplication overall.
- Strengthening customer ties.
- Enhancing product offerings by increasing the ability of employers to design the continuum of care they wish to offer, especially for the self-insured organization.

Shortell et al. (1993) defined an organized delivery system as a "network of organizations that provides or arranges to provide a coordinated continuum of servic-es to a defined population and is willing to be held clinically and fiscally accountable for the outcomes and the health status of the population served." They also identified three key elements of integration: functional, physician-systems, and clinical. Functional integration is understood as adding value to a system by coordinating financial management, human resources, information systems, strategic planning, and total quality management. Physician-systems integration refers to the alignment of economic incentives between physicians and the components of an organization, based on the extent to which physicians use the organizational facilities and the extent to which they participate in planning, management, and governance. Clinical integration refers to the extent of continuity of care in all areas of the continuum of care.

Integration can be further defined as horizontal and vertical. Horizontal integration refers to the coordination of organizations, providers, and services at the same level of care (e.g., acute care). Vertical integration implies coordination of various levels of care (e.g., hospitals with outpatient clinics, or hospitals with physicians). Integration can also be labeled as virtual, reflecting a certain reality rather than a formal legal structure. Most organizations, no matter how large or well financed, can rarely offer all required services under a single structure. Several organizations will link with one another to form a virtual integration or a network of closely allied organizations.

Throughout the United States, many organizations have engaged in expensive, time-consuming, and controversial integration efforts. By and large, behavioral health has lagged behind, mostly letting management companies create carve-outs, virtual organizations or networks that are controlled tightly through utilization management. Yet researchers investigating integrated models have pointed to behavioral health as particularly well suited to integration and its benefits. Other areas suitable for integration include cardiovascular, orthopedics, and women's health (Greene 1995). The integration progress has been slow and has required extensive resources. Research also shows that total quality management is an important tool in integrative efforts (Shortell et al. 1993).

The choice of integration tools is wide, and the best fit is often an elusive goal. This section provides several examples of models to adapt, avoiding the blind adoption of highly touted models that may not offer the most appropriate and adequate solution to local conditions. Each organization must choose from an array of integration tools. Figure 1 summarizes the use

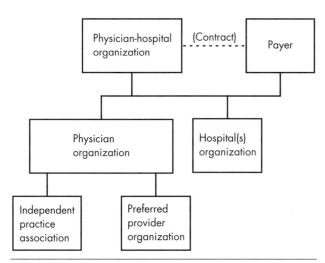

FIGURE 1. Physician-hospital organization.

of a physician-hospital organization as a tool for integration, as discussed by Liptzin in Chapter 27.

Figure 2 and Table 1 show how a management service organization can be used to integrate several components of a network.

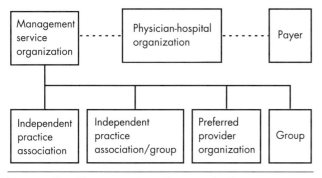

FIGURE 2. Management service organization.

TABLE 1. Management service organization function

1. Marketing
2. Provider relations
3. Insurance
    Eligibility
    Claims
4. Medical management
    UM
    Quality assurance (credentialing)
    Pharmacy/lab
    Protocols
5. Physician practice management
    (May own assets)
    (May employ physicians)

Finally, academic centers face a particularly arduous task in attempting to combine cost effectiveness, efficiency, teaching, and research (Figure 3).

Several integrative options available to behavioral health organizations are reviewed in this section. In Chapter 21, Sharfstein, Stoline, and Szpak address the many challenges in integration for private psychiatric hospitals. In Chapter 22, Shaffer and Hullett describe the evolution of managed behavioral health organizations in a climate of integration strategies.

Godleski, Vadnal, and Tasman (Chapter 23) and Giannandrea, Larson, and McDuff (Chapter 24) tackle the unique challenges faced by the Veterans Administration (VA) and the military, respectively. By definition, these organizations have the greatest potential in being integrated systems. The authors of these chapters describe specific efforts directed toward improving their systems and the attempts at creating proper incentives.

Integrating state and county agencies, at the other end of the spectrum, is a daunting task. In Chapter 25, Hogan reviews the successful transition from fragmented to integrated public systems of care in states such as Ohio. In Chapter 26, McFarland reminds us of the HMO perspective on integration. In Chapter 27, Liptzin describes how a joint venture between physicians and hospitals can constitute an integrated system of care and a productive contracting structure.

Psychiatrists need to look at horizontal integration to retain or even expand their market share and their contracting clout. In Chapter 28, Axelson and Freeman review a useful model that is currently in operation. Finally, in Chapter 29, Vallani proposes a model of clinical integration particularly well suited for children's services.

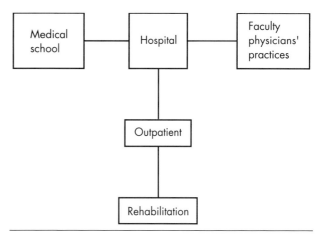

FIGURE 3. Academic model.

Will the integration efforts deployed in healthcare in general and in behavioral health in particular yield the touted benefits? Several considerations require cautious appraisal. First, collaborative efforts are fraught with legal pitfalls. Antitrust considerations require careful review of the Sherman Act of 1980 and the Clayton Act of 1914. In part, the Sherman Act "prohibits contracts, combinations, and conspiracies that unreasonably restrain trade." The Clayton Act "deals with price discrimination, exclusive dealing, and tying arrangements and with mergers and acquisitions." Legal consultation is required when engaging in collaborate ventures.

Several problems may be encountered in efforts at integration. Cost efficiency is difficult to achieve because consolidation most often implies a loser: one of at least two organizations must be willing to close a service to achieve cost-cutting, which is a difficult endeavor. Payers have looked at integrative efforts as defensive maneuvers by providers to avoid price reduction and loss of market share. They are thus more inclined to contract directly with individual hospitals, physicians, and outpatient facilities to avoid power plays, unless they can pass on most of the risk. Providers have not demonstrated the necessary capacity and competency to assume and manage risk. Payers are reviewing their current strategy of offering cradle-to-grave coverage. Populations do not necessarily accept that the responsibility for health status, including behavioral health status, is bestowed on an integrated delivery system. Instead, the general public seems to be more inclined to use services when sick; assume responsibility for, including neglect of, their health when well; and perhaps seek complementary healing as a source of wellness. Under this cost scenario, vertical integration is favored at the expense of horizontal integration. A single specialty integration such as psychiatry becomes much more cost effective and efficient to operate than is an integrated delivery system that offers the whole continuum of care that few want to buy as a whole. For psychiatry, the challenge is particularly difficult because the carve-out approach has definite drawbacks: a further marginalization from the rest of medicine.

Employers and employees are looking at choice rather than the closed panels found in many integrated delivery systems. Also, a difficulty resides in aligning physicians' and providers' incentives when risk is assumed by large organizations where governance is at the top, far removed from clinical practices. A clear example is the VA, where a large integrated system already exists. The challenge for the VA is to create incentives for physicians and other providers in order to modify behavior toward better outcomes and better efficiencies.

Despite these challenges, systems of behavioral healthcare must evolve and prepare for the changing healthcare scene. When the emphasis on cost diminishes, as it does in highly penetrated managed care areas where prices have bottomed out and leveled off, clinical outcomes, functional levels, and patient satisfaction will become the prominent and differentiating variables. Organizations capable of assuming responsibility and accountability for cost and quality will then be in a position to add value to patients. Integration may then be the tool of choice, and those who began the long, arduous process may well benefit.

References

Coddington DC, Moore KD, Fischer EA: Making integrated health care work. The Physician Executive 22:24–28, 1996
Greene J: Clinical integration increases profitability, efficiency study. Modern Health Care, February 6, 1995, pp 39
Hammer M, Champy J: Reengineering the Corporation: A Manifesto for Business Revolution. New York, HarperCollins, 1993
Shortell SM, Gillies RR, Anderson DA, et al: Creating organized delivery systems: the barriers and facilitators. Hospital and Health Services Administration 38:447–466, 1993

❖ 21 ❖

Private Psychiatric Hospitals

Steven S. Sharfstein, M.D.

Anne Stoline, M.D.

Carole Szpak

Perhaps at no time in the history of mental healthcare in the United States has change been as rapid as it has in recent years. This is particularly true for one key segment of the mental health delivery system: private psychiatric hospitals.

Coming from a rich tradition of providing "asylum"[1] for the mentally ill since 1751, private specialty hospitals have navigated a changing course that has come from philosophical, clinical, political, and economic perspectives. The facilities that we categorize today as private psychiatric hospitals remain a vital and important part of the overall mental health and substance abuse delivery system; however, the terminology may already be antiquated. Although useful within the context of studying evolving systems, the language we use to identify such institutions is likely to undergo further changes. For example, in January 1993 the primary association that had represented this constituency since 1933 officially changed its name from the National Association of Private Psychiatric Hospitals to the National Association of Psychiatric Health Systems (NAPHS),

in recognition of trends that continue to sweep the field (National Association of Psychiatric Health Systems 1993). These trends include the evolution from hospitals to systems of care, from independent organizations to integrated delivery systems, and from a philosophy of treating illness to one of maintaining healthy communities. Although we conceptualize this chapter around "hospitals," many facilities that can best be described as hospitals have evolved into *systems* (and changed their names to incorporate that concept), offering a wide array of services that are not limited to inpatient care.

The terminology *behavioral healthcare* is also often used by today's facilities to encompass the variety of treatment settings for both psychiatric and addictive disorders (Shueman et al. 1994). In fact, many members of the NAPHS by 1996 include the term *behavioral* in their facilities' names.

Defining the private psychiatric hospital has been a challenge over the years (Kanno 1966). Because researchers—and hospitals themselves—have often used different criteria to determine what constitutes a pri-

---

[1]The term *asylum* came into vogue at the end of the nineteenth century.

vate psychiatric hospital, the Joint Information Service of the American Psychiatric Association worked with the National Association of Private Psychiatric Hospitals in 1966 to develop the following working definition:

> A private psychiatric hospital is an active treatment institution that admits patients with a wide range of psychiatric diagnoses, provides continuous 24-hour service, and has an organized medical staff. It is operated under non-government auspices either on a nonprofit or proprietary basis and, if associated in some way with a larger institutional complex, it has enough administrative and/or physical independence to be recognized as a separate entity by its officers and the public. (Kanno 1966)

Although definitions and terminology to describe private psychiatric hospitals have been as varied over the years as the services offered, this chapter focuses on those organizations that—even today—have the following characteristics in common:

- They are focused specifically (and most exclusively) on providing specialty care for individuals with psychiatric and addictive disorders.
- The majority of their funding comes from insurance (both public and private), rather than from direct federal, state, or local governmental grants.

History of Private Psychiatric Hospitals

Private psychiatric hospitals have been in operation in the United States for well over 200 years. The Institute of Pennsylvania Hospital, the nation's oldest, was founded as an independent organization in 1751. Table 21–1 lists other early private psychiatric hospitals in the United States.

These first private-sector facilities had several things in common. As independent organizations (whether supported by charitable donations, family fortunes, or community volunteers/service), they relied primarily on nongovernmental funding for support. They were "specialty" hospitals or services that focused exclusively on mental disorders. They reflected the morals, experiences, and political realities of the times. For example, some of the earliest hospitals were chartered as a result of public appeals to counteract the abuses and neglect that resulted when families were

TABLE 21–1. Early private psychiatric hospitals

The New York Hospital-Cornell Medical Center, Westchester Division, New York (1771)
Friends Hospital, Pennsylvania (1813)
McLean Hospital, Massachusetts (1818)
The Institute of Living, Connecticut (1822)
Brattleboro Retreat, Vermont (1834)
Butler Hospital, Rhode Island (1847)
Sheppard and Enoch Pratt Hospital, Maryland (incorporated 1853, opened 1891)
DePaul Hospital, Louisiana (1861)
Emerson A. North Hospital, Ohio (1873)
St. Vincent's Hospital and Medical Center of NY, Westchester Branch, New York (1879)
South Oaks Hospital, New York (1882)
Milwaukee Psychiatric Hospital, Wisconsin (1884)

Source. National Association of Private Psychiatric Hospitals internal fact sheet/memo undated.

permitted to take patients under home care (Deutsch 1937).

Since earliest times, hospitals have focused on safety and security for one of our most vulnerable populations. They have worked to serve populations of all ages (with varying degrees of success and specialization over the years) and to improve the lives of the patients they serve (within changing views of the causes of mental illness, the role of the family, and the best treatment approaches). Throughout their evolution, there have been significant variations in the services that various hospitals offer, reflecting differing treatment philosophies and populations seen.

Changes Over the Decades

From the foundation begun by the earliest private psychiatric hospitals in the mid-1700s, there have been several growth periods in hospital development. With significant advances occurring in psychiatry by the late 1930s, "treatment programs for the first time became, to a much greater extent, active treatment for hospitalized psychiatric patients" (Herman 1983). According to a 1966 American Psychiatric Association survey, the majority of private psychiatric hospitals began operating since 1930. "Between 1910 and 1939 the rate of hospital openings was fairly regular—from 16 to 20 in each of the three decades," according to the survey. "In the 10 years after World War II the number of openings jumped to 35. Between 1955 and 1964...the number decreased to the pre-war rate" (Kanno 1966). However, another growth period for private psychiatric hospitals was to follow as the private sector responded to changes occurring within the marketplace—particularly within public institutions serving the severely mentally ill. From the 1850s through the 1950s, public-sector hospitals dominated as the public came to believe that care of the poor and mentally ill was a responsibility of the state. By 1955 the population served by state and county institutions in the United States peaked at 550,000. However, new approaches and ideas were evolving that put emphasis on community-based care. The 1963 passage of the Mental Retardation Facilities and Community Mental Health Centers Construction Act "officially marked the end of the preeminence of state hospitals in America's mental health system and the beginning of the era of deinstitutionalization" (Breakey 1996).

The Shift From Public to Private Sector Services

With the movement toward deinstitutionalization in the 1960s, there was heavy pressure to rely less on publicly funded institutional care for the mentally ill and more on community-based alternatives. Although this movement held promise, few community-based alternatives materialized, and deinstitutionalization came under significant attack for failing to adequately care for the mentally ill and contributing to a growing homeless population (Foley and Sharfstein 1983). State and county mental hospitals accounted for about four-fifths of all psychiatric beds available in the United States in 1970; by 1990 they represented only about one-third (Center for Mental Health Services 1994).

As the public system began to dismantle its services, the private sector stepped in to provide new services—particularly for populations that had been underserved. The number of private psychiatric hospitals increased slowly but steadily from 150 in 1970 to 184 by 1980 (Figure 21–1). Beginning in 1980, however, the number grew rapidly, climbing to 444 hospitals by 1988. All of these hospitals provided inpatient care (Center for Mental Health Services and National Institute of Mental Health 1992). Specialty services evolved, such as adolescent units, eating disorder programs, and chemical dependency treatment programs, to respond to concerns about the unavailability or lack of specialization of services for specific populations. For example, as recently as 1987, the U.S. Office of Technology Assessment estimated that "from 70 to 80% of children in need may not be getting appropriate mental health services" (U.S. Office of Technology Assessment 1987, p. 4). Several other factors led to this growth spurt of specialty psychiatric hospitals in the 1970s and 1980s. One key factor was the remarkable progress being made in the science of treating mental illnesses. New medications were rapidly becoming available to help manage a variety of disorders, and research was demonstrating the effectiveness of psychotherapeutic techniques. These breakthroughs helped create an environment in which new technologies were available to serve individuals with the most severe mental illnesses.

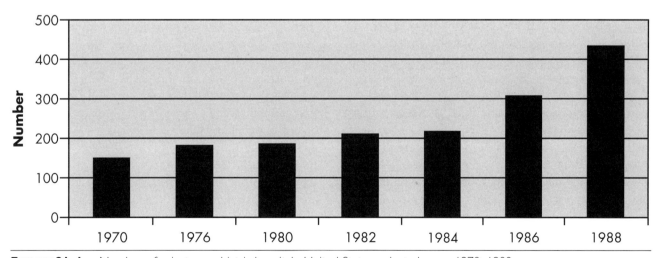

FIGURE 21–1. Number of private psychiatric hospitals: United States, selected years, 1970–1988.
Sources. Center for Mental Health Services 1994; Center for Mental Health Services and National Institute of Mental Health 1992.

During this period, employers—who had become the primary payers for healthcare services for millions of Americans—began to recognize the impact of mental and addictive disorders on their workers and, ultimately, on their bottom lines. As employers recognized the potential value of treatment, they began to take a hard look at the coverage they provided for these services and found it wanting. Employers worked to improve the benefits they offered. Employee assistance programs began to develop. The public also began to talk about once-taboo subjects (such as addiction, child abuse, and depression). With a growing overall acceptance of the role that early intervention and treatment could play, the demand for—and utilization of—mental health services grew. Proprietary hospitals, which had the capital to move quickly to respond to this demand, accounted for substantial growth during this period.

Because state-of-the-art benefit design of this era had been modeled after benefit design for general healthcare, coverage tended to be focused on the potential of catastrophic illness and to be heavily weighted in favor of inpatient care. Increased utilization of expensive inpatient care, coupled with the rapid and uneven growth of private psychiatric hospitals and other mental health providers, including psychiatric units, led not only to an oversupply of inpatient beds but also to a significant increase in costs—a problem mirrored in general healthcare.

An important contributor to this rise in mental healthcare costs was the rapid growth of inpatient treatment for substance abuse. In addition, many parts of the country had a similar increase in inpatient treatment for children and adolescents. These increases were noted with concern by third-party payers, especially employers, and led to an examination of inappropriate hospitalizations. Scandals arising from unethical marketing by some private psychiatric hospitals, especially in Texas and elsewhere, magnified the problem and gave it urgency. Lawsuits proliferated, with large settlements negotiated between private psychiatric hospital corporations and private third parties as well as the government (Frank et al. 1991). In 1994, National Medical Enterprises, Inc. (NME) settled a case with the U.S. Justice Department by paying a record $379 million in fines. NME agreed to a permanent injunction against future violations and to a groundbreaking agreement that implemented a program designed to ensure its corporate integrity in its relations with the government and its quality of care (Stern 1994).

As rising healthcare costs throughout the 1980s became alarming, employers began quickly to develop ways to reduce costs. Managed care was a major factor

in the stabilization of the number of private psychiatric hospitals, with a decline in the number of days of inpatient care delivered by 1995. For example, an estimated 5,646,550 inpatient days of service (estimate adjusted upward to account for total NAPHS hospital membership) were delivered in 1995, compared with an estimated 8,625,884 days in 1988 (National Association of Psychiatric Health Systems 1990, 1996).

A combination of factors—including managed care, changing incentives in benefit design that began to emphasize non-inpatient coverage, exciting scientific breakthroughs that improved medication management for mental illnesses, and technologies that enabled hospital administrators to track and better manage limited resources—played a role in the reshaping of private psychiatric hospitals that continues today.

The Shift From Long-Term Inpatient Care to Acute Care

Among the fundamental changes in private psychiatric hospitals has been a rethinking of the very nature of their core service—inpatient care. Whereas inpatient services had once concentrated on long-term treatment of severe mental illness, the medical model in use in the 1980s shifted inpatient treatment away from traditional long-term care to acute care services (Lion et al. 1988; Thienhause 1995). Stabilization, with rapid transition to less restrictive levels of care, became the goal of many inpatient treatment programs. This goal became achievable for more patients as psychiatric hospitals broadened into systems of care (see next section), as services along the continuum of care (including, for example, partial hospitalization and intensive outpatient therapy) were increasingly covered by health plans, and as new psychotropic medications became available. Clinicians' skills have evolved to put increasing emphasis on short-term treatment approaches (Schreter 1997).

As inpatient services have increasingly come to focus on stabilization, lengths of stay have declined significantly in private psychiatric hospitals. In 1987 an average hospital length of stay in a private psychiatric hospital was 30.5 days (trimmed at 90 days—that is, removing "outlier" cases with stays greater than 90 days), and many patients' stays were substantially longer (National Association of Psychiatric Health Systems 1990). By 1995 the average length of stay was just 11.7 days (trimmed at 30 days)—a drop of 61.6% in just 8 years. Reductions in lengths of stay have been even more dramatic in some specialty programs. For example, the average length of stay in child programs dropped from

48.1 days in 1987 to 14.6 days in 1995—a 69.6% drop. The average length of stay in adolescent programs dropped from 43.8 days in 1987 to 12.2 days in 1995—a 72.1% drop. Finally, the average length of stay in alcohol and drug use programs declined by 62.1% from 22.7 days in 1987 to 8.6 days in 1995.

Declining lengths of stay have continued in recent years, with average lengths of stay (trimmed at 30 days) declining one-third (33.8%) in the 7-year period from 1993 through 1999, from an average of 16.2 days in 1993 to just 10.2 days in 1999 (National Association of Psychiatric Health Systems 2000; Figure 21–2). By 1999, three-quarters of all patients in NAPHS member hospitals had very brief stays (12.2 days or fewer). Over a 5-year period the median length of stay dropped 19.2%, declining from 11.4 days in 1995 to 9.2 days in 1999.

The Shift From Hospital to Health System

Perhaps the most striking trend in recent years has been the dramatic and rapid evolution of private psychiatric hospitals into systems of care. Until the 1980s, hospitals, by their very definition, tended to focus primarily—if not exclusively—on inpatient care. Today both inpatient care and the mix of services offered by private psychiatric hospitals have evolved.

Admission

From Inpatient to Continuum

As recently as 1992 nearly all hospital services delivered by organizations belonging to the NAPHS were inpatient services. According to the NAPHS, 89.1% of all psychiatric admissions to its member hospitals in 1992 were for inpatient care (National Association of Psychiatric Health Systems 1994). By 1995 nearly 3 in 10 admissions (28.8%) within organizations belonging to the NAPHS were to services other than inpatient hospitalization, compared with just over 1 in 10 admissions (10.9%) in 1992 (Figures 21–3 and 21–4) (National Association of Psychiatric Health Systems 1996).

These changes mirror the dramatic shift that has occurred within mental healthcare overall. "Over the past 35 years, the locus of mental health care in the United States has shifted from inpatient to ambulatory services, as measured by the number of patient care episodes," according to the Center for Mental Health Services (1993, p. 1). In 1955, 77% of 1.7 million patient-care episodes were in inpatient settings and 23% were in outpatient settings. By 1990 the percentages were nearly reversed, with 67% of 8.6 million episodes in outpatient services, 7% in partial care services, and only 26% in inpatient services (Center for Mental Health Services 1993).

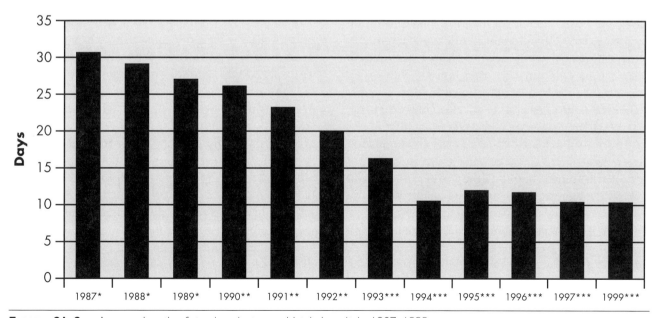

FIGURE 21–2. Average length of stay in private psychiatric hospitals, 1987–1999.
* trimmed at 90 days; ** trimmed at 60 days; *** trimmed at 30 days.
Source. Reprinted from National Association of Psychiatric Health Systems: *Trends in Psychiatric Health Systems: 2000 Annual Survey Report.* Washington, DC, NAPHS, 2000. Used with permission.

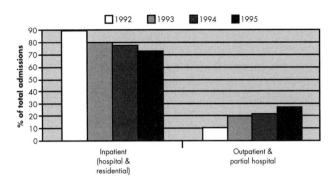

FIGURE 21–3. Change in inpatient versus outpatient admissions, 1992–1995.
Source. Reprinted from National Association of Psychiatric Health Systems: *Trends in Psychiatric Health Systems: 2000 Annual Survey Report.* Washington, DC, NAPHS, 2000. Used with permission.

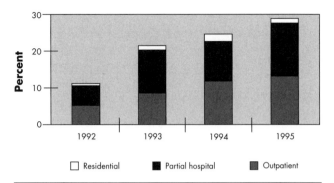

FIGURE 21–4. Outpatient, partial, and residential as a percentage of total admissions.
Source. Reprinted from National Association of Psychiatric Health Systems: *Trends in Psychiatric Health Systems: 1996 Annual Survey Report.* Washington, DC, NAPHS, 1996. Used with permission.

The significant shift in service mix has been attributed to a number of factors. One factor is the growing scientific understanding of the role—and the cost effectiveness—of a wide variety of approaches along the continuum of care, including partial hospitalization and residential treatment (Cuyler 1991; National Association of Psychiatric Health Systems 1991). These advances were occurring at a time when employers were seeking strategies for controlling skyrocketing health benefit costs. Until then, insurance plans typically covered either inpatient or outpatient services, but few—if any—reimbursed for services along the continuum, such as partial hospitalization or residential treatment. Employers and insurers began to change incentives in benefit design and began to turn to new strategies, such as managed care and flexible benefit design, for controlling costs. Other factors in the changing service mix have been the proliferation of medications available to treat various psychiatric disorders, greater consumer involvement in treatment planning, and the pressure of cost constraints that favor the least restrictive and least costly treatment settings.

Impact of Managed Care on Behavioral Health

Today managed care screens the appropriateness of mental health services for the vast majority of Americans. According to the Institute of Medicine, half of all insured Americans (110.9 million) receive insurance coverage through specialty managed behavioral healthcare programs, and millions more are in health main-

tenance organizations (HMOs) that manage their mental health benefits (Institute of Medicine 1996). When these two populations are combined, an estimated 78.1% of insured Americans have their behavioral health benefits managed (Open Minds 1996). Utilization review and precertification are virtually universal tools used to determine whether inpatient psychiatric services are necessary and, if so, which types of treatment will be authorized.

Managed care market penetration is higher for behavioral healthcare services than for general healthcare services. This difference has occurred as many employers have carved out mental health benefits and treated them separately from general health benefits with special gatekeeping and triaging structures. Although up to 78% of insured Americans are covered by managed behavioral healthcare arrangements and HMOs (Open Minds 1996), only 26% (58.2 million) of insured Americans are enrolled in HMOs for general healthcare (Institute of Medicine 1996).

As these managed care systems have taken hold in behavioral health, private psychiatric hospitals have developed services to meet these purchasers' demands for speed and cost savings. At the same time, private psychiatric hospitals have intensified their own efforts to control costs and improve care through more aggressive management of care, using mechanisms such as case management and utilization review. Regardless of whether the oversight function is an internal or external one, this type of proactive management of costs and care will remain an integral feature of private psychiatric hospitals.

Shift From Fee-for-Service to At-Risk Contracting

Financial incentives are changing. Psychiatric hospitals—along with other types of organizational providers—are increasingly sharing in the risk for maintaining the health of populations. By 1995 nearly three-quarters of respondents to the NAPHS's annual survey had entered into global rate contracting, in which a flat amount is paid per episode of illness. This approach allows the provider to determine the best clinical interventions within a fixed number of dollars, compared with a micromanagement approach in which an insurance company or managed care organization determines the site of care and length of treatment in each site of care. By 1995 more than 37.2% of respondents had entered into capitated and other at-risk arrangements (National Association of Psychiatric Health Systems 1996). These changing financial incentives help to prevent unnecessary and costly hospitalizations. They also offer challenges for administrators, including managing what can be substantial financial risk when caring for severely ill populations. At-risk arrangements require sound actuarial analyses and understanding of the population being served. If the population has higher utilization of services than anticipated, financial ruin can occur.

Blurring of Public-Private Distinctions

The reliance on private funding sources has traditionally been a fundamental feature of private psychiatric hospitals, but even this distinction began to blur in the 1990s. Within their own walls, private psychiatric hospitals are increasingly serving populations covered by federal programs, including Medicare and Medicaid. For example, financial responsibility for patients seen in private psychiatric hospitals shifted dramatically from 1991 to 1999. NAPHS members began serving more Medicaid patients, who—combined with Medicare patients—accounted for 40.9% of all inpatient admissions in 1999. In contrast, only 29.6% of all inpatient admissions in 1991 were from Medicaid and Medicare (National Association of Psychiatric Health Systems 1994, 2000). A total of 24.9% of admissions was covered by commercial insurers (including BlueCross BlueShield) in 1995, down from the 31.1% of admissions in 1994.

At the same time, private psychiatric hospitals are also increasingly working side-by-side with the public sector to coordinate care and to develop strategies for serving community needs. These public-private part-nerships are evolving to meet the challenges posed by the combination of limited resources (human and financial) and a high prevalence of mental and addictive disorders.

At Sheppard Pratt in Baltimore, a rapid decline in length of stay due to managed care led to a dramatic shift in the mission of this not-for-profit institution. A broad reinvestment in the continuum of care, a "hospital without walls," led to expansion of programs off campus in a variety of community-based settings. The state of Maryland at the same time began to privatize its public community mental health centers, and Sheppard Pratt took the lead in bidding for and winning contracts to provide community mental health in several areas throughout the state. Emphasizing accessibility, early intervention, mobile treatment, and aggressive aftercare of patients who had been hospitalized, these mental health programs are true public-private partnerships (Frank and Sharfstein 1993).

Challenges Facing Today's Administrator: Internal and External Implications

From Independent to Interdependent

Some people still have an image of the private psychiatric hospital as an isolated retreat on a hill. The reality today is very different. Today's private hospitals are operating—and must operate—as integral parts of their community if they are to remain viable entities offering effective treatment services.

Interdependence and open communication help to dispel stigma, which—though reduced—remains a problem. With short lengths of stay and growing reliance on community-based services, a key goal of treatment is to help people reconnect with their daily routines as quickly and smoothly as possible.

Interdependence is increasingly a financial reality as well. Hospitals are serving and reporting not only to patients and families but also to the employers, insurers, or managed care companies that are paying the hospital bills.

Administrators must be aware of and anticipate shifting financial realities and demands. For example, the proportion of patients covered by private insurance is shrinking, and the proportion covered by government programs is growing (Figure 21–5). The

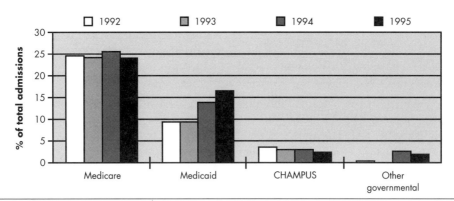

FIGURE 21–5. Psychiatric inpatient admissions: governmental, 1992–1995. CHAMPUS = Civilian Health and Medical Program of the Uniformed Services.

Source. Reprinted from National Association of Psychiatric Health Systems: *Trends in Psychiatric Health Systems: 1996 Annual Survey Report.* Washington, DC, NAPHS, 1996. Used with permission.

proportion of care covered through contractual arrangements (such as HMOs and preferred provider organizations) jumped 31.6% between 1994 and 1995, covering 17.7% of admissions in 1994 and 23.3% of admissions in 1995.

As the payers of care have shifted, private psychiatric hospitals have found creative ways to work with others. In Baltimore, Sheppard Pratt bid on and won the behavioral health carve-out for all Maryland residents covered by Kaiser Permanente (except for the Washington, D.C., area). This at-risk contract brought Sheppard Pratt into the mainstream of managed care with a heavy emphasis on cost-effectiveness, including brief hospitalization and the use of day treatment and residential alternatives. Another strategic partnership was the merger of Sheppard Pratt with the University of Maryland for the training of future psychiatrists. Two programs of outstanding reputation realized that with the market for psychiatrists and the available training dollars shrinking, their merger provided the best marketplace solution.

Identity Challenges: To Merge or Not to Merge?

Sooner or later, administrators in private psychiatric hospitals will face the toughest question of all for their institutions: Who are we? This can be a wrenching exercise, particularly for institutions with long-standing traditions and strategies rooted in successful histories. Should we jump on the bandwagon to merge with other organizations? And if so, which partnerships make sense for our organization? If we do merge, to what extent should we maintain separation?

Some private psychiatric hospitals have answered these challenges with creative and unique solutions. For example, private psychiatric hospitals are increasingly involved with joint ventures and mergers.

Joint Ventures

In Nebraska, a private psychiatric hospital (Methodist Richard Young) has formed a regional partnership called Family Connections with Catholic Charities, Child Saving Institute, Salvation Army, and Family Services to undertake contracts with private and public organizations that require a comprehensive range of services to address their clients' needs. Family Connections is a contracting agency only. It retains no income after administrative expenses, and all service income is channeled to the member agencies. According to Sandra Carson, chief executive officer of Methodist Richard Young, the partnership not only creates contract opportunities and economic stability for member agencies but also helps to establish and ensure a reputation for quality within the community and facilitates communication and coordination. The partnership is also, says Ms. Carson, a role model for other agencies in shaping delivery systems for the future. Participating agencies gain additional bargaining power, leverage, and contract access, while sharing risk through capitated contracts. Administrative cost-sharing leads to operational efficiency. Contracting agencies gain "one-stop shopping" that eliminates political concerns about favoritism in contract awards. A single service payment covers a broad community spectrum, and administrative services are coordinated. Contracting agencies also benefit from a formal, organized, and consolidated quality assurance mechanism.

Mergers

Mergers may occur when organizations decide to integrate services either horizontally or vertically. Mergers can be between like facilities (e.g., when two private psychiatric hospitals agree to form a single operational entity). Mergers may also occur between former competitors (e.g., when a specialty hospital joins with a medical center offering a psychiatric unit). In the future, mergers that unite different components of the overall delivery system are increasingly likely.

Horizontal integration of services creates an opportunity for economies of scale through administrative consolidation. It also increases accessibility to care by expanding the service base. Creation of specialized centers of excellence within the system provides for improved quality of care (e.g., eating disorder programs) and cost savings through elimination of duplicative services.

Vertical integration of services increases the spectrum of care offered by the system. Opportunities are created for economies of scale and administrative efficiencies. Systems with a full continuum of care are attractive to insurers and employees seeking "one-stop shopping." Patients, too, appreciate the coordination of services provided by smooth-running systems of care. Improved quality of care should be expected when the administrators and clinicians within such systems are knowledgeable about the system's mission and share a vision for its activity and implementation.

Whatever type of integration is attempted, the importance of dual clinician-administrator leadership in such systems should not be underestimated. Their potential is best realized when clinicians and administrators work with mutual respect within clear organizational structure and decision-making roles. This marriage of clinical and administrative expertise creates the setting for the successful integration of healthcare organizations.

Market Challenges: The Importance of Skill With Business Tools and Concepts

Administrators of private psychiatric hospitals will also find that their institutions demand new skills from them. They must be adept at

- Contracts (negotiating at-risk contracts)
- Reimbursement issues
- Cost control/efficiencies of care
- Marketing, balance sheets, cash flow, and real estate/land leases
- Regulatory and data-reporting issues

An example of a challenge that uniquely affects private psychiatric hospitals is the Institutions for Mental Diseases (IMD) exclusion that bars federal Medicaid coverage for persons aged 22 and 64 years in private psychiatric hospitals. Private psychiatric hospitals are working hard at the federal level to remove this exclusion and create a level playing field for all behavioral health organizations—a concept that on its face seems simple but that is enmeshed in a host of political issues. The IMD issue is a classic example of how important it is for the leadership within private psychiatric hospitals to understand and play an active role in advocacy.

Role of Data in Integration

Administrators must be prepared to help their facilities evolve within a world of regulatory and data-reporting challenges. Complex financing mechanisms are only one reason that data have become a key factor in a facility's ability to move forward. Understanding the cost, utilization, and effectiveness of various treatment approaches is essential in order to be able to assume financial risk.

At the same time, employers, insurers, managed care organizations, and patients themselves are demanding increasingly complex assessments of the care they are purchasing. Accrediting bodies, such as the Joint Commission on Accreditation of Healthcare Organizations, are requiring facilities to benchmark their services against others. Private psychiatric hospitals have responded to these challenges by developing a wide range of outcome studies (Docherty and Dewan 1995; Mirin et al. 1991; Sederer and Dickey 1996). Quality, continuous quality improvement, or performance improvement teams are an integral part of today's private psychiatric hospitals. Their purpose is to drive the process that monitors and strives to improve the quality of services delivered to patients. Usually interdisciplinary in composition, these teams identify opportunities for performance improvement, design methods to achieve that improvement, and monitor the sustained progress.

Implementing a Strategic Vision

An overriding challenge for the administrator of a private psychiatric hospital is to understand the fundamental business of the institution (i.e., patient care) and to develop a vision that will help the organization remain cohesive, effective, and on track. Pressures of costs and limited resources in the 1980s forced the field of psychiatry to rethink how mental health services should be delivered and forced many in the field to re-train. Clinicians are developing new skills with respect to short-term treatment, stabilization in hospital settings, and greater use of outpatient care (Schreter 1997). Administrators are changing their focus from filling beds to managing a continuum of care. But the rapid changes in psychiatry continue to raise tough questions. What is the role of the physician? As hospitals assume greater risk, financial realities are encouraging a changing work force that relies on fewer physicians and more flexible staffing. To what extent can and should other professions control or be involved in treatment decisions? How will this control or involvement affect medical staff relationships? These are all issues with which psychiatry as a profession continues to grapple.

And how can the physical space of the psychiatric hospital, once focused exclusively on inpatient care, be better used to respond to the clear need for flexible programming (such as outpatient services and partial hospitalization)? For example, are beds necessary, or would satellite clinics be a better approach? Should you downsize hospital beds and use space for outpatient treatment, group homes, halfway houses, or quarter-way housing? Should you relocate your inpatient beds to other sites (e.g., a general hospital) and use your site for alternatives to inpatient care?

Change is never easy, and the answers to these types of questions have a direct—and sometimes painful—impact not only on hospital staffs but also on the communities in which they operate. Will a hospital close? Will jobs be lost or consolidated? If issues fester unanswered, an organization will flounder. By developing a clear strategy, mission, and direction for an organization, an administrator can facilitate effective management and lead an organization into the twenty-first century.

References

Breakey WR: The rise and fall of the state hospital in integrated mental health services, in Modern Community Psychiatry. Edited by Breakey WR, New York, Oxford University Press 1996, pp 15–28

Center for Mental Health Services: Data highlights the evolution and expansion of mental health care in the United States between 1955 and 1990. Mental Health Statistical Note 210 (DHHS Publ No SMA-94-2085). Edited by Redick RW, Witkin MJ, Atay JE, Manderscheid RW. Washington, DC, U.S. Government Printing Office, 1993

Center for Mental Health Services: Mental Health, United States (DHHS Publ No SMA-94-3000). Edited by Manderscheid RW, Sonnenschein MA. Washington, DC, U.S. Government Printing Office, 1994

Center for Mental Health Services and National Institute of Mental Health: Mental Health, United States (DHHS Publ No SMA-92-1942). Edited by Manderscheid RW, Sonnenschein MA, Washington, DC, U.S. Government Printing Office, 1992

Charter Medical Corporation: News release. Charter medical forms first fully integrated national behavioral healthcare system through strategic alliance with green spring health services; Charter renamed Magellan Health Services; Magellan Public Solutions formed as subsidiary to focus on opportunities in the emerging public sector market. Atlanta, GA, Charter Medical Corporation, October 19, 1995

Cuyler RN: The Challenge of Partial Hospitalization in the 90s. Alexandria, VA, American Association for Partial Hospitalization (now Association for Ambulatory Behavioral Healthcare), 1991

Deutsch A: The Mentally Ill in America. New York, Columbia University Press, 1937

Docherty J, Dewan N: Outcomes Assessment Monograph. Washington, DC, National Association of Psychiatric Health Systems, 1995

Foley HA, Sharfstein SS: Madness and Government: Who Cares for the Mentally Ill? Washington, DC, American Psychiatric Press, 1983

Frank L, Sharfstein SS: Dramatic changes in care: the experience of one psychiatric hospital. The Psychiatric Hospital 24(1–2):19–24, 1993

Frank RG, Salkever DS, Sharfstein SS: DataWatch: a new look at rising mental health insurance costs. Health Affairs 10(2):116–123, 1991

Herman M: The NAPPH tradition. The Psychiatric Hospital 14(1):39–44, 1983

Institute of Medicine: Managing Managed Care: Quality Improvement in Behavioral Health, prepublication copy. Edited by Edmunds M, Frank R, Hogan M, et al. Institute of Medicine, Committee on Quality Assurance and Accreditation Guidelines for Managed Behavioral Health Care, Division of Neuroscience and Behavioral Health, Division of Health Care Services. Washington, DC, National Academy Press, November 20, 1996

Kanno CK: Private Psychiatric Hospitals: A National Survey. Joint Information Service monograph. Washington, DC, American Psychiatric Association, 1966

Lion JR, Adler WN, Webb Jr. WL (eds): Modern Hospital Psychiatry. New York, WW Norton, 1988

Mirin SM, Gossett J, Grob M: Psychiatric Treatment: Advances in Outcome. Washington, DC, American Psychiatric Press, 1991

National Association of Psychiatric Health Systems: 1989 Annual Survey, final report. Washington, DC, National Association of Psychiatric Health Systems (formerly National Association of Private Psychiatric Hospitals), 1990

National Association of Psychiatric Health Systems: Partial Hospitalization, special edition. The Psychiatric Hospital 22(2):47–80, 1991

National Association of Psychiatric Health Systems: News release. NAPPH name change, membership expansion reflect evolution of hospital-based psychiatric services. Washington, DC, National Association of Psychiatric Health Systems, February 4, 1993

National Association of Psychiatric Health Systems: 1993 Annual Survey Report. Washington, DC, National Association of Psychiatric Health Systems, 1994

National Association of Psychiatric Health Systems: Trends in Psychiatric Health Systems: 1996 Annual Survey Report. Washington, DC, National Association of Psychiatric Health Systems, 1996

National Association of Psychiatric Health Systems: 2000 Annual Survey Report: Trends in Behavioral Healthcare Systems—A Benchmarking Report. Washington, DC, National Association of Psychiatric Health Systems, 2000

Open Minds: HMOs and Their Behavioral Health Program Arrangements. Gettysburg, PA, August 1996

Schreter RK: Essential skills for managed behavioral health care. Psychiatr Serv 48:653–658, 1997

Sederer LI, Dickey B (eds): Outcomes Assessment in Clinical Practice. Baltimore, MD, Williams & Wilkins, 1996

Shueman SA, Troy WG, Mayhugh SL (eds): Managed Behavioral Health Care: An Industry Perspective. Springfield, IL, Charles C. Thomas, 1994

Stern GM: Statement of Gerald M. Stern, special counsel, Health Care Fraud, U.S. Department of Justice. Before the Subcommittee on Crime and Criminal Justice, Committee on the Judiciary, U.S. House of Representatives July 19, 1994

Thienhause OJ (ed): Manual of Clinical Psychiatry. Washington, DC, American Psychiatric Press, 1995

U.S. Office of Technology Assessment: Children's Mental Health: Problems and Services. Durham, NC, Duke University Press, 1987

❖22❖

Managed Behavioral Healthcare Organizations

Ian A. Shaffer, M.D.

F. Joseph Hullett, M.D.

Managed behavioral healthcare organizations (MBHOs) began in the early 1980s in response to a dramatic increase in mental health/substance abuse (MH/SA) treatment costs. MBHOs now manage the behavioral healthcare of more than 124 million Americans (Open Minds 1996). Adding those covered directly through health maintenance organizations (HMOs), over 160 million Americans receive MH/SA treatment through managed care programs. In this chapter, we discuss the structure and operation of MBHOs and predict activities that may engage MBHOs in the near future.

Historical Overview

The American healthcare economy is rapidly evolving from a loose-knit, laissez-faire cottage industry to one of corporate concentration and centralized management. The cultural upheaval created by this economic revolution threatens to foment a populist counterrevolution akin to that sparked by the demise of the family farm.

Although problems caused by managed care continue to fuel a debate out of which further change is inevitable, MBHOs are a necessary and successful stage in the development of a new synthesis.

The unique social role of "medicine men"—specialized priests commanding the arcana of life and death—has generally exempted physicians from direct control. Inherently unequal trade relationships were instead regulated by a strong moral code steeped in personal trust. As long as healthcare provision remained dyadic, with transactions regulated by the wealth or wages of the healthcare purchaser, its economic base could be ignored.

Beginning with the New Deal, unions and industrial corporations seeking a nontaxed wage equivalent found common ground. Their combined efforts solidly established the institution of employer-paid healthcare insurance. Healthcare, thus, changed from a personally purchased service to a benefit bestowed by others. Inherent in the concept of insurance for healthcare, however, were contradictions that crumbled the ignored economic base of physician-patient relationships and made MBHOs inevitable.

Unpredictable individual loss can be insured only when large population pooled loss is historically predictable. Because one need not be sick to get better, healthcare losses are intrinsically demanded and, hence, unpredictable. By attenuating recipient-perceived cost of service, third-party payment removes price constraints from healthcare purchase decisions, inflates demand, raises prices, stimulates supply, and increases total cost. Such a spiral is particularly likely with MH/SA services because they are generally less risky and more gratifying than medical-surgical services and because illness and normalcy—Freud's "neurotic suffering" and "normal human misery"—is a distinction difficult to draw.

Initially, demand for MH/SA services was restricted by stigmatization and paucity of providers. As stigma diminished and third-party reimbursement became possible, demand increased, giving rise to new cadres of providers whose supply created additional demand. In a fee-for-service system in which price had become no obstacle, alternative allocation mechanisms were inevitable.

A simple way to understand MBHO evolution and function is to consider three basic equations that illustrate relationships between elements of direct cost, total cost, and value (Figure 22–1). Faced with spiraling MH/SA costs, payers first sought methods to control direct costs. Direct costs are a simple function of penetration rate (the number of persons utilizing a service) multiplied by the average number of service units multiplied by the unit cost to which is added the administrative cost.

Initially unwilling to change the traditional fee-for-service framework of healthcare provision, payers adopted only rudimentary supply-side cost-control strategies. Reasonable and customary fee schedules lowered unit costs while provider limitations (e.g., MD-only rules, certificates of need) reduced penetration rates.

Payers eagerly eliminated MH/SA benefit parity, however, and pursued the demand-side strategies of benefit management. MH/SA benefit exclusions incurred no administrative fee and yielded a penetration rate of zero, thus eliminating direct costs. Benefit limitations reduced penetration rates in a Procrustean fashion by lopping off outliers (day, dollar, and visit limits). Such limits, while excluding the sickest persons from coverage, encouraged those not in need to access services up to the maximum, which, in effect, became a minimum.

Recognizing these third-party payment problems, payers reintroduced cost into purchase decisions via differential co-payments and deductibles. Such limitations directly lowered unit costs, encouraged consumption of fewer units of service, and established a "first-dollar" access barrier to reduce penetration rates. Although almost all employer-paid healthcare plans continued to include some MH/SA benefits, a minuscule fraction paid and administered MH/SA benefits in the same fashion as medical-surgical benefits.

Paradoxically, some benefit limitations significantly increased unit costs (e.g., by shifting treatment from outpatient to inpatient settings). Others drove up total costs by shifting mental health treatment into potentially less effective, more expensive medical settings. Ill-conceived limitations aimed at reducing unnecessary treatment also reduced effective treatment, presumably increasing indirect costs such as absenteeism, disability, poor productivity, and recruitment. Finally, treatment for essential but noncovered services was shifted from plans onto community agencies and public-sector providers of last resort, thus increasing both taxes and indirect social costs.

As costs continued to mount despite benefit limits, noninsurer payers (i.e., those not protected by the safety net of claims-based premium adjustment) clamored for new methods of cost control. Large manufacturing concerns, increasingly plunged into a global economy to compete with firms to whom healthcare was not a balance sheet item, saw bottom lines reduced by healthcare costs. More important, the federal government had assumed astronomical healthcare costs through Medicare and Medicaid.

As the saying goes, who pays the piper calls the tune. Amendments to the Social Security Act in 1972 mandated professional standards review organizations (PSRO), which heralded external professional accountability for cost and quality of care. The 1982 Peer Review Improvement Act replaced PSROs with utiliza-

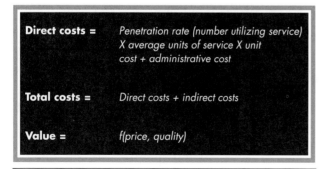

FIGURE 22–1. The basic equations.

tion and quality control peer review organizations (PROs) and required Medicare providers to release patient information to PROs for review. These provisions opened the door for private payers to review individual requests for care and deny or reduce reimbursement prior to payment.

Simultaneously, supply-side management was finally embraced in the rediscovery of the prepaid capitated model of service delivery. In such models, fee-for-service supply incentives are replaced by supervisory control (staff model) and/or interposition of a third-party dual agency into the physician-patient dyad (i.e., risk sharing). Demonstrably successful in limiting costs, particularly MH/SA costs, HMO options (spurred by government mandate) burgeoned.

Utilization Review

First-generation utilization review agencies developed primarily to serve self-funded, non-HMO-based plans. They combined benefit restrictions with medical necessity rationing of individual case resources. Charged to achieve direct cost stability, little incentive existed for such agencies to focus on total cost or value equations.

Simple utilization review uses several tools, easily understood in terms of the direct cost equation (Table 22–1). Precertification reduces penetration rate by preventing unnecessary utilization. It also decreases unit cost by diverting patients from higher cost service to lower cost service (e.g., inpatient to partial hospitalization). Continuing-stay review reduces average number of service units. Case management accomplishes unit cost reduction by arranging for less expensive alternative levels of care and by negotiating point-of-service discounted fees.

MBHO Formation

A niche market obviously existed for specialized MH/SA utilization review. Quality of care considerations demanded specialist-based review standards and experienced teams. Specialist case managers and physician reviewers were better equipped to draw fine distinctions between medical necessity and medical appropriateness. These new companies quickly realized that HMO-like incentives could be built into a service delivery network. Referral volume and other reimbursement strategies

TABLE 22–1. The spectrum of psychiatric/substance abuse cost-control methods

Benefit limitations
Dollar/co-pay
Day/session
Service
Diagnosis/condition

Managed care demand management
Precertification
Continuing-stay review
Level of care management (acute, subacute, outpatient)
Case management

Managed care supply management
Fee negotiation (contracting)
Risk sharing (capitation, case rates)
Provider limitation (preferred provider organization, exclusive provider organization, flex plans)
Access control (directed access)

Quality management

Care management

could move independent providers to accept managed care standards up front. Compatible providers would directly reduce penetration rate and units of service without noncertification. Provider networks also allowed for significant unit cost reduction by means of competitively established deep discount rates. Moreover, contracts established provider management, enforced participation in the review process, prevented balance billing, and allowed for quality assurance and profiling. MBHOs thus incorporated not only the tools of utilization review but also staff models or managed network service provisions, approaching (and sometimes achieving) the status of virtual HMOs (Table 22–2).

Healthcare Integration

MBHOs focus critically on the third of the basic equations (see Figure 22–1). Clients turn to comprehensive MBHO management not only for cost control or for quality of care but also for value, which is a function of both. Driven by the value equation, old style carve-out MBHOs are evolving into sophisticated integrated systems that take full advantage of the economies of healthcare integration (e.g., medical-surgical, MH/SA, pharmacy integration). Benefit limitations are recognized as both unnecessary and counterproductive

TABLE 22–2. The healthcare management spectrum

1. No precertification (PC). No continuing-stay review (CSR). Free provider access to any licensed provider. No benefit limitations.
2. No PC. No CSR. Free provider access to any licensed provider. Benefit limitations.
3. Acute care PC/CSR (without outpatient [OPT] PC/CSR). Free provider access to any licensed provider. Benefit limitations.
4. Acute and subacute PC/CSR (without OPT PC/CSR). Free provider access. Benefit limits. Case management. Limited fee negotiation/contracting.
5. Acute and subacute PC/CSR (without OPT PC/CSR). Benefit limitations allow free provider access or preferred provider organization (PPO) access (i.e., flex plans). Case management. Increased contracting.
6. Acute and subacute PC/CSR (some OPT PC/CSR—may have nonreviewed initial visits). Free exclusive provider organization (EPO) access. Case management. Full network contracting.
7. Acute and subacute PC/CSR (increasing OPT PC/CSR). Directed access EPO. Case management. Network management.
8. Acute, subacute, and OPT PC/CSR. Directed access EPO. Case management.
9. Health maintenance organization (HMO) models (prepayment/capitation) without walls.
10. Staff model HMO. Salaried staff.

when viewed in a context of effective care management, total cost control, and value assurance.

The final and perhaps most important evolution within the healthcare system is the shift from episode-of-care treatment to patient-centered care. MBHOs are focusing on this shift as they move into the public sector and increasingly manage individuals who have long-term mental illness. This change in approach may improve treatment. Patient-centered care leads to enhanced coordination with other elements of the healthcare system; to integration with other benefit programs such as disability management; and, in the public sector, to linkages with human services, judicial, and other agencies.

Integrated healthcare delivery is a system of care that facilitates coordination of care and provider interaction to ensure that all providers of care are aware of necessary elements of ongoing treatment. Integration encompasses not only coordination of behavioral and physical health treatments but also pharmacy, disability, workers' compensation, employee benefit, and utilization management elements. Effective communication among elements of the healthcare system ensures that new components of healthcare are built on those already delivered. An ultimate goal would be a single patient record, available in real-time to all providers. Integrated healthcare reduces harmful treatment interactions, leverages synergies of mixed treatments, and eliminates wasteful duplication.

Integration also facilitates strategic alliances among providers that allow for more global risk sharing, thus encouraging effective treatment coordination to avoid cost shifting. Globally capitated, strategically aligned provider partners will more rapidly refer to effective treatment resources and follow up on patients connected to other caregivers within the integrated system.

Such integration goes beyond a vertical, continuum-of-care model of integration, envisioning instead a hub-and-spoke, patient-centered model of care delivery in which the spokes are the panoply of treatment resources held together and coordinated by the wheel rim of the overall employer or government health plan.

Modern MBHOs generally combine a broad geographic network anchored by high-volume group practice partners who provide cost-effective coordination of care, quality of care oversight, outcomes management, quality improvement, and ease of access. These features are subsumed by a shared philosophy of practice guided by aligned reimbursement incentives such as capitation, case rates, quality bonuses, and the like.

MBHO Models

There are several current MBHO models, both for-profit and not-for-profit. The most common is the carve-out, in which benefits for MH/SA treatment are carved away from other benefits and managed by a separate vendor. Carve-out organizations provide a network of caregivers, arrange for referrals, review cases for benefit authorization, and in many cases pay claims. Interaction with the rest of the benefit program varies. Most commonly, an interface is developed between the MBHO and employee assistance programs (EAPs). Another interface to the general medical benefit involves MBHOs developing procedures to ensure that both programs effectively monitor patients with comorbid conditions. Such procedures usually involve an easily accessed interface between their care management services. Another aspect of the MBHO/general medical plan interface involves a mixed service protocol. Here, both plans determine the level of responsibility for various aspects of care. Decisions are made as to which program will provide benefits for which services and how those services will be monitored. MBHOs work closely with clients to ensure that these interfaces are developed during the implementation phase of a new contract, thereby minimizing operational problems.

Another MBHO model is the carve-in. Several versions exist, and lines between carve-in and carve-out are blurred. In the carve-in, the MBHO generally works closely with another health plan such that beneficiaries experience an integrated service delivery system while still receiving the specialty focus an MBHO offers. In one version, the MBHO, a component of the HMO, provides the behavioral healthcare program for the HMO's population. Close linkages between the HMO and MBHO are important. Shared information systems are desirable so that data can readily flow in order to coordinate treatment effectively. At the same time, both programs must be careful to protect confidential and sensitive medical and psychiatric information.

Another version of the carve-in involves an independent MBHO placing MBHO staff and administrative personnel within the health plan itself, most frequently within the same building. This approach has been extended to the placement of MBHO network providers into health plan medical group offices.

A final model involves behavioral healthcare within health plans provided by health plan staff. Although this is not a true MBHO, many of these behavioral health departments are struggling to develop an identity that recognizes their special value. A key challenge in this model is the need to avoid complete assimilation of the behavioral group within the larger health plan with subsequent diminution of MH/SA treatment importance.

Clients

Each of the models described in the preceding section can have a variety of clients. Many of the early MBHOs provided utilization review to health plans. Problems related to benefit restriction generated negative press. Many MBHOs found such programs unrewarding and discontinued them. During the 1990s most new clients

purchasing MBHO programs were self-insured employers. Through Employee Retirement Income Security Act (ERISA) provisions, these companies developed self-insured benefit programs. They contracted with medical plans and then with MBHOs to make certification decisions and pay claims. MBHOs are generally reimbursed for administrative services and are not at risk for delivering care. In some cases, however, MBHOs were asked to share risk or savings for a percentage of care costs above or below an estimated claims target. Although some critics asserted that potential windfalls motivated MBHOs to deny care, the overall program belonged to the self-insured company and many performance standards had to be met. With such standards and the client's corporate culture in mind, MBHOs carefully determined reasonable claim cost estimates. Large bonus savings were neither common nor expected by MBHOs. Today, few self-insured plans continue to offer bonus arrangements for claims targets. In essence, the self-insured company purchases the MBHO's network, care management expertise, and claims payment services.

As HMOs increasingly recognize the value of effective behavioral healthcare, they are becoming a larger percentage of MBHO clients. Previously, many HMOs were accused of providing insufficient and poor quality MH/SA care. Several HMOs (e.g., Kaiser Permanente and Group Health Cooperative of Puget Sound) have developed high-quality programs that are maintained within the health plan. Data indicate that less than 50% of HMOs manage their own behavioral health benefits (Open Minds 1996). Other HMOs have recognized the value of specialization in this area and have chosen to work with MBHOs in either a carve-in or a carve-out model. Most commonly, the MBHO receives capitation, a per-member, per-month fee, from which all the MBHO services, including costs of care, are provided. Capitation arrangements are under continuing study as pricing pressures early in this process threatened to turn behavioral healthcare into a commodity. Such pressures are strongly resisted by reputable MBHOs, which look to clinicians to point out the value of behavioral healthcare both in direct services and medical cost offset. Less commonly, HMOs reimburse MBHOs for administrative services only, retaining responsibility for claims costs while still providing MH/SA treatment through a specialty organization.

Recently, CHAMPUS and Medicaid moved to carve out behavioral health programs. After a utilization review program, CHAMPUS adopted a more formal managed care program which has been rolled out nationwide. Also, a number of states have moved their behavioral health Medicaid programs to MBHOs. Here again, a wide variety of programs are taking shape. At one end, MH/SA programs are completely carved away from other aspects of the Medicaid health benefit (e.g., Massachusetts and Iowa models). At the other end, managed care technology is integrated into community mental health centers and county mental health departments that manage care. Numerous variations are found in between. One common variation is the provision of health benefits through HMOs that subcontract with MBHOs for the behavioral health component. Another variation is the provision of managed care programs by community or county mental health systems that partner with an MBHO to provide the unfamiliar technology necessary to operate their programs.

MBHO Services

MBHOs offer a variety of services that can be purchased as components. The most common package includes a behavioral healthcare provider network, referral services, and care management. In this basic model, the MBHO contracts with clinicians, programs, and facilities. Clinician contracts generally involve a discounted fee for service and include expectations that providers will seek certification prior to service. Evolution of reimbursement has moved toward capitation contracts and case rates. Program and facility contracts are generally made on an all-inclusive per-diem basis. Major MBHOs provide access to their care managers for referral services (American Managed Behavioral Health Association 1996). Patients can access these clinicians 24 hours a day through an 800 number. MBHO clinicians provide telephonic crisis services as well as triage of individuals to appropriate treatment resources. During treatment, the care management process certifies care, monitors quality, and helps to optimize treatment within the available benefit framework.

MBHOs maintain customer service and provider relations departments to answer questions from members and providers. This service is extremely important because recent studies have indicated that many individuals misunderstand managed care and how their own MH/SA programs work.

Claims payment for clinicians may also be a component of the MBHO. MBHOs prefer to pay claims for services rendered through their program. Alternatively, the MBHO receives and processes claims to determine claims payment amounts and forwards them to the health plan claims payer. In other instances, claims are sent directly to the health plan and the MBHO regularly forwards certification data to allow the health plan to determine appropriate payment.

MBHOs also offer additional services. Occasionally, MBHOs rent their networks to other companies for use in those companies' programs. In this model, the MBHO is responsible for maintenance of its behavioral healthcare network but has no direct involvement with the program. Conversely, an MBHO may provide the services described in the basic managed care program while using a client's network rather than its own. One rapidly disappearing product is simple utilization review. Here, the MBHO provides certification decisions with no network, fee schedule, or claims payment. Finally, MBHOs have entered the EAP arena to offer stand-alone EAP services or EAP services as a component of an overall managed behavioral healthcare program in which individuals may be referred for either EAP or managed MH/SA treatment. This integrated EAP-MH/SA model has been successful in enabling individuals to access a variety of services to meet their various needs.

The mission of MBHOs is to ensure that beneficiaries receive appropriate, cost-efficient care. As has been described, primary MBHO activities involve access to treatment and monitoring care. At the same time, MBHOs are involved in a variety of other activities that will ultimately shape care delivery. At the beginning of this chapter, we referenced the interfaces among health plans, EAPs, clients, and MBHOs. Such external relationships are important to the overall functioning of both physical and behavioral components of the health plan. The client interface is managed by an account executive charged with working with the clients to maximize the efficiency and effectiveness of the plan.

Interface With Employee Assistance Programs

The interface between EAPs and the managed MH/SA care program is vital. In some cases, employers require beneficiaries to access the EAP first and then receive a referral to the MBHO if necessary. The MBHO manages behavioral components, whereas the EAP deals with work-related and personal issues such as job concerns, legal issues, and financial problems. Both programs often collaborate to deal with substance abuse and emotional disorders that directly affect an employee's ability to function on the job. The method of interaction, referral, and information flow is clearly delineated in order for the beneficiary to receive optimal benefit from both programs. Often MH/SA providers are insufficiently attuned to workplace issues. As a result, EAPs become frustrated with providers when necessary employee issues are not addressed. Examples include a requirement that the EAP be notified of any treatment for substance abuse for job protection or that the EAP be informed of treatment progress as an individual approaches return to work. A provider's failure to address these job protection and return-to-work issues can jeopardize an employee's job. Another key interface is between the medical and behavioral components of the plan. This interface is critical to administering the plan and to coordinating care among providers. Historically, behavioral health clinicians have tended to function in an isolated manner, often neglecting to coordinate care with other providers. This has created fragmented care within the healthcare delivery system. MBHOs are working with health plans to improve coordination between behavioral healthcare providers and primary care physicians. The increasing role of primary care providers as treatment coordinators makes it important for behavioral health clinicians to understand the interface and integrate treatment with other caregivers.

Behavioral Healthcare Parity

MBHOs have been active in enhancing MH/SA benefits and access by decreasing co-payments and deductibles. Another significant benefit limitation has been the restriction of services to either inpatient care or outpatient providers. The managed behavioral healthcare industry has successfully championed acceptance of alternative levels of care such as partial hospitalization and intensive structured outpatient programs. MBHOs through the American Managed Behavioral Healthcare Association (AMBHA) have been active in the parity movement. A coalition of organizations, including AMBHA, the American Psychiatric Association, the American Psychological Association, the National Alliance for the Mentally Ill, the National Mental Health Association, and the National Association of Psychiatric Health Systems, has been formed to advocate on behalf of parity treatment for behavioral healthcare. A small but highly significant inroad was made in 1996 when President Clinton signed into law a parity provision.

This provision prohibits differential annual and lifetime financial limits on behavioral healthcare. Although the parity amendment retains many possible benefit disparities, the law recognizes the validity of mental illnesses and the need for those afflicted to have the same care access as those with physical illnesses.

Behavioral Healthcare Accountability

At a conference in 1996, Donna Shalala, secretary of the Department of Health and Human Services, described important aspects of managed care (U.S. Department of Health and Human Services 1996). Among them she pointed out the need for accountability within behavioral healthcare. MBHOs continue to push for accountability on multiple levels. MBHOs are accountable to their clients to ensure that the behavioral healthcare plan is administered in a fair and high-quality fashion. They also are accountable to the membership to ensure that there is appropriate access to desired clinicians. Through a number of organizations, MBHOs have worked actively to develop methods to measure accountability. The National Committee for Quality Assurance (NCQA) is a leading organization in this area. NCQA has developed the Health Plan Employer Data and Information Set (HEDIS) (National Committee for Quality Assurance 1996b) to monitor aspects of managed care activity. As this report card evolves (current version is HEDIS 2000), employers, members, and providers will be able to judge MBHOs on a variety of measures. HEDIS 2000 measures include effectiveness of care, accessibility to/availability of care, satisfaction with the experience of care, health plan stability, use of services, cost of care, informed health choices, and health plan descriptive information. Accompanying this at NCQA is the accreditation process, which initially applied only to full-service HMOs but now applies to MBHOs (National Committee for Quality Assurance 1996a). The categories for MBHO accreditation include quality management and improvement, accessibility, availability, referral and triage, utilization management, credentialing and re-credentialing, members' rights and responsibilities, preventive behavioral healthcare services, and clinical evaluation and treatment records.

Other organizations are also active in developing accreditation surveys and report cards. The Joint Commission on Accreditation of Healthcare Organizations, to date accrediting hospitals, programs, and networks, has created its own MBHO accreditation process. The Utilization Review Accreditation Commission (URAC), initially active in the accreditation of utilization review organizations, has also turned to the development of standards to accredit full MBHOs.

The Center for Mental Health Services has been working with a number of public-sector programs to develop the Mental Health Statistics Improvement Program (MHSIP) report card (Center for Mental Health Services 1996). Incorporating design input from providers and consumers, this report card is intended to focus more on public-sector care than other report cards. Organizations active in promoting report cards are attempting to include more functional outcomes measures. Generally, report cards review measures of process, which are used as proxies for outcome. Over the next several years an explosion of data is likely. The ability to efficiently collect this data and convert it to meaningful information is a challenge to MBHOs and providers of treatment.

Disease Management

MBHOs are also involved in the development of disease management protocols. In these protocols, patients with specific long-term illnesses such as depression can receive treatment in a program that looks not only at treatment required at presentation but also at case finding, patient education, family education, and long-term treatment planning and follow-up (Dubois et al. 1995). This patient-centered approach moves us away from focusing on episodes of care as they occur toward comprehensive consideration of long-term management.

Delivery System

The behavioral healthcare delivery system in the United States continues to evolve. We have moved from a time when care was provided by clinicians and reimbursed by recipients through a time when unquestioning third-party reimbursement motivated providers and patients to overutilize services to the modern era of managed behavioral healthcare. Beginning as utilization reviewers, MBHOs have become organizations that provide a complete managed care program. The initial driver for these programs was cost reduction. With costs now better controlled, payers are requiring better definitions of quality and value in treatment. MBHOs have begun to focus on data that will demonstrate the value of treatment services by the positive outcomes achieved. There will be increasing interest in this information and, along with it, sophistication in data collection systems to create readily available data sets to monitor for quality of services and results. Providers will need to demonstrate positive outcomes that can be formulated as measurable data elements to be used for comparison purposes.

Another shift involves the locus of decision making. Although treatment decisions remained with providers and beneficiaries, third-party payers, to ensure provider accountability, had managed care organizations decide the medical necessity of the treatment, creating significant tension between providers and managers. The decision-making process is also evolving. In part, it is shifting back to the provider of care who, in working more closely with MBHOs to provide overall quality management data, retains the utilization management decision. At the same time, however, patients and their families have become more vocal. No longer content to be passive recipients of care, they expect, and in fact, demand that they be included in treatment-planning decisions.

Data Collection and Analysis

Data are becoming increasingly important. Demographic and diagnostic data, symptom clusters, signs of illness, and specific treatment interventions must be collected and readily available. Data sets must be analyzed to improve our understanding of population health needs and trends. This analysis will lead to effective treatments for specific types of problems and improve the quality of treatment rendered by various providers. It is estimated that well over 2 million beneficiaries per year receive treatment for depression through MBHOs. Narrative data that cannot be analyzed (the type of data most commonly collected) shed little light on effective treatments for depression. Health services research is crucial to improving overall healthcare delivery. MBHOs can be at the forefront of this information revolution. Working closely with their providers, MBHOs can learn a significant amount of information about effective treatments for diverse populations.

Another aspect of outcomes information involves the need for accountability to payers and recipients of care. Providers and MBHOs must demonstrate the value of services provided, particularly if benefit parity is to be accomplished. MBHO data may well demonstrate the importance of behavioral healthcare both in improving individual function and in reducing medical care costs.

Collection and analysis of meaningful data will also allow for improved care coordination. Currently, disparate data reside with each treating practitioner, and limited amounts are merged as required for coordinated treatment. Although it is important to recognize the right to confidentiality of sensitive information, privacy must be balanced by the need to coordinate treatment. Symptoms described, results of examinations, diagnosis, and treatment planning must be shared with other healthcare providers. Failing this, patients risk having treatments work against one another with the potential for harm. At the same time, all parties must understand the type of information to be shared and the value gained through coordination of treatment. MBHOs must assist in educating the public about the need for collection and sharing of data. They must work with patients, families, and providers to ensure that data elements are necessary and that access to information is limited to those who need to know.

Another component of data coordination involves the development of what has been called virtual healthcare. In these models, multiple providers may contribute to the treatment of a given individual. The ability to access and add data to the system is crucial. In such a model, multiple providers maintain a single medical record that is available to all caregivers who may simultaneously access the information. This model allows for multiple experts to coordinate healthcare. MBHOs have worked for years to coordinate activities with medical carriers and EAPs. This experience, shared with other components of the delivery system, can enhance data coordination.

Summary

MBHOs began as utilization managers to assist in cost containment of behavioral healthcare. Since the mid-1980s they have become overall managers of care in a network model in which micromanagement of provider care decisions is supplanted by macromanagement of quality and analysis of outcomes. The next step in this evolution will be for MBHOs to become information managers, a step that will require appropriate safeguards for sensitive information while fostering data sharing that allows for care coordination. Finally, MBHOs are joining with others in moving from episode-of-care treatment to a longer-term patient-centered focus that recognizes the need to coordinate all aspects of care over time.

References

American Managed Behavioral Health Association: Case Manager Qualifications in AMBHA Member Companies. Washington, DC, American Managed Behavioral Health Association, 1996

Center for Mental Health Services: Mental Health Statistics Improvement Program (MHSIP). Washington, DC, Center for Mental Health Services, 1996

Dubois RW, Kosecoff J, Michelson L: Disease management: the maturation and application of health sciences research. Compensation and Benefits Management, Summer 1995, pp 20–26

National Committee for Quality Assurance: Accreditation for Managed Behavioral Healthcare Organizations. Washington, DC, National Committee for Quality Assurance, 1996a

National Committee for Quality Assurance: Health Plan Employer Data and Information Set (HEDIS). Washington, DC, National Committee for Quality Assurance, 1996b

Open Minds 10(2):entire issue, 1996

U.S. Department of Health and Human Services: National Leadership Conference on Managed Behavioral Healthcare. Washington, DC, U.S. Department of Health and Human Services, 1996

❖ 23 ❖

Psychiatric Services in the Veterans Health Administration

Linda S. Godleski, M.D.

Robert Vadnal, M.D.

Allan Tasman, M.D.

The Veterans Health Administration (VHA) is the largest integrated healthcare network in the United States and ranks among the largest in the world (Fonesca et al. 1996). Furthermore, the VHA is the largest trainer of healthcare professionals and is a major research support in the United States (Kizer 1995). In this national role of service, education, and research provider, the VHA has the capacity and potential to significantly influence changing practices of medical care, with broad implications for mental health and psychiatry.

In 1999, more than 3.6 million people were treated in approximately 1,200 VHA healthcare facilities, including 172 medical centers, 650 ambulatory care and community-based outpatient clinics, 206 counseling centers, more than 100 nursing home care united, and 40 domiciliary facilities (Department of Veterans Affairs State Summaries 2000). That same year, specialty mental health services were provided to more than 650,000 veterans at a cost of almost $2 billion (Rosenheck 2000).

As the largest U.S. health education system, the VHA trains more than 100,000 health science students annually (Fonesca et al. 1996). A total of 132 VHA facilities are affiliated with 107 medical schools and more than 1,000 educational institutions (Petersdorf 1996). The VHA has a budget of more than $300 million (Fisher and Welch 1995) to train more than 33,000 medical residents and 21,000 medical students (Kizer 1996). The VHA funded a total of 850 general psychiatry residency positions and 19 geriatric psychiatry slots during academic year 1995–1996 (Petersdorf 1996). This academic interface led the VHA to develop a strong investment in research. In FY 1994, the VHA research budget was $252 million, supporting approximately 2,000 grants and more than 7,200 investigators (Academic Medicine 1994).

Although the VHA has a profound impact on medical care as a result of its age and size, it is also significantly affected by factors that are dramatically influencing the healthcare industry. Advances in technology, forces of economics, changes in demographics, and the rise of managed care continue to change the complexion of medical care in the United States. In response to these factors, Kenneth W. Kizer, former U.S. undersecretary for health, originated a reorganization of the veterans healthcare system and a profound shift in the way the VHA provides service to veterans (Kizer 1995, 1996). While still capitalizing and building on major accomplishments and successful aspects of the VHA, he instituted programs aimed at improving quality and efficiency, initiating an era of change at the VHA designed to place the VHA competitively at the forefront of medical care.

VHA psychiatry operates within the organizational context of this oldest, largest, and most politically sensitive megasystem, which is affected by powerful and industrywide dynamics. The vast magnitude and duration of VHA involvement in mental health services have significantly affected psychiatry in the United States. Trends of psychiatric service delivery, training, and research have evolved over the years, and new models emerged as the twentieth century ended.

Historical Perspective

Medical care for wounded soldiers and public support for disabled veterans dates back to ancient Greece. Not until many centuries later, however, was the prototype established for today's U.S. veterans' benefits policies. Adkins (1967) identified the 1593 English "Acte for the Reliefe of Souldiours," which outlined treatment for those who served in the British defeat of the Spanish Armada, as providing the cornerstone for the later American compensation and pension system and for federal care for disabled veterans. Since the inception of the United States, attempts were made to reward veterans in appreciation of their military service. The first American veterans benefit law, initiated in 1624 by the Virginia colony, was never ratified. The first law on record followed shortly thereafter, created by the Pilgrims in 1636. Most of the colonial laws provided for veterans' pensions, but New Hampshire was the first colony to specify payment of medical care in 1718. Cash payments and land grants were made to those who served in the Revolutionary War, and national veterans' homes were established after the Civil War. From as far back as the first wars of this country, the need was recognized to provide medical care for those wounded, to treat combat-related injuries, and to rehabilitate veterans with disabilities resulting from their military service. Not until the 1920s, however, was this philosophy expanded to include healthcare benefits for all veterans (Adkins 1967).

The medical system of the Veterans Bureau in the 1920s officially became the Veterans Administration (VA) in 1930, with the mandate to hire physicians through the civil service system to care for the nation's 4.7 million veterans in 54 hospitals. In January 1946, less than 6 months after the end of World War II, Public Law 79-293 designated the VA Department of Medicine and Surgery as a separate entity, with a chief medical director and its own personnel system. That same year, the collaboration between Northwestern University School of Medicine and the Hines VA Hospital initiated 50 years of VA hospital affiliation with national medical schools, strengthening national resources for medical education and research. In 1989 the Veterans Administration was renamed the U.S. Department of Veterans Affairs as it became the 14th cabinet-level department. The VA Department of Medicine and Surgery ultimately became the Veterans Healthcare Administration in 1991 (Fonesca et al. 1996).

Psychiatric care was provided for veterans long before the establishment of the VA. St. Elizabeth's Hospital, founded in 1855 as The Government Hospital for the Insane, became the first psychiatric hospital to provide treatment for veterans. Though it was never a part of the Veterans Bureau or VA, it set aside a number of beds for veterans' care. Psychiatrists were later recruited to provide veterans' mental health services specifically for the Veterans Bureau medical system in the 1920s and the VA in the 1930s. The trend after World War II was to include medical, surgical, and psychiatric services in the same hospitals rather than to develop psychiatric hospitals similar to state mental institutes. General Paul Hawley, post–World War II chief medical director, initiated this policy in order to avoid the stigma for the veteran's family members that he felt might result if their relative was in an "insane asylum." The VA later developed innovations in psychiatric service delivery, including the creation of the unit system for inpatient treatment, pioneered in 1958. At that time, patients were first admitted to an observation unit, progressed to an acute treatment area, and then advanced to higher functioning wards (Adkins 1967). By 1985, however, Paul Errera, the director of the mental health and behavioral science service at the VA central office, began to identify problems with the VA national mental health delivery network, including budgetary squeezes, a relatively weak power base for mental health service within the VHA, criticism of the long inpatient stays for a large number of psychiatric patients, and problematic diagnosis-related groups (Errera 1992).

Veterans' healthcare benefits were developed in response to social and political forces rather than economic or healthcare needs (Rosenheck 1986). The veteran population is recognized as a powerful lobby. In 1990, 27.2 million of the 248.7 million U.S. residents were veterans (Fonesca et al. 1996). Along with their immediate families, they made up 40% of the population (Pittman 1995). This makes the VHA exquisitely sensitive to political initiatives.

The VHA differs from private sector medical care because of the special characteristics of the populations it serves. Combat-related injuries led to advances in the study of spinal cord injuries, rehabilitation programs, and treatment of posttraumatic stress disorder (PTSD) in psychiatric patients. In addition, the VHA has evolved to serve the older, sicker, and poorer populations (Kizer 1995). This has led to special services for the homeless, those needing long-term care, and patients with substance abuse and chronic mental illness.

Before 1995 the VHA focused on hospital-based, specialty-oriented care. Meanwhile, private practice and managed care initiatives have moved toward an ambulatory care, generalist-driven model. The VHA has lagged in making this change. Historically, it has operated as an independent entity, removed from the rest of U.S. healthcare (Meadows 1991), but in the 1990s it was thrust into the competitive healthcare arena as a result of fiscal constraints and economic scrutiny (Drucker 1995).

A number of other factors, in addition to economic forces, have driven a reassessment of the need for change within the VHA. Following President Clinton's ill-fated healthcare reform initiative, reexamination of the federal veterans' healthcare system was encouraged. In September 1994, Kizer became under secretary for health and initiated a national reorganization of the VHA.

Dr. Kizer's Prescription for Change

In 1995, Kizer submitted his Vision for Change document to Congress (Kizer 1995) followed by his Prescription for Change the next year (Kizer 1996). These plans delineated his belief that the VHA needed to fun-

damentally change its approach in order to remain a viable provider of excellence in healthcare. He proposed a major reorganization, emphasizing integration defined as a more efficient and effective unification and coordination of medical services. His goals addressed integration on three levels: integration of specialty medical services with primary care delivery, integration of inpatient and outpatient resources, and administrative integration of the regional medical centers through a top-down reorganizational approach. Closing the previous central and regional office hierarchy, he established 22 Veterans Integrated Service Networks (VISN), each consisting of 5 to 11 medical centers, which became operational by May 1996. This decentralization resulted in substantial monetary savings and was designed to move administration closer to the centers, to encourage coordination and cooperation within each VISN, and to eliminate costly redundancy of services within a given region.

Healthcare value was emphasized as a priority, consisting of four aspects of economic performance: 1) cost/price, 2) technical quality, 3) customer satisfaction, and 4) access (Kizer 1996; Sunshine 1995). Specific customer requirements that were addressed included bringing clinical services closer to the patient, decreasing waiting times for appointments, and improving continuity of care. Although psychiatric services had always addressed quality of care, they were now mandated to establish cost justification for level and intensity of services. In addition, psychiatric patients now rated their services as consumers, so that it became a challenge to develop accurate customer ratings, especially if patients had severe psychiatric disorders that altered their perceptions.

Kizer stated that in 1996 the VHA was at a crossroads, moving away from hospital-centric specialty-based medical services into the uncharted path toward a coordinated national healthcare system emphasizing ambulatory and primary care (Kizer 1997). Every patient was to be assigned his or her own primary care physician rather than being seen by whoever was on duty in the clinic on the day of the appointment. Patients were to be referred to specialists only after screening by their primary care physician. Although this arrangement was the norm in most managed healthcare systems, it represented a major transformation in the way most VHA facilities operated. VHA studies illustrated that 88% of all patient encounters were for primary care services (Graning et al. 1994). In 1994 only 10%–20% of patients were enrolled in primary care VHA clinics, but by January 1997 this percentage increased to more than 70% (Kizer 1997).

The reorganization was designed to shift away from expensive inpatient programs while increasing emphasis on less expensive outpatient services aimed at preventing hospitalizations. From FY 1993 to FY 1995, admissions dropped by 100,000, and ambulatory visits increased by more than 5 million. In FY 1995 alone, outpatient visits increased by 2.44 million (9.2%) to an annual total of 28,939,000 visits. From 1980 to 1995, outpatient visits increased by 60% (10,735,000 visits in 1995, compared to the 18,207,000 visits in 1980). During the same time, the VHA closed 34,934 (42%) of its beds, 2,409 beds in FY 1995 alone, and another 2,255 beds in the first half of FY 1996, freeing up outpatient dollars (Kizer 1996). This also meant that a number of intensive and costly inpatient psychiatry programs, such as many inpatient substance abuse and inpatient PTSD units, were scrutinized or abolished (Burda et al. 1991).

Kizer stated that in order to be compared accurately with other U.S. healthcare providers, the VHA needed to account for outcomes in the same manner as the rest of the industry (Kizer 1996). The new VHA system requires uniform treatment and accountability as the focus shifts to outcome measures. Clinical pathways have been developed for all specialties, including psychiatry, to standardize treatment nationwide and eliminate regional variations, such as those identified in the past in inpatient psychiatric care (Rosenheck and Astrachan 1990). Psychiatric rating scales have become nationwide VHA performance monitors requiring mandatory incorporation into clinical visits to more objectively document treatment outcomes. In addition, psychiatric utilization criteria for admissions are being nationally employed as the VHA moves away from a fee-for-service model to a capitation model. Expanding on the utilization review program established in 1993, Kizer mandated that each network establish hospital admission, utilization, and length-of-stay criteria, encompassing preadmission screening and discharge planning programs (Kizer 1996).

Cost effectiveness accountability has been difficult in the VHA because treatment was not previously standardized and symptoms are often subjective (Taylor and Dees 1993), especially in psychiatry. Swindle et al. (1996) further discussed how difficult it is to obtain reliable and accurate costing data under the current VHA cost accounting system, which was designed for management responsibility and control rather than determining the cost of services. Froelicher (1996) described the VHA as an umbrella of socialized healthcare for the indigent and the sickest people in society and questioned whether it was applicable to imitate the HMO model at all, which he believed was designed to treat relatively well people. He pointed out that the sickest patients will continue to utilize the VA so that cost efficacy will never equal that required in managed care, which is particularly relevant to psychiatric patients with chronic mental illnesses (Liberthson 1994). The VHA is still in the process of establishing incentives and risks for those delivering care in an effort to further optimize efficiency and accountability.

Although the total veteran population is decreasing as World War II veterans are dying, more veterans are more likely to use the VHA system if congressional legislation decreases Medicare benefits, with cost shifts and uncompensated private healthcare; if private insurance co-payments, deductibles, and premiums increase; and if state-level rationing increases (Paralyzed Veterans of America Strategy 2000 [1992]). In addition, the VHA faces the challenge of treating an increasingly diverse veteran population, including patients with special needs such as spinal cord injuries and PTSD (Kizer 1996). Services for women have expanded to include treatment for women who experienced PTSD from war or sexual trauma during military duty (Liberthson 1994). Additionally, as the VHA increases its contracts with the Department of Defense (Schwartz 1996), it will be serving more women and children than in the past, when the patient population was predominantly male (Sunshine et al. 1991).

Administration and Organization of Integrated Psychiatric Services at the Local Level

To provide an example of VHA organization, we discuss the Department of Veterans Affairs Medical Center in Louisville, Kentucky. Before 1995 this medical center was one of 12 hospitals in the central VHA region. Each hospital operated in a relatively independent manner. With Kizer's initiation of the VISNs, this Louisville facility became one of seven VHA medical centers within the local VISN. These seven VHA hospitals are more geographically cohesive than those in the previous administrative structure. As a group, all seven medical centers in the VISN are financially and administratively accountable to the VISN director and are clinically accountable to the VISN chief clinical manager, a physician.

At the Department of Veterans Affairs Medical Center at Louisville, as well as at each medical center within the VISN, the medical center director and associate director are responsible for administrative services, and the medical center chief of staff oversees all clinical affairs. Answering to the chief of staff are the chiefs of the various services. In 1995 the psychiatry service combined with the psychology service and was renamed the mental health and behavioral sciences service. This incorporation of the psychiatry and psychology departments under the chief of mental health and behavioral sciences appears to echo a nationwide trend to consolidate mental health services.

Each VISN has a budget established by the national central office, and each VISN director designates the financial allowance for individual medical centers within the network. In the early 1990s the amount of funding each medical center received was based on an estimate of the cost of actual and projected patient visits. In the later 1990s the money began to be allotted by a capitated disbursement model. The medical centers are reimbursed based on the number of patients rather than on the number of treatments. At most facilities, the mental health and behavioral sciences service budget is derived from the general hospital budget at the discretion of the medical center director and from funds designated for specific programs (e.g., homeless, substance abuse, PTSD, day treatment program). Staffing recommendations from the chief of mental health and behavioral sciences are presented for approval to the resource management committee under the direction of the medical center associate director.

The Department of Veterans Affairs Medical Center at Louisville has a working collaboration with the University of Louisville, similar to the medical school collaborations of most other VA medical centers. Physicians on the Louisville VA Medical Center staff have joint appointments with the University of Louisville Medical School. In the mental health and behavioral sciences service, all psychiatrists are on the faculty of the University of Louisville Department of Psychiatry and many are tenured or tenure track. University of Louisville medical students and residents rotate at the Louisville VA Medical Center during their psychiatry clerkships and residency rotations on both inpatient and outpatient services.

VHA National Trends of Inpatient-Outpatient Psychiatric Services

From 1955 to 1975, VA inpatient psychiatric episodes increased by 143% in contrast to a 37% decrease in inpatient episodes in state and county mental hospitals. These inpatient increases occurred despite the concurrent psychiatric deinstitutionalization movement in which the VA participated actively. VA deinstitutionalization initiatives started as far back as 1954 with VA community residential placements, expanding to include VA day care programs beginning in 1959 and VA halfway houses in 1961. Neff and McFall (1990) discussed the possibility that the increased number of VA inpatients reflects the admission of those previously hospitalized at state and county facilities prior to state and county deinstitutionalization.

From 1963 to 1984, the use of inpatient psychiatric services increased overall by 194%. From 1963 to 1978, VA neuropsychiatric hospital patients were shifted to psychiatric beds in general medical hospitals, resulting in a dramatic 210% increase in inpatient usage during that time. From 1976 to 1981, psychiatric inpatient usage remained about the same, dropping only slightly during the 1980s (Neff and McFall 1990).

With the onset of the economic pressures of the 1990s, along with Kizer's reorganization, the emphasis began to shift from inpatient to outpatient psychiatric services. During fiscal year (FY) 1999, there were 671,287 veterans who received specialized mental health service in the VHA system. This represented a 3.3% increase in workload over FY 1998. The average length of stay on 4,402 general psychiatry beds in FY 1999 was 15.9 days, an 8.2% decrease from FY 1998. The number of beds also decreased by 15.2% from FY 1998. The average cost of mental health care per treated veteran during FY 1999 was $2,673 (down from $3,558 in FY 1995). Although 59.2% of the VHA resources were spent on inpatient care as opposed to outpatient care in FY 1999, this percentage was down from 63.1% in FY 1998 and from 77% in FY 1995 (Rosenheck 2000).

Innovative Models for Delivering VHA Psychiatric Services

The Traditional Model

Many previous hospital-based mental health delivery systems utilized separate inpatient and outpatient services. Historically, the community mental health centers were created as separate entities from the state mental hospitals. This traditional model of discrete inpatient and outpatient treatment has been adopted in many VHA and academic environments.

Traditionally at the VHA, psychiatrists were assigned to either an inpatient or an outpatient position. The outpatient psychiatrist cared for each patient until he or she needed hospitalization. The patient's care was then transferred to a different inpatient psychiatrist, who often was unfamiliar with the patient and the treatment background. Once the patient was hospitalized, the inpatient psychiatrist could make treatment changes that were not necessarily consistent with ongoing outpatient treatment planning. When hospitalization was no longer necessary, the patient was discharged to a different psychiatrist for outpatient care at the next available appointment, which was often several weeks later.

The Louisville VA Medical Center Model

In an effort to provide the best possible psychiatric care in the most cost-effective manner, Robert Vadnal, chief of the psychiatry service at the Louisville VA Medical Center, initiated a program to integrate inpatient and outpatient services into a number of continuous treatment teams (Godleski et al. 1996). This new model of psychiatric service delivery was designed to facilitate patient movement through the treatment process and subsequently prevent and minimize costly inpatient hospitalization.

Prior to this reorganization of services, each mental health clinician was assigned to a single separate program. Inpatient and outpatient services were disjointed and poorly coordinated. The inpatient wards were nearly always full. The outpatient services had lengthy waiting periods for appointments, and outpatient emergencies were handled in the emergency room.

On October 1, 1995, the Louisville VA Medical Center reorganized from the traditional model described in the preceding section by integrating all inpatient and outpatient psychiatric services. The reorganization created cohesive teams that were responsible for inpatient, outpatient, and crisis management of a cohort of patients. Patients were reassigned to a single multidisciplinary treatment team headed by a psychiatrist; the team provided all aspects of mental healthcare, including crisis intervention, outpatient psychotherapy and pharmacotherapy, and inpatient management. Emphasis was placed on outpatient services; all crises were managed with intensive outpatient interventions whenever possible. The same treatment team facilitated the transition from outpatient to inpatient for those who required hospitalization and directed the inpatient treatment while following the patient during his or her hospital stay. On the patient's discharge, outpatient services were immediately resumed with the same clinicians.

When the statistics from the first full year of this reorganization (October 1, 1995 to September 30, 1996 [FY 1996]) were compared with the year immediately prior to the reorganization (FY 1995), we found that

- Inpatient average daily census decreased 32% (from 49.8 in FY 1995 to 33.9 in FY 1996).
- Admissions declined 19% (from 1,345 in FY 1995 to 1,094 in FY 1996).
- Average length of stay diminished by 22% (from 12.9 in FY 1995 to 10.1 in FY 1996).
- Bed occupancy rate decreased by 32% (from 87.0 in FY 1995 to 59.5 in FY 1996).
- Total annual bed-days of care were 32% less (18,176 in FY 1995 to 12,421 in FY 1996).

We found that costly inpatient admissions could be prevented with less expensive intensive outpatient interventions by the comprehensive service team. Furthermore, inpatients could be discharged earlier because, at the moment of admission, the comprehensive service team was already familiar with the patient and the treatment plan. Continuity of care increased because the team cared for the patient both as an inpatient and as an outpatient. Discharge planning and follow-up improved because the same team followed the patient immediately after release from the hospital. With a decrease in needed clinician time for inpatient services, additional clinician time was available for outpatients, resulting in a significant decrease in length of time from discharge to follow-up appointment. Patients often were seen the day or week after discharge when necessary. Patient satisfaction increased once patients no longer had to switch clinicians depending on whether they were in or out of the hospital.

The Bridge Model

The Extend Team at the University of Texas Southwestern Medical School in Dallas developed a team-based, postdischarge strategy to provide a treatment bridge from inpatient to outpatient (Goldman 1997). The Extend Team members initiate care for patients while they are in the hospital preparing for discharge, and then provide intensive posthospitalization follow-up. In some cases, the Extend Team provides daily visits and may even escort patients to 12-step programs, support groups, or other follow-up services. As the patient adjusts to life as an outpatient, contact with the Extend Team is tapered. The clinicians are in the process of demonstrating the cost efficiency of this labor-intensive program in terms of hospital days, relapse prevention, jail time, family burden, and loss of productivity.

The Product Line Model

VHA headquarters dissolved discipline-specific services and reorganized along 10 product lines aimed at being multidisciplinary and transdimensional (Kizer 1996). These strategic healthcare groups, or product lines, include primary and ambulatory care, mental health and behavioral medicine, acute care hospital-based services, geriatrics and extended care, diagnostics, pharmacy, prosthetics, rehabilitation, nursing, and allied clinical services. An increasing number of VISNs are proposing and implementing similar clinical, and sometimes budgetary, reorganizations along product lines. Under this model, VHA psychiatry is no longer a discrete department but rather is part of a product line that can include psychiatry, psychology, readjustment counseling, and other disciplines that provide mental health service (nursing, social work, and occupational and recreational therapies). As a product line, mental health and behavioral medicine is one of several strategic healthcare groups based on types or lengths of services (e.g., acute care, extended care) rather than a discipline-specific specialty as in the past (e.g., surgery, medicine, radiology). These other specialties are subsumed under similar, non-discipline-specific lines.

VHA Residency Training

VHA residency training policy must be examined in the context of national residency and specialty trends. In 1961, half of all U.S. physicians were generalists, but by 1990 generalists declined to 33.5%. Relevant to psychiatry, 10% of medical students chose psychiatric residencies in the late 1960s; this percentage declined in the 1970s, increased during the 1980s, and then decreased to 5.5% in the mid-1990s (Beigel 1995; Martini and Grenhom 1993; Rivo and Satcher 1993). The VHA residency training programs find themselves in the midst of the current national emphasis on primary care training and residency reduction (by attrition as in psychiatry or by policy as in other specialties).

In 1995 the VHA Residency Realignment Review Committee was established to make recommendations for a possible realignment in the VHA's residency programs that would affect resource allocation and residency education. Under the chairmanship of Robert G. Petersdorf, this committee strongly advocated that the VHA have a continued role in graduate medical education based on its value to the nation, its quality of care at a reasonable cost, and its impact on physician recruitment and retention (Petersdorf 1996). In 1996 about 30%–40% of the 8,900 VHA residency positions at 132 affiliated medical schools were in primary care, as a result of programs such as the Primary Care Education Program, created in 1993. The committee based its recommendations on the assumption that there is a national oversupply of physicians, especially in nongeneralist disciplines. The committee proposed the elimination of 1,000 non-primary-care VHA residency training positions. This reduction would be accomplished by returning to the 1987 resident totals, which would cut 250 residency positions in non-primary-care specialties. In addition, the committee recommended a shift of 750 positions from specialties to primary care. This shift would restore a 49% primary care composition to the total VHA residency slots. These changes were to be phased in over a 3- to 5-year period from 1997 to 2001, depending on the number of years of the residency. Of the 869 VHA psychiatry and geriatric psychiatry positions in 1996, 71 residencies (8%) would be eliminated.

The committee also proposed the total number of non-primary-care residency positions that could potentially be eliminated in the future. For psychiatry, they recommended that ultimately up to 289 VHA psychiatry residency slots could be eliminated. Although the actual and proposed decrease in the number of psychiatric residency positions supported by the VHA is quite significant, its overall effect is modulated by the currently decreasing number of applicants to psychiatric residency training programs.

Aside from the number of psychiatry residents, the training experience has also changed appreciably on the local level with the institution of the Louisville VA Medical Center Model of service delivery described earlier in this chapter. Residents actively participated in the integrated inpatient-outpatient system, being assigned to a team of patients to follow through all aspects of their care. This approach gave the residents a greater continuity of teaching experiences and enabled them to get to know a variety of patients throughout the continuum of their illnesses.

VHA Research

The U.S. Department of Veterans Affairs has supported research in the following three general areas: 1) medical research, 2) rehabilitation research and development, 3) health services research and development, and 4) cooperative studies programs.

The largest service within the Office of Research and Development is the Medical Research Service. The Merit Review program is this service's main mechanism for funding peer-reviewed biomedical research. Each specialty area has its own review board, with psychiatry and psychology under the mental health and behavioral sciences board. In addition to the merit review grants, the Medical Research Service provides support for Designated Research Centers for specific diagnoses, including schizophrenia and alcohol-related disorders.

The Health Services Research and development Service supports research at the interface of health care systems and outcomes. It funds peer-reviewed research through its Health Economics Resource Center (HERC), Management Decision and Research Center (MDRC), VA Information Resource Center (VIREC), and 11 Centers of Excellence.

As an example of local-level structure, the Louisville VA Medical Center has appointed an associate chief of staff for research and development to oversee the research service that facilitates and coordinates all ongoing research and grants at the medical center. The research service works closely with the University of Louisville because most VA staff are also University of Louisville faculty members. In addition, the research service coordinates its efforts with the Clinical Research Foundation, a state-chartered nonprofit corporation established in 1988 to administrate extramural funding. Congress has permitted the implementation of

such nonprofit corporations to facilitate research at VA medical centers. The institution of psychiatric services under the Louisville VA Medical Center Model has further facilitated clinical research within the Department of Psychiatry. Because the psychiatrists follow their patients through all aspects of their clinical care, accurate pharmaco-economic data are more easily obtained for current research protocols.

Conclusion

The VHA system has changed dramatically in recent years, positioning it to meet the demands of the marketplace but retaining its commitment to education and research. The new mandate for major structural improvements in the delivery of clinical care will increase, with an emphasis on primary care and the team approach. New affiliation agreements will be forthcoming with medical schools, and a significant challenge will exist to maintain the education and clinician-investigator missions within the VHA. So far, the VHA remains distinct from the managed care industry in supporting a combination of quality healthcare, the education of future doctors, and research programs on disorders that affect veterans. The new VHA has the potential to become a national model for healthcare systems in the future (Holsinger 1991; Simpson 1995).

References

Academic Medicine: The Veterans Health Administration: options for the future. Acad Med 69:516–518, 1994

Adkins RE (ed): Medical Care of Veterans. Washington, DC, U.S. Government Printing Office, 1967

Beigel A: A proposed vision for psychiatry at the turn of the century. Compr Psychiatry 36:31–39, 1995

Burda PC, Starkey TW, Dominguez F, et al.: A biopsychosocial approach to the chronic psychiatric patient. VA Practitioner, December 1991, pp 55–60

Department of Veterans Affairs State Summaries. Washington, DC, Department of Veterans Affairs, Office of Public Affairs, Media Relations, October 2000, pp 1–6

Drucker J: Resetting the course of VA psychiatric services. Federal Practitioner, 12(10):28–32, 1995

Errera P: Psychiatry programs at VACO: the intertwining of plan and happening. VA Practitioner, July 1992, pp 41–50

Fisher ES, Welch HG: The future of the Department of Veterans Affairs health care system. JAMA 273:651–655, 1995

Fonesca ML, Smith ME, Klein RE, et al: The Department of Veterans Affairs medical care system and the people it serves. Med Care 34(3 suppl):MS9–MS19, 1996

Froelicher VF: How academic medicine and the VA are being influenced by changes in health-care delivery. Chest 110:239–242, 1996

Godleski LS, Vadnal RE, Tasman A: Integration of inpatient and outpatient mental health services. American Psychiatric Association 48th Institute on Psychiatric Services Institute Proceedings and Syllabus Summary 124, Washington, DC, 1996

Goldman EL: Extended contact can cut psychotic relapse. Clinical Psychiatry News, January 33, 1997

Graning K, Walters K, Headley J: A bold new world in VA health care reform. VA Practitioner, June 1994, pp 33–35

Holsinger Jr. JW: The Veterans Health Administration: a health care model for the nation. Acad Med 66:674–675, 1991

Kizer K: Vision for change. VA government document submitted to Congress. March 17, 1995

Kizer K: Prescription for change, the guiding principles and strategic objectives underlying the transformation of the veterans healthcare system. VA government document, March 1996

Kizer K: VA becomes true "system" of care. US Medicine 33:10–11, 1997

Liberthson D: Palo Alto VAMC: the women's trauma recovery program. VA Practitioner, December 1994, pp 59–64

Martini CJM, Grenhom G: Institutional responsibility in graduate medical education and highlights of historical data. JAMA 270:1053–1060, 1993

Meadows OE: The Department of Veterans Affairs health care system and national health care. Acad Med 66:744–745, 1991

Neff JA, McFall SL: Explaining trends in use of VA inpatient psychiatric services. Health Serv Res 25:257–268, 1990

Paralyzed Veterans of America Strategy 2000: The VA responsibility in tomorrow's national health care system. Washington, DC, Paralyzed Veterans of America, 1992

Petersdorf RG: Report of the Residency Realignment Review Committee 1-19. Submitted to the Under Secretary for Health, Veterans Health Administration, Department of Veterans Affairs, Washington, DC, 1996

Pittman Jr. JA: The future of the VA. Centralization, costs, politics and presentism. JAMA 273:667–668, 1995

Rivo ML, Satcher D: Improving access to health care through physician workforce reform. JAMA 270: 1074–1078, 1993

Rosenheck R: Professionalism, bureaucracy and patriotism: the VA as a health care megasystem. Psychiatr Q 58:77–90, 1986

Rosenheck R: National mental health program performance monitoring system: fiscal year 1995 report. VHA government document from Northeast Program Evaluation Center, West Haven, CT, 1995

Rosenheck R, Astrachan B: Regional variation in patterns of inpatient psychiatric care. Am J Psychiatry 147:1180–1183, 1990

Rosenheck R: Department of Veterans Affairs National Mental Health Program Performance Monitoring System, Fiscal Year 1999 Report. West Haven, CT, Department of Veterans Affairs, Northeast Program Evaluation Center, 2000

Schwartz S: Dallas VAMC: a new health care option for DoD. Federal Practitioner 13(8):30–37, 1996

Simpson AK: The future of veterans' health care. Acad Med 70:700–701, 1995

Sunshine JH: Dr. Kizer's vision for transforming VA health care. Federal Practitioner 12(8):73–75, 1995

Sunshine JH, Witkin MJ, Atay JE, et al: Mental health services of the Veterans Administration United States 1986 (Mental Health Statistical Note 197:1-17). Washington, DC, U.S. Department of Health and Human Services, 1991

Swindle RW Jr, Beattie MC, Barnett PG: The quality of cost data. A caution from the Department of Veterans Affairs experience. Med Care 34 (3 suppl):MS83–MS90, 1996

Taylor JR, Dees JP: How to design a mental health system. American Association of Occupational Health Nurses Journal 41:330–336, 1993

❖ 24 ❖

Psychiatric Services in the Military

Paul F. Giannandrea, M.D.
Susan G. Larson, M.D., M.P.A.
David McDuff, M.D.

One usually considers the birth of the health maintenance organization (HMO) to be the development of Kaiser Permanente in Southern California in the late 1960s. However, quietly operating for decades before Kaiser was the largest and most diverse managed care organization (MCO) and healthcare delivery system—that operated by the U.S. military. In today's parlance, military medicine represents the first integrated delivery system to have merged the MCO and delivery system into one organization. It is also the first example of the merger of managed behavioral health with the other medical disciplines and their delivery systems, having never been carved out from those services to begin with. It is the only managed care system that can claim massive resource expenditures for preventive medicine initiatives, a primary focus on maintenance of the health of its target population, and economic incentives as not the first and foremost factor shaping its methodology and operations.

Although current fiscal concerns have affected the military as they have its civilian counterparts, the primary mission of the armed services' medical corps has been the health, well-being, and physical and mental readiness of its active duty population. Through an evolution of experience and research emanating from that mission came timely initiatives to serve the dependent family members of that active duty force. Out of the concerns and needs to better retain well-trained and healthy service members, there began a focus on the retiree and Veterans Administration (VA) services made available to service members upon leaving military service. Thus, three major target populations evolved in the armed services and related Department of Defense delivery systems—active duty members, their families, and veteran/retiree populations. As a result of the armed services' success in their focus, tradition, and mission, their medical delivery systems have much to offer the civilian community in this age of MCOs and

The opinions expressed in this chapter are those of the authors and do not necessarily reflect those of the United States armed services.

the management of care delivery during a time of limited economic resources. One can consider the U.S. military medical corps of the three military services to be the only true HMOs in existence.

The military medical system has greatly, but relatively silently, contributed to the arena of community health and civilian medicine (Debakey 1996). In psychiatry alone, the modalities of milieu and group therapies and assessment have drawn substantially from the military. The concept of psychologically screening populations for fitness, for example, in the occupational and corporate worlds, as well as the modalities of hypnotherapy and eye movement desensitization, reintegration (EMDR) have borrowed from the military medical experience (Davidson et al. 1990). Our understanding of specific disorders, such as posttraumatic stress disorder (PTSD), conversion disorders, and chronic pain disorders, has advanced as a result of military medicine and psychiatry (Fitzgerald et al. 1993).

Concepts now being considered and developed as novel from the most recent wave of managed care have their precursors in the military medical system. Stratified treatment or echelons of care (Jones 1995a) predate the diversified levels of care that have developed in the past decade. The contingency approach to treatment decision making predates the current critical pathways, practice guidelines, and clinical decision algorithms. Albeit most prominently displayed in the area of trauma care, these precursors also have been present in military psychiatry. Combat triage has been a topic in battle stress casualty management since World Wars I and II. Community programs that focus on the well-being of abused children and spouses have roots in military advocacy programs. The current public health concerns regarding drug abuse in the community have only to look to the no-tolerance military policy and structure for the first international drug use detection and treatment program in a work force and its surrounding communities.

Because the need for flexibility, reproducibility, and efficiency is high, the military services have made great inroads to establish a stable and standardized delivery system for all three services. Thus, the military offers a diverse, yet standard, level of care designed to be reproducible anywhere in the world. This delivery system is supported and stabilized through medical personnel management, standardized medical records, and a highly sophisticated and professional training and education process. System flexibility, stabilization, and efficiency are thereby preserved. A common criticism of civilian MCOs is that the quality and satisfaction of individual treatment will be sacrificed as provider continuity diminishes. This potential problem and realistic concern has been functionally and successfully managed for many years in the military medical system. Individual treatment has been preserved successfully without provider continuity. The managed care and customer satisfaction puzzle that plagues MCOs in the civilian community has been resolved generally and successfully in the uniformed services.

Service Delivery System: The Past

From an historical perspective, the military integration of the organized practice of psychiatry with that of the practice of general medicine and surgery had its roots in the enlightened and visionary organization of the Army's and Navy's medical corps during World War II. During the early months of that conflict, medical planners heeded the battlefield lessons of World War I. It was clear from the experiences of early trench warfare that rapid, early intervention in forward positioned medical units could return to the front a large percentage of the soldiers with shell shock or battle fatigue, representing 30%–75% of the casualties from all causes (Beebe and Debakey 1952).

Because of shortages of fully trained psychiatrists during World War II, many general medical officers (i.e., general practitioners) were trained in abbreviated 6-week courses to function as triage-and-treatment mental health providers stationed in the front echelon units. Medical evacuation for the patients unable to be returned to combat, whether for medical or psychiatric reasons, followed the same pathways to the rear echelon treatment, with the same levels-of-care approach. That is, the farther from the front lines the medical echelon was positioned, the more sophisticated the care, support, and treatment modalities became. Eventually, of course, those patients who needed long-term or inpatient care were transported to the continental United States, where the tertiary care military medical centers and eventually the VA hospitals provided care.

The military system of echelons of care (Table 24–1) predated the integrated vertical levels of care of the MCO of today (Jones 1995b), with its dispersed network of primary care providers referring selectively to specialty care, and then with even greater care to tertia-

TABLE 24–1. Psychiatric echelon care

Site	Level	Holding time
Battle	Self/buddy	4 hours
	Small unit leader; medical aid/corpsman	4 hours
Forward areas	Battalion aid station	8 hours
	Brigade clearing station	3 days
Rear areas	Division clearing station	4 days
	Special treatment hospital	1–2 weeks
	Evacuation hospital	1–2 weeks
Communication zone	Hospital outside combat zone	1 week to 1 month
Continental United States	Medical center in United States	Indefinite

ry care, followed by graduated "step down" of care from greater intensity to less (Dickey et al. 1989). It also predated by many years—by sheer necessity—the system of vertical integration of medical and psychiatric services and, in effect, clinical pathways. Patients who could receive rapid treatment, and be returned to duty at the front, were so managed. Patients not responding to initial treatment were moved along the clinical pathway, or echelon care, to a medical station to the rear, and so on, depending on their clinical response. The absence of case managers to facilitate this flow, or written clinical pathways, has never been problematic in the military triage system. There is wholehearted, universal acceptance by the care providers, the patients, and the line commands of both the wisdom and the necessity of the echelon approach. Because there is broad support for the mission, those who are not healthy enough to participate want to assist by using the fewest resources for their own needs. A rapid decision on clinical matters is to everyone's advantage, and clinicians who cannot meet the challenge of decisiveness despite inadequate information are quickly indoctrinated or sent to the rear.

Within this historic and classic military medical framework, the practice of both administrative and clinical psychiatry arose and developed in the uniformed services. Out of necessity, many of the principles of practice useful in management of medical and surgical cases were adapted to the practice of psychiatry. As a result, within the global HMO of the military medical system, the practice of psychiatry was standardized to a degree that would be considered extraordinary in any privatized mental health system. Examples include triage of psychiatric cases by diagnosis into clinical pathways and transport to appropriate levels of

care based on response to treatment; rapid stabilization and return to duty whenever possible; use of physician extenders (field corpsmen) in mental health; allegiance to corporate priorities (combat readiness) for both the practitioner and all of the patient population; emphasis on short-term treatments, limited interventions, and group therapy; time-limited treatments and expected outcomes (an early form of case management); and application of principles of combat psychiatry (proximity, immediacy, expectancy) to the practice of both medicine and psychiatry in the occupational setting (U.S. Department of the Army 1984).

The practice of psychiatry within the military HMO setting gave rise to manpower-conserving innovations in the practice of population-based medicine that have yet to be applied on a large scale in the private sector. These innovations include psychological screening for high-stress and isolated assignments (U.S. Department of the Air Force 1994); 100% screening and zero tolerance for drug use; aggressive intervention for alcohol abuse and family dysfunction; medical/psychological screening of family members prior to overseas transfer; 100% training of personnel in suicide prevention, sexually transmitted disease prevention, and sexual harassment prevention; mandatory weight requirements and physical fitness programs; widespread smoking cessation programs; 100% immunization rates for active duty; and 100% dental health.

The practice of preventive psychiatry is integrated into day-to-day military operations, and training is on a scale unheard of anywhere in the private sector. For example, the principle of unit cohesiveness, so essential to combat effectiveness, is also one of the strongest deterrents to battle fatigue. Building unit cohesiveness is fundamental in the process of basic training, especially in the elite units of the Army and Navy. It is close to being a religion in the daily life of the U.S. Marines Corps (Drucker and Brandt 1952). In addition, ample evidence indicates that the process of debriefing has a preventive effect against PTSD (National Institute of Mental Health 1988). Debriefing, a standard military process involving a focused inquiry into the specifics of a recent event, was initially practiced with aviators and others involved in high-risk, specialty missions. The process of verbalizing emotionally charged material, and receiving tacit organizational recognition, defuses some of the emotions and provide a means of mastery over the event. Thus, debriefing (Table 24–2) has become an integral part of the work of Critical Incident Stress Debriefing teams, widely used for trauma and tragedy in both civilian and military settings worldwide (Raphael 1986; U.S. Department of the Army 1994b).

The military has broken ground elsewhere in the practice of administrative psychiatry. The military psychiatrist has struggled for years with issues of patient privacy and confidentiality, experiencing competing loyalties to both the patient and the employer. A body of psychiatric literature and administrative orders detail the often difficult position of the uniformed psychiatrist as he or she deals with a military patient. Both members are subject to the articles of the Uniform Code of Military Justice. Both members owe primary allegiance to the military, which supersedes any individual or civil rights. This unique and often difficult arrangement has implications for those who practice within a managed care setting, in which a patient's behavior is no longer a matter solely between the patient and the clinician. With the entry of the third party—the HMO—into the medical decision-making picture, the issue of confidentiality in psychiatry as well as the rest of medicine is sure to become controversial. The military psychiatrist is an expert at meeting the needs of the patient within the larger framework of the needs of the system.

Similarly, the huge challenge of meeting the patient's clinical needs within the framework of limited resources—capitation-based practice—has been the experience of the military psychiatrist since the 1950s. The need to keep providers at the battlefront has always been in competition with the need to provide care for those moved to higher echelons of care. Pioneering work in milieu psychiatry, group evaluation and treatment, and behavioral medicine resulted from such constraints. In addition, less visible but equally innovative treatment approaches have long been accepted prac-

TABLE 24–2. Key steps in an after-action debriefing

Explain at the outset the purpose and ground rules to be used during the debriefing.
Involve everyone in verbally reconstructing the event in precise detail.
Achieve a group consensus, resolving individual misinterpretations and misunderstandings and restoring perspective about true responsibility.
Encourage expression (ventilation) of thoughts and feelings about the event.
Validate feelings about the event as normal and work toward how they can be accepted, lived with, and atoned for.
Prevent scapegoating and verbal abuse.
Talk about the normal (but unpleasant) stress symptoms that unit members experience and that recur for a while, so that they too can be accepted without surprise or fear of permanence.
Summarize the lessons learned and any positive aspects of the experience.

tice in the worldwide HMOs of the Army, Navy, and Air Force. Use of an administrative tool known throughout the military medical system as the limited duty medical board is one such vehicle. Through use of the written prescription of a board, the treating physician can give the patient a strong incentive to complete treatment within a prescribed (3-month to 6-month) period of time, spell out the exact limitations of the condition to his or her employer, allow the patient to continue in some work, and enable the patient to proceed along a clinical path to recovery—or chronic care—based on both clinical criteria and objective work-based criteria, since the employer has input into the final evaluation.

The cooperative relationship between the employer and the military psychiatrist works to the advantage of all. In many if not most psychiatric cases, input is available from the individual's supervisor or the family member's supervisor regarding current and previous work performance, unusual circumstances or behavior, alcohol use, and unusual occupational demands or stressors. Likewise, cooperation between the therapist and the supervisor enhances the patient's response to treatment and provides objective information on observable progress. The patient receives treatment with the advantage of support at work, and the employer's needs are met in that potential dangerousness due to occupational demands can be considered during treatment, and reassignment, as necessary, can be accomplished. This is also the case when legal issues complicate management. Rather than experiencing a mutually adversarial relationship, the mental health provider, the patient, the patient's legal representative, and command resources all come together to provide family and social support for the patient.

The most visible evidence of the benefits of employer–mental health cooperation in treatment is that of the military's alcohol rehabilitation programs. Command representatives remain in frequent contact with the individual in treatment. Aftercare programs developed during the course of treatment are shared with the sponsoring command, and sponsors for the patient's sobriety program are arranged within the command whenever possible. Each command has a command alcohol counselor, a trained layperson who tracks the patient's work in his or her aftercare program for a year following formal treatment. Long-term follow-up of substance abuse treatment within this cooperative network with the employer substantiates less than a 40% recidivism rate for alcohol use, a figure considered extraordinary in the mental health literature (Grodin, personal communication, summer 1994).

Service Delivery System: Present and Future

The day-to-day integration of the mental health provider with the so-called line is a key element in successful management of competing demands. In military parlance a line command is an operational unit, part of the structure. It may be a squadron, a ship, an infantry battalion, a special forces unit, or any of the warfare-oriented portions of the armed services. But working closely with the providers of medical and surgical care (physical collocation in all instances), and with legal, social work, financial, and other support services, the line has been invaluable in assisting the provider with managing the conflicting roles that have become problematic in the private sector.

For military psychiatrists, it has long been a fact of life that they must juggle the competing demands for resources, manage the needs of competing customers, handle the shifting priorities of divergent roles, and reassess priorities, values, and political realities. Out of necessity, those trained to work in the military mental health system have learned to manage these conflicting roles by the process of prioritization. Working with a contingency model, just as the line commands do, priorities are pre-decided, agreed-upon, and well under-

stood by all (U.S. Department of the Army 1994a). The role of the healthcare providers—including mental health workers—in meeting those priorities within the military HMO is clear. In times of crisis and forced rapid response, all participants revert to the priorities, and there is unified support for necessary sacrifices. For example, during the Desert Storm conflict, large numbers of psychiatrists and psychologists were deployed from clinics and hospitals in the continental United States and reassigned to combatant units in the Middle East. Those who stayed at the hospitals of origin enacted contingency plans to deal with the remaining workload. The patient population, for the most part, understood inconveniences and delays and supported efforts to provide care for those deployed. Line commands adjusted their demands to take into account personnel shortages at the hospitals. Politicians supported efforts by mobilizing reserve personnel. Everyone worked harder and worked together to support the top priority. It was absolutely critical to have agreed, well in advance, on what that priority should be (Ursano and Norwood 1996).

A paradoxical advantage of this contingency-based prioritization system for both providers and beneficiaries is that the system is stable at the expense of individual continuity and one-on-one patient-provider relationships. The beneficiaries, who understand the system and its priorities, accept the mobility and interchangeable roles of the providers. The providers accept the necessity of adaptability and the challenge of mastering not only individual therapy techniques but also techniques of group therapy, industrial psychiatry, systems theory, preventive psychiatry, community psychiatry, advocacy, and administrative medicine. This arrangement is a win-win situation for management, providing the flexibility needed to match personnel assignments with the training, skills, and abilities demonstrated by various providers as they tackle differing roles.

A bedrock value throughout the military managed care system has been fidelity and commitment to the service member. The system is dedicated to maintaining the optimal health of the "covered lives" rather than to managing the cost of those covered lives. This approach has given rise to the claim that administration and delivery of medical care within the military HMO is prohibitively expensive and massively inefficient. This notion parallels the propagated civilian MCO ideology that to provide comprehensive medical care, including mental health and substance abuse treatment, would be too expensive. The only thing that is thus far quite clear in the business setting of providing care is that the less paid out, the more profit is experienced. Without a clear commitment to keeping subscriber membership healthy, as with the military healthcare delivery system, all claims by MCOs that they provide adequate care show no apparent benefit. Rather, these MCOs' major commitment has been to keep the company's stockholders happy and profit margins high. Unfortunately, the claim of the exorbitant expense of maintaining adequate healthcare has been borne out by the early private-sector managed care initiatives. The cost per-member per-month consistently declined in highly penetrated markets, and the number of visits and the cost of subspecialty care likewise plummeted where managed care prevailed.

Commitments to the health of covered lives and to the cost of that health are not necessarily mutually exclusive. In fact, reliable data have demonstrated that the cost of operation for military tertiary care centers—benchmarked against civilian standards for length of stay, morbidity, staff-to-patient ratio, and the like—is comparable with competitive institutions throughout the country. Indeed, the cost of operation of the military medical departments has held steady or declined since the 1990s, while that of the nation as a whole, measured as a percentage of gross national product, has continued to climb (Koenig 1996). Other measures of efficiency and quality of medical facilities also are comparable. Virtually all military hospitals seek Joint Commission on Accreditation of Healthcare Organizations accreditation and boast an extraordinary record. In fiscal year 1996, for example, 60% of the Navy's teaching hospitals boasted "accreditation with commendation," as did 100% of the tertiary care centers in the U.S. Army.

Factors in the private sector that lend this issue more urgency, especially in the arena of mental health, are those that are forcing the evolution of MCOs more and more into quasi-public-health agencies. As HMOs move into subcontracting of Medicare and Medicaid populations, the ability to screen out enrollees, to avoid preexisting conditions, and to shift costs is bound to become more problematic. The politics of public opinion will begin to exert major influence over the decisions of MCOs. Competing demands by the sponsoring contractors, the covered lives, political forces, judicial decisions, and congressional mandates will become the rule. Meeting the physical and emotional needs of the patients—including a lot of chronically ill patients—in such an environment will be a challenge of awesome proportions.

The answer to all such difficulties lies in effective leadership not only in the military but also in all of medicine. Leadership must first embrace a commitment to the values of medicine, above those of economics, if any form of organized medical structure is to gain and maintain public acceptance. Leadership must then formulate a vision of the future and evolve a clear sense of what the system ought to be, rather than allow it to grow in whatever direction cost avoidance dictates. Finally, leadership must keep a commitment to both the covered lives and the cost of achieving the best possible outcomes.

For this reason, the leadership of military psychiatry has moved forward in recent times to re-engineer the delivery of mental healthcare so that all of the covered lives receive the necessary care, with measurable and reproducible outcomes, at a cost lower than that of previous care in the military and private sector combined. The re-engineering began in the northeast region of the United States and will be a model for other regions to emulate as more data become available.

In the National Capital Mental Health Alliance model, patients receive the right level of care at the right time by the right provider, within an organized framework, integrated with the delivery of primary care. In a system familiar to the military psychiatrist, patients are triaged at the primary care center sites, given diagnoses, and then referred to the proper echelon of care. Those who need acute inpatient stabilization or emergency intervention are referred to one of three possible inpatient centers, located in the tertiary care medical facilities. By the use of clinical pathways, those patients are rapidly stabilized and moved along to day treatment, long-term group therapy, short-term outpatient treatment, adolescent care, or other appropriate care. Psychiatrists, psychologists, social workers, occupational and mental health therapists, chaplains, nurses, psychiatric technicians, and other specialists all have roles and participate in the clinical pathways, which are formatted for an automated system. Concomitant utilization review is designed to be an integral part of the pathways. Outcomes are measurable and negotiated with the patients in advance and at appropriate points along the treatment pathways. In brief, all of the participants agree to the goals and landmarks at every point in the diagnostic and treatment process. Because the population is captured—that is, disenrollment and denial of other services is not possible because of the system's commitment to the patients' health above all else—it is to everyone's strong advantage to work toward actual improvement and toward a satisfactory outcome during the first encounter. Recycling of patients, which is common in community-based mental health systems, works against the fixed costs of healthcare and is inefficient for everyone. This is as true for the patient as it is for all of the involved providers. Clarifying a realistic and desired outcome in advance is key. Along with rapid and accurate initial diagnosis, that negotiation with the patient is the sine qua non of the mental health clinical pathways (American Psychological Association 1996).

Initial results from the clinical operation of this integrated military mental health system were promising. Significant cost avoidance was achieved in the first year, during which shifts of personnel from the tertiary care centers to the peripheral primary care centers were not yet completed (Mental Health Alliance Board of Governors Report 1996). The total savings have yet to be reached, but the lessons are there for the managed care systems of the future. Clarity of purpose, concrete written goals and pathways, and interspecialty cooperation in achieving those goals can clearly allow the healthcare system to place fidelity to the patients' heath needs as its top priority, while achieving savings in resources.

The real future of managed care and of healthcare in general depends on the character and vision of leadership. If a commitment is made—in fact, in deed, and in principle—to the ongoing health of the covered lives with whom we enter into partnership, then the next step beyond fixing clear goals and partnering with those beneficiaries is that of entering into a cooperative campaign of prevention. Prevention is as applicable to long-term mental and physical health as it is to discrete disease entities such as lung cancer or hypertension. Before today's medical leadership is willing to embrace this obvious and fundamental measure of cost avoidance, however, it needs to rediscover and adhere to an old-fashioned principle of medical ethics, embedded in the Hippocratic Oath: "I will prescribe regimens for the good of my patients according to my ability and my judgment and never do harm to anyone... If I keep this oath faithfully may I enjoy my life and practice my art, respected by all men and in all times; but if I swerve from it or violate it, may the reverse be my lot" (Hippocratic Oath 1997).

The Military Psychiatrist/ Administrator

A good administrator, civilian or military, must possess an admixture of skills that typify good leadership and management, the percentage composition of each to be determined specifically by the system that one administers. A fine balance of wisdom and action must be honed in the crucible of life experiences. The timely actions of courage and perseverance must be tempered by the sober quiet of meditation and scholarly knowledge. There have been multiple perspectives on leadership throughout modern history (Zaher 1996); traditional military leadership is but one representation of leadership. The spiritual and corporate arenas promote two other diverse versions of what leadership is about (Zaleznik 1989).

What component parts make up a good administrator? Zaleznik (1989) discussed in much detail the difference between managers and leaders (Table 24–3). He described a contrasting image of these two dichotomous poles of typical administrative personnel. In essence, the common characteristic of the leadership pole is the ability to face situations actively rather than passively, to overcome and transform conditions, and not to simply react and adapt to them. As Figure 24–1 depicts, the good administrator, either military or civilian, must maintain a set of traits that represent a balance between these two sets of characteristics. To fall too far to one side or the other of this polarity upsets the fine balance of the system. Descriptions of management skills are legion (Pascale and Athos 1981; Sloan 1964). Easily usable descriptions of leadership skills, in contrast, are not. Perhaps this difference is because of the types of characteristics that management skills offer, that is, the more compulsive, calculating, and content-driven orientation that minimizes creativity, affect, and passion. In other words, it is the stuff of which manuals and texts are made, unlike the less descriptive and expansive leadership qualities described in Table 24–3. Because medical delivery systems resemble corporate businesses, the tendency is to err in the same way that businesses do. Zaleznik (1989) made important points regarding how businesses operate and how administrator leadership has been undermined much to its detriment because of the excessive focus on management skills in administrator training programs. We should look to the military for help in determining the characteristics that make a leader because military administrators represent an admixture of the two sets of characteristics. In the military setting we can best observe and learn about the leadership component of administration.

Further description of these contrasting sets of characteristics is useful. The vocabulary of a leader in-

TABLE 24–3. Leader versus manager traits

Leader	Manager
Affectively directed	Cognitively directed
Commitment oriented	Cooperation oriented
Values creativity in subordinates	Values reliability in subordinates
Focuses on ideals	Focuses on process and structure
People oriented	Technique oriented
Has vision	Projects self-centered needs
Substance, humanity, and morality approach	Team approach over individual approach
Faces situations actively	Faces situations passively
Confronts to overcome and transform conditions	Reacts and adapts to situations
Strikes out into unexplored areas	Navigates only in chartered territory
Extrapolates data	Interpolates data
Discusses mutual obligations and responsibilities	Concerned only with narrow self-interests
Learns how to lead	Learns how to follow
Talks about compacts and covenants	Talks about contracts and the letter of the law
Focuses on *what* decisions get made	Focuses on *how* decisions are made
Focuses on what is communicated (substance)	Focuses on how communication flows (style)
"Good people produce good results"	"Solid methods produce good results"
In conflicts, targets winning and losing	In conflicts, targets reconciliation, compromise, and balance of power
Values clearly stated messages	Uses signals (indirect messages)
Will risk ferment in order to produce and perform	Sacrifices performance and clarity in order to avoid challenges
Relates empathically to the person	Relates to the role the person occupies
Encourages local decision making	Encourages efficient coordination
Asks for the hearts and minds of subordinates	Asks only for the performance of subordinates

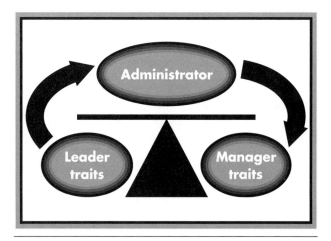

FIGURE 24–1. The balance of the successful administrator.

cludes "compacts" and "covenants," whereas the manager speaks of "contracts" and the "letter of the law." Managers are more concerned about how decisions get made and how communications flow, whereas a leader is concerned with what decisions get made and what he or she communicates. Thus, managers exhibit style over substance and process over reality (Zaleznik 1989). In the *Managerial Mystique*, Zaleznik (1989) indicated that the belief in authority and the support of one's boss must be constantly questioned and demonstrated. Therefore, allegiances cannot just be programmed into subordinates through training exercises or more Orwellian tactics. Those who wish to be leaders must welcome these challenges and demonstrate by example their value and the value of their administrative position to their organization. They should contribute substance to their jobs and add value beyond superficial symbols and good intentions. This adds another dimension to leadership: accountability. The administrator who does not provide accountability merely reflects the latest Dilbert cartoon (Adams 1996) and thus becomes a tragic, ineffective, corporate automaton as opposed to an effective and productive leader. Leaders are people centered verses technique centered. Managers often believe "solid methods will produce good results." This belief perpetuates the fantasy that a sound policy and procedure manual and a cadre of techniques for control will overcome all human frailties. In contrast, a leader knows that "good and bad substantive decisions are directly related to the strengths and weaknesses of the individuals involved." To the technocrat this stance is perhaps anxiety provoking but nevertheless true. Leaders stimulate and drive others to work hard and create reality out of ideas. When substance no longer is the focus, politics come into play. This leads to the discouragement of assertiveness, individual responsibility, and creativity. "When they [workers] lose sight of their work, when they become insecure as a result of poor leadership, or when they are asked to do what they are not capable of doing and therefore must endure the humiliation of poor performance, they turn to process, which becomes equivalent to politics. As a result of these distortions, the lesson people (workers) learn is how to be devious." No matter what its form it leads to "detaching work from authority relations and the consequent encouragement of irrationality" (Zaleznik 1989, p. 37). This leads to unwieldy bureaucratic systems mired in their own red tape.

The military is not immune to this bureaucratic process of over-management at the expense of leadership. In fact, General Edward C. Myer, former chief of staff for the Army, pointed to a decline in the leadership ideal in the military as it moved away from command and toward bureaucratic politics (Myer 1983). When General Myer stated that there were two careers in the military—the field and Washington—he implied that when military leaders moved toward Washington, they simultaneously moved away from their field commands along with their commitments to responsibility, accountability to their subordinates, and dedication to their superiors; in Washington these commitments were replaced by self-interest and political adeptness (Gabriel and Savage 1978).

In summary, a bipolarity exists in the components of a good administrator. On one pole are leadership qualities that propel one toward a direction of change, in contrast to and counterbalanced by the alternate pole of management skills, which tend to stabilize one about a mean and tend to direct away from change. Military administrators have a higher component percentage of leadership skills directly as a result of the military's need to prepare for spontaneous, abrupt, and extreme changes, but this need is somewhat neutralized by the simultaneous need for stabilization during peacetime. In addition, the military service is still the most typical arena for the development of leadership qualities. Although other arenas exist, leadership is created most often in the military system. Consider the high proportion of military representation in the history of the office of the presidency of the United States.

Clearly, however, military leaders and commanders in chief require a very different admixture of skills.

Conclusion

In the age of sophisticated models of managed care and in a time of developing large healthcare delivery systems, we only have to look to the military to observe an evolved and true HMO whose primary mission has been to preserve the optimal health of its members. New and efficient levels and modalities of care have also come from its ranks, some of which have become standards of practice in the medical community. The modern-day military HMO has worked on efficiency and cost-of-care issues to a degree of success that rivals any civilian MCO. Finally, medical leadership has a time-honored tradition in the military system. We would do well to look to the armed services to learn how to develop leadership skills and mentor young leaders so that we could then inculcate them into our administrative psychiatry training programs.

References

Adams S: The Dilbert Principle. Kansas City, MO, Universal Press Syndicate Company, 1996

American Psychological Association: NCS Assessments. National Capital Area Mental Health Alliance Conference, Outcomes Management Plan, January 1996. Washington, DC, American Psychological Association, 1996

Beebe GW, Debakey ME: Incidence of Hits and Wounds in Battle Casualties: Incidence, Mortality, and Logistic Considerations. Springfield, IL, Charles C. Thomas, 1952

Davidson JT, Kudler HS, Smith RD: Assessment and pharmacotherapy of post-traumatic stress disorder, in Biological Assessment and Treatment of Post-Traumatic Stress Disorder. Edited by Giller EL. Washington, DC, APA Press, 1990, pp 203–221

Debakey ME: History, the torch that illuminates: lessons from military medicine. Military Medicine, 161:711–715, 1996

Dickey B, Binner P, Leff S, et al: Containing mental health treatment cost through program design. Am J Public Health 79:863–867, 1989

Drucker AJ, Brandt KH: A survey of options of officers and senior NCOs in Korea: factors contributing to maintenance of morale under combat conditions. Army Project Number 29535100, PRS Report 951, April 1, 1952

Fitzgerald ML, Braudaway CA, Leeks D, et al: Debriefing: a therapeutic intervention. Military Medicine 1158(8), 1993

Gabriel RA, Savage PL: Crisis in Command: Mismanagement in the Army. New York, Hill & Wang, 1978

Hippocratic Oath: Microsoft Encarta Online Encyclopedia 2000. http://encarta.msn.com/find/concise.asp?ti=015B2000

Jones FD: Traditional warfare combat stress casualties, in Textbook of Military Medicine, Part I. Edited by Jones FD. Washington, DC, Borden Institute, 1995, pp 43–45

Koenig, H: Address to the TRICARE lead agent conference. Washington, DC, January 1996

Mental Health Alliance Board of Governors Report. Washington, DC, 1996

Myer EC: Executive form: leadership—a soldier's view. Washington Quarterly 6(3), 1983

National Institute of Mental Health, Division of Education and Service Systems Liaison, Emergency Services Branch: Prevention and Control of Stress Among Emergency Workers: a Pamphlet for Team Managers. Rockville, MD, U.S. Department of Health and Human Services, 1988

Pascale RT, Athos AG: The Art of Japanese Management: Applications for American Executives. New York, Simon & Schuster, 1981

Raphael B: When Disaster Strikes. New York, Basic Books, 1986

Sloan AP: My Years With General Motors. New York, Doubleday, 1964

Ursano RJ, Norwood A: Emotional Aftermath of the Persian Gulf War. Washington, DC, APA Press, 1996, pp 251–281

U.S. Department of the Air Force: Medical Examinations and Standards (Air Force Instruction 48-123, Attachment 6). Washington, DC, U.S. Government Printing Office, November 1994

U.S. Department of the Army: Neuropsychiatry and Mental Health (Army Regulation 40-216). Washington, DC, U.S. Government Printing Office, 1984

U.S. Department of the Army: Combat Stress Control in a Theater of Operations (Field Manual 8-51). Washington, DC, U.S. Government Printing Office, September 1994a

U.S. Department of the Army: Leaders' manual for combat stress control (Field Manual 22-51:6-7). Washington, DC, U.S. Government Printing Office, September 1994b

Zaher CA: Learning to be a leader. The Physician Executive 22(9):10–17, 1996

Zaleznik A: The Managerial Mystique: Restoring Leadership in Business. New York, Harper & Row, 1989

❖ 25 ❖

State and County Agencies

Michael F. Hogan, Ph.D.

State and county governments coordinate a substantial mental health delivery system that has no parallel in healthcare. For virtually all other health problems, care is paid for by health insurance (employer based, or Medicare and Medicaid) and provided through a single complex system of hospitals and other providers. Some general healthcare providers (e.g., inner city hospitals) care for a high proportion of indigent or uninsured individuals, and others (e.g., physician practices in suburbia) care for few uninsured patients. However, the basic structure and financing of the U.S. healthcare system relies on private and nonprofit providers, with funding from health insurance. The mainstream health system serves both the insured and the uninsured, although access to care is uneven, and worse for the uninsured.

As a significant exception to this pattern, this separate mental health delivery system has existed as a safety net since the origins of the public mental health system in nineteenth-century state-sponsored asylums. This separate and publicly funded and administered system has provided care for persons with the most serious mental illnesses and for those without adequate commercial health insurance coverage for mental healthcare. No other substantial category of illness, since tuberculosis was controlled, has been treated through a distinct governmentally financed and managed delivery system.

The existence of this separate and publicly managed system has broad and pervasive consequences. On the one hand, the public mental health system functions as an essential safety net for the most seriously mentally ill individuals in our society. On the other hand, it is increasingly apparent that eligibility for care in the public system is poverty based—and dependence on this system for care may unintentionally keep individuals in poverty. Additionally, the presence of a safety net system may militate against achieving more equitable insurance coverage for mental healthcare. It is timely to critically examine the successes and limitations of public mental healthcare, in the light of recent progress and considering developments in healthcare generally. In this chapter I describe the state- and county-managed public mental health systems that play this unique role in healthcare and identify some of the leading trends in these systems.

Mental Health's Unique Structure

Several unique aspects of the organization and financing of mental healthcare help explain why mental healthcare—especially in the public sector—is poorly understood in mainstream health policy circles. These same factors may also help explain why mental health policy perspectives may be limited in scope and poorly informed by trends in the larger health system.

The first anomaly in mental healthcare is the unusual division of labor between insurance-financed and publicly managed care: A much higher proportion of mental healthcare is governmentally paid and managed, compared with healthcare in general (National Advisory Mental Health Council 1993). The second structural factor that contributes to poor understanding of mental health by health policymakers is the fact that public mental health systems are orchestrated and financed primarily at the state and county levels rather than by the federal government. In healthcare in general, government health programs that do exist (e.g., Medicare, Medicaid) are national in scope and similar to commercial health insurance in many respects. It follows that most analyses of health policy have a national perspective—although they may be mindful of regional variances such as the degree of managed care penetration in the health marketplace. Mental health is an exception to this pattern, with a dominant state and county role in the financing, policymaking, and management of public care systems—in addition to the deep divisions between private and public responsibilities.

Most analyses of a perceived stepchild status for mental health (from within the field) focus on factors such as the stigma attached to mental illness but do not consider the pervasive effects of system structure and financing. Similarly, mainstream health biases about how mental health is different from the rest of healthcare tend to emphasize perceived clinical differences between health and mental health such as treatment efficacy or diagnostic accuracy. Ironically, these perceptions of differential (poorer) diagnostic accuracy in mental health are generally outdated and no longer accurate based on the evolving research evidence (National Advisory Mental Health Council 1993), but the fundamental underlying differences related to the structure and financing of care are often not recognized.

Roots and Evolution of Public and Private Mental Health Systems

The landscape of healthcare today is dominated by employer-financed group health insurance, the huge

Medicare and Medicaid programs, and controversy over managed care. Remarkably, each of these dominant systems is a relatively recent development. In contrast, the state mental health programs had their roots in the asylums founded in the middle of the nineteenth century during a first cycle of reform of public mental healthcare (Morrissey and Goldman 1984). Since the origins of U.S. mental healthcare in these state psychiatric hospitals, the states have played a leadership role in mental health.

A brief history of mental health policy sets the stage for understanding the challenges that states and counties are wrestling with today. Although the public mental health system has existed for well over a century, the dominant mainstream healthcare system has evolved much more recently. Employer-paid group health insurance is today the dominant form of healthcare financing, but the first prepaid group health insurance plan in the United States was not initiated until 1929 (Bodenheimer 1994). Medicaid and Medicare have also become dominant forces in healthcare, but these large public insurance programs are also relatively young. Both were initiated as part of President Johnson's Great Society initiatives of the mid-1960s. Managed care may be the most dominant and controversial trend in healthcare today, but federal health maintenance organization (HMO) legislation was not enacted until 1973. Thus, the mainstream U.S. healthcare system is very young compared with the public mental health system.

Development of Mental Health Services and Coverage in Commercial and Public Insurance Programs

For a variety of reasons, coverage for treatment of mental disorders is limited in most commercially issued health insurance plans. It is impossible to assess the relative impact of factors limiting this coverage. They certainly include the stigma of seeking mental healthcare, a failure by both consumers and health providers to see mental disorders as illnesses, payer concerns about costs, and the fact that the public sector provides catastrophic care—making coverage less essential.

Inclusion of mental health benefits was not particularly popular or necessary during and after World War II when employer-paid coverage grew rapidly. Mental health concerns did not resonate with the mainstream health professionals and hospitals that advocated—and benefited from—expanded health insurance coverage. These factors also contributed to the low mental health benefits included in Medicare, Medicaid (as originally enacted), and the 1973 HMO Act. Medicare included an outpatient benefit capped annually by costs and an inpatient benefit with a low lifetime limit, the HMO Act required HMOs to offer only limited coverage, and Medicaid included only office-based and inpatient services.

Expansion of Mental Health Coverage in Commercial Health Insurance

Coverage for mental healthcare in health insurance expanded in an accelerating fashion in the 1970s and 1980s. Mental disorders were increasingly seen as illnesses rather than adjustment or social problems, due in large part to the advocacy efforts of the National Alliance for the Mentally Ill. Research demonstrated the efficacy of mental health treatments. Mental health benefits (albeit as a state option) were added to Medicaid in response to criticisms of an inadequate federal government role in deinstitutionalization (Government Accounting Office 1977) and recommendations of the President's Commission on Mental Health, established by President Carter.

Expansion of Mental Health Services and Managed Care

The expansion of benefits and the decreased stigma of seeking care led to an explosion in the costs of providing mental health benefits. In the late 1980s the cost of providing mental health coverage grew at an annual rate of about 20% (Martinsons 1988). These cost pressures led to the development and rapid expansion of managed care approaches, particularly among plans sponsored by large employers. Managed care quickly demonstrated the capability to contain treatment costs in a commercially insured population, largely through reducing levels of hospitalization and also by negotiating fee discounts (Freeman and Trabin 1994). As a result, by 1996, managed behavioral health organizations were responsible for managing the care of 57% of Americans (Open Minds 1997).

Reform Patterns in Public Mental Healthcare

While mental healthcare patterns within mainstream healthcare were changing, public mental health systems were also undergoing transformational change.

The total census of the nation's state psychiatric hospitals peaked at about 550,000 in 1954 and began a slow decline (Kiesler and Sibulkin 1987). However, the sea changes in public systems did not begin until the 1960s—when changes in mental health policy (e.g., community mental health and deinstitutionalization) followed broader societal changes (e.g., the civil rights movement). The 1963 Community Mental Health Act was flawed from an implementation viewpoint. Consistent with the federal "policy chauvinism" of the time, community mental health centers (CMHCs) were granted directly from the federal government to local entities, all but bypassing the state governments that ran the public psychiatric hospitals and the county governments that managed other human services. This unconscious dechaining undermined coordinated deinstitutionalization from state hospitals.

Another design flaw resulted from the historic ambivalence of the federal government to commit to a national mental health program. This ambivalence had old roots. By the middle of the nineteenth century, reformer Dorothea Dix had visited every state legislature east of the Mississippi and convinced most states to found state hospitals. Flushed by this success, Dix advocated for federal land grant legislation that would make federal funds available for state hospital construction. In a short-lived high watermark of national responsibility for mental health, Congress passed legislation in 1854 providing for this program, but the legislation was then vetoed by President Pierce as an unwarranted assumption of federal responsibility. This same reluctance to assume responsibility for a state program shaped CMHC legislation a century later. First, federal funding was limited to a 7-year start-up period, locking the fledgling centers into a search for paying customers (and services for destitute, formerly state hospitalized individuals were hardly likely to pay the bills). Second, although about 2,600 CMHCs would have been required to cover the country, only about 700 were funded by the time the program was slowed by President Nixon's impounding of mental health funding and later eliminated in favor of President Reagan's "new federalism" block grant approach.

The New Imperative of Community Care

Despite these structural limits, the strong policy message favoring community care that was at the heart of the CMHC initiative signaled the beginning of the end for the century-old, hospital-dominated and state-operated system. Change was accelerated by other developments: reforms suggested by the President's Commission on Mental Health led by Rosalyn Carter (especially reforms in Social Security, federal housing programs, and Medicaid [Koyanagi and Goldman 1991]); the strong national leadership provided by a small community support program (CSP) office at the National Institute of Mental Health (Turner and Ten-Hoor 1978); and, ironically, by President Reagan's new federalism philosophy.

These developments came together in a curious way. By the early 1980s, states were reeling from public and media criticism of the failures of deinstitutionalization and were eager to try better approaches. The CSP approach provided direction, inspiration, and small capacity-building grants to the states to leverage change. The reforms in Social Security and housing programs provided a means to address the basic community survival needs of disabled individuals with mental illnesses. As Morrissey and Goldman (1994) pointed out, these basic and functional needs had never been addressed before in mental health reforms, which historically emphasized reforms of acute treatment services rather than long-term support. Adding reimbursement for functional mental health services (e.g., case management) to Medicaid provided another means to finance community care programs—especially the kinds of practical services called for by the CSP emphasis on longitudinal community support. Finally, President Reagan's new federalism gave states a period of respite from federal policy directives and placed CMHC resources back under state control—albeit with a 35% reduction in funding levels. This curious combination of factors led to a quiet revitalization of public mental health systems at the state and local levels.

Community Mental Health: Devolution Before Its Time

The 1980s and 1990s saw a gradual shift in U.S. politics from an emphasis on federal initiatives toward state and local efforts. The term *devolution,* describing the return of leadership and responsibility to state and local governments, has been coined to describe this trend. Applied frequently to welfare reform, devolution implies a preference for and reliance on local decision making rather than federal control. The community mental health movement (and the dominant state and local leadership role that it implied) is generally described as a reform in mental health policy. However, given the strong commitment to locally managed services that has been built into these reforms, community mental health can equally well be described as an early experiment in political devolution—particularly in states where local mental health systems are managed by governmental units. During the 1980s and 1990s, development of capacities at the local level was a consistent theme in reforming public mental health systems in every state.

Management and Government of Community Mental Health Systems

The movement from hospital to community in public mental health is both universal and variable. The movement is universal in that the shift has been substantial and has affected every state. For example, the census of state hospitals dropped from a high of over 550,000 in 1954 to 69,177 in 1995 (Atay et al. 1997; Kiesler and Sibulkin 1987). In 1993, for the first time since data on state mental health budgets were collected, a higher proportion of resources controlled by state mental health authorities (SMHAs) was devoted to community care than to state hospitals (Lutterman et al. 1995). Yet considerable variance exists on almost every dimension of state mental health operations. Table 25–1 illustrates this variance with reference to state hospital use. Some states had 10 persons or fewer in state hospitals per 100,000 population, whereas others had over 50 persons hospitalized per 100,000 population. This variance is also reflected in the size and scope of state hospital operations. In 1995, 10 states had state hospital populations of less than 200, whereas 11 states had more than 2,000 persons hospitalized (Atay et al. 1997). This variability reflects many factors, including state size, resource levels, SMHA leadership, and whether a large hospital system was established in the past century (typical in the Northeast and Midwest) or never substantially developed (as in some western states).

Variance also exists in levels and patterns of funding (Tables 25–2 and 25–3). Per capita funding controlled by the SMHAs in 1997 ranged from $23 in Tennessee and West Virginia to $99 in Connecticut and $113 in New York. The percentage of funds devoted to

TABLE 25–1. Variable state hospital per capita use rates, 1995 (resident patients per 100,000 population)

Mean	High use states		Low use states	
26.3	Delaware	73.6	Rhode Island	5.5
	Virginia	63.0	Arkansas	5.8
	New York	56.7	Nevada	6.3
	Kansas	51.9	West Virginia	9.8
	Mississippi	45.4	Alaska	10.4

Source.   Data from Atay et al. 1997.

TABLE 25–2. Variable state mental health agency (SMHA) funding levels per capita, 1993

Mean	High expenditure states		Low expenditure states	
$44	New York	$113	Tennessee	$23
	Connecticut	$99	West Virginia	$23
	New Hampshire	$99	Utah	$28
	Montana	$93	Iowa	$29
	Vermont	$92	Idaho	$29

Source.   Data from Lutterman et al. 1999.

TABLE 25–3. Variable SMHA expenditures for inpatient care as a percentage of budget, 1993

Mean	High use states		Low use states	
49%	West Virginia	77%	Arizona	15%
	Georgia	77%	Vermont	25%
	Virginia	75%	California	26%
	Nebraska	74%	Massachusetts	29%
	Wyoming	73%	Wisconsin	32%

Source.   Data from Lutterman et al. 1999.

hospital care in 1997 ranged from 77% in West Virginia and Georgia to 15% in Arizona and 25% in Vermont (Lutterman et al. 1999). Thus, wide variability is found in the levels of state mental health expenditures and in how resources are spent.

Considerable variability exists among the states in how community care is organized and funded. Two dominant patterns are found: 1) funding counties or county-based organizations and 2) funding nonprofit agencies such as CMHCs to orchestrate or provide local services. In half of the states, and typically in larger states, the dominant pattern is that the SMHA funds a local government-based entity, which is responsible for managing a system of care (National Association of State Mental Health Program Directors, unpublished material, 1997).

The Dominant Role of County-Based Mental Healthcare Systems

In about half of the states, county government (or local boards or authorities with strong ties to county government) are charged with managing public community mental healthcare. Yet this picture does not adequately capture what is increasingly a dominant role for counties in the public mental health system. County government tends to be more influential in larger states, and mental health tends to be a county responsibility in these states. The 25 states relying on local governmental units to orchestrate community care have an average population of 7.9 million people (National Association of State Mental Health Program Directors, unpublished material, 1997). Local government therefore manages public mental healthcare in areas covering approximately two-thirds of the country's population. The fact that this is a dominant approach—especially when coupled with the politics of local control and the ideologies of community mental health—makes county-managed mental healthcare a significant enterprise.

Challenges Confronting State and County Mental Health Systems: Ohio as a Case Study

Although larger than most states, Ohio, with a population of about 11 million people, in many ways is quite representative of the rest of the country. Often thought of as an urban industrial state, Ohio is largely rural: Its largest business is agribusiness, and 29 of the state's 88 counties are part of Appalachia. Ohio is politically moderate, with a tendency to alternate Republican and Democrat governors and a history of being a decisive state in presidential elections. As an index of effort in mental health, Ohio ranked 25th among the states in per capita SMHA spending in 1993 (Lutterman et al. 1995), although county contributions make Ohio's total public mental health spending somewhat higher than average.

None of this is to suggest that Ohio is completely typical. But the variance among states—in culture, wealth, politics, governmental organization, and patterns of mental health reform—is so idiosyncratic that, to quote a weary managed care executive, "If you've seen one state…you've seen one state." Ohio has enough in common with many states in terms of patterns of mental healthcare and reform to serve as a useful example.

The headline of the story of public mental health reform in Ohio—like that in many states—is that the wrenching structural reforms of the past generation are by and large completed, but new issues, tensions, and challenges have emerged. The processes of deinstitutionalization and developing a community mental health infrastructure are essentially completed. From a high of over 20,000 patients in the mid-1950s, the census of state hospitals in Ohio had been reduced to about 3,800 when 1988 reform legislation was enacted and was further reduced to under 1,200 patients in 1997 (Ohio Department of Mental Health, unpublished statistics, 1997). As in other states, the precipitous declines in state hospital use in the 1960s and 1970s were largely due to nursing home placements and the discharge of patients to marginal community settings—not to the development of well-structured community care. Since the mid-1980s, however, uneven

local community care systems were consistently upgraded. The major elements of improvement included 1) increased funding as illustrated in Figure 25–1 (increased local levies, additional state funding, and increased Medicaid revenues), 2) the introduction and refinement of CSP service models (e.g., case management, assertive community treatment teams), and 3) fixing service planning and management responsibility at the local level (including financial risk for state hospital utilization).

Downsizing of the State Hospital System

A powerful set of economic, clinical, and political forces contributed to remarkable reductions in levels of state hospital utilization in Ohio. The primary economic force was contained in the 1988 reform legislation—the gradual movement of state hospital resources to local boards, allowing them to choose where and how to invest these resources. Primary clinical tools included a parallel reform in civil commitment law requiring that commitments be made to the board rather than the state hospital. From a political perspective, fixing the responsibility and fiscal liability for state hospital care at the board level made managing utilization a high priority of local government. This priority led to increased local investments in mental healthcare and higher prominence for the local mental health system.

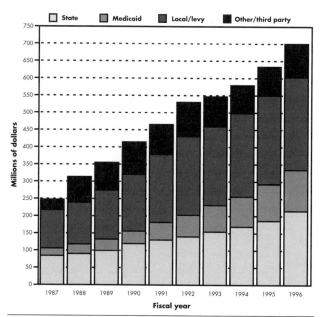

FIGURE 25–1. State of Ohio community mental health funding, 1987–1996.
Source. Ohio Department of Mental Health, unpublished data, 1997. Used with permission.

Figure 25–2 illustrates the patterns of the decline in the use of state hospitals. As the data indicate, the decline is largely attributable to reductions in long-term, nonforensic hospitalization. This pattern fits the general conception of the role of hospitals; there is little evidence of clinical benefit from long hospital stays, and reserving scarce resources for patients who clearly need the intensive resources and controlled environment of a hospital makes sense.

Building a Community Support Service Portfolio

As the responsibility for planning and managing public mental health services was shifted to county-based boards, increased funding was also available—from reallocated hospital resources, increased local levy support, and the ability to claim Medicaid reimbursement. These resources were invested in systems of care that had the capability to minimize use of hospitalization (because the 1988 law required boards to develop community support systems, preventing hospitalization was clinically desirable, and the county-based boards were now financially at risk for the costs of state hospital care). Figure 25–3 illustrates the total resource portfolio in Ohio's public mental health system.

As these data illustrate, the costs of inpatient care within Ohio's public mental health system absorb only about one-third of the roughly $1 billion in annual expenses. The array of other services is broad and arguably begins to approach the balance envisioned or idealized by the community mental health reformers of a generation ago. This is not to suggest that the quality, consistency, or responsiveness of this system is ideal. But the structural aspects of changing from a hospital-dominated to a community-oriented and locally managed system are largely complete.

New Challenges in Public Mental Healthcare

Several broad challenges occupy the new public mental health landscape. These challenges reflect past progress and emerging realities. The emerging concerns of state and local mental health authorities include 1) managing care systems in a postinstitutional era, 2) adapting to emerging financial constraints and determining the right role for managed care in public systems, 3) adjusting to the second-order demands of community-centered and community-managed care, and 4) dealing with the reality of two-tiered mental health delivery as healthcare and financing continue to evolve.

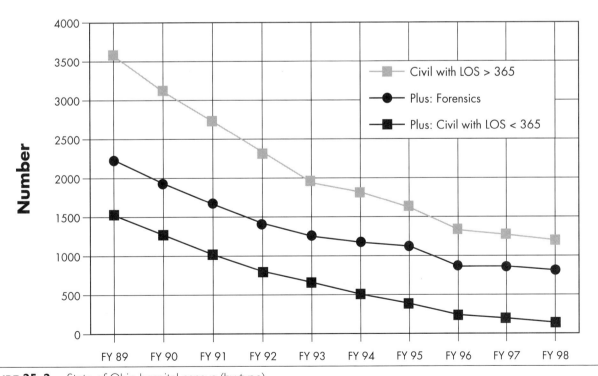

FIGURE 25–2. State of Ohio hospital census (by type).

Source. Ohio Department of Mental Health, unpublished data, 1999. Used with permission.

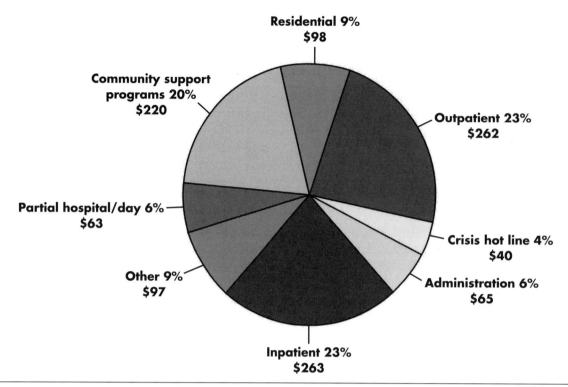

FIGURE 25–3. State of Ohio total resource portfolio, mental health, fiscal year 1996 ($994.5 million).
Source. Ohio Department of Mental Health, unpublished data, 1997. Used with permission.

Managing Care Systems in a Postinstitutional Era

The concept of a postinstitutional mental health system, perhaps first articulated by Minkoff (1987), fits in many Ohio communities and in many communities around the country. At the level of the entire state, only about 10 state hospital beds are occupied per 100,000 population, including forensic patients. When Ohio's 50 local service systems are ranked in terms of levels of nonforensic state hospital bed utilization, the median local system uses fewer than five state hospital beds (Ohio Department of Mental Health, unpublished statistics, 1997). These low levels of state hospital use have not been achieved primarily by transferring inpatient treatment to Medicaid. Although use of Medicaid-paid psychiatric hospitalization has increased somewhat in Ohio as state hospital use has decreased, only about 350 individuals are in Medicaid-paid psychiatric unit beds at any one time (Ohio Department of Mental Health, unpublished statistics, 1997).

These low levels of hospital use are not unique to Ohio. Data from 1995 show that 18 states had state psychiatric hospital use rates below 20 beds per 100,000 population (Atay et al. 1997). Hospitalization has be-

come an exceedingly rare event in current public mental health systems.

There are many implications and consequences of managing systems of care with such low levels of hospital use—and managing hospitals at such a reduced level. Ohio's approach to this problem has involved community care adaptations (e.g., developing alternatives to hospitalization for both acutely ill and disabled populations) and adaptations in inpatient care—conceiving the role of the hospital as akin to a critical care unit in general medicine, and providing inpatient care for individuals with high-acuity needs only (Ohio Department of Mental Health 1994). Managing a system in this fashion is arguably the right thing to do from economic, clinical, and consumer perspectives. But it is continually challenging for consumers and family members, clinicians, and administrators. Challenges in community care include developing hospital-like services in nonhospital settings (e.g., crisis intervention centers), managing care for acutely disoriented individuals in community settings, ensuring access to clinical competence in a decentralized system, and managing boundaries with other systems that deal with aberrant behavior (e.g., law enforcement, child welfare, adult and juvenile corrections). The challenges in hospital care are similarly daunting. They include providing quality care to diverse high-acuity patients while limiting costs. The emerging reality in comparatively well-funded and experienced public systems such as in Ohio is that these issues and tensions are being managed every day, but the challenge of managing a mature public system is no less complex than the task of building it.

Adapting to Emerging Financial Constraints and Exploring Managed Care

On the surface, it appears that SMHAs are rushing to embrace private-sector managed care approaches (e.g., Essock and Goldman 1995); however, this trend must be examined closely. The trend in states toward managed care contracting appears to be slowing and almost certainly does not reflect the infatuation with managed care that some critics have suggested. A close examination of managed care trends in the states will reveal that the vast majority of managed care contracts are focused solely on Medicaid. Because states are moving Medicaid healthcare services in general toward HMOs, the trend toward managed care in public mental health may be more reflective of cost-control issues in Medicaid than of a mental health policy initiative.

Structured as an entitlement program for providers as well as consumers (i.e., no qualified provider, under Medicaid law and in the absence of waivers or these provisions, can be denied a contract), Medicaid poses an extreme budgetary challenge for states. In many states, including Ohio, Medicaid is the largest item in the state budget, bigger than primary and secondary education, the state university system, and even the growing prison system. In 1994–1995, when the congressional debate about federal deficit reduction was most intense, proposals to cap Medicaid costs—and perhaps to turn the program into a block grant—were openly discussed.

These developments had a chilling effect in state and local mental health circles. Ever since new optional service categories were added to Medicaid in the early 1980s—precisely to help underwrite the emerging community support programs that were then being developed—the open-ended Medicaid funding stream has been a major mental health funding source. In Ohio, federal Medicaid revenues to community mental health programs grew by more than $100 million from 1982 to 1997 (Ohio Department of Mental Health, unpublished statistics, 1997). In most states, Medicaid now provides about one-third of the revenues for community mental healthcare. The prospect of capping or cutting this source of revenue is what really sparked state exploration of managed care. This is evident in the fact that most states exploring managed care are applying it first—or only—to Medicaid.

At the same time, understanding managed care experimentation in the public mental health sector as primarily an attempt to gain control of Medicaid costs does not imply that managed care should not be taken seriously. Precisely because Medicaid has become such a significant payer of public-sector mental health costs, the trend is significant. In states like Ohio, considerations of managed care have raised serious concerns and tensions, including new conflicts over resource control, with the old and familiar conflicts over who will control state hospital funds replaced by new conflicts over controlling Medicaid. Because Medicaid is managed by designated state agencies (usually the state welfare agency rather than the SMHA), this tension occurs between state agencies as well as between the state and local levels, and between traditional providers such as hospitals and community mental health agencies. Furthermore, because Medicaid is primarily a payer of basic heath care and long-term care services, and because Medicaid health services are being moved into HMOs, tension exists between the desire to integrate mental healthcare within the primary healthcare delivery (HMOs) and the goal of integrating all public mental healthcare within the local mental health system. Finally, all the usual tensions about managed care (provider concerns versus payer concerns, fears that consumers will be lost in the shuffle, fears about excess profits on the one hand and excess costs on the other) are part of the mix.

Despite the complexity of these interrelated issues, some evidence indicates that patterns are emerging. Most statewide, large-scale efforts to manage mental health Medicaid costs have been exceedingly complex at best and marked by delays, problems, and setbacks at worst. Although lessons have been learned from these major efforts (e.g., in Tennessee, Massachusetts, and Oregon), the emerging pattern is for incremental solutions. These solutions may involve partnerships between levels of government rather than radical centralization or decentralization, and importing private administration systems (e.g., information systems, claims payment) to the public system rather than transferring public risk and responsibilities to the private sector. Adaptation and experimentation with these challenges will continue to mark the landscape of public mental healthcare for some time.

Adjusting to the Second-Order Dynamics of Community Care

The community mental health approach is no longer new or experimental in the public mental health system. It has been emerging as the dominant paradigm since the mid-1970s, and many programs and executives in local systems have been doing their jobs since the late 1980s. As a result, the emerging challenges often reflect local problems and partnerships rather than the historic state-level challenges of mental health system change. Thus, for local mental health executives, horizontal relationships with other county human service systems are often more significant on a day-to-day basis than the vertical relationships with the SMHA. This trend—coupled with the fact that concerns about financing have shifted from the relatively simple state mental health budget to the labyrinthine and politically complex Medicaid program—has significantly changed relationships and focus in public mental health systems.

Another way to describe this trend is to paraphrase former Speaker of the House Tip O'Neill, who said that "all politics are local." In the emerging public mental health system, postdevolution as well as postinstitutional, all policies—as well as most politics—are ultimately local. Like the trend toward handling clinical care in a postinstitutional system, this trend leads to many challenges (e.g., achieving equitable access to care, maintaining a balance between local and state governments). The important dynamic is that the framework for public mental health policy—just like the framework for care—is irrevocably changed. The new issues, challenges, and tensions will be as much about local dynamics and politics as about state or national issues.

Dealing With the Mixed Legacy of a Two-Tiered Mental Health System

For most of the 1980s and 1990s, the dominant reform issues in mental health were largely centered within the separate public system. The debacles of institutional abuses and deinstitutionalization occasionally became front-page news and certainly focused national attention. At times, public interest in mental health issues extended to broader concerns about managed care, the use or overuse of Prozac, and other matters. In general, however, concerns about public-sector problems have been dominant.

The experience in Ohio and a number of other states with well-developed community systems and relatively adequate funding is that the wrenching structural changes required to address the serious public-sector problems are largely completed. Community-centered and managed care systems are in place. The state hospital system has been downsized to the lowest levels that are practicable given current treatment technologies and resource levels. New challenges abound, but the old problems have been substantially solved.

In this context, a sober examination of the social and economic role of the private and public mental health systems is disquieting. On the one hand, the worst problems of prior neglect and abuse in the public system have been addressed. On the other hand, it is increasingly clear that the function of the public system is to care for poor people—and the system tends to keep them poor. This is not precisely the fault of anyone in the public mental health system. Rather, the links between mental health services, Medicaid eligibility, Social Security and supplemental security income rules, and a poor focus on employment outcomes create an unintended web from which it is very hard for people to escape. The problem is compounded by the exclusions and restrictions on mental health coverage that are found in most health insurance plans. Once people have lost their health insurance (whether due to lost employment or to exceeding coverage limits) and tumbled into the public system, they have a preexisting condition that makes coverage either impossible to obtain or unaffordable. Faced with this hurdle, staying poor so that Medicaid will cover treatment costs is a rational choice.

An alternative to this dilemma was envisioned in President Clinton's proposed and ill-fated Health Security Act. Architects of the mental health section of the plan—led by Tipper Gore—realized the problematic nature of the current two-tiered system and proposed a conceptually simple but radical solution. At its core, the proposal was 1) to extend mental health insurance coverage to essentially the entire population, 2) to contain the costs of this expanded coverage through broader use of managed care, and 3) to finance the extension of coverage to the uninsured by using some of the resources now spent in the public sector to pay for the same services.

A view of the implications of this proposal might be, for example, that resources now spent on inpatient and outpatient care and medications would be used to purchase coverage—not requiring poverty status for eligibility—for these same services. Presumably, care would continue to be delivered by many current providers, and locally managed CSP systems would be sustained to manage and provide the many services that are not amenable to inclusion in a health insurance package. The complexities of this transition cannot be underestimated—just as the conversion from a hospital-based to a community-based system proved complex. However, the structural problems in the current two-tiered system—one that delivers improved care but unwittingly sustains lifelong poverty for its members—must now be attended to.

Conclusion

State- and county-managed mental health systems have no analogue in mainstream healthcare. They manage care for millions of Americans who formerly might have been consigned to long-term institutionalization. In many states like Ohio, these systems have emerged from several decades of change as diverse and vibrant organizations, having mastered not only the clinical and organizational challenges of community care but also the political challenges of devolution.

New challenges are emerging. These challenges include the ongoing realities of managing care for people with serious, episodic, and acute illnesses in ambulatory settings and the need to develop and master relationships with many other health, welfare, and social service systems. Broad and pervasive differences exist in how various states and local communities address these problems, and the adequacy, quality, and financing of care vary widely. Even so, the transition from a system dominated by state hospitals and centralized administration is largely complete.

The next broad challenge in mental health reform may be even more daunting. The public system has been reformed in many locations, but it remains a system for poor people, with adequate commercial health insurance unavailable to most seriously mentally ill people. In many states and counties, we have largely mastered the task or reform within the public system. The next challenge will be to create a single system that provides care without regard to income, and one in which people can afford to not stay poor.

References

Atay JE, Witkin MJ, Mandersheid RW: Additions and resident patients at end of year, state and county mental hospitals, by age and diagnosis, by state, United States, 1995. Washington, DC, U.S. Department of Health and Human Services, Center for Mental Health Services, 1997

Bodenheimer T, Grumbach K: Paying for health care. JAMA 272:634–639, 1994

Essock SM, Goldman HH: States' embrace of managed mental health care. Health Affairs 14:34–44, 1995

Freeman MA, Trabin T: Managed behavioral health care: history, models, key issues and future course. Washington, DC, U.S. Department of Health and Human Services, Substance Abuse and Mental Health Services Administration, 1994

Government Accounting Office: Deinstitutionalization: government needs to do more. Washington, DC, Government Accounting Office, 1977

Kiesler CA, Sibulkin AE: Mental Hospitalization: Myths and Facts About a National Crisis. Newbury Park, CA, Sage, 1987

Koyanagi C, Goldman HH: The quiet success of the national plan for the chronically mentally ill. Hosp Community Psychiatry 42:899–905, 1991

Lutterman T, Hirad A, Poindexter B: Funding sources and expenditures of state mental health agencies: study results fiscal year 1997. Alexandria, VA, National Association of State Mental Health Program Directors, 1999

Martinsons JN: Are hospitals slamming the door on psych treatment? Hospitals 1988:62:50–56, 1988

Minkoff K: Beyond deinstitutionalization: a new ideology for the post-institutional era. Hosp Community Psychiatry 38:945–950, 1987

Morrissey JP, Goldman HH: Cycles of reform in the care of the chronically mentally ill. Hosp Community Psychiatry 35:785–793, 1984

National Advisory Mental Health Council: Health care reform for Americans with severe mental illnesses: report of the National Advisory Mental Health Council. Am J Psychiatry 150:1447–1465, 1993

Ohio Department of Mental Health: Community Care and Inpatient Treatment: Solutions for the Next Century. Columbus, OH, Ohio Department of Mental Health, 1994

Open Minds: Managed care enrollment continues to rise. Open Minds 11(8):12, 1997

Turner J, TenHoor W: The National Institute of Mental Health Community Support Program: pilot approach to a needed social reform. Schizophr Bull 4:319–348, 1978

❖ 26 ❖

Health Maintenance Organizations

Bentson H. McFarland, M.D., Ph.D.

In this chapter I review the types of health maintenance organizations (HMOs) and describe their growth in enrollment. Behavioral health service delivery in HMOs is discussed in relationship to the benefit structure, and issues surrounding quality of behavioral healthcare in HMOs are addressed.

Historical Evolution

HMOs may be defined as systems that are prepaid on a per-capita basis to deliver medically necessary health services to their enrollees (McFarland and George 1995). Programs of this type have been available in the United States at least since 1910 (Greenlick et al. 1988; Zieman 1995). Enrollment in HMOs increased dramatically during the 1990s but appears now to have peaked (Rojas-Burke 2000). Roughly 65 million Americans were enrolled in HMOs during 1998, representing about a quarter of the population (U.S. Census Bureau 1999). Enrollment in HMOs equals if not exceeds enrollment in traditional indemnity (fee-for-service) programs for people with employer-purchased insurance (Jacob 1997; KPMG Peat Marwick 1996). Roughly half of the people with employer-purchased health insurance have but one choice of health plan—and that

choice is often an HMO (KPMG Peat Marwick 1996). State Medicaid agencies are rapidly converting their fee-for-service programs into capitated systems that extensively involve HMOs (McFarland 1996, 2000). About half of the Medicaid population is enrolled in managed care systems that are often HMOs (Mechanic et al. 1998). About 5 million Medicare beneficiaries (about 13% of the total) are enrolled in HMOs (Jacob 1997). Table 26–1 illustrates the growth in HMO participation by physicians—including psychiatrists (American Medical Association 1996).

Why HMO Enrollment Grew

The growth in HMO enrollment was not surprising. First, during the 1990s, HMOs typically cost less than fee-for-service or preferred provider plans that offer comparable benefits. Second, the rate of growth in premiums for HMOs was less than that for competing systems (such as indemnity plans or preferred provider programs) for several years (KPMG Peat Marwick 1996). In 1996, HMOs' premiums generally remained constant or even declined (KPMG Peat Marwick 1996). Furthermore, the reduction in the growth of healthcare

281

expenditures during the 1990s was due in large measure to the shift of enrollees from fee-for-service programs into HMOs. The low cost of HMOs attracted employers that compete with industries in other countries where employees' healthcare is financed by government programs. In a recent survey, business executives ranked "rising cost of healthcare" third on their list of concerns for the nation—far below "crime and lawlessness" but close to "breakdown of the family" (Siegel and Gale 1996). Similarly, state governments see HMOs as a solution to their problems of rising Medicaid expenditures (McFarland 1996, 2000). Finally, the predictability of prepaid healthcare expenditures is of great interest to self-insured payers. Large employers that are self-insured (or, for that matter, state Medicaid agencies) were unable to forecast healthcare expenditures under the fee-for-service system. Capitation (i.e., the HMO system) removed that uncertainty. Purchasers of prepaid healthcare can negotiate with provider systems much as they bargain with any other vendor. For better or worse, prepaid healthcare can easily be treated as a commodity (Woolhandler and Himmelstein 1996). In response to this demand for prepaid healthcare systems, the healthcare industry has experienced numerous structural changes—not the least of which is integration.

Horizontal and Vertical Integration

The term *integration* is used in several contexts and can have numerous meanings. In the economic context one often distinguishes between horizontal and vertical integration (Freudenheim 1996). Horizontal integration refers to the amalgamation or merger of similar firms. For example, Kaiser Permanente for many years purchased or merged with smaller HMOs (some of which were subsequently sold owing to financial losses). The recent affiliation between Group Health Cooperative of Puget Sound and the Northwest Division of Kaiser Permanente is an example of horizontal integration.

TABLE 26–1. Physicians with HMO contracts

Category	1990	1995
All physicians	36%	64%
Psychiatrists	14%	40%

Source. Adapted from American Medical Association 1996.

The chief aim of horizontal integration is to bring economies of scale to the combined organization. Indeed, horizontal integration has been used to save smaller HMOs from bankruptcy. Furthermore, organizations that wish to assume financial risk (i.e., to become capitated) must be large enough to have financial viability. An additional objective is to increase the geographic scope of the healthcare delivery system. Large employers, for example, increasingly wish to contract with a sole vendor of healthcare services for all their employees. Horizontal integration enables HMOs to expand their geographic service areas.

Vertical integration is the amalgamation or affiliation of the firms necessary to produce a given product or deliver a given service. For example, the Sisters of Providence (a religious organization) began its healthcare operations in the nineteenth century by establishing hospitals throughout the western United States. During the 1980s the Sisters of Providence system expanded to include health insurance (e.g., an HMO), outpatient programs, residential treatment, and the like. In the 1990s the organization expanded further and began employing primary care providers. At present, the Sisters of Providence is a vertically integrated system that encompasses virtually all the components necessary to deliver healthcare, including physicians (chiefly primary care providers), other clinicians, hospitals, outpatient clinics, and health insurance programs. Of course, older HMOs such as Kaiser Permanente were designed originally to be vertically integrated systems. Vertical integration among for-profit enterprises such as that involving the Columbia hospital system and the Value Health family of managed care companies yielded enormous organizations that theoretically have substantial economic clout.

The transition from amorphous fee-for-service to vertically integrated capitation carries with it both benefits and risks. The older HMOs have for many years cited benefits of vertical integration such as having all services under one roof, a unified medical record, simplified financial systems, straightforward billing for payers and consumers, and the like. It is often stated that integrated systems (such as Kaiser Permanente) have administrative costs on the order of 5% of revenue, in contrast to the 10%–15% for disaggregated systems (such as the BlueCross HMOs). Administrative savings from vertical integration (not to mention economies of scale from horizontal integration) could be used to reduce payers' premiums, to expand or improve services, to increase "cash generation" (for nonprofit programs), or to raise stockholder dividends (in the for-profit sector).

Nevertheless, vertical integration can be quite challenging for both consumers and providers. Consumers may find that their long-standing provider has not been included in the vertically integrated system, or the integrated system may have few providers, limiting the choice of provider and limiting opportunities for second opinions. Managers of newly integrated systems may well discover that information needed for decision making is difficult to obtain. Often, integrated systems find that substantial investment must be made in communications and information systems in order to be competitive. Clinicians may need to change their loyalties. Rather than working solely on behalf of their own patients, clinicians may need to consider the overall needs of the HMO's enrolled population. Physicians sometimes find themselves having to convert from being the owner and operator of a small business to being a staff member of a large organization.

A question of considerable interest is whether clinicians should be employees or contractors of integrated healthcare delivery systems. Traditional HMOs (in which clinicians are, for all practical purposes, employees) can find themselves at a competitive disadvantage in that they are obliged to pay salaries (plus benefits) and have limited flexibility in the work force. Salaried employees might not be as productive as contractors paid on a fee-for-service basis. In contrast, salaried employees may well have more loyalty to the integrated organization than contractors (who could be affiliated with several competing healthcare delivery systems). The notion of provider loyalty raises additional questions about exclusive contracting between clinicians and an integrated delivery system. In this regard, health systems that rely on contractors may be able to reduce expenditures by lowering reimbursement schedules, but in so doing they might also compromise quality of care.

HMO Features

The modern era of HMOs began with the federal Health Maintenance Organization Act of 1973 (Dial et al. 1996; Ellwood and Lundberg 1996). The HMO Act required federally qualified HMOs to provide 10 basic benefits: physician services, hospitalizations, well child care, emergency care, diagnostic tests, rehabilitation, physical and occupational therapy, outpatient mental health, detoxification, and home healthcare (Gabel et al. 1994).

Many of these benefits are limited. For example, rehabilitation is limited to short-term treatment, and physical and occupational therapy are limited to 2 months (if the patient shows improvement). Behavioral health benefits in HMOs are addressed later in this chapter.

Types of HMOs

Students of HMOs usually divide these organizations into several types or models (Dial et al. 1996; Edmunds et al. 1997; U.S. Bureau of the Census 1996). In the staff model HMO, the physicians (and other healthcare providers) are employees of the organization. Prior to its merger with Kaiser Permanente, Group Health Cooperative of Puget Sound was a prominent example of this model. The group model HMO signs a sole source contract with a physician organization for the provision of medical services. The Kaiser Permanente program is a group model. In this system, the physicians are organized into professional corporations (known as Permanente medical groups). These medical groups provide capitated medical services to the HMO (called the Kaiser Foundation Health Plan or some variation thereof). In the group model, the nonphysician clinicians are employees of the HMO. In both the staff and the group models, full-time clinicians provide treatment only to HMO members. Finances are straightforward in these programs. Physicians are paid a salary in the staff model or a salary with bonus in the group model; nonphysician clinicians are salaried in both models. Many staff and group model HMOs have been in operation for decades. Most of the research on HMO behavioral healthcare has been conducted in staff or group model HMOs (Johnson and McFarland 1994; Johnson et al. 1997; Katon et al. 1995, 1999McFarland et al. 1996; Simon et al. 1994, 1996; Wells et al. 1986, 1989a, 1990).

Much newer and much different are independent practice association (IPA) model HMOs. Under this arrangement the HMO contracts with a physician organization that, in turn, contracts with individual physicians (Edmunds et al. 1997). In this situation, the physicians see both HMO and non-HMO patients. Innumerable financing mechanisms are possible in the IPA model. The physician organization may well be capitated while the physicians themselves are paid on a fee-for-service plus withhold basis. In some IPAs, individual physicians (usually primary care providers) are capitated. Generally speaking, IPA panel sizes (i.e., numbers of providers) are much larger than those in group or staff model

HMOs. Not surprisingly, there can be combinations of HMO types (including mixed and network models).

The growth in HMO enrollment was due in large measure to a dramatic surge in IPA membership (Table 26–2). The traditional staff and group models grew to some extent during the 1980s but stayed more or less constant in the 1990s. Conversely, IPAs increased substantially since 1990. With some exceptions (Rogers et al. 1993; Wells et al. 2000), little research has examined behavioral healthcare provided by IPA model HMOs.

Concerns About HMOs

Accompanying the growth in HMO membership has been a storm of protest about access to and quality of care in these prepaid systems (Bodenheimer 1996; Consumer Reports 1996; Eist 1997; Woolhandler and Himmelstein 1996). Though the concerns are many, they can be summarized as issues of access to, satisfaction with, and quality of care. Here quality of care is defined as "the degree to which health services for individuals and populations increase the likelihood of desired health outcomes and are consistent with current professional knowledge" (Edmunds et al. 1997, p. 17).

Many anecdotes exist about denial of services—for either physical or behavioral healthcare (Consumer Reports 1996). In response, HMOs have undertaken a variety of strategies to address payer (usually employer) and enrollee concerns. For example, many HMOs have commissioned enrollee satisfaction surveys. Employers indicate that enrollee satisfaction is often the chief (if not the only) measure they use to determine value received for their healthcare dollars (Burns 1996; Rost et al. 2000). However, HMO-sponsored satisfaction surveys raise several questions about subject selection and question authorship, response rate, and so forth. In particular, one can wonder if these surveys should focus on enrollees who have used (or attempted to use) HMO services. This issue is especially pertinent in the behavioral health arena where only a minority (typically less than 10%) of enrollees will use specialty mental health or chemical dependency services in a given year (Teich and Melek 2000).

Quality Assurance in HMOs

The Institute of Medicine report on managed behavioral healthcare (Edmunds et al. 1997) lists several

TABLE 26–2. Type of HMO and millions of enrollees

Year	Staff	Group	Independent practice association
1980	1.67	5.73	1.69
1985	2.69	6.49	4.65
1990	3.58	9.54	13.88
1995	0.73	9.18	17.37

Source. U.S. Bureau of the Census: *Statistical Abstract of the United States 1996.* Washington, DC, Bureau of the Census, 1996.

approaches to quality assurance ranging from traditional accreditation organizations (e.g., the Joint Commission on Accreditation of Healthcare Organizations [JCAHO]) to a report card on behavioral healthcare designed in large part by consumers of behavioral health services (Mental Health Statistics Improvement Program 1996). However, to date, only a few of these methodologies appear to have influenced HMOs.

The National Committee for Quality Assurance (NCQA) represents one approach to dealing with purchaser and enrollee concerns about HMO quality of care as well as access and satisfaction (O'Kane 1991; Zablocki 1992). The NCQA provides accreditation to HMOs that satisfy a variety of criteria somewhat analogous to those utilized by the JCAHO in its evaluations of hospitals. As with the JCAHO, the NCQA is heavily influenced (if not dominated) by the organizations it is accrediting. Nonetheless, HMOs that have been NCQA accredited make considerable use of that fact in their marketing (especially to employer-purchasers). The relevance of NCQA accreditation to enrollees remains to be seen.

The NCQA has developed definitions for a package of information known as the Health Plan Employer Data Information Set (HEDIS) that may be of value to healthcare purchasers and, perhaps, to enrollees (National Committee for Quality Assurance 1996). The HEDIS (currently in version 2001) contains a variety of measures such as fraction of women over age 52 in the health plan who have had a mammogram in the previous two calendar years (National Committee for Quality Assurance 1996). To date, there is little evidence that employer-purchasers use HEDIS data when making decisions about HMOs. Behavioral health in HMOs is addressed in the next section.

Another approach to HMO quality assurance has been taken by the Foundation for Accountability (FACCT). This organization sees itself as independent of the HMO industry. FACCT has focused to a large extent on the outcomes of treatment for particular conditions—

including major depressive disorder—in HMO members (Foundation for Accountability 1996). The implications of this approach are discussed in the next section.

Behavioral Health Benefits in HMOs

It is worthwhile examining in some detail the mental health and substance abuse benefits found in typical HMO contracts signed by purchasers (such as employers). Based on the HMO Act, outpatient mental health benefits are usually limited to 20 visits (typically within a 1-year time period). The HMO Act itself does not require HMOs to provide inpatient mental healthcare. However, 94% of HMO programs do offer inpatient psychiatric care, which is typically limited to 30 days (Dial et al. 1996). About half of all HMO enrollees are members of federally qualified HMOs (Gabel et al. 1994), and most of the rest are in programs that offer benefit packages comparable with the federally required services (Peterson et al. 1992).

Generally speaking, HMO contracts are limited to provision of mental health services for conditions that in the judgment of the provider can benefit from acute treatment, or similar language (Mechanic et al. 1995). There are widely varying interpretations of this contract language. For example, some HMOs exclude conduct disorder or personality disorder from the list of covered conditions (Dana et al. 1996). In contrast, some HMOs appear to provide considerable mental healthcare to members with chronic conditions such as schizophrenia (McFarland et al. 1996).

The HMO mental health benefits can be quite complicated (Peterson et al. 1992). For example, there is usually a co-payment. The typical outpatient co-payment is $20, although there is wide variation (Gabel et al. 1994). Nearly half (49%) of HMO enrollees had no outpatient mental health co-payment in 1990, whereas the current figure is 29% (Gabel et al. 1994). Higher co-payments appear to reduce the probability of mental health service use—regardless of the severity of the enrollee's mental disorder (Simon et al 1996). Also, the co-payment structure can vary, with higher payment for individual treatment than for group treatment (Peterson et al. 1992). The inpatient co-payment can be either (or both) a daily rate ($50 is typical) or a fraction of the hospital charges (20% is common but 50% is not unusual). Some HMOs allow for benefit flexibility in which, for example, the inpatient benefit can be used for residential (rather than hospital) care. Chemical

dependency benefits can be equally complex.

Surveys of HMOs show that considerable variation exists in the nature of the behavioral health benefit package (Gabel et al. 1994). Purchasers, typically employers, can buy virtually whatever set of behavioral health benefits they wish. In practice, however, most enrollees are covered by the standard package (20 visits with co-pay and 30 days at 80% coverage). These benefit limitations generally pertain to a time period of either 1 or 2 years. Recent state and federal mental health parity legislation has had little impact on HMO behavioral health benefits (Sturm and Pacula 2000).

Behavioral Health Integration Versus Carve-Out

Yet another domain of integration pertains to the linkage between physical healthcare and behavioral health. Indeed, a key feature of an HMO is the way in which the organization provides for behavioral healthcare. By and large, two systems have emerged—the integrated approach and the carve-out approach.

Figure 26–1 illustrates the flow of funds in integrated and carve-out systems. Under an integrated model, funding flows from the payer to the HMO, which is charged with providing or arranging for mental health services. Conversely, in the carve-out approach, funding flows in two parallel streams from payer to the health and mental health providers, respectively. These two idealized systems might be considered opposite ends of a continuum. Intermediate systems can exist that represent a blended approach. Although exact figures are not available, data provided by the Institute of Medicine can be used to estimate that about 29% of HMO enrollees are in integrated systems (Edmunds et al. 1997).

Advocates of an integrated approach argue that major mental conditions such as schizophrenia and bipolar disorder are diseases that are more properly addressed in the healthcare system. It has also been suggested that integrating physical and mental health services may bring benefits in terms of screening and early intervention. A powerful argument for integrating health and mental health systems is the fact that large segments of the population prefer to obtain (at least some of) their mental healthcare in the general medical sector (Edmunds et al. 1997; Strosahl and Quirk 1994).

There is a fear that the general healthcare system will consume funds earmarked for the mentally ill while directing resources to other populations. Indeed, the

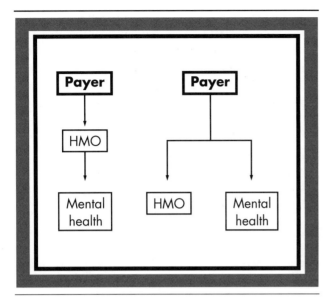

FIGURE 26–1. Flow of funds in integrated (*left*) versus carve-out (*right*) systems.

essence of the carve-out view is that integrated programs deflect resources away from mental health and toward other aspects of the HMO such as physical healthcare, administration, or profits (S. Feldman 1994). Gatekeeping by primary care providers in integrated HMOs could be one mechanism to reduce specialty behavioral health expenditures.

In this context it is worthwhile examining the fraction of the healthcare dollar allocated to behavioral health (Table 26–3). Although current data are not available, the Institute of Medicine reported that capitated behavioral health programs covering some 22 million enrollees in 1995 had an average premium of $60 per person per year (Edmunds et al. 1997). The average HMO premium at that time was roughly $1,800 per person per year (Gabel et al. 1994). The implication here is that somewhere around 3% of the HMO premium dollar goes to mental health. Table 26–3 suggests that (at least in 1990) private-sector behavioral health spending was roughly 5% of the healthcare dollar. The U.S. Substance Abuse and Mental Health Services Administration estimates that in 1987 some 6.6% of the private healthcare dollar was devoted to behavioral health; figures for 1992 were 5.4% and for 1997 were 6.0% (Coffey et al. 2000). It appears, then, that HMO spending on behavioral health is a bit less than in the rest of the private sector. The difference between HMO and other private-sector behavioral health spending was said to be much greater (3%–5% of the HMO healthcare dollar versus 10% of the healthcare dollar in fee for service) during the 1980s (Edmunds et al.

1996). It should also be noted that people with chronic mental disorders such as schizophrenia are underrepresented in HMOs (Johnson and McFarland 1994). Furthermore, the limited data available on HMO behavioral health expenditures may or may not include the provision of behavioral health services by primary care providers. In any event, it seems that HMOs may devote a bit less of their resources to behavioral health than do other private-sector health systems.

Those who favor the integration approach accuse carve-out proponents of erecting barriers (or interposing complicated referral pathways) between enrollees and mental healthcare (Strosahl and Quirk 1994). The implication is that carve-out programs thrive by using these barriers to reduce mental health service utilization. This reduced utilization translates into higher profits for the carve-out program. Also, integration supporters argue that carve-out proponents ignore the fact that much mental healthcare is delivered by primary care providers (with the implication that some patients might prefer to have their mental health problems addressed in the primary care sector). Carve-out advocates respond by depicting primary care mental health service as second rate at best. The counter-argument is that tighter integration might lead to improved primary care mental health services. Conversely, sophisticated carve-out programs emphasize the delivery of a full range of mental health services with close linkages between employee assistance programs and mental health triage specialists.

By and large, the traditional staff and group model HMOs appear to have adopted the integrated model, whereas many IPA programs are pursuing the carve-out approach. Indeed, more than 170 million people are enrolled in carve-out behavioral health plans (Oss and Cleary 1999). IPA model HMOs wishing to be NCQA accredited may need to ensure that their affiliated behavioral health carve-out programs also qualify for accreditation.

TABLE 26–3. Total and behavioral healthcare spending ($billions), 1990

Population	Total healthcare	Behavioral health (percent of total)
Privately insured	450.8	22.2 (4.9%)
Medicaid	64.8	9.5 (14.7%)
Medicare	111.0	2.2 (2.0%)

Source. Total healthcare expenditures are from U.S. Bureau of the Census 1996. Behavioral health expenditures are from Edmunds et al.1997 and Frank and McGuire 1996.

Primary Care Behavioral Health Services in HMOs

Considerable research has been conducted on the provision of behavioral health services by primary care clinicians in HMOs. At least in integrated HMOs, primary care providers deliver a substantial fraction of the behavioral health services. For example, in one large HMO, the vast majority of antidepressant prescriptions were written by nonpsychiatric physicians in the 1990s (Johnson et al. 1997). Observational data from the Rand Corporation's Medical Outcomes Study suggested that capitated primary care providers did less well than their fee-for-service counterparts at detecting major depressive disorder in patients (Wells et al. 1989a). In contrast, the treatment of major depressive disorder by primary care providers resulted in similar outcomes when fee for service was compared with capitation (Rogers et al. 1993). Primary care providers' treatment for depression was less expensive than that of mental health specialists but also less effective (Sturm and Wells 1995). However, randomized trials have suggested that primary care treatment of depression can be improved in HMOs by extensive collaboration with mental health specialists (Katon et al. 1995, 1999).

A key issue in integrated HMOs is the division of labor between primary care and the specialty mental health department (Brown et al. 1995). Who provides which service for which patients is a matter of considerable interest to HMO consumers and providers. Indeed, the role of psychiatric versus nonpsychiatric physicians in this highly competitive and rapidly changing environment remains to be determined. For better or worse, the ratio of psychiatrists to members is typically much lower in HMOs than in the general population (Weiner 1994).

Behavioral Health Quality in HMOs

Enrollee concerns about quality of care in HMOs pertain to behavioral as well as physical healthcare (Consumer Reports 1996; Eist 1997). Interesting data in this regard were provided by fluoxetine manufacturer Eli Lilly, which financed a survey of some 10,000 HMO members enrolled in about 40 health plans located in Connecticut, Cleveland, Houston, New Jersey, and Southern California (Eli Lilly 1996). Over 20% of respondents described themselves as being familiar with their HMO's mental health treatment program. About one-fifth of these "mental health aware" members were receiving mental health treatment, but the majority were family members, friends, co-workers, or employee benefits managers. Some 35% of these individuals rated their HMO's mental healthcare as "not adequate"; in contrast, only 14% gave a "not adequate" rating to the HMO's asthma, pregnancy, and high blood pressure treatment programs. Whereas 85% of people rating the HMO's mental health program as excellent would reenroll, only 58% of those rating the mental health program as inadequate would reenroll. This finding has implications for selection bias (i.e., "cream skimming"). In theory, individuals who use HMO mental health services and are dissatisfied will disenroll. The implication is that the remaining enrollees may be the healthier fraction of the population. In contrast, evidence suggests that at least some HMO members with severe mental illness tend to remain enrolled longer than members who are not mentally ill (McFarland et al. 1996), regardless of dissatisfaction (Druss et al. 1999).

National accreditation standards may be a vehicle for ensuring that HMOs deliver high-quality behavioral healthcare. The current version of HEDIS does include behavioral health. However, the measures have traditionally emphasized utilization statistics such as the fraction of patients discharged from an inpatient psychiatry unit who have an outpatient mental health visit within the subsequent 30 days (National Committee for Quality Assurance 1996). The American Managed Behavioral Healthcare Association's performance measurement system is quite similar to that developed by the NCQA (American Managed Behavioral Healthcare Association 1995). Although these measures are crude, anecdotal reports suggest that they have had an impact on provision of behavioral health services in at least some large HMOs.

Although the original HEDIS measures pertaining to behavioral health were primitive, more sophisticated approaches have been examined by the NCQA. For example, HEDIS 2001 includes an item pertaining to duration of antidepressant use. Whether the NCQA will adopt more sophisticated behavioral healthcare quality measures remains to be seen.

At least one large employer has collaborated with an insurer to develop its own standards for behavioral healthcare quality. Digital Equipment Corporation's behavioral health standards (developed with John Hancock) are comprehensive in that they include measurements of level of functioning. The Digital Equipment Corporation approach appears to have had an impact on at least some HMOs (J. Feldman 1996). Nonetheless, Digital Equipment corporation fared poorly and was purchased by Compaq.

As noted earlier, the FACCT approach to accreditation has focused on treatment outcomes for HMO enrollees with major depressive disorder (Foundation for Accountability 1996). The original FACCT system involved patients completing questionnaires at the time of diagnosis and 6 months later. The notion of rating HMOs based on treatment outcomes raises a number of issues that are discussed in depth in the next section.

Outcomes of HMO Behavioral Healthcare

During the 1970s and much of the 1980s the Rand Corporation conducted a randomized trial known as the Health Insurance Experiment, in which subjects were assigned to either fee-for-service or prepaid healthcare (Wells et al. 1986). The HMO arm of the protocol was Group Health Cooperative of Puget Sound. The study showed that, by and large, fee-for-service subjects used more specialty mental healthcare than did people in the HMO (Wells et al. 1989b, 1990). Nonetheless, mental health outcomes for the population in the fee-for-service arm of the protocol were about the same as those for subjects enrolled in the HMO (Wells et al. 1990).

Conversely, the Rand Corporation's observational Medical Outcomes Study from the late 1980s (Rogers et al. 1993) suggested that depressed psychiatric patients in fee-for-service systems benefited from the additional psychiatrist hours they received (as contrasted with comparable HMO psychiatric patients who received fewer hours of care and had poorer outcomes). Although the two Rand Corporation studies differed in several ways, at first glance these results seem to be contradictory. A simplified numerical example will help reconcile the two Rand Corporation studies and will illuminate the challenges involved in reporting outcomes data from HMOs.

Suppose one were comparing two HMOs and that the cases of interest are persons with major depressive disorder or dysthymia. Suppose further that the outcome of interest is depressive symptoms, which will be rated as unimproved or better. Here, better implies that one has converted from being a case (i.e., satisfying DSM-IV criteria) to being a noncase. Suppose too that HMO Number One offers high-intensity mental health services whose effectiveness is comparable with the efficacy found in clinical trials. Imagine that treatment in HMO Number One will lead to better outcomes for about 60% of treated cases (Bech 1993).

Conversely, imagine that HMO Number Two provides low-intensity treatment that yields better outcomes in 40% of cases. Also suppose that about 20% of cases will spontaneously become better (Bech 1993). One important question is the sample size needed to demonstrate that HMO Number One is superior to HMO Number Two in terms of outcomes.

Table 26–4 shows expected outcomes for the two HMOs. Round numbers are chosen for convenience, but the percentages in Table 26–4 are close to those suggested by the Epidemiologic Catchment Area project (Regier et al. 1993). Notice that in both HMOs, some individuals who are noncases receive treatment—as would be expected from national data (Regier et al. 1993).

The percentages in Table 26–4 can then be related to the sample size needed to show (with a P value of 0.05 and a statistical power of 0.80) that HMO Number One is superior to HMO Number Two (Table 26–5). If one focuses on the population as the denominator, the difference between the two HMOs is rather small (4% in HMO Number One got better versus 3% in HMO Number Two). The problem here is the large number of unimproved enrollees. Using the cases as the denominator points out the differences between the HMOs (40% better versus 30%). Comparing the users (including the users who were not cases) the percentages are 30% better versus 20%. The most powerful comparison is obtained by contrasting the user cases (60% versus 40%).

The point here is that it may not be realistic for purchasers to expect that mental health services will have an impact on population outcomes large enough to be measurable in most HMOs. Indeed, the "no difference between prepaid and fee for service" results from the Rand Corporation's earlier Health Insurance Experiment may well be due to the choice of the overall population as the denominator. Conversely, the findings from the later Medical Outcomes Study that more intensive psychiatric care (in the fee-for-service sub-

TABLE 26–4. Data for HMO outcomes comparisons

	HMO 1		HMO 2	
Subjects	**Unimproved**	**Better**	**Unimproved**	**Better**
Noncases				
Nonusers	85%	0%	85%	0%
Users	5%	0%	5%	0%
Cases				
Nonusers	4%	1%	4%	1%
Users	2%	3%	3%	2%

Source. Adapted from Bech 1993; Regier et al. 1993.

TABLE 26–5. Sample sizes for HMO outcomes comparisons

Population	HMO 1	HMO 2	Total N needed
User cases	60%	40%	214
All cases	40%	30%	752
All users	30%	20%	626
All enrollees	4%	3%	11,004

Source. Adapted from Fleiss 1981.

jects) leads to improved outcomes (in comparison with prepaid care) is likely related to the focus on the user-cases.

This numerical example also illustrates the impact of choosing one lumping algorithm over another when aggregating outcome measures. Notice that the unimproved category combines "no change" with "worse." The cases can get better or can be unimproved. However, the noncases can only stay in the unimproved category. Implicitly this lumping algorithm suppresses information on incident cases arising in the population.

Notice, too, that this example takes a longitudinal perspective. In other words, enrollees in the HMOs are compared with themselves (in order to measure the outcomes as unimproved or better). Suppose instead that one were to take a cross-sectional perspective. In both HMO Number One and HMO Number Two, the cases are much more likely to use mental health services than are noncases (50% use versus 5.6% use). Also, in cross-section the cases (by definition) have poorer mental health status than the noncases. If one were to consider the cross-sectional case versus noncase status as the outcome measure, then the noncases would be plotted in the upper left-hand corner of the graph of

outcomes versus resource use (since these people have good, i.e., noncase, outcome status but use few mental health resources). Conversely, the cases would be (in cross-section) plotted in the lower right-hand corner (since they have poor outcomes but high resource use). Connecting these two points would show a downsloping curve suggesting that more resources lead to poorer outcomes.

This problem pertains to physical as well as mental health. Admission to an intensive care unit is a powerful predictor of death but, presumably, does not in and of itself hasten one's demise. Indeed, if the outcome is "walked out of hospital" versus "other," then for medical-surgical cases a negative relationship exists between resource expenditure and outcomes. In epidemiologic terms the problem is that the relationship between outcome and expenditure is confounded by severity (Kleinbaum et al. 1982). The adjustment for severity that a longitudinal design makes possible can minimize this spurious correlation problem.

The HMOs shown in Table 26–4 may be expected to change over time. Suppose HMO Number One is regarded as the baseline, and imagine that it is in equilibrium. Recall that 4% of the enrollees are cases who get better within a unit of time (e.g., 1 year). If one defines getting better as losing one's "caseness," then 4% of the enrollees must become cases within a unit of time. According to the two-wave Epidemiologic Catchment Area project data, this 4% incidence figure is about the number of new affective disorder cases expected to arise in a population during 1 year (Regier et al. 1993). Now consider HMO Number Two, where only 3% of the enrollees get better per unit of time. Assuming that HMO Number Two also has an incidence of 4% per time unit, then clearly this HMO is not in equilibrium. Perhaps HMO Number Two was at one time equivalent to HMO Number One but has had a perturbation (such as a reduction in resources allocated to mental health). In any event, over time the prevalence of cases within HMO Number Two will rise from 10% (at baseline) to 13.3%. With a P value of 0.05 and statistical power of 0.8 this difference in prevalences of depression in the HMOs could be detected if the total sample size were 3,064 (Fleiss 1981). HMO Number Two will be halfway to its equilibrium (i.e., maximum) prevalence after 2.3 time units (i.e., years) have passed. The point here is that generous sample sizes and appropriate time periods are needed to show differences in the dynamic aspects of population-based outcome measures.

Medicaid and Behavioral Health in HMOs

There have been and will continue to be debates about the role of HMOs in the delivery of behavioral healthcare to Medicaid clients (McFarland 1996, 2000). Yet another definition of integration refers to the connection (if any) between private-sector healthcare systems (such as HMOs) and the public sector. In the medical-surgical area, most states are rapidly enrolling their Medicaid clients in HMOs. However, public and private integration for behavioral health (if it is to take place) needs to address the traditional public mental health system (i.e., community mental health programs and state mental hospitals). The role for HMOs in this process remains to be seen (McFarland 1994, 1996). Certainly, the replacement of fee-for-service Medicaid with capitation has inspired considerable discussion about HMOs and people with severe mental illness (McFarland 1994; Riggs 1996). Randomized trial data from Minnesota's Medicaid project in the 1980s suggested that HMOs may not necessarily be deleterious for people with severe mental illness (Lurie et al. 1992), but the evidence is incomplete (McFarland 1994, 2000). More information will be provided from natural experiments in which states provide a variety of prepaid behavioral health programs (some involving HMOs) for Medicaid patients (Deck et al. 2000; McFarland et al. 1997). Issues of resource allocation, quality of care, access to services, and consumer satisfaction will need to be addressed anew as private and public health systems learn to work with each other.

References

American Managed Behavioral Healthcare Association: Performance Measures for Managed Behavioral Healthcare Programs. Washington, DC, American Managed Behavioral Healthcare Association, 1995

American Medical Association: Socioeconomic Characteristics of Medical Practice 1996. Chicago, IL, American Medical Association, 1996

Bech P: Acute therapy of depression. J Clin Psychiatry 54 (8 suppl):18–27, 1993

Bodenheimer T: The HMO backlash—righteous or reactionary? N Engl J Med 335:1601–1604, 1996

Brown JB, Shye D, McFarland B: The paradox of guideline implementation: how AHCPR's depression guideline was adapted at Kaiser Permanente, Northwest Region. Joint Commission Journal on Quality Improvement 21:5–21, 1995

Burns J: Measuring health care quality. Medical Benefits, Special Report No 2. New York, Panel Publishers (Aspen Publishers Inc.), 1996

Coffey RM, Mark T, King E, et al: National Estimates of Expenditures for Mental Health and Substance Abuse Treatment, 1997. SAMHSA Publication No SMA-00-3499. Rockville, MD, Center for Substance Abuse Treatment and Center for Mental Health Services, Substance Abuse and Mental Health Services Administration, July 2000

Consumer Reports: How good is your health plan? Consumer Reports, August 1996, pp 28–42

Dana RH, Conner MG, Allen J: Quality of care and cost-containment in managed mental health: policy, education, research, advocacy. Psychol Rep 79(3 part 2):1395–1422, 1996

Deck DD, McFarland BH, Titus JM, et al: Access to substance abuse treatment services under the Oregon Health Plan. JAMA 284:2093–2099, 2000

Dial TH, Bergsten C, Kantor A, et al: Behavioral health care in HMOs, in Mental Health, United States (DHHS Publ No SMA-96-3098). Edited by Manderscheid RW, Sonnenschein MA. Washington, DC, U.S. Government Printing Office, 1996, pp 45–58

Druss D, Schlesinger M, Thomas T, et al: Depressive symptoms and plan switching under managed care. Am J Psychiatry 156:697-701, 1999

Edmunds M, Frank R, Hogan M, et al: Managing Managed Care: Quality Improvement in Behavioral Health. Washington, DC, Institute of Medicine, National Academy of Sciences, National Academy Press, 1997

Eist HI: The HMO M.O. Psychiatric News, January 3, 1997, p 3

Eli Lilly: 1996 CareData Report on How Mental Health Care Services Impact HMO Member Satisfaction. New York, CareData Reports, 1996

Ellwood Jr. PM, Lundberg GD: Managed care: a work in progress. JAMA 276:1083–1086, 1996

Feldman J: How will mental health outcomes data be used in private systems? in Using Client Outcomes Information to Improve Mental Health and Substance Abuse Treatment. Edited by Steinwachs DM, Flynn LM, Norquist GS, et al. New Directions for Mental Health Services, No 71. San Francisco, CA, Jossey-Bass, 1996, pp103–109

Feldman S: Dialogue: integrated or carved out: the future of behavioral health programs. A marriage unconsummated. Behavioral Healthcare Tomorrow 3(6):41–48 1994

Fleiss JL: Statistical Methods for Rates and Proportion, 2nd Edition. New York, Wiley, 1981

Foundation for Accountability: Synopses of Measures to Assess Quality of Care. Portland, OR, Foundation for Accountability, 1996

Frank RG, McGuire TG: Introduction to the economics of mental health payment systems, in Mental Health Services: A Public Health Perspective. Edited by Levin BL, Petrilla J. New York, Oxford University Press, 1996, pp 23–37

Freudenheim E: Healthspeak: A Complete Dictionary of America's Health Care System. New York, Facts On File, 1996

Gabel JR, Dial TH, Hobart J, et al: HMO Industry Profile, 1994 Edition. Washington, DC, Group Health Association of America, 1994

Greenlick MR, Freeborn DK, Pope CR: Health Care Research in an HMO: Two Decades of Discovery. Baltimore, MD, Johns Hopkins University Press, 1988

Jacob JA: Local health plans could top big HMOs in '97. American Medical News 40(3):28–29, 1997

Johnson RE, McFarland BH: Treated prevalence rates of severe mental illness among HMO members. Hosp Community Psychiatry 45:919–924, 1994

Johnson RE, McFarland BH, Nichols G: Changing patterns of antidepressant use in an HMO. Pharmacoeconomics 11:274–286, 1997

Katon W, Von Korff M, Lin E, et al: Collaborative management to achieve treatment guidelines: impact on depression in primary care. JAMA 273:1026–1031, 1995

Katon W, Von Korff M, Lin E, et al: Stepped collaborative care for primary care patients with persistent symptoms of depression. Arch Gen Psychiatry 56:1109–1115, 1999

Kleinbaum DG, Kupper LL, Morgenstern H: Epidemiologic Research: Principles and Quantitative Methods. Belmont, CA, Lifetime Learning Publications, 1982

KPMG Peat Marwick: Health benefits in 1996. Medical Benefits 13(21):1–2, 1996

Lurie N, Moscovice I, Finch M, et al: Does capitation affect the health of the chronically mentally ill? Results from a randomized trial. JAMA 267:3300–3304, 1992

McFarland BH: Health maintenance organizations and persons with severe mental illness. Community Ment Health J 30:221–242, 1994

McFarland BH: Ending the millennium (editorial). Community Ment Health J 32:219–222, 1996

McFarland BH, George RA: Ethics and managed care. Child Adolesc Psychiatr Clin N Am 4:885–901, 1995

McFarland BH: Overview of Medicaid managed behavioral health care, in What the Oregon Health Plan Can Teach Us About Managed Mental Health Care. Edited by Goetz RR, McFarland BH, Ross KV. New Directions for Mental Health Services, No 85. San Francisco, CA, Jossey-Bass, 2000, pp 17–22

McFarland BH, Johnson RE, Hornbrook MC: Enrollment duration, service use, and costs of care for severely mentally ill members of a health maintenance organization. Arch Gen Psychiatry 53:938–944, 1996

McFarland BH, Winthrop K, Cutler DL: Integrating mental health into the Oregon Health Plan. Psychiatr Serv 48:191–193, 1997

Mechanic D, Schlesinger M, McAlpine DD: Management of mental health and substance abuse services: state of the art and early results. Milbank Q 73:19–55, 1995

Mechanic D, McAlpine DD, Olfson M: Changing patterns of psychiatric inpatient care in the United States, 1988–1994. Arch Gen Psychiatry 55:785–791, 1998

Mental Health Statistics Improvement Program: Consumer-Oriented Mental Health Report Card. Rockville, MD, Substance Abuse and Mental Health Services Administration, Center for Mental Health Services, 1996

National Committee for Quality Assurance: Health Plan Employer Data and Information Set (HEDIS 3.0). Washington, DC, National Committee for Quality Assurance, 1996

O'Kane ME: A new approach to accreditation of HMOs. Journal of Health Care Benefits, Sept/Oct 1991, pp 40–43

Oss ME, Clary JH: The 20 largest specialty managed behavioral health programs, by 1999 enrollment. Gettysburg, PA, Open Minds, 1999

Peterson MS, Christianson JB, Wholey D: National Survey of Mental Health, Alcohol, and Drug Abuse Treatment in HMOs: 1989 Chartbook. Excelsior, MN, Interstudy Center for Managed Care Research, 1992

Regier DA, Narrow WE, Rae DS, et al: The defacto US mental and addictive disorder service system: Epidemiologic Catchment Area prospective 1-year prevalence rates of disorders and service. Arch Gen Psychiatry 50:85–94, 1993

Riggs RT: HMOs and the seriously mentally ill—a view from the trenches. Community Ment Health J 32:219–222, 1996

Rogers WH, Wells KB, Meredith LS, et al: Outcomes for adult outpatients with depression under prepaid or fee-for-service financing. Arch Gen Psychiatry 50:517–525, 1993

Rojas-Burke J: Firms grapple with tough choices. Portland Oregonian, October 29, 2000 page C-1

Rost K, Smith J, Fortney J: Large employers' selection criteria in purchasing behavioral health benefits. J Behav Health Serv Res 27:334–338, 2000

Siegel and Gale: Executive Voice: Listening to the Business Executive on Health Care. New York, Siegel & Gale, 1996

Simon GE, VonKorff M, Durham ML: Predictors of outpatient mental health utilization by primary care patients in a health maintenance organization. Am J Psychiatry 151:908–913, 1994

Simon GE, Grothaus L, Durham ML, et al: Impact of visit co-payments on outpatient mental health utilization by members of a health maintenance organization. Am J Psychiatry 153:331–338, 1996

Strosahl K, Quirk M: The trouble with carve outs: separate behavioral health plans drive up costs because most patients seek mental health care from primary care doctors. Business and Health 12(7):52, 1994

Sturm R, Pacula RL: Mental health parity and employer-sponsored health insurance in 1999-2000, I: limits. Psychiatr Serv 51:1361, 2000

Sturm R, Wells KB: How can care for depression become more cost-effective? JAMA 273:51–58, 1995

Teich JL, Melek SP: Characteristics of managed behavioral health care organizations in 1996. Psychiatr Serv 51:1422–1427, 2000

U.S. Bureau of the Census: Statistical Abstract of the United States 1996. Washington, DC, Bureau of the Census, 1996

U.S. Census Bureau: Statistical Abstract of the United States, 1999, 119th Ed. Washington, DC, U.S. Census Bureau, 1999

Weiner JP: Forecasting the effects of health reform on US physician workforce requirements: evidence from HMO staffing patterns. JAMA 272:222–230, 1994

Wells KB, Manning Jr. WG, Benjamin B: Use of outpatient mental health services in HMO and fee-for-service plans: results from a randomized controlled trial. Health Serv Res 21:453–474, 1986

Wells KB, Hays RD, Burnam MA, et al: Detection of depressive disorder for patients receiving prepaid or fee-for-service care: results from the Medical Outcomes Study. JAMA 262:3298–3302, 1989a

Wells KB, Manning WG, Valdez RB: The Effects of Insurance Generosity on the Psychological Distress and Well-Being of a General Population. Santa Monica, CA, Rand Corporation, 1989b

Wells KB, Manning Jr. WG, Valdez RB: The effects of a prepaid group practice on mental health outcomes. Health Serv Res 25:615–625, 1990

Wells KB, Sherbourne C, Schoenbaum M, et al: Impact of disseminating quality improvement programs for depression in managed primary care: a randomized controlled trial. JAMA 283:212–220, 2000

Woolhandler S, Himmelstein DU: Annotation: patients on the auction block. Am J Public Health 86:1699–1700, 1996

Zablocki E: Is accreditation in your future? HMO Magazine, July/Aug 1992, pp 48–53

Zieman GL: Nearly a century of capitation: how and why, in The Complete Capitation Handbook: How to Design and Implement At-Risk Contracts for Behavioral Healthcare. Tiburon, CA, CentraLink Publications, 1995, pp 1–9

❖ 27 ❖

Physician-Hospital Organizations

Benjamin Liptzin, M.D.

Physician-hospital organizations (PHOs) have received increasing attention in recent years. The principal factor in the emergence of this entity is the restructuring of the U.S. healthcare system, which has accelerated since the failure of President Clinton's health plan legislation in 1994. The original impetus for the restructuring was the perception that healthcare expenditures could not continue to increase at double-digit rates without doing major damage to the U.S. economy. These expenditure increases were making it increasingly difficult for U.S. corporations to compete in the global marketplace. In addition, the increasing expenditures for Medicare and Medicaid were straining the budgets of federal and state governments. In response to these economic pressures, the private sector (and more recently governmental healthcare financing programs) turned to managed care as a way to control costs. Some have questioned whether this has really changed the way care is managed or has primarily managed costs and "mangled care" (Sharfstein 1990) by demanding and obtaining discounts from providers and instituting prior authorization procedures for expensive care such as hospitalization.

Perhaps no area of healthcare has been affected as dramatically as behavioral healthcare, the generic term for treatment of mental health and substance abuse problems (see Chapter 22). In the early 1990s, many

corporations noted rapid increases in their expenditures for behavioral healthcare. This increase resulted in part from improved insurance coverage for such services, which led to increased demand and the development of greatly increased system capacity including the development of for-profit psychiatric hospitals and freestanding substance abuse facilities. This spiral caught the attention of benefits managers and other corporate executives who turned to behavioral health carve-out companies to slow the increases or reduce their overall costs. In the late 1990s, these companies were consolidated into just a few major national players (e.g., Magellan or Value/Options), which themselves have been bought (and sometimes sold) by Fortune 500 companies (e.g., Merck or Columbia/HCA).

While these dramatic changes were occurring with behavioral healthcare, hospitals and physicians in private practice were feeling the effects of managed care. Large health insurers began consolidating and moving away from open-ended indemnity insurance and instead set up preferred networks of hospitals and practitioners. These insurers demanded deep discounts from hospitals and practitioners with the threat of taking their subscribers (or covered lives) to other competing providers if cost and quality standards were not met. In response to these threats to their survival, hospitals and practitioners on their medical staff (employed or in private practice) have increasingly joined together into PHOs. The rest of this chapter discusses the rationale and structure of a PHO, issues involved in operationalizing the concept, and special considerations for psychiatrists and other mental health practitioners.

Why Form a PHO and What Does It Look Like?

Figure 27–1 illustrates the structure of a typical PHO. A hospital or health system joins with its affiliated physicians either through an independent practice association or through agreements with individual physicians or group practices. The hospital and the physicians jointly own or control the organization and appoint the board members. The PHO then negotiates contracts on behalf of the hospital and physicians usually within the boundaries of terms that have previously been agreed upon.

PHOs have been formed in response to the changes in the healthcare marketplace. According to Straley (1995, p. 1),

> A PHO is a vehicle that enables hospitals and physicians to work cooperatively toward accomplishing several objectives. Primary purposes for forming a PHO include contracting with managed care organizations with joint risk sharing, developing standards of care, and building trust between hospitals and independent physicians. Secondary purposes may include developing improved methods of health care delivery; overseeing integration of physicians and hospitals into health care delivery networks; assisting in voluntary group formation; and collecting, analyzing, and disseminating information.

In this context, integration means joining together with shared incentives to make the organization successful.

The impetus for PHO formation is usually a current or projected increase in managed care penetration in a geographic region. Hospital chief executive officers anticipate pressures to reduce prices and inpatient utilization and worry about losing market share to their competitors. Physicians experience similar pressures; specialist physicians are usually more threatened than primary care physicians. For specialists the threats are loss of market share and volume if they are cut out of particular contracts and reduced fees if they choose to participate. Most geographic areas still have a rela-

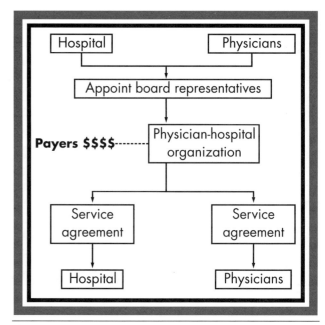

FIGURE 27–1. Structure of a physician-hospital organization.

tive shortage of primary care physicians so that their concerns are usually about the terms of their contracts and the nature of the network that will be available for their patients. The network will usually include a limited number of hospitals or specialists to which patients can be referred.

Against this backdrop, hospitals see the PHO as a way to preserve market share and their competitive position by aligning with physician referral sources. Physicians see the PHO as a vehicle for obtaining expertise in analyzing and negotiating contracts. This is particularly important for physicians in solo or small group practices who may be overwhelmed by the complexity and volume of paperwork involved in managed care contracting. In some markets, physicians may choose to form a physician organization that will negotiate just on their behalf, in contrast to a PHO, which also represents a hospital. Once a contract is obtained, physicians may benefit from access to capital and the expertise needed to develop the information systems that will support the financial and medical management systems necessary to be successful. In a PHO, the hospital may bring these strengths to the partnership. For a payer, a PHO is attractive if it can simplify the contracting process and deliver a geographically dispersed and comprehensive range of services that the payer can then market to employers and other purchasers of healthcare. The alternative would be for the payer to individually negotiate with a hospital and small groups of physicians. The latter alternative may be more attractive to a payer if the market is oversupplied with hospital beds and specialist physicians, in which case the payer can get lower rates by playing one group against another.

Staff of the PHO negotiate with payers to try to achieve the best overall contract. Some payers insist on using their own standard contracts, which may differ from the contract preferred by the PHO. A PHO usually sets up a contracts review committee, which analyzes each contract from the point of view of primary care physicians, each specialty, and the hospital. The committee can either reject the contract and recommend further negotiation or approve the contract and send it forward for the individual physician members to make an individual decision on participation. The whole area of contract negotiations is complex and subject to antitrust laws that carry severe penalties if it is concluded that physicians have taken collective action to boycott a particular payer. Unless there is substantial risk sharing, the PHO may share information on fees only through a "messenger model" that does not allow individual physicians to make joint decisions. With substantial risk sharing, physicians are more likely to be protected from antitrust violations if they discuss fees. A PHO will need to consult with a lawyer knowledgeable in the area of antitrust law to avoid any potentially serious problems. Once the contract is finalized, the PHO develops service agreements with the hospital and with physicians to provide the services required under the contract. Often a PHO will try to negotiate an exclusive contract with a payer because that guarantees the largest number of covered lives for the hospital and physicians.

Developing a PHO

In order to begin the discussions that lead to formation of a PHO, some level of trust is needed between the physicians and the hospital. This level of trust varies in each geographic area and community as hospitals have pursued different strategies of partnering with their medical staffs or setting up competing primary care or specialist practices. Given at least some history of cooperation, a task force should be formed with representation from the medical staff and from hospital management. The size of the task force is determined by the competing interests of having broad representation from the physician community and having a manageable size so that the task force can accomplish its work.

In choosing the physician members, it is generally desirable to include both primary care physicians and specialists, private practice and employed physicians, and hospital-based and office-based practitioners.

As members of a hospital medical staff, psychiatrists should volunteer to get involved in such a task force. In addition to protecting their own interests, psychiatrists have often had more experience with managed care than most other physicians because of the rapid development of behavioral health carve-out companies. This experience has generally led most psychiatrists to prefer the option of working with their local hospital and physicians to the alternative of dealing with a for-profit national company headquartered in another state. As a result, psychiatrists can often be effective advocates for moving forward with formation of a PHO.

The task force must first address the strategic feasibility of proceeding with development of a PHO. Is there a perceived need in the local market? Is there an alternative to developing a PHO? Does sufficient trust exist among the different parties, and are the parties willing to proceed? The answers to these questions will determine whether it makes sense to proceed to the next step of designing the organizational structure of the PHO. This step includes clarifying what the PHO will do and how it will relate to its members. Decisions will have to be made regarding which physicians will be invited to join. Will the PHO include all members of the medical staff or only those who are closely aligned with and refer to the hospital? The legal organization and structure will have to be defined with legal counsel. How will the PHO be financed initially before having any contracts? Generally, an application fee or a contribution that may include a stock ownership interest will be needed if the PHO is set up as a for-profit entity. Stock ownership may be voluntary or mandatory as a condition of participating in the service agreements and voting on contract or other issues. A PHO may choose to associate with a venture capital company in anticipation of a later public offering or sale to a larger corporate entity.

When these issues are satisfactorily resolved, the next step is to develop a plan for implementing the PHO. This step involves extensive planning regarding the application and credentialing process, financial arrangements, contracting structure, medical management system, and information systems. (For more details on the process of developing a PHO, refer to Straley 1995.)

Implementing a PHO—Issues for Psychiatrists and Other Mental Health Professionals

When should psychiatrists and other mental health professionals get involved with a PHO?

The answer to this question depends in part on the mental health practitioner's relationship to the hospital partner and how dominant that hospital is in the local market. Hospital-based psychiatrists have a clear stake in the success of the hospital where they practice or are employed; however, community-based office practitioners also have a strong interest in the future of a PHO if it is likely to result in managed care contracts that include behavioral health services. In some markets, such carve-in arrangements will integrate behavioral healthcare into general medical care and eliminate the need for carve-out networks of care. Furthermore, as part of networks of care, office practitioners need to ensure that patients have access to high-quality, cost-efficient inpatient services if they require that level of care. In general, it is a good idea to be involved as early as possible to help shape the process. That involvement includes membership on any planning groups such as the one outlined above.

Who should be invited to join the PHO in order to ensure an adequate network of mental health providers?

It is important to have an adequate number of mental health practitioners who are geographically dispersed throughout the region likely to be served by the PHO. They should also represent various subspecialties including child, geriatric, and addiction psychiatry. In forming a PHO, the interest of having broad participation is balanced by the desire to include practitioners who will be closely aligned and provide cost-effective and high-quality care. With respect to psychiatric participation, generally all active members of the medical staff are invited to join. Nonphysician mental health practitioners may also have appointments as members of the hospital's associate professional staff, which could be the basis for inviting them to join. In addition, existing referral relationships between nonphysician practitioners and psychiatrists in the PHO should be maintained. Participating psychiatrists could also nominate other practitioners for inclusion in the network.

In general it is much easier to add practitioners as the volume expands than it is to drop practitioners who are not needed. The criteria for inclusion and the process for choosing the network members will vary depending on the political situation in any given community. In addition, psychiatrists are usually full voting members of the PHO, whereas nonphysician practitioners may be full members, nonmembers, or some intermediate category.

How should the mental health practitioners be organized into a network?

Various models have been used including a centralized triage system that assigns patients to individual clinicians, authorizes a limited number of visits, and then carefully reviews requests for additional visits based on specific guidelines. This is the usual model of behavioral health carve-out companies. Another model is that of professional affiliation groups (Pomerantz et al. 1994, 1995, 1996). In this model, nonphysician mental health clinicians are organized into groups with a managing psychiatrist who collaborates with the nonphysician practitioners and authorizes sessions as needed. This model has the advantage of tying fiscal and clinical accountability together because the psychiatrist will also have a treatment relationship with the patient if psychopharmacologic consultation or treatment is necessary. This model also helps move the whole network toward focused briefer treatments based on clinical discussions. It is important for these groups and the practitioners in them to take responsibility for seeing emergency or urgent cases to avoid hospitalization if possible or to reduce the length of stay if admission is necessary.

How will the budget for mental health services be set?

The PHO may negotiate contracts that pay practitioners on a fee-for-service basis, although the PHO will more likely prefer to accept contracts that share risk with the payer. This approach allows the PHO to benefit from any savings achieved by cost-effective case management. Under capitated contracts, the payer usually keeps a percentage of the premium dollar for its administrative costs including marketing, sales, and general plan administration. For-profit plans also keep as much as they can as profit to be retained or distributed to their shareholders. The remainder (sometimes called the medical loss ratio) is allocated to a health ser-

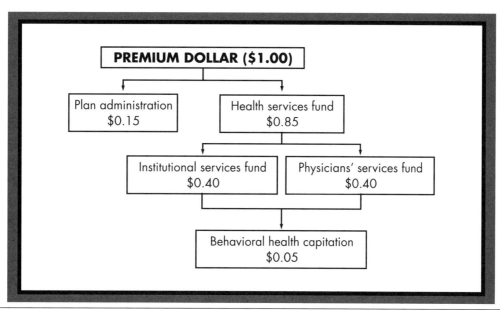

FIGURE 27–2. Hypothetical example of how premium dollars are divided.

vices fund. Generally it is up to the PHO to determine how much of this fund will be spent on hospital-based inpatient or outpatient care and how much will go into a physicians' service fund. Figure 27–2 illustrates how the premium dollar is divided.

The PHO may also separate other services, including behavioral health, for subcapitation. It is extremely important for psychiatrist members of the PHO to strongly advocate for adequate resources to support behavioral health services. Currently the per-member per-month (PMPM) capitation rate in various plans for commercial populations ranges from over $6 PMPM to as low as $0.80 PMPM. As a percentage of premiums, behavioral health services range from 1% to 5% of the total medical expense budget. Clearly the same quality or number of services cannot be provided if the capitation rate is set at the lower figure rather than at the higher figure.

How does the capitation rate affect utilization rates?

The total budget for behavioral health services consists of the capitation rate multiplied by the number of members in the plan each month. Thus, if the specific PHO contract has 10,000 members and a PMPM of $6, the total budget for behavioral health for the year is $720,000. In order to function within this budget, estimates need to be made of utilization rates for the various types and levels of service including inpatient, par-

tial hospital, and outpatient mental health and substance abuse services. The utilization rates initially should be based on historical rates for the enrolled population, if possible. Those rates can be adjusted based on the aggressiveness of the case management system. For example, inpatient utilization rates may historically be 100 days per 1,000 subscribers but should be relatively easy to reduce to less than 50 days per 1,000 subscribers. Very aggressive plans have utilization rates in the range of 10–15 days per 1,000 subscribers. Similarly, outpatient utilization rates vary from over 700 visits per 1,000 subscribers to under 300 visits per 1,000 subscribers. Some plans keep their outpatient utilization low by restricting access to a very limited network of providers and thereby encouraging patients to seek care out of the network and pay for it out of their own pocket.

Total costs also depend on price per unit of service whether for an inpatient day or an outpatient visit. The cost per visit generally varies according to the discipline of the provider and the mix of disciplines providing the services. As a result, most plans try to make use of the lowest cost provider who is qualified to deliver the service. For the overall plan, it is important to provide treatment at the lowest intensity level of care consistent with the patient's clinical needs. In order to minimize the use of expensive inpatient or partial hospital care, the plan may develop a continuum of services that include acute residential services, respite services, in-home follow-up, or intensive outpatient services. Outpatient providers also need to be comfortable providing treatment to distressed patients, as the level of acuity will increase at every level of the continuum as the capitation rate is ratcheted down. The utilization needs to be carefully tracked to ensure that all providers are using resources responsibly. Such provider profiling is still in the early stages of development and requires sophisticated stratification of risk by severity of illness and other parameters that affect utilization. The structure of the PHO allows hospital-based and community practitioners to work together to manage utilization effectively and negotiate how the available dollars will be allocated.

What is the role of psychiatrists?

In general, psychiatrists in such plans are responsible for psychopharmacologic management but may also provide psychotherapy for complicated cases, for which it makes sense to integrate the psychotherapy and medication management. For less complicated cases (or for less impaired patients), the psychiatrist may consult with the outpatient psychotherapist and the patient's primary care physician, who will be the principal prescriber. In plans in which the primary care physicians have large numbers of patients, the capitation rate for behavioral health services may be higher so that psychiatrists can provide the psychopharmacologic management. Primary care physicians may also decide that they are not knowledgeable or skilled enough in the treatment of mental and substance use disorders and allocate more money to the behavioral health program.

How will practitioners be paid?

Once the budget is determined, various methods are used to pay individual practitioners. A fairly common method is to pay practitioners using a fee schedule that is often based on the resource-based relative value scale developed for Medicare. In order to protect the plan from the risk of high utilization leading to budget overruns, many plans withhold 10%–20% of each fee, which is returned at the end of the year only if the budget is met. Some plans also have an end-of-year bonus if utilization comes in under budget. This bonus rewards practitioners for being cost effective but also raises ethical concerns about treatment being withheld for the financial benefit of practitioners instead of the well-being of patients. Generally speaking, fee-for-service

payments reward practitioners for doing more for patients and the bonus arrangement rewards them for doing less. This arrangement is probably a good balance of conflicting incentives for practitioners.

What other PHO activities should psychiatrists participate in?

Many PHO activities will require input and oversight by physician members. The development of appropriate information systems is critical to the success of a PHO and will require significant investments of capital and staff time. Practitioners need to make sure that the systems implemented meet their needs and are user friendly. Similarly, case management systems, including the development of practice guidelines or critical pathways, require extensive input from practitioners. Expenditures on pharmaceuticals are often a significant expense, and psychiatrists should serve on the PHO's pharmacy and therapeutics committee to ensure that any restrictions to the drug formulary are clinically sound. Psychiatrists should participate in decisions about medical management, including the development of treatment protocols for depression in primary care. Psychiatrists also should have input into decisions about credentialing (i.e., which practitioners are allowed to join the network) because such decisions can determine the network's effectiveness and efficiency. The PHO will face strategic decisions about whether to accept certain contracts even if the rates are too low or the terms are problematic (e.g., using a behavioral health carve-out company). Participation in the overall governance of the organization will improve the chances that the needs of mental health practitioners and their patients will be met.

Summary

PHOs are relatively new organizations being set up to help hospitals and physicians cope with the sweeping changes in healthcare brought about by managed care. In order to accept contracts that involve financial risk, systems must be developed to set budgets, monitor utilization, and manage patients in the most cost-effective way at the most appropriate level of care. Psychiatrists and other mental health practitioners can be influential in a PHO because of their extensive experience with managed care.

References

Pomerantz JM, Liptzin B, Carter AH, et al: The professional affiliation group: a new model for managed mental health care. Hosp Community Psychiatry 45:308–310, 1994

Pomerantz JM, Liptzin B, Carter A, et al: Forming practice groups to deal with managed care: two views. How to develop a virtual group practice. Journal of Practical Psychiatry and Behavioral Health 1:232–235, 1995

Pomerantz JM, Liptzin B, Carter A, et al: The multidisciplinary team: cotreatment in the professional affiliation group (PAG) model for private practice. Journal of Practical Psychiatry and Behavioral Health 2:247–250, 1996

Sharfstein SS: Utilization management: managed or mangled psychiatric care? Am J Psychiatry 147:965–966, 1990

Straley PF (ed): Developing a Successful Physician-Hospital Organization. Chicago, IL, American Hospital Publishing, 1995

❖ 28 ❖

Behavioral Group Practice

Alan A. Axelson, M.D.
Michael A. Freeman, M.D., D.M.H.

Hiring the ball players is easy. It's getting them to work together that's the hard part.

Casey Stengel

In this chapter we review the characteristics, competency requirements, and challenges of a new setting for administrative psychiatry: behavioral group practices. Trends related to group practice growth in medicine are reviewed, and the emergence of single-specialty behavioral groups is described. Information about the Institute for Behavioral Healthcare's Council of Behavioral Group Practices is presented as a framework for describing the characteristics of owner-operated and wholly owned behavioral groups. Administrative and leadership challenges during the start-up phase of group development, and beyond, are considered. The chapter concludes with a review of group practice approaches to contracting for and providing clinical services within the context of horizontally and vertically integrated delivery systems and the administrative competencies required in order to succeed in this endeavor.

Trends in Medical Group Practice Development

Group practice has become a fixture in the landscape of psychiatric practice settings, as is true throughout the practice of medicine. The 1996 report of the American Medical Association Council on Medical Service documents the movement of physicians from solo practice to employment and group practice. In 1983, 25% of practicing physicians identified themselves as employed. By 1995 that number had grown to 45% of physicians. At the same time the proportion of physicians in practice with two or more doctors increased from 46% to 60%. Groups of 5 or more rose from 18% to 32%, and groups of 10 or more jumped from 8% to 16% (Mitka 1997). The solo practitioner category experienced a concomitant decrease.

The transition from solo to group practice is a popular subject in the medical and psychiatric press. Articles are often based on interviews with physicians who have either made or not made the transition. Generally, physicians who made the move to group practice refer to the needs to meet the demands of a more competitive local market; to gain access to information systems that can provide efficient billing, inpatient tracking, and contract management; and to secure an opportunity to provide a broader range of clinical services.

Group practice physicians see the need to combine the revenue-generating power of a number of professionals to better distribute fixed overhead costs and to secure capable professional practice management infrastructure and services. Clinicians in behavioral group practices recognize that they have more favorable opportunities to secure managed care contracts and obtain access to much needed capital (Goldstein 1997). They give up the type of autonomy experienced by the solo practitioner in favor of the collegiality and mutual support of the group practice. The ideal may still be the solo practitioner who sees cash-paying patients in an office located in his or her own home in an area where demand is high. Unfortunately, this situation is only rarely available as a full-time practice opportunity. Economic and administrative demands seem to be favoring a trend toward organized practice.

Practices that have gone through such a process of evolution include Mesa Mental Health of Albuquerque, New Mexico; NoVaPsy, in the Washington, D.C., area; and InterCare Behavioral Health, my own group (A.A.A.) in Pittsburgh, Pennsylvania. The senior clinical leadership of each group can, with some ambivalence, trace the development of the group's extensive behavioral health delivery system.

As the medical financing, reimbursement, care management, and regulatory system becomes increasingly complex and organized, the clinical and administrative complexity of medical practice increases. The establishment of group practices is one way of meeting these demands.

In the general medical sector, group practices have a long and distinguished history. In some parts of the United States, they constitute a substantial component of regional delivery systems and they have developed financial and clinical operations and management systems that establish consistency, quality, and efficiency of care. Medical group practices are represented by their own professional associations, such as the Medical Group Management Association and the American Medical Group Association, and they publish a robust

professional literature in their own journal, *Group Practice Journal*, and elsewhere. These are all indications of the strength, stability, and vitality of this type of service organization.

The Emergence of Single-Specialty Behavioral Group Practice

Reflecting the experience of other medical specialties, the behavioral healthcare field is also experiencing rapid growth of multidisciplinary group practices. In most competitive urban markets, solo practitioners are aggregating into professional organizations that vary in size and complexity. These groups are typically started by clinicians who believe that together, behavioral healthcare providers can respond effectively to market changes that make solo practice less viable. Founders of behavioral groups are motivated by the assumption that they can accomplish more by practicing in a group than they can by practicing as individuals.

The emergence of behavioral group practices parallels the growth of managed behavioral healthcare companies and health maintenance organizations (HMOs) and the consolidation of regional healthcare markets. The dramatic growth of the managed behavioral healthcare industry and the subsequent contracting and management of behavioral healthcare services have created an interplay between national managed care organizations and clinicians who are interested in participating in organized systems of care.

Behavioral groups that form in order to participate in managed care systems must struggle to develop and master new administrative and organizational processes that are required for efficient operations within a managed care context. Behavioral group practices are experimenting with new ways of organizing services and delivery systems, managing quality, allocating resource utilization, and measuring outcomes. The group practice develops and supports the increased organization of providers within a continuum of care that can provide integrated service delivery. In a well-functioning, integrated system, patients receive care at the most appropriate level and for no longer than is necessary. The transition to the next level of care is smoothly managed by the internal system. Integrated systems can track and evaluate their outcomes and costs. They can use this information to negotiate larger and more favorable contracts with healthcare payment systems.

The consolidation and increased sophistication of healthcare payers and managed care networks support the trend from solo to group practice. As an opening strategy, managed care companies contracted with a number of solo practitioners. As it has become more costly to manage these networks, managed care companies have begun to contract with group practices, downloading certain administrative, quality, and utilization management functions to the group's administrative structure. As managed care companies are required to meet more extensive regulatory requirements measuring quality and outcome, partnership relationships with group practices will likely increase.

The Institute for Behavioral Healthcare's Council of Behavioral Group Practices

This rapid transition from loosely affiliated professionals to well-organized and integrated delivery systems has been encouraged by a commitment to group practice and support for their development by the Institute for Behavioral Healthcare (IBH), a nonprofit national center of excellence for managed behavioral healthcare leadership development and industry education. This support from IBH has resulted in the provision of continuous training and technical assistance for groups since 1989 at the IBH annual national meeting and also in regional meetings where group practice development has been a specific focus.

Interest in the growth of behavioral group practices was sufficiently intense that, in 1991, behavioral health professionals, including social workers, psychologists, nurses, general psychiatrists, and child and adolescent psychiatrists, met to organize the Council of Behavioral Group Practices (CBGP). This was done with the encouragement of the authors and the IBH. Since 1991 the IBH has provided staff support and services for the development of the CBGP, which in 1997 included over 65 full and affiliate members. The IBH also maintains a database containing the names of approximately 500 additional behavioral group practices, many of which participate in educational programs supported by the IBH and the CBGP.

The CBGP has established membership criteria, a governance system, and goals and objectives. It has developed cooperative programs for mutual consultation and education. The council has benchmarked and pub-

lished administrative management tools, initiated a national system of quality management and outcomes measurement, established a data warehouse for comparative health services research in partnership with the University of Cincinnati, and implemented national comparative performance-based benchmarking studies. It is committed to the development of an award-winning outcomes management system. The CBGP, with its annual retreats and program tracks at the annual Behavioral Healthcare Tomorrow conference, is clearly the national forum for the development of behavioral group practices.

Structural Characteristics of Behavioral Group Practices

Any discussion of administrative issues as they relate to group practices must first consider the organizational, operational, and administrative characteristics that define a behavioral group practice. How are groups differentiated from other organizations that deliver behavioral health services? For the American Medical Association's census purposes, a group practice is defined as two or more physicians who practice together. Complex federal legislation and regulations have established legal boundaries requiring special organizational structures and shared economic risk to differentiate group practices from an aggregation of independent professionals working together for economic benefit and other forms of affiliation that may constitute a violation of antitrust regulations.

Although formal structural characteristics can be identified, group practice is also a state of mind in some respects. In the prototypical behavioral groups of today, the members of the leadership team are committed to the principles and philosophy of group practice, and they identify with the group practice model. In the prototype group practice represented by CBGP members, clinician executives rise to positions of administrative authority, often by virtue of their willingness to take risk and to invest in an ownership interest in the group. This owner-operator structure ensures that generally a close correspondence exists between the clinical and business mission of the group and its leadership. Although this alignment communicates the impression of an equity interest, in many instances the investment in the group by its professional staff may be emotional rather than financial.

Essential to the success of a group practice is the ability of the entity to legitimately present itself to the public as an organized set of professionals providing medical, psychological, psychosocial, and other therapeutic services. The structure and operations of this entity must meet state and professional liability insurance requirements and must be configured appropriately so as to bear some legal responsibility for its employees' actions.

In the prototype, the health professionals may be organized in a variety of corporate structures such as a professional corporation, a partnership, or a limited liability company. Choice of business structure is a complex matter. Consult a lawyer!

Professional Corporation

A professional corporation is an entity organized under the corporate laws of a state. The corporation's primary purpose is to deliver professional services. Its ownership (stockholders) is limited to members of one professional group. For federal and state tax purposes it may be a C corporation, paying income taxes at the corporate level, or an S corporation, in which case income is passed through to the shareholders according to their proportions of ownership. Corporate shareholders, in general, are not liable for acts of the corporation.

Professional Partnership

A professional partnership is an organization of two or more persons or entities joined for a common purpose. Tax liability passes to the partners based on their shares of ownership. Each partner can be held responsible for the acts of the other.

Professional Limited Liability Company

A professional limited liability company is an organizational structure available in some states that combines the tax structure of a partnership with the liability protections of a professional corporation. In addition, it usually does not require the extensive legal and organizational structure of a corporation.

The owner-operators bear personal financial risk and experience an immediate sense of professional responsibility for the services and quality of care provided by the group. Typically, group practice providers whose professional reputations and financial stability are at stake through their signatures on a bank obligation are sharply focused on the clinical and business missions of their organizations. Solo practitioners are often in the

same situation regarding professional and financial responsibility, but often the group practice's scope of services and contractual obligations are more complex. In addition, their goals must be accomplished through group effort rather than the productivity of one individual who has more direct and immediate control.

Wholly Owned Behavioral Groups

Another type of group practice exists that meets the legal definitions of a group practice but, from the perspective of its operations, is much different. This is the professional group that is part of a regional healthcare system, a physician practice management business, an insurance company or managed care plan, or an academic medical center. As regional healthcare markets consolidate, and as access to capital and management expertise becomes more important for the viability of groups, practices tend to become parts of consolidated ventures and are more likely to be wholly owned subsidiaries of parent organizations.

In the past, some states were concerned that corporations with a purely business purpose and not owned by physicians could enter the practice of medicine by hiring physicians and other healthcare personnel. In states that have and enforce laws that prohibit the corporate practice of medicine, a business-owned healthcare group might sponsor a professional corporation whose sole owner is a physician who is the group's employee. That physician hires and manages physicians and other professionals who work for the sponsored professional corporation. In this situation, the healthcare professional/owner is in that position because he or she is an employee of the sponsoring entity. The business direction, strategic planning, administrative staff, and start-up capital may all come from the sponsoring organization.

Experience and performance data suggest that clinicians who work in wholly owned group practices tend to have lower productivity and to behave as employees without truly demonstrating the responsibility and motivation that occurs when clinicians have significant financial risk associated with their participation in the group. Even the method of compensation affects the group's performance and character. Kralewski et al. (1996) has discerned attitudinal differences between employed and self-employed group practice providers. These differences, identified in a 35-item questionnaire, accurately identify physicians who draw a salary from a prepaid group practice and those affiliated with fee-for-service practices.

Common Characteristics of Owner-Operated and Wholly Owned Behavioral Groups

The membership of the CBGP includes both owner-operated and wholly owned groups. Examples of sponsored or wholly owned groups include mental health departments of large multi-specialty medical group practices, professional practice plans of university medical school departments of psychiatry, the psychiatry departments of large general hospitals, and community-based clinics. Although these groups have a variety of ownership structures that are either taxable or tax exempt, each has to meet criteria that provide a good outline for the major administrative issues of concern to group practices. Table 28–1 sets forth CBGP membership requirements.

Despite varying organizational and ownership structures, groups that have demonstrated long-term viability tend to be composed of psychiatrists or other mental health professionals with roots in office-based outpatient practice settings. These groups add to their capabilities by employing additional professionals and widening their range of services to provide more diverse types of care and sometimes higher intensity outpatient services. Other than the combination of psychiatrists and other mental health professionals working together, there is no correct mix of professionals. The ideal mix depends on the needs and desires of patients and payment sources and the capabilities of the specific professionals.

Similarly, competitive and viable behavioral groups often pursue local and regional growth. They expand their service capacity by opening intensive care services, larger facilities, or service centers in multiple locations. The development of affiliated provider networks helps the groups cover a broader geographic area. Over time, these groups tend to attract capitation and at-risk contracts, develop cost-accounting and risk-management capabilities, and subsequently internalize many functions formerly assumed by managed care organizations such as intake assessment and triage, level-of-care determination, case management, and utilization review.

TABLE 28–1. Characteristics of members of the Council of Behavioral Group Practices

Administrative characteristics

Full economic and operational integration

Structured as a leading single-specialty behavioral group or the mental health department within a multi-specialty medical group

Professional management and administration in place to facilitate claims

Computerized management and medical information systems

A strong commitment to advanced training and leadership in managed behavioral healthcare

Clinical characteristics

10 or more equivalent behavioral health practitioners with psychiatrists fully integrated into the practice

Active involvement in the provision of managed behavioral healthcare services

Cost-effective and flexible treatment programs that use multidisciplinary treatment teams linked to a continuum-of-care delivery system

24-hour access and an emergency response system

An active quality assurance and/or quality management program

An active care management or continuity-of-care system

Source. Institute for Behavioral Healthcare, Council of Behavioral Group Practices. Used with permission.

Common key characteristics of group practices, at least as envisioned by the founders of the CBGP, are related to the development of systems of behavioral healthcare through integration of various clinical and administrative components. Group practices recognize the need to bring together key clinical elements, including continuous responsibility for clinical access and the availability of appropriate levels of care. They are able to provide appropriate care to a wider range of patients by having a critical mass of essential clinicians who are able to work together as a team and provide continuity of care through a continuum of clinical services.

A similar qualification exists on the administrative side, namely, full economic and operational integration. Specific administrative tasks required of groups include communication with patients, payers, and contractors; processing of all financial transactions; development and operation of programs to meet clinical and administrative needs; and management of resources and infrastructure required in order to take advantage of business opportunities.

CBGP administrative benchmark studies (Kramer et al. 1996) indicated that a group of 10 or more professionals is the minimum size required to achieve this level of systems integration efficiently and to be viable in competitive local markets. The group must be large enough to support professional administration and management. It is the administrators' job to determine and implement organizational structures and administrative processes that accomplish operational objectives while facilitating and supporting the clinical and business mission of the group practice.

Administrative and Clinical Leadership During Start-Up and Beyond

A key to group practice administration is reliability and consistency of leadership, tempered with the flexibility required to adjust to a rapidly changing environment. Through flexible operations and evolving organizational structures, and through business process development and continuous clinical process improvement, the groups move from relying solely on the energy and creativity of the founding individuals to establishing policies and programs that bring consistency to the group's operations and services.

The establishment of new administrative structures requires leadership and has a cost that can be justified only if the volume of services rendered is sufficient. Leadership during the start-up phases of many groups must focus on marketing and business development as well as clinical and operations issues in order to ensure that services rendered by the organized group substantiate the expenditures of time and effort required to make the endeavor worthwhile. This point is important because only when a basis of consistent practice and operations exists can variations in clinical services and outcomes be appropriately evaluated against standardized benchmarks.

During the start-up phase, the group initiates or maintains its organization for a purpose. Group leaders establish an assessment of needs or opportunities regarding professional practice, and they create a mission statement that defines the scope of the group practice's response to its local clinical service needs and opportunities and its vision for itself. The mission statement is translated into a strategic plan, setting forth a pattern for resource application, development of new services, and necessary support structures.

In some locations, this process of environmental and market needs assessment, articulation of the mission, and vision and implementation of strategic plans is reasonably straightforward. However, in most metropolitan areas, the penetration of managed behavioral healthcare companies, HMOs, and provider-based integrated delivery systems has made this a more complex process.

The leadership team has another core responsibility: development and implementation of a continuing process of assessing the national and local environment and developing strategic plans consistent with the vision and mission of the group practice and the resource capabilities of the group. A corollary is that the leadership team must develop and organize the administrative and clinical resources of the group practice to accomplish the objectives of the strategic plan. Being able to flexibly utilize the clinical resources of more than a few clinicians to consistently meet the needs of patients requesting services, and delivering those services within the boundaries of the patients' clinical needs and economic resources, is often a central aspect of the group's mission.

Group practice leadership responsibility clearly has both clinical and administrative aspects. Early in the process of formation, a clinician with administrative experience may serve in both roles, but the demands of a fully functioning group practice require specific attention to each leadership area. Clinical and administrative leaders have complementary but different objectives. The processes of office organization, telephone communication, billing, and financial management are quite different from ensuring quality clinical care and allocating clinical resources appropriately. The continuing success of a group as a viable clinical and economic entity is often related to the clear definition of boundaries and mutual respect.

The differentiating asset of the group practice is the depth and breadth of its services. Multiple clinicians mean open access and clinical diversity. Multiple locations broaden the patient base by satisfying the patients' and payers' interests in easy geographic access. Other important features include office space management, personnel administration, handling of patient accounts and the group's financial structure, as well as regulatory compliance.

Group Approaches to Contracting for the Provision of Clinical Services

Unlike community mental health centers and nonprofit community-based organizations, groups have rarely been financed on a cost-plus basis by public-sector funding streams. Contracting for the provision of clinical services has distinguished behavioral groups from both solo practice clinicians and nonprofit community-based organizations. Because entrepreneurial savvy is required to function within this context, recruitment and supervision of staff have been critical tasks of group practices, particularly in the 1970s and early 1980s, before capitation contracting became as prevalent as it is today. In the past the group's accessibility, availability, and clinical reputation were often sufficient to ensure consistent fee-for-service patient flow in a system in which referring professionals and patients established individual treatment contracts with free choice of clinician. With the development of managed care organizations and organized health plans, payers have increasingly contracted with groups and the organized healthcare system to which they belong. These contemporary contracts specify a set of behavioral healthcare benefits. When such contracts specify different services for different beneficiaries, and when they are coupled with financial incentives and disincentives for the group, a complex management system is required. This type of management is typically not available for solo practice clinicians. In contrast, community mental health centers and nonprofit community-based organizations have extensive management structures that have been directed toward fulfilling bureaucratic and regulatory requirements. In many agencies these administrative resources are now being refocused on meeting the competitive aspect of today's contracting environment. With new productivity requirements and incentives, these restructured organizations resemble group practices.

Behavioral healthcare benefits and services are increasingly being purchased through the intermediary of managed care organizations or organized health plans. In the past, patients took responsibility for securing their own care, either paying for it themselves or obtaining reimbursement for their payment from indemnity insurance plans. Purchasing entities, such as an employer, a business coalition, or a state department of medical assistance, had only limited requirements for participation in the payment process. Insurers would accept invoices from any licensed provider. This level of contracting was easily accommodated by solo practice clinicians.

In the late 1980s, payers became increasingly aware of the high variability of services, uncertainty about quality, and waste generated by fee-for-service reimbursement systems. Given the need and desire to control costs, the business opportunity for the development of managed care organizations created a commensurate opportunity for the development of behavioral groups. Managed care organizations must ensure that the services provided are both affordable and consistent with what the benefit plan covers. They must ensure that costs are controlled through the elimination of unnecessary, inappropriate, or high-cost services. The managed care organization must also interface with providers who can help them address quality of care concerns.

These performance requirements of managed care organizations establish their need to contract with behavioral group practices. Managed care organizations' obligations to their customers initiate a cycle of interaction with providers who are called on to fulfill the managed care organization's promise to deliver services according to contracted specifications.

As managed behavioral healthcare organizations developed national management structures and provider networks, the advantages of contracting with behavioral groups became apparent. Employers and other customers of managed care organizations require assurance that managed care companies are delivering services as specified in the contracts. These payer requirements have resulted in a broad quality and accountability mandate for the field, exemplified by the National Committee for Quality Assurance (NCQA), a managed care accrediting organization that now has specific accreditation standards and criteria for behavioral health (National Committee on Quality Assurance 1996).

The behavioral healthcare marketplace continues to be favorable to behavioral group practice as it evolves more sophisticated requirements to demonstrate the value of services, to meet contract expectations, and to manage the clinical and functional outcomes of care. Managed care companies also respond to another aspect of competitive market pressures, the mandate for lower price. Group practices have been one component of the behavioral health delivery system that has actively responded to these shifting market forces. Because of their accumulation of resources that can be flexibly deployed and their experience in sharing responsibility for the quality of services, behavioral group practices are naturally adapted to the managed care environment. In this environment, providers and care managers are obligated to do much more than deliver a unit of professional service to a particular patient.

Horizontal Integration, Vertical Integration, and Strategic Alliances

As managed care plans and regional health systems consolidate, the independent behavioral group practice experiences a variety of pressures to affiliate with larger regional or national organizations. In response to these competitive pressures, horizontal integration, vertical integration, and strategic alliances are increasingly popular among groups. In a horizontally integrated structure, groups that provide similar services such as outpatient care may join to increase geographic coverage, reduce administrative overhead, or share a common referral access system. In contrast, vertical integration brings together different system components such as assessment, crisis intervention, outpatient treatment, day hospital treatment, and inpatient treatment. In such a system, patients can move from one level of care to another. One important differentiation is that services may have working relationships developed to fulfill a business purpose. These strategic alliances are often a step on the way to an integrated services system but do not have the economic and organizational structure that characterizes a truly integrated system.

Development of integrated behavioral health delivery systems involves a substantial cost. The costs are related to administrative processes, information systems, communication systems, financial services, consultation fees, legal fees, and transition costs, some hard to quantify. Many hospitals have joined with their medical staff organizations to form physician-hospital organizations (PHOs). Sometimes considerable time and money are spent without considering how a particular integrated delivery system will recoup the resources spent in organization and operation. Important questions to consider include the following:

- How will the PHO improve the quality of care? Will staff be willing to share information about utilization and outcome so that best practices can be rewarded?

- Will the PHO be able to develop new and needed services, making them accessible to patients and financially attractive to payers?
- Can the PHO take a hard look at redundant services, making the necessary changes to improve efficiency and reduce unit cost?
- Can the physician and the administrative members of the PHO work together, responding to the requirements of the market when necessary, standing firm when quality of care is threatened if long-term economic benefit does not justify a decision?

Administrative structure and information systems will not be of much assistance unless an integrated delivery system is ready to address these questions and a local healthcare market is ready to contract with provider-based organizations.

Another type of system integration arrangement that is becoming more common is the professional corporation that is in partnership with a hospital, healthcare company, insurance company, other group within a region, or other health-related business such as a physician practice management company. The affiliated or partnering entity may own or be responsible for most or all of the physical resources of the practice (i.e., furniture, computers, office equipment, office leases, and the like) and may also employ a number of the staff, sometimes all but the physicians or key clinicians. The structure is often based on a partnership between a professional corporation and a management service organization, a business corporation that provides management services.

Even within this particular partnership or joint venture structure, arrangements vary regarding governance, administration, financial risks, and incentives. At one end of the spectrum is the professional corporation shell, in which all the stock is owned by a physician employee of a business corporation. This physician owes his or her continued employment to the business corporation. This arrangement involves no financial risk to the physician. Of course the owner's continued employment depends on how he or she leads or manages the corporation. At the other end of the spectrum can be a strong professional group practice owned by practicing professionals, each of whom can be either an equal or a dominant component in the partnership arrangement. As in any business endeavor, what each partner brings and sustains in terms of capital (financial and in-kind), creativity, and expertise will determine the success of the partnership.

Group practices and partnership relationships are set out in written agreements and contracts that legally establish relationships. The contracts set forth arrangements that seem equitable and appropriate when the contracts are signed but may not endure over time, in response to changes within the organizations that make up the partnership or changes in the surrounding environment. The group practice and its institutional partner may have excellent alignment of vision and incentives at the initiation of the partnership but may find themselves unable to sustain the partnership over time because of dramatic changes in the external environment. For example, a joint venture between a hospital and a group practice to develop and run a residential substance abuse treatment center may have been an appropriate response to local market characteristics in 1980 but could not have been sustained unless an effective process was in place to change the vision, mission, and responsibilities as patterns of practice and payment changed. The group practice that is a professional shell, owned by the healthcare institution, will follow the objectives and priorities of its institutional owner. The co-equal or strong group practice will have more mutual participation and also more responsibility in evaluating the changing situation and making decisions to effectively respond to those changes. In any case, the organization's success is likely to depend on the capacity of the leadership to get the buy-in of the key people who make up the group practice.

Building Core Competencies for Business and Service Development

A critical function of the leadership of group practices is to get information about national and regional changes or trends that may affect the group. The leadership evaluates the significance of this information and determines a course of action for the group. The solo practitioner does this through a process of continuing clinical education that incorporates new diagnostic skills for therapeutic capabilities. As solo practice clinicians gain new clinical skills and information, they appreciate new clinical service opportunities. The solo practitioner may be limited by insufficient clinical opportunity or resources to utilize a treatment innovation effectively. Successful group practices have a clinical ad-

ministrative structure that facilitates the transfer of new clinical understandings derived from external sources, lectures, readings, professional meetings and training, and the group's internal experience.

The interaction of multiple professionals with their partners more rapidly and consistently brings new research and insights to bear on clinical treatment. Therapeutic and psychoeducational groups; evaluation and decision making; clinical records assisted by forms, questionnaires, and computer software; more rapid and broad experience with innovations in the use of psychopharmacologic agents; and presentation of organized clinical data are some examples of effective clinical and administrative processes that facilitate clinical change. These clinical development resources are well established, easily accessible, and generally of reasonable cost. The process of this clinical information is often as available to the solo practicing and institutionally practicing professional as it is to those in group practices.

Information that relates to business processes and management services is less familiar, less available, and more unusual, depending on practice setting and structure. Since 1990 a whole information industry has developed to address the need for information and administrative tools to deal with changing healthcare economics and structures. A multitude of books, audiotapes, workshops, conferences, and consultants address the desire to structure healthcare delivery systems and, specifically, behavioral healthcare delivery systems that will survive the healthcare economic revolution.

Although many resources are available to behavioral group practices, the most focused resources are those provided by the IBH at its annual Behavioral Healthcare Tomorrow conference. This meeting provides special focused professional education for groups, supplemented by an intensive full-day retreat for behavioral group practices. The agenda for the annual retreat and a large part of the group practice track of the conference are determined by the steering committee of the CBGP, informed by an educational needs assessment survey of the council's member group practices. Excerpts from the survey completed in early 1997 provide insight into the concerns, competency development needs, questions, and educational requirements of behavioral group practice leaders and administrators (Table 28–2). The respondents' ratings and suggestions indicate the challenges that behavioral healthcare groups face in today's dynamic market (Table 28–3 and Table 28–4).

TABLE 28–2. Competency development objectives for behavioral group practices in 1997

High priority

Cost management and efficiency strategies

How to form linkages with primary care provider settings

Medical cost offset services

Managing capitated services

Implementing and using performance indicators

New product and service innovations for groups

Intermediate priority

Benchmarking clinical and quality performance

Benchmarking administrative performance

Provider and group practice productivity measurement

Clinical process improvement

Quality assurance

Marketing group practices to primary care and the general medical sector

Management information systems improvement, procurement, and administration

Outcomes management

Marketing groups directly to employers

Source.   Institute for Behavioral Healthcare 1997. Used with permission.

Analysis of the survey responses on educational needs and the accompanying comments makes clear that a primary concern of these group practice leaders is cost-management and operating-efficiency strategies, particularly incentive compensation for employed clinical or administrative staff. Another objective of behavioral healthcare groups is learning how to form linkages with primary care provider settings and how to develop medical cost offset services that work. The overall theme is the desire for educational experiences that can be translated directly into practices that will promptly improve operations.

Establishing Excellence in a Changing Environment

According to Peter Schultz, chief executive officer of Porsche from 1981 to 1987,

> [T]he only purpose of management is to deal with change. One of the most important roles of a chief executive officer is to make sure that people understand in the clearest and simplest possible terms what...we are trying to do around here. There are three pieces to being a manager: people, process,

TABLE 28–3. Council of Behavioral Group Practices (CBGP) Institute for Behavioral Healthcare retreat and symposium educational needs assessment

Survey question: Please rate how important it is for your organization to receive focused, skill building education about:	Average rating[a]
Cost management and efficiency strategies	2.61
Medical cost offset services that work	2.55
Managing capitated services effectively	2.52
Performance indicators for group practices	2.48
New product and service innovations for groups	2.48
Benchmarking clinical and quality performance indicators	2.40
Performance measurement in groups	2.38
Benchmarking administrative performance indicators	2.37
Clinical process improvement	2.34
Quality assurance	2.34
Utilization and case management systems	2.26
Group psychotherapy and other cost-effective services	2.24
Measuring patient satisfaction	2.10
Intensive case management	1.98
Risk management and re-insurance	1.96
Capital formation for behavioral groups	1.78

[a]Ratings: 3=very important; 0=not important.

and structure. Success does not depend on finding a group of superstars. The secret to the success is to get extraordinary results out of ordinary people in the process and structure of the organization appropriate for what you are trying to do. (Schultz 1996)

The purpose of behavioral group practices is to deliver accessible, affordable, appropriate, and effective behavioral health services in a changing environment. Group practice professionals establish an organization with the belief that delivering behavioral health services consistent with the vision of the group's leadership requires a combination of resources, structure, and processes that are different from those available, either in solo practices or in the various types of institutional delivery systems. In the purest form of behavioral group practice, the ownership and governance are vested in health professionals who are, or at least have been, involved in clinical practice. This feature is changing as business corporations, insurance companies, and healthcare organizations—both not-for-profit and investor owned—purchase clinical practices. Critical to the success of the organization are the extent to which

TABLE 28–4.   Results of Council of Behavioral Group Practices (CBGP) Institute for Behavioral Healthcare educational needs assessment

Survey question: Please rate the importance of including each of the following topics:	Average rating[a]
How to form linkages with primary care provider settings	2.57
How to measure practice performance and provider productivity	2.36
How to market your group to primary care and the general medical sector	2.34
Management information systems products for behavioral group practices	2.32
Outcomes management: providing tools for evaluation and improvement	2.32
How to market your group directly to large regional employers	2.31
How to develop and effectively price capitated contracts	2.27
How to identify high-risk, high-cost cohorts and develop targeted interventions	2.21
High-performance behavioral group practices: interpreting CBGP benchmarking study data	2.20
How to form linkages with integrated delivery systems	2.18
How to subcapitate mental health from medical groups and delivery systems	2.14
Group practice consolidation and implications for behavioral group practices	2.13
How to prepare for accreditation by NCQA and the Joint Commission on Accreditation of Healthcare Organizations	2.05
How to market your groups to Medicare behavioral health purchasers and serve Medicare recipients	2.05
How to form and market provider-sponsored networks	2.02
How to manage burnout and stress in group practice providers	2.02
How to market your groups to Medicaid and serve Medicaid recipients	1.98
How to market your groups to child and family services purchasers and serve child and family service recipients	1.96
Downloading case management: mutual expectations between groups and managed care organizations	1.96
How to form linkages with nonprofit, community-based providers	1.95
How to market your groups to public substance abuse payers and serve public substance abuse service recipients	1.86
How to market your groups to criminal justice purchasers and serve criminal justice recipients	1.75
Other: developing non-managed-care products and services to round out a group's financial portfolio	

[a]Ratings: 3=very important; 0=not important.

the people that make up the organization buy into the organization's mission and how those tasked with leading and managing the organization implement that mission in a changing environment.

References

Goldstein D: Group practice revolution: leading the way in restructuring health care delivery. Group Practice Journal 46(1):12–28, 1997

Institute for Behavioral Healthcare: Educational Needs Assessment. Tiburon, CA, Council of Behavioral Group Practices, Institute for Behavioral Healthcare, 1997

Kralewski JE, Wingert TD, Barbouche MH: Assessing the culture of medical group practices. Med Care 34:377–388, 1996

Kramer T, Daniels A, Mahesh N: National Leadership Council on Performance Indicators in Behavioral Healthcare: Measures of Access, Appropriateness, Quality, Outcomes and Prevention. Tiburon, CA, Institute for Behavioral Healthcare, 1996

Mitka M: Doctors opt for employment, larger groups. American Medical News 40(3):1, 1997

National Committee on Quality Assurance: 1997 Standards for Accreditation of Managed Behavioral Healthcare Organizations. Washington, DC, National Committee on Quality Assurance, 1996

Schultz P: The Porsche Story: Implementing Decisions. CEO speaker series on audiotape, 1996. San Diego, CA, The Executive Committee, 1996

Resources for Behavioral Group Practices

Group Practice Journal, 1422 Duke St., Alexandria, VA 22308

Institute for Behavioral Healthcare, 1110 Mar West Street, Suite E, Tiburon, CA 94920

National Committee for Quality Assurance, 2000 L St., Suite 500, Washington, DC 20036

The Executive Committee, 5469 Kearny Villa Rd., San Diego, CA 92123-1159; 800-274-2367; fax 800-934-4540

Daniels A, Dickman N, Zieman G: The Comprehensive Group Practice Tool Kit: A Manual for Behavioral Group Practice Development and Management. Tiburon, CA, CentraLink Publications, 1995.

Use this resource to help establish, operate, and improve integrated behavioral group practice. The Tool Kit includes a diskette containing working policies, procedures, and forms currently used in behavioral group practices with models, templates, and examples related to staffing and personnel, patient accounts, clinical records, intake and clinical pathways, and quality improvement.

Daniels A, Dickman N, Zieman G: The Comprehensive Managed Care Tool Kit: A Manual for Capitated and Managed Behavioral Healthcare Delivery Systems. Tiburon, CA, CentraLink Publications, 1996.

Use this resource to give your behavioral healthcare organization the policies, procedures, protocols, and proven tools it needs to develop the appropriate infrastructure to enter capitated contracting; cost out a capitation bid and write a full capitation proposal; set up the intake and utilization review staff to make capitation profitable; increase your readiness for NCQA accreditation; and benchmark your organization's systems against three successful delivery systems.

Daniels A, Kramer T, Mahesh N: Behavioral Group Practice Performance Characteristics: IBH's Council of Behavioral Group Practices Benchmarking Study. Tiburon, CA, CentraLink Publications, 1995.

This tool will show you how to establish benchmarking standards for the operation and development of your behavioral group practice. This resource includes benchmarking data regarding practice size and location, revenue sources, budget allocations, credentialing and peer review, clinical staffing, and compensation.

Daniels A, Zieman G, Kramer T, et al: The Behavioral Healthcare Quality and Accountability Tool Kit. Tiburon, CA, CentraLink Publications, 1997.

This comprehensive resource guide is designed to serve as a framework for the implementation of quality programs throughout your organization. It provides currently used policies, procedures, and other resources in the areas of performance measurement, practice guidelines, outcomes management, quality improvement, and accreditation standards compliance.

Kramer T, Daniels A, Mahesh N: National Leadership Council on Performance Indicators in Behavioral Healthcare: Measures of Access, Appropriateness, Quality, Outcomes and Prevention. Tiburon, CA, Institute for Behavioral Healthcare, 1996.

Review the results of the national survey of behavioral healthcare organizations' performance indicators in action today. Performance indicators address access, clinical appropriateness, quality, outcomes, and prevention.

Zieman G: The Complete Capitation Handbook: How to Design and Implement At-Risk Contracts for Behavioral Healthcare. Tiburon, CA, CentraLink Publications, 1995.

More than 20 pioneering providers tell you how they succeeded with capitation contracting. Includes sections on writing, negotiating, and implementing at-risk contracts; designing outcomes studies; designing total quality management initiatives; understanding ethical issues related to capitation; and learning from case studies.

❖ 29 ❖

Children's Services

V. Susan Villani, M.D.

Child and adolescent mental health services have undergone rapid and all-encompassing changes. Major forces that have affected children's services include the sweeping changes of managed care and mandates at the level of state government to change how services are provided to severely disturbed children and adolescents, who have traditionally received care in the public sector. In some states these forces have converged, resulting in the closing of state hospitals for children and adolescents and the shifting of care to managed medical assistance provided by general hospitals and private psychiatric hospitals.

Administrators of children's services have always been challenged to provide care that integrates the best interests of the child across the biopsychosocial spectrum, from both short-term and longitudinal perspectives. Treatment services have ideally been inclusive of, but not dominated by, the interests of the parents and family, while still operating within the financial limits set by societal imperatives. The recent shift in societal imperatives (i.e., demanding lower costs) has led to the sweeping changes in how care is delivered. According to Geraty et al. (1992, p. 398), "Managed care represents more than a new approach to healthcare; it represents a new shift in societal values. Society is declaring

that there are limits to healthcare spending and that employers, the government, and individuals are reaching the extent of their resources."

Such changes have required administrators to be creative with service system design, relying less on restrictive and costly levels of care while caring for a population that is associated with an increasing number of risk management factors and that requires different services at different ages and stages of development. Amidst such sweeping developments is great potential for children's growth and development to be optimized through care that is less restrictive and more normalizing, if the focus can be maintained on the integration of care and long-term positive outcomes.

In the first section of this chapter I describe the administrative impact of the special and unique needs of children. The implications of developmental level and behavioral functioning on treatment planning, program design, and staffing are outlined. In the second section I describe the movement away from the dichotomous thinking of outpatient versus inpatient care to a more complex approach that utilizes services across a full continuum of care. In the third section I elaborate on the risk management factors now operant in the delivery of child and adolescent mental health services.

Each of these sections includes examples of common administrative problems. In the final section I summarize how the changes under consideration will affect the management and financing of child and adolescent services. Ethical questions about the future of sharing what is now considered proprietary outcome data are also posed for the reader's consideration. Whether care is delivered through health maintenance organizations (HMOs) or carved-out managed care entities, administrators will likely face the challenge of integrating the complex biopsychosocial needs of children while delivering less costly services and maximizing the child's potential for long-term gains and for healthy adult life functioning.

Administrative Impact of the Special and Unique Needs of Children and Adolescents

Providing care for children has traditionally been recognized as labor intensive, with the general axiom prevailing that the younger the child the more staff necessary to ensure safety, daily care, and feeding. A survey of members of the National Association of Private Psychiatric Hospitals found that child programs typically average close to twice the staff required in adult programs (1.7 full-time equivalents of direct-care staff per child) (Gibson 1981). The developmental level of the population being served also requires psychiatric milieu programming and staffing that is appropriate for the child's age and level. Services geared toward very young children (e.g., under age 5 years) usually consist of therapeutic nursery-based programs or outpatient treatment that is parent-child focused. In milieu-based programs such as hospital units, group homes, or residential facilities, the program design needs to take into account whether the program will be serving school-age children, preadolescents, or adolescents. It has generally been considered unsafe for adolescents and school-age children to reside together, given the potential for the younger children's needs to be overwhelmed by the adolescents' or for the younger children to be victimized by the adolescents. Thus, the usually recommended age groupings in children's services programs are ages 3 to 5, ages 6 to 12, and ages 13 through 17. See Table 29–1 for a list of treatment components that need to be included, but adapted accordingly, regardless of age.

TABLE 29–1. Areas of milieu treatment that must be adapted to developmental level

Daily schedule, including bedtime and wake-up time
Number of staff necessary for activities of daily living such as bathing, dressing, and eating
Therapeutic groups—the focus of the group and the length of time that the group lasts
Arts and crafts groups—materials used
Music groups—kind of music listened to
Activity-based groups such as dance, gym, and athletics
Behavioral management programming, including privilege-level system
Space design and furnishings

Whatever the specific age group, clinical staff need to be well versed in the developmental tasks for the index client age and must know what constitutes age-appropriate behavior. The Joint Commission on Accreditation of Healthcare Organizations (1990) added standards developed by nationally recognized multidisciplinary experts on child and adolescent services. These standards emphasized the clinical privileging of staff based on competence; patient rights; comfortable and safe physical and social environment; family involvement in assessment; treatment and continuing care; patient records that include a complete physical health assessment, immunization status, psychosocial assessment, and growth and developmental history; play and daily activities; and a physical health assessment that includes motor development and function, sensorimotor functioning, and visual functioning. Compliance with such specific child competency standards necessitates that staff training begins with the orientation process and uses more than one developmental paradigm. For example, a facility may choose to focus on Erikson's stages of psychosocial development (Erikson 1963) combined with some basic knowledge regarding the development of cognitive capacity as described by Piaget (1963). Staff training usually should also include milieu treatment principles as elaborated by Aichhorn (1935), Bettelheim (1974), Stanton and Schwartz (1954), and Redl and Wineman (1957). Generally speaking, the more advanced the staff role, from child care worker to board-certified child and adolescent clinician, the greater the knowledge and expertise about child and adolescent development. The paradox, however, for administrators of children's services, is that the time actually spent with the patient for a given clinical role is usually inversely proportional to the place of that clinical role in the clinical staff hierarchy. Thus, the child care worker with the least training in developmental issues is often spending the most time directly with the patient. This reality means that administrators of children's services must pay close attention to staff training on child and adolescent development and must provide ongoing staff supervision at all levels.

The amount and degree of parent and family involvement also varies with the child's age. Younger children need much closer involvement from one or both parents. This is not to minimize the importance of family treatment for older children and adolescents. Parents must be closely aligned with the treatment plan and the treatment team's goals and methods, in order for the plan to be effective. Administratively, achieving this partnership requires staffing that includes skilled social workers who possess solid understanding of the manifestations and treatment of mental illness in children and adolescents. These clinicians must also be knowledgeable about the psychodynamics of families and informed about modern-day societal issues.

In addition to staff and program differences with children, space needs are also different for adolescents in a number of ways. Play space, both indoor and outdoor, is essential not only for the patients being served but also for the activity needs of siblings, who may be brought along to the identified patient's treatment or who may be present for family therapy sessions. The treatment unit's or outpatient clinic's space must be cheerful, should be furnished with indestructible furniture, and should contain toys and reading material for all developmental levels and ages. When it comes to destructive potential, children and adolescents are often very creative and also potentially dangerous to themselves or others. Youngsters might climb on chairs and tables, dismantle furniture or electrical sockets, write or draw on walls, and in general wreak a degree of havoc that is not usually the case in treatment settings with adult patients.

Lessons From the Lion's Den (Cotton 1993), a comprehensive book that addresses these issues, is filled with abundant examples that illustrate the useful and well-organized considerations of children's inpatient treatment. This book effectively imparts the author's wisdom and knowledge and is a valuable reference for administrators of any kind of milieu-based program along the continuum of child and adolescent services.

Consider the following examples of problems that commonly occur during the typical work week of an administrator of children's services:

Problem #1

An 8-year-old male was admitted at 8 P.M. to an inpatient psychiatric unit for safety and containment following a serious suicide attempt by hanging. The patient was described as being very close to his mother, having trouble leaving the house to go to school, and becoming easily overwhelmed in new situations. After the decision was made to hospitalize the child, he became tearful and began to cry loudly, pleading for his mother not to leave him. The mother became very displeased with the staff who were trying to help her leave the unit, and she insisted that the director of the hospital be called.

Formulation and solution. The child in this example was experiencing separation anxiety and panic superimposed on his suicidal condition. Problems like this are common in this age group. The child might not have slept away from home before, let alone spent a night in a hospital setting. Staff who are well trained in developmental issues would recognize this and be able to engage the mother in helping the child to settle. The mother needed to feel that the unit was a friendly, safe place for her young child and that the staff were not judging her. She needed to believe that they would be able to comfort her son and not punish him for his behavior. Useful and necessary responses to be used by the staff in helping this parent and her distraught child to separate successfully include suggesting to the mother that she bring a special stuffed animal or other transitional object from home, call the child at regular prescheduled times to reassure him, and be clear about when she will return to visit. When not approached in a developmentally enlightened manner, this kind of situation is almost certain to escalate, and a valuable opportunity to strengthen an essential family treatment alliance will have been lost.

Problem #2

A 16-year-old female was seen by a male social work therapist in weekly outpatient treatment for depressed mood and irritability and for refusing to cooperate with family rules, listening to loud "shock rock" music, and insisting on dressing in black. The therapist had not met with the parents and had not returned their calls. They angrily called the clinic administrator. When approached by the administrator, the therapist insisted that if he spoke with the parents he would be violating his patient's right to confidentiality.

Formulation and solution. The therapist's concern about confidentiality was at the expense of a more complete evaluation of the patient within her family context. The evaluation phase of treatment must almost always include meeting with the parents. The patient in this situation may have successfully enlisted the unwitting therapist in her adolescent rebellion. Although such rebellion can be a normal developmental phase during adolescence, this particular patient could be in danger. The therapist could have been unaware of this because of his failure to develop a treatment alliance with the parents, from whom further important collateral information could have been obtained. Of note in this example is the importance of keeping abreast of current music trends when providing treatment to adolescents. The music chosen by this adolescent, so-called shock rock, is among the most offensive currently on the market, in its mingling of casual sex with violence in an overtly gruesome, macabre manner. Given the other symptoms exhibited by this adolescent, her attraction to this particular style of music may indicate that she is at greater risk for self-harm than if her musical preferences were otherwise.

Developing and Utilizing the Full Continuum of Care

The increasing application of medical necessity criteria to the utilization of inpatient hospitalization has resulted in shorter length of stays and greater reliance on less restrictive levels of care in the treatment of psychiatric disorders in youth. The focus of hospitalization has changed from one of comprehensive evaluation and treatment to an approach that emphasizes focal treatment as described first by Nurcombe (1987) and further modified by Harper (1989). In a focal approach the goal of treatment is often limited to getting the patient out of the hospital by stabilization of the specific crisis that precipitated the need for a hospital level of care. Further treatment goals are then addressed in partial hospital programs, respite programs, and home-based treatment services as components of the continuum of care for children and adolescents. Such treatment contexts can serve as both step-down and diversion from the hospital setting. This decreased reliance on inpatient treatment has been a major impetus both for developing creative alternative services and for combining services in unique ways. The combination of services to specifically meet complex, often chronic, patient needs is sometimes referred to as *wraparound services,* a term that derives from providers of clinical programs endeavoring to wrap treatment services around the child and family (England and Cole 1992).

Coincident with the development of services along the continuum of clinical care has been significant growth of special educational settings that combine educational services provided to psychiatrically impaired youth with individual, group, and family treatment. Many special education schools have doubled the number of youth served, with particular expansion at the high school/adolescent level. In some states the number of children and adolescents in group homes and residential treatment centers has increased. The number of children with severe emotional disturbances who need comprehensive treatment has not decreased, but this treatment no longer occurs in psychiatric inpatient units.

Table 29–2 lists the levels of care typically present in a modern-day continuum of care (Villani and Fassler 1995). As healthcare systems mature, it is anticipated that more systems will offer services at all levels of the continuum, each connected to the other through clinical philosophy and with the availability of continuity of caregivers, as patients move seamlessly from one level of care to another.

Consider the following examples of problems that arise from this rapid expansion of the continuum:

Problem #1

A child and adolescent day hospital had operated well for several years under the leadership of a program director whose background was nonclinical but who was a talented, trained recreational therapist. With the changing marketplace, however, came the need to expand the continuum of care to include a respite program. The respite program would be used as diversion to prevent hospitalization and also as a step-down from inpatient treatment. In either case, patients would receive clinical care through the day hospital, and the respite program would be under the umbrella of the day hospital and its program director. Although the written narrative and planning phases of the new program proceeded easily, when implementation got under way, the program director began to experience major problems. He was unable to successfully recruit child care workers to staff the program on nights and weekends and did not successfully manage the interface with the inpatient units. Management consultation through a higher level administrator sought to clarify the problem and consider alternatives.

Formulation and solution. After multiple attempts to help the program director improve his administrative performance, a decision was made to change the leadership of the respite program. The leader of such a program clearly needed to be comfortable with operating a program 24 hours a day, seven days a week. The individual to be recruited could be a nurse, a social worker, or a psychologist. The successful candidate needed to be someone

TABLE 29–2. Levels of care in a comprehensive continuum

Outpatient
Intensive outpatient
Home-based services
Mobile emergency service
Crisis stabilization
Observation bed
Respite
Acute residential
Partial hospital program
Therapeutic group home
Therapeutic foster care
Acute inpatient program
Residential

with clinical skills, solid inpatient experience, and an understanding of staffing needs for a program where patients would be living.

Problem #2

An experienced child psychiatrist called the director of child and adolescent services to discuss the referral of a 14-year-old female for inpatient hospitalization. The patient was described as depressed and argumentative with her mother on a daily basis about going to school, yet she was not suicidal. During individual sessions over the preceding two weeks, the patient had become more sullen and essentially now came to therapy and spoke very little. She was also refusing to take medication. The treating clinician felt there was little choice but to hospitalize this increasingly unstable patient.

Formulation and solution. Although this patient was clearly not getting better with standard outpatient treatment, she did not meet medical necessity criteria for inpatient hospitalization. The director discussed with the referring psychiatrist the possibility of having the patient admitted to the day hospital program. On further discussion of what such a program could provide, this indeed seemed to make the most sense. This option had simply not occurred to the referring clinician because he had trained 10 years earlier, when there were no day hospitals. He remembered treating on inpatient units many patients like the one he was referring.

The patient and her family were scheduled for an intake meeting at the day hospital the next day. At the conclusion of that meeting, the family's insurance company was called, the case reviewed, and authorization for admission given. After 2 days in the day hospital program and hearing several other adolescents in group therapy discuss how medication had been helpful to them, the patient agreed to a trial of an antidepressant. Within 1 week she was

responding positively to the medication, actively participating in groups, and concentrating better as reflected in her schoolwork in the classroom located within the day hospital. She had begun to talk more openly to her therapist. She was discharged, much improved, to the care of her outpatient therapist after 12 days of day hospital treatment.

Risk Management Issues

As patients move more quickly through less restrictive settings, coupled with dramatic advancements in the use of psychopharmacology, combined with societal trends and changes, risk management issues relevant to child and adolescent psychiatry have increased significantly. Regarding psychopharmacology alone, child psychiatrists are initiating medications earlier in treatment in order to achieve faster alleviation of symptoms and shorten the time necessary for treatment. A child or adolescent may be discharged, after a brief hospitalization of less than 1 week, with prescriptions for two or three different medications. The tradition in child psychiatry has been for community standards of practice regarding the use of medications to precede the research literature. This has become even more striking with the increase in the number and kinds of medications marketed; the relatively low side effect profiles of the newer medications; and managed care's insistence on brief, symptom-focused treatment.

As for the impact of societal trends and changes, children by their very nature of being dependent on adults for care and shelter, are most vulnerable. Factors that affect children include the increased number of children living in single-parent homes, the continued rise in domestic and family violence, and the increased incidence of sexual abuse and sexually transmitted diseases within younger and younger children. Administrators of children's services often feel beleaguered by the management of cases complicated by psychosocial factors, which have increased short- and long-term risk. Table 29–3 lists some of the factors that complicate treatment and increase risk. Several factors are discussed in more depth in the sections that follow.

Divorcing Parents

Parents engaged in high-conflict divorce frequently cannot agree on the treatment needs of their children. Their reporting of behaviors and vegetative symptoms is often different, resulting in disagreements about psychopharmacologic recommendations and compliance

TABLE 29–3. Factors that complicate treatment and increase risk

Divorcing parents engaged in high-conflict divorce[a]
One or both parents drug addicted or incarcerated
One or both parents with AIDS
Child with history of physical or sexual abuse
Child in temporary or permanent custody of the state department of social services
Child or adolescent with sexually transmitted disease
Child or adolescent with AIDS[a]
Child or adolescent with history of violence or threats of violence[a]
Child or adolescent with history of sexually predatory threats or behaviors[a]

[a]Discussed in more depth in this chapter.

problems. The medical record must contain a copy of the separation agreement as soon as it exists and, later, a copy of the final divorce agreement as it pertains to custody and the ability of the custodial parent to make medical decisions, with or without the input of the noncustodial parent. If custody is joint and disagreements about treatment persist, it may be necessary to request that the court appoint a guardian to act in the best interest of the child.

Children With AIDS

The impact of the AIDS epidemic is now felt in child and adolescent psychiatry. Sometimes children with AIDS are psychiatrically hospitalized, and sometimes several children on a unit have one or both parents dying from AIDS. The tragedy of the disease itself is compounded by the difficult and life-threatening behaviors that children with AIDS sometimes exhibit. They may attempt to bite staff when being physically restrained or to spit at them with particular aim toward the eyes or mouth. The pervasive anger and rage that these children exhibit, which underlie their behaviors, are particularly difficult for staff to manage given the life-threatening actions that are aimed at them. Staff must receive regular, up-to-date training from infectious disease staff about universal precautions and about what to do if precautions are violated.

Children With a History of Violence or Threats of Violence

Although the general incidence of violence has been reported to be decreasing, in many areas of the United States it continues to increase in the adolescent population. Violent patients previously contained in safe, locked inpatient units now receive treatment at various levels of care in the continuum. The concerns that arise in treatment settings essentially parallel those present in large, urban public school settings where more and more children and adolescents bring weapons to school and a greater number of children use violence as a way to resolve conflicts with peers and adults. Staff need to be well trained in the assessment of a child's or adolescent's potential for violence, in aggression prevention and management techniques and skills, and in determining when to seek forensic consultation regarding a patient's potential for dangerousness. Being attuned to violence in the media and music is also particularly important and requires continual attention (Strasburger and Dietz 1991). This issue extends to the management of television and video watching, computer access, and the kinds of music that are permitted in various treatment settings. For clinical staff, taking a media history has become increasingly important as a way to assess the patient's inner world and his or her potential for violence.

Children With a History of Sexually Predatory Threats or Behaviors

This area has many similarities to the issue of children with a history of violence. Staff training and the availability of consultation from forensic specialists with expertise in this area are important. Although these cases are less frequent than are cases involving violent adolescents, when they occur they are particularly worrisome, whether the child is evaluated and treated as an inpatient, outpatient, or at any level of care in between. Again, it is important for staff to be well versed in the current trends of sex and violence as portrayed in all forms of media.

Summary

The general risk management principles of thorough evaluation, good documentation, and consultation or second opinions when indicated are the mainstays of each of the risk management issues described in the preceding sections. The additional emphasis on thorough staff training that is tailored to children and adolescents and regularly updated to include changing societal issues, new laws, and precedent-setting court rulings is key to risk management for the institution and for the individual clinician.

Consider the following examples of problems relevant to these risk factors:

Problem #1

A 10-year-old boy was brought to an outpatient evaluation appointment by his father's live-in girlfriend for assessment of attention problems in school; poor academic performance that had worsened since his parents' separation 3 months earlier; and angry, oppositional behavior at home. The biological parents had not been able to reach a separation agreement because they disagreed on almost everything, including the child's behavior and responsiveness to redirection. The girlfriend was adamant that the boy needed medication because she had seen how effective it was with her adolescent son when he was younger.

Formulation and solution. Unfortunately, whoever scheduled this appointment either did not know the correct questions to ask or was misled regarding who needed to accompany this child to the appointment. The girlfriend had no legal status in this child's life and could not be assumed to be a reliable or nonpartial historian. The evaluation must include the presence of one or both of the parents. It may be necessary to have separate meetings with each parent, and then with the child, if the parents cannot be respectful of each other when together.

Problem #2

A 15-year-old male living in foster care was admitted to the inpatient service after threatening to blow up his biology teacher's truck. He had a history of one previous violent episode toward another foster child 2 years earlier but otherwise was doing well in school, was active in swimming and karate, and had good peer relationships. His goal in life was to become a Marine. Although he settled well on the unit, his initial presentation of bravado—including bragging about his karate training and expertise—had made many staff members uncomfortable and fearful of him. He was started on Depakote, tolerated it well, and began to minimize the reason he was hospitalized, saying that he would never really do anything.

Formulation and solution. Given the risk posed by this patient, and the concerns of people in his community, an outside consultation from a forensic expert was obtained regarding the patient's potential for dangerousness. This kind of second opinion by someone not a part of the hospital-based treatment team provided an additional opportunity for the patient to reveal information that he might have been hiding and also offered a structured way of thinking about a potentially dangerous individual. Because this consultation confirmed that the patient was in a low-risk category as long as ongoing

treatment was in place, it was much easier for the hospital clinician to effect a discharge plan of return to the foster home and intensive outpatient services. The discharge plan would include a safety plan specifying the early signs that might indicate that the patient needed additional attention and support.

The Future: Management Concerns, Financial Imperatives, and Ethical Considerations

Management Concerns and Financial Imperatives

Administrators of children' services face the daunting task of managing more complicated patients with greater risk in less structured, less restrictive settings, with ever decreasing financial resources. Most child and adolescent systems prior to the 1990s were to a large extent funded from the profit created by inpatient services. Outpatient clinics, particularly those that provided services for the severely emotionally disturbed, have historically not been profit centers because of the labor-intensive nature of child outpatient work. This includes time spent communicating with parents, schools, and pediatricians, most of which is not reimbursed by third-party payers. Although the private practice of child psychiatry has flourished, this has been in part due to the referral of complicated, labor-intensive cases to clinics that are part of a system of care in which clinical costs could be offset by the larger system.

The financial pressures caused by low-profit-margin inpatient care have forced administrators to closely monitor and manage for both cost containment and revenue enhancement. On the cost-containment side, administrators look for efficiencies wherever they might be found in order to make at least a small profit on each encounter, whether inpatient, outpatient, or at a level of care in between. Given that labor costs are the single most costly item in a psychiatric budget, this area is often targeted for cost savings. The following strategies are increasingly used in cost-saving efforts:

- Staff and clinicians with less professional training who are therefore paid less
- Employees hired part time in order to decrease the cost of benefit packages
- Less administrative time for clinicians

- Clinician reimbursement linked to clinician productivity
- Business-oriented staff to monitor clinician productivity
- Flexible staffing models that can be adjusted to correspond to census

The issue of variable census is a particular problem for child and adolescent services. The summer months when school is not in session are notoriously low inpatient census months, whereas the winter months can be very busy. For example, a large system with a 56 inpatient bed capacity averaged only 26 patients for an entire summer; 6 months later, the system averaged 52 patients for the winter months and at times was at 58 patients.

Revenue-enhancement strategies must also be put in place. Key to these strategies is the development of new services in the continuum that can be operated in a cost-efficient manner, applying the strategies described earlier, from the program design stage, through implementation of the new service. Careful attention to staff costs, including the gradual phase-in of new staff during the start-up of a new program, is essential in today's healthcare environment.

Marketing of new services with attention to all possible purchasers is another important component for administrators of children's services. This component often translates into having the service appeal to many payers: managed care companies specific to mental healthcare; HMOs, including capitation-oriented systems; medical assistance for the severely impaired; and social service agencies that are often entrusted with providing care to children for whom they are the guardian or custodian. Successful services must appeal to more than one payer, not a narrowly defined payer niche, and they must be actively marketed.

The administration of children's services requires considerable creative integrative ability, which combines knowledge about the local mental healthcare marketplace—including the local state-operated social service agency structure and funding opportunities—with knowledge about state regulations regarding funding of educational services. Increasingly, the penetration of managed care into a particular area is openly discussed. For adult psychiatrists, this is the factor that most affects their work to an increasing degree. Child psychiatrists and administrators of children's services must also negotiate the social agency structure and the educational service delivery system in order to provide services.

The most difficult challenges often occur at the interface of these systems. With regard to educational services, for example, a state's implementation plan for Public Law 94-142 interfaces most significantly with children's services. Passed in 1975, and interpreted in 1982 by the U.S. Supreme Court in a landmark decision, this law requires that a state provide educational services for all children and adolescents, regardless of emotional or physical impairment. Each state has designed its own plan to comply with this law in a way that is consistent with local school agency bureaucracy and budgetary constraints.

The following problems illustrate the importance of integrating this information in order to successfully deliver child and adolescent mental health services:

Problem #1

A state made the financial decision to convert children on medical assistance to plans managed by several private managed care companies over a 4-month period. In preparation for this conversion, a large health system decided to begin a respite service to use for diversion and step-down from more costly hospital care. As the new service opened, it became apparent that some of the adolescents in need of the day hospital component of the service had no family or other residential care service where they could reside. Although the state social service agency central office had been encouraging the development of the service throughout the licensing procedure, once the program was licensed there was considerable delay in getting it reimbursed.

Formulation and solution. An understanding of this problem lies in knowing that in this particular state the social service budget is completely decentralized. Although the central office handles licensing, it does not deal with reimbursement. Each county has its own budget and therefore develops its own individual service reimbursement contracts. The delay in getting the residential component paid could have been avoided if the relevance of this fact had been better appreciated so that contracts to each county were immediately available at the time of licensure.

Problem #2

A 15-year-old male with a history of sexual abuse as a young child was admitted for his fourth psychiatric hospitalization after setting a fire in the family home. His history revealed symptoms of attention-deficit/hyperactivity disorder dating back to his preschool years, specific learning disabilities, conduct disorder symptoms, and an increasing preoccupation with sexual predatory fantasies. The later fantasies and emerging related behaviors of exposing himself, making lewd phone calls, and threatening to rape accompanied the fire setting at the time of admission. After an extensive hospital stay, including various medication trials that were only somewhat effective, a decision was made that residential treatment was indicated. The process for such a placement in this particular state included a special school meeting to present the case and advocate for the local school district to cover the cost of the educational component. Despite the clinical team's efforts, the recommendation for residential placement was made at the first meeting the parents attended, but the school denied payment, stating that prior to hospitalization the patient's educational needs were being adequately met in the school system.

Formulation and solution. Although the school system's point was somewhat valid, it denied the potential danger to other students and the need for intensive treatment for this disturbed youth. The patient's parents were encouraged to obtain legal counsel from a specialty group that deals locally with disability law. In addition, with permission from the parents, the hospital reports were carefully written to include the sexual fantasies and predatory behaviors in a manner sensitive to a school meeting setting. Information from a forensic consultation was also referenced in the reports. An appeal of the initial funding denial decision was successful, when preceded by telephone calls from the family's legal counsel and the rewritten hospital reports.

As these examples illustrate, issues that are often a part of providing services for emotionally disturbed children and adolescents are not typically encountered with adults. Administrators of children's services must actively integrate information from the child's living situation and the child's educational needs with an enlightened understanding of the child's clinical status.

Ethical Considerations

Issues raised in efforts to integrate treatment modalities sometimes give rise to ethical dilemmas that challenge administrators of children's services. If one narrowly approaches psychiatric illness in a youngster in ways akin to the medical model of managing acute illness, then treatment of children is not significantly different from treatment of adults. However, if one acknowledges that most children who experience the onset of mental illness early in life are at increased risk of more serious long-term impairments, then the problems of cost-containment-bound treatment become more ethically challenging. A frequent concern is that

the least costly treatments in the short term may render the child with less ability to learn in school and therefore with less chance of being able to support himself or herself as an adult. Particularly with serious emotional disturbances, what may look like cost savings during the treatment of mental illness in children and adolescents may create a generation of undertreated young adults with few if any adult life skills. Similarly, the undertreatment of the disruptive disorders of childhood can lead to an increased need for juvenile justice programs. This essentially amounts to cost shifting from mental health to social services and juvenile justice programs.

Long-term outcome studies that look at cost-effective treatments clearly are needed. Studies of this kind are complicated and expensive and require the use of multiple evaluation and treatment sites. In the current model of marketplace-driven, short-term profit-oriented care, these costly studies are unlikely to be undertaken by managed care companies or HMOs, because they will detract from bottom-line profitability. Furthermore, if such studies are done, the data may be viewed as proprietary and thus not shared with other professionals. The funding of studies could be remedied if state or national regulations required that a percentage of profits be set aside to fund outcome research and specified that the results of the research be designated as public domain. Otherwise, studies will need to be funded on the national level and designed to be relevant to the delivery systems and practices of care being delivered in the for-profit marketplace.

Outcomes-based research was not previously performed with cost containment as a parameter; therefore, recommendations for diagnostic evaluations and for subsequent treatment have not been consistent with the reality of what could be delivered in a cost-effective way in the for-profit marketplace. For example, research on the diagnosis and treatment of attention-deficit/hyperactivity disorders, largely funded by research grants, emphasizes a diagnostic workup that involves behavior checklists, collateral information from schools, and a detailed family history. This kind of rigorous, accurate evaluation is labor intensive and costly and, therefore, is not possible in clinical settings reimbursed by fees determined by managed care reimbursement parameters. Yet without such evaluation, either overdiagnosis or underdiagnosis of the syndrome may result, with concomitant improper treatment and poor outcome. The continued discrepancy between practice parameters developed by outcomes-based research and the community standards of practice guided by time and reimbursement constraints is an ethical challenge for administrators and clinicians that must be addressed in the future.

How these issues will be presented to consumers will likely determine the method of resolution, but government regulation will likely enter the picture in the near future. If the issues become manifest to consumers through untoward outcomes in large numbers of underserved poor individuals, consent decrees that mandate court involvement will likely result. This situation has occurred when children were poorly served (e.g., Willie M. v. VS Hunt; Lisa L. decree). Another possible scenario will be regulatory interventions at the national level imposed as part of a larger reexamination of the need for healthcare reform. Regardless of the method, administrators of children's services will need to provide data about the care they deliver, with corresponding outcome data, in order to further the cause of improving services to children. Administrators of services will also need to work closely with the professional organizations of clinicians, social workers and psychologists specifically trained to evaluate and treat children, and child psychiatrists; in addition, administrators will need to join forces with educators and, especially, parent advocacy groups. What may ultimately unite previously guild-oriented member organizations with parents and payers may be the recognition that providing integrated care for children is the most sensible way to preserve the future for society.

References

Aichhorn A: Wayward Youth. New York, Viking, 1935

Bettelheim B: A Home for the Heart. New York, Knopf, 1974

Cotton N: Lessons From the Lion's Den. New York, Jossey-Bass, 1993

England MJ, Cole R F: Building systems of care for youth with serious mental illness. Hospital Comm Psychiatry 43:630–633, 1992

Erikson EH: Childhood and Society. New York, Norton, 1963

Geraty RD, Hendren RL, Flaa CJ: Ethical perspectives on managed care as it relates to child and adolescent psychiatry. J Am Acad Child Adolesc Psychiatry 31:398–402, 1992

Gibson RW: Staffing pattern survey. National Association of Private Psychiatric Hospitals Research Memo No 512. Washington, DC, National Association of Private Psychiatric Hospitals, 1981

Harper G: Focal inpatient treatment planning. J Am Acad Child Adolesc Psychiatry 28:31–37, 1989

Joint Commission on Accreditation of Healthcare Organizations: Primer on Indicator Development and Application: Measuring Quality in Health Care. Oakbrook Terrace, IL, Joint Commission on Accreditation of Healthcare Organizations, 1990

Lisa L. decree: U.S. District Court, Maryland, K87-138

Nurcombe B: Diagnostic reasoning and treatment planning. Aust N Z J Psychiatry 21:477–499, 1987

Piaget J: The Developmental Psychology. New York, Van Nostrand, 1963

Redl F, Wineman D: The Aggressive Child. Glencoe, IL, Free Press, 1957

Stanton AH, Schwartz JS: The Mental Hospital: A Study of Institutional Participation in Psychiatric Illness and Treatment. New York, Basic Books, 1954

Strasburger VC, Dietz WH: Children, adolescents, and television. Curr Probl Pediatr 21:8–31, 1991

Villani S, Fassler D: Systems of care. AACAP News, No 30, 1995

Willie M. v VS Hunt: Federal Ruling Cit No 564F2363 and 90FRD601

❖ Section VI ❖

Law and Ethics

Donald H. Williams, M.D., Section Editor

Introduction

Donald H. Williams, M.D.

Psychiatry, like the rest of medicine, is undergoing the greatest transformation of its practice within the memory of current practitioners. As Starr forecast, the last decades of the twentieth century were "a time of diminishing resources and autonomy for many physicians, voluntary hospitals, and medical schools" (Starr 1982). The sovereignty of the medical profession over the provision of American healthcare has ended. Governments and employers are determined to control the costs of healthcare. To achieve such cost controls, medical practice has become organized. Individual, fee-for-service physicians are becoming members of organized groups. These practitioners have experienced a profound loss of autonomy. Physicians are losing control over the rules and standards of practice and their level of income. Many components of the provision of healthcare are being transferred from highly skilled, expensive health professionals to limited-skilled, lower paid paraprofessional employees. Physicians and laypersons alike are greatly concerned that these changes are eroding the patient-physician relationship.

Psychiatrists in private, individual practices have been particularly affected by the corporatization of medical care. Some psychiatrists are questioning whether psychiatry will survive as a medical specialty. It is important to remember that since the inception of psychiatry as a specialty, a significant portion of psychiatric practice and administration has occurred in private and publicly financed organized settings. Legal, fiscal, and organizational constraints have been realities of psychiatric practice from the beginning. Psychiatric administrators have always had to face the moral and ethical challenges of rationing psychiatric services to medically indigent populations. In the past, psychiatric administrators dealt primarily with state, local, and federal governmental agencies and third-party payers. Managed care organizations and consumer groups have become important participants in determining the allocation of psychiatric services. The issues of providing rationed mental health services in a professionally ethical manner and preserving the patient-physician relationship are the same as in the past. Therefore, it is more useful for readers of this section to regard the discussion of the legal and ethical issues in the following chapters, not as further evidence of our diminished professional autonomy, but as guidelines for clarifying and preserving psychiatry's professional authority. With such knowledge, the psychiatric administrator will be better able to influence psychiatric managed care systems to become less of a threat and more of an opportunity for improved care.

In Chapter 30, Simon reviews relevant legal decisions that pertain to civil liability of institutions and their staffs for substandard care of psychiatric patients.

In Chapter 31, Miller discusses how criminal law pertains to psychiatric care. Psychiatric administrators must familiarize themselves with this area because increasing numbers of mentally ill persons are also involved with the criminal justice system at some point in their lives. (In some public mental health clinics, over 40% of current patients have criminal records.) Miller also highlights the need for psychiatric administrators to be knowledgeable about relevant laws and regulations and the appropriate interventions to protect clinicians and their patients from illegal or inappropriate judicial actions by criminal court justices unaware of the laws and regulations that protect psychiatric care.

In Chapter 32, Gunnings, Giampa, and I present an overview of the administration of psychiatric programs in American prisons, including three broad areas. First, we summarize a history of the attempts to establish treatment and rehabilitative programs in American prisons and the sociopolitical and professional issues that led to the demise of these programs. Following is a discussion of the issues of treatment and custody within the framework of an open-systems theory of organizations. Finally, we discuss the organizational factors, including managed care, necessary for creating and administering an efficient, effective, and humane mental healthcare system in the twenty-first century.

In Chapter 33, Lazarus discusses ethical psychiatric practices, based on the seven principles of medical ethics contained in the American Medical Association's Code of Medical Ethics. He emphasizes that both the American Psychiatric Association and the American Medical Association hold that a physician's primary obligation is to the individual patient, no matter what role the physician might have in healthcare organizations. Lazarus discusses each of the seven principles in the context of psychiatric administrative practices and then provides clinical vignettes illustrating their application in organizational settings.

References

Starr P: The Social Transformation of American Medicine. New York, Basic Books, 1982, pp 444–449

❖ 30 ❖

Administrative Psychiatry

Practice and Legal Regulation

Robert I. Simon, M.D.

Since the 1970s, an ever-increasing number of medical malpractice lawsuits have been brought against all medical professionals. Hospitals also face a variety of malpractice actions (1). In this chapter I present a brief overview of some of the major legal issues facing hospitals, institutions, and other facilities providing services to psychiatric patients. These issues may serve as the basis for holding psychiatric care providers legally liable for substandard medical care. No single chapter, however, can adequately address all of the potential scenarios that might lead to a lawsuit. Nor can one chapter fully explain the many applicable legal theories and doctrines. For example, Table 30–1 provides a reasonably comprehensive outline of many potential areas of liability associated with psychiatric, institutional, and hospital care. Not even this table is exhaustive. Readers interested in a detailed explanation of the law governing hospital care and liability issues are referred to numerous sources that provide general information about hospital law (2) and hospital liability case law (3) and specific information regarding legal issues that affect psychiatric hospital care (4).

As reflected in Table 30–1, with no less than 75 potential areas of liability associated with the care of hospitalized psychiatric patients, the number of lawsuits is thought to be extensive. Unfortunately, no reliable data are readily available that detail the number of lawsuits filed against psychiatric facilities annually. Many of these cases are settled out of court or are dismissed. It stands to reason, however, that the increasing expansion of litigation against psychiatrists is a minimum reflection of what is occurring with hospitals (5). As illustrated in Table 30–2, the amount of monetary damages awarded to psychiatric patients in lawsuits against hospitals and their staffs is no less significant.

Theories of Liability and Defenses

Liability Theories

The liability of a hospital institution for the acts committed or omitted by an employee or person using the facility is evolving and not nationally uniform. Many of the legal principles that govern the liability of individual physicians are applicable to hospitals as well. Because

TABLE 30–1. Potential areas of liability: institution

Admission
1. Failure to admit patient
2. Negligent evaluation—inappropriate treatment
3. False imprisonment: negligent commitment

Treatment
1. Generally
   a. abandonment
   b. inadequate care or treatment
   c. negligent treatment
   d. failure to obtain informed consent
   e. breach of confidentiality
   f. breach of contract
2. Electroconvulsive therapy
   a. negligent assessment—wrongful use
   b. improper administration
   c. failure to supervise properly (posttreatment)
   d. informed consent
   e. failure to follow up (posttreatment)
   f. civil rights claim: "right to refuse" violation
3. Medication
   a. informed consent
   b. negligent assessment—improper selection
      1) medication in general
      2) specific medication
   c. failure to supervise (post–drug treatment)
   d. improper administration
   e. improper use
   f. failure to monitor treatment
   g. failure to monitor side effects
      1) tardive dyskinesia
      2) lithium toxicity
      3) other side effects
   h. negligent treatment of side effects
   i. civil rights claim: "right to refuse" violation
   j. experimental drugs
      1) informed consent
      2) negligent or inappropriate use
4. Psychotherapy
   a. assault and battery: "innovative treatment"
   b. sexual exploitation of patient
   c. defamation
   d. negligent supervision (residents, nonmedical professionals)
   e. failure to protect or warn
   f. breach of confidentiality

Patient management
1. Patient abuse: failure to protect
   a. other patient attack
   b. staff abuse
2. Restraint and seclusion
   a. improper application
   b. negligent supervision
   c. punitive use ("chemical restraint")

Special patients
1. Suicide potential
   a. diagnosis
      1) suicide not known but foreseeable: failure to assess records properly
      2) suicide known: failure to document
      3) suicide known: improper diagnosis—failure to treat
   b. treatment
      1) failure to supervise properly
      2) failure to restrain (high-risk patients)
      3) premature release
      4) negligent discharge
      5) unjustified freedom of movement (negligent use of open-door policy)
      6) inadequate or negligent follow-up (outpatient treatment)
2. Dangerous patient
   a. negligent release
   b. negligent discharge
   c. failure to warn or protect
3. Elopement
   a. failure to assess risk
   b. failure to supervise or control

Patient records
1. Breach of confidentiality
2. Negligent release: invasion of privacy
3. Failure to release on proper authorization
4. Libel

Discharge
1. Failure to release pursuant to statute (false imprisonment)
2. Wrongful release (discharge or pass)
   a. harm to third party
   b. harm to patient
      1) suicide
      2) patient's condition deteriorates

Staff relations
1. Peer review
2. Hospital privileges
3. Physician discipline
   a. impaired professional
   b. incompetent professional
   c. professional misconduct

Miscellaneous issues
1. Dual interests: professional-patient
2. Useless treatment
3. Vicarious liability
4. Team treatment
5. Outpatient treatment
   a. failure to supervise
   b. negligent placement (inappropriate patient)
   c. failure to control
6. Patient with acquired immunodeficiency syndrome

TABLE 30–2. Institutional liability and damage awards: a sample

Area of liability	Citation	Judgment/ settlement ($)
Admission		
Failure to admit	*Clark v. State* (NY 1985)	700,000
Negligent evaluation	*Salinas v. Goldin* (MI 1976)	240,000
False imprisonment: commitment procedures	*Gonzalez v. New York* (NY 1983)	10,000
Treatment		
Generally		
Inadequate care	*Pursley v. County of Rensselaer* (NY 1985)	40,000
Wrong treatment	*Smith v. University Medical Center* (FL 1987)	1,048,986
Breach of contract	*Lovelace v. York-Adams Mental Health-Mental Retardation Program* (PA 1986)	40,000
Electroconvulsive therapy		
Wrongful use	*Monty v. Natchaug Hospital* (CT 1982)	270,000 (S)
Failure to supervise	*Strong v. Methodist Hospital* (IN 1975)	750,000
Negligent follow-up	*Pettis v. State Department of Hospitals* (LA 1976)	35,000
Medication		
Informed consent	*Urbani v. Yale University School of Medicine* (CT 1986)	25,000 (S)
Negligent assessment	*Blanchard v. Levine* (GA 1986)	80,000 (S)
Failure to supervise	*Bucklew v. Washington Adventist Hospital* (MD 1984)	1,531,225
Improper use: polypharmacology	*Katz v. Oakland Medical* (MI 1982)	1,000,000
Failure to monitor treatment	*Kilgore v. County of Santa Clara* (CA 1982)	230,000 (S)
Tardive dyskinesia	*Hedin v. United States* (MN 1985)	2,100,000
Lithium toxicity	*Wright v. State* (LA 1986)	456,000 (S)
Other side effects	*Blanchard v. Levine* (GA 1985)	80,000 (S)
Experimental drugs	*Putnam v. Schultz* (VA 1985)	175,000 (S)
Psychotherapy		
Sexual exploitation	*Lewis v. Wilhoil* (FL 1980)	375,000
Negligent supervision (resident/ nonmedical professional)	*Andrews v. United States* (9th Cir 1984)	100,000
Patient management		
Patient abuse		
Other patient	*Estate of Vaillancourt v. United States* (D.CA 1976)	373,431
Staff abuse	*Newman v. Glendale Adventist Medical Center* (CA 1986)	350,000
Restraint and seclusion		
Improper application	*Jansen v. University Hospital* (WA 1982)	75,000
No supervision	*Zamora v. State* (NY 1985)	53,317
Special patients		
Suicide		
Foreseeable: failure to assess	*Wormbly v. United States* (IL 1987)	152,277
Improper assessment	*Wagner v. Shamsi* (CT 1982)	225,345
Treatment/supervision	*Lasley v. Jackson Park Hospital* (IL 1984)	2,400,000
Failure to restrain	*Goldstein v. Providence Hospital* (MI 1981)	236,000
Negligent pass	*Uphoff v. DePaul Hospital Corp.* (LA 1987)	625,000 (S)
Negligent discharge	*Dunn v. Howard University Hospital* (DC 1981)	500,000
Negligent open-door policy	*Gaskill v. Doe* (KY 1984)	1,200,000
Negligent follow-up outpatient treatment	*Perry v. Seekunger* (PA 1983)	696,000
Dangerous patient		
Failure to warn	*Moskowitz v. MIT* (NY 1982)	5,000,000
Negligent release (pass)	*Estate of Berwid v. New York* (NY 1983)	600,000
Elopement		
Negligent supervision	*Radzikowski v. Metcalfe* (NY 1978)	1,600,000

TABLE 30–2. Institutional liability and damage awards: a sample *(continued)*

Area of liability	Citation	Judgment/ settlement ($)
Discharge		
Wrongful release	*Martin v. Washington Hospital Center* (DC 1980)	202,967
Wrongful harm to third party	*McDonald v. County of Nassau* (NY 1985)	425,000
Wrongful suicide	*Bell v. New York City Health & Hospital* (NY 1982)	564,000
Staff relations		
Negligent termination of privileges	*Laje v. R. E. Thomason General Hospital* (TX 1980)	52,400
Miscellaneous issues		
Negligent team treatment	*Sibley v. Board of Supervisors of LSU* (LA 1985)	500,000
Wrongful supervision	*Clark v. State* (NY 1985)	700,000
Negligent placement	*Desaussure v. New York* (NY 1985)	153,007

Note. (S) = settlement.

a hospital is essentially the sum of the many individuals that participate for the single purpose of caring for patients, the primary source of hospital liability is *vicarious liability.*

Vicarious liability arises from the individual actions of specific hospital employees who are alleged to have injured a patient. Under the doctrine of *respondeat superior,* meaning "let the master answer," vicarious liability may be imposed on hospitals for negligent acts of employees under their supervision. Traditionally, hospitals were deemed liable under the doctrine of respondeat superior for the negligence of their residents, interns, and other employees—but not for the actions of staff physicians and nurses (6). In a landmark case, *Bing v. Thunig* (7), the hospital exception to the theory of respondeat superior was overturned by New York's highest court. The court found that physicians and nurses were "servants" for purposes of the doctrine of respondeat superior.

Courts in recent years have adopted a theory of "corporate negligence," which enables patients to sue the hospital as a corporate entity for the acts or omissions of its employees, administrators, and staff acting collectively on behalf of the corporation (8). A problem facing many patient-plaintiffs desiring to add the hospital, and its "deep pockets" or corporate wealth, to their lawsuit is that the alleged negligence is committed by a private attending physician who is merely an independent contractor exercising hospital privileges. As a general rule, employers are not vicariously liable for the torts of an independent contractor (9). This is because most physicians possessing staff privileges are not employed by the hospital but, rather, are entitled to use hospital facilities for treatment of their patients. Thus,

in most hospitals two classes of physician staff members exist: those merely holding staff privileges and those who are employees of the hospital. Interns and residents are among the most common of the latter group. The threshold difference between the two classes in imposing vicarious liability on a hospital is the amount of control the hospital exerts over the physician. There are, however, exceptions to the rule of nonliability. One exception is if some direct economic relationship exists between the hospital and the physician. For example, in some situations, a psychiatrist or other physician who is not technically an employee may share an economic relationship with a hospital. These cases typically involve physicians who have agreed to provide support services to the hospital through anesthesiology, pathology, radiology, psychiatry, emergency room, or other departments.

Whether doctors are independent contractors or servants of the hospital is generally a factual determination. The determining factor typically is the amount of authority or control that the hospital has or is implied to have over the physician (10). Some courts have concluded that, as a matter of public policy, it is unduly burdensome to require patients to determine whether their treating physician was a hospital employee or an independent contractor (11). Some courts have applied the theory of *ostensible agency,* which holds the hospital vicariously liable for the physician's conduct when a hospital causes a patient to assume, justifiably, that a physician is a hospital employee (12).

Another exception to hospital liability is the *borrowed servant doctrine* (13). The treating physician or staff psychiatrist is sometimes supported by other physicians (including interns and residents), medical technicians, various therapists, and nurses. Most of these individuals will either be hospital employees or self-employed (e.g., independent contractors), but few, if any, will be employees of the treating physician or psychiatrist.

This raises a significant question regarding liability. An individual's status as a "borrowed servant" will greatly depend on a finding that the "master" (e.g., the treating psychiatrist) possessed a requisite degree of control over the assistant. The question of control can be controversial; consequently, courts are particularly sensitive in analyzing the evidence. For a plaintiff to prevail under the borrowed servant doctrine, he or she must prove that 1) the person assisting the treating physician was negligent, 2) the physician possessed a requisite degree of control over the assistant, and 3) the assistant acted within the scope of his or her role as an assistant. Direct negligence on the part of the treating physician need not be proved. Thus, based on the borrowed servant theory of vicarious liability, a plaintiff may obtain a judgment against the physician although only proving the negligence of an assistant (14).

A final exception to hospital nonliability is based on the negligent selection of independent contractor, private attending physicians (15). This exception was expanded further in *Darling v. Charleston Memorial Hospital* (16). In *Darling*, the Illinois Supreme Court held that a hospital (via its employees and nonemployee professional staff) must supervise the care administered by nonemployee physicians holding hospital staff privileges. Specifically, the court stated that the hospital was independently liable for negligently failing to "require consultation with or examination by members of the hospital surgical staff skilled in such treatments; or to review the treatment rendered to the plaintiff and to require consultants to be called in as needed" (17). Following the *Darling* decision, other courts have expanded this concept and imposed liability on a hospital for the negligent supervision of an attending physician's professional acts (18) and for negligently granting medical staff privileges to physicians who were later judged incompetent to practice medicine (19).

Defenses and Limitations

An allegation of negligence made by a patient can be countered by a number of defenses that can be asserted to bar recovery altogether, to have the lawsuit thrown out before the trial, or to reduce the overall amount of liability (and hence damages to be recovered).

Although too numerous to detail, some of the more common defenses deserve mention.

All civil lawsuits have a *statute of limitations*, which requires that an action be commenced within a prescribed time period following the discovery or occurrence of the allegedly negligent act. If no lawsuit is filed within the requisite time period, the suit will be barred (20) unless a recognized exception that suspends the statute of limitation exists. These limitations are procedural and are usually governed by the laws of the state in which the suit is being brought (21).

The use of *reasonable professional judgment* is a mainstay defense (22). The credibility of this defense depends on the compliance with the standard of care as documented by the physician's own records. The law does not require psychiatrists and other physicians to provide perfect care. For example, in *Centeno v. New York* (23), the court ruled that the decision to release a patient from the hospital and place the patient on convalescent outpatient status prior to the patient's suicide was not a negligent act but was based on reasonable medical judgment.

Several defenses are based on the plaintiff's conduct potentially available to hospitals. For example, in some situations and jurisdictions, a person may be prohibited from recovering for negligence when that person's own carelessness contributed to the injuries. This is known as *contributory negligence*. In *Johnston v. Ward* (24), an action brought against several physicians and hospitals for the salicylate poisoning death of a patient, the jury found that one of the physicians was negligent. The jury, however, also found the patient was contributorily negligent by ingesting the overdose of the aspirin-like substance. There was no evidence that the physicians knew or had reason to know of the true nature of the substances ingested until the plaintiff told the physician the facts. Unfortunately, by that time, it was too late to save the patient's life.

Similarly, there has been judicial recognition of the *patient noncompliance defense*. In *Skar v. City of Lincoln* (25), the patient failed to cooperate in any manner, which prevented the psychiatrist from obtaining a case history and from assessing the actual suicide risk. The patient subsequently injured his spine after attempting to jump out of a window. The court denied the claim of liability and stated that the patient had a duty to cooperate with the psychiatrist to the extent he was able.

Most states adopt the alternative theory of *comparative negligence*, which reduces the plaintiff's damages to be recovered according to the comparative percentage of negligence attributable to each of the parties, rather than barring the action altogether. Comparative negligence is exemplified in the case of *Peck v. Counseling Service of Addison County, Inc.* (26), in which the parents of a counseling center patient sued the center for the therapist's failure to warn them that their son had threatened to burn down the family barn. Evidence supported the trial court's finding that the parents were 50% negligent because they had been aware of their son's proclivity for violent behavior. The father suggested that the patient lie to Social Security to receive benefits to which he was not entitled. When the patient angrily refused, the father told the patient he was sick and belonged in a hospital. The parents knew or should have known that their actions would cause their son to become angry, and that their son was capable of violent acts when angry.

A lawsuit may be barred when the plaintiff voluntarily "assumes" the risk of another's negligence. This is known as *assumption of the risk* (27). In other words, persons may not recover for an injury when they voluntarily expose themselves to a known and appreciated danger. In some cases of assumption of the risk, damages may be reduced instead of barred using a comparative negligence approach.

Although minors and mentally disabled people have traditionally been held liable for their torts (28), in contributory negligence cases, the mentally disturbed person is usually held only to the standard that he or she can personally meet (29). Moreover, in medical malpractice cases involving minors and persons of unclear mind (e.g., those who are mentally disturbed), the courts rarely sustain a defense of assumption of the risk because of the disparity in knowledge that exists between the patient and the physician. The defense is likely to be upheld, however, in cases where patients are repeatedly warned about engaging in an activity that is understood to be potentially harmful and the warnings are disregarded. For instance, patients who are repeatedly warned not to leave the bed without assistance and who competently acknowledge this precaution assume the risk of falling.

According to Perlin (30), assumption of the risk "has apparently not been litigated squarely in cases involving mental health professionals." The defense may be applicable, however, to patients who competently waive informed consent despite a clinician's diligent effort to warn of a treatment's serious side effects. Similarly, this defense may be applied to competent patients who exercise their constitutional right to refuse treatment but later bring suit for alleged harm suffered as a consequence of not being treated.

Despite reasonable care provided for a suicidal patient, an unforeseen or extraordinary circumstance may arise that enables the patient to commit suicide. When this occurs, it is theorized that the unforeseen event is an intervening act that supersedes the care or lack of care provided by the defendant, even if it was indeed negligent. In *Paddock v. Chacko* (31), a Florida appellate court concluded that the psychiatrist who had only seen the patient once was not liable for that patient's self-inflicted injuries. The patient placed herself in her parents' care and custody, but the parents disregarded the psychiatrist's recommendation that their daughter be hospitalized. This unwillingness to heed the psychiatrist's recommendation represented a superseding factor that intervened between the patient's injuries and the psychiatrist's care.

A final area of defense that may be available to hospitals and their employees is *immunity* (32). Some individual defendants who are government employees may be entitled to assert official immunity (33). Similarly, some institutional defendants, such as hospitals, may be eligible for *charitable immunity* if run by a charitable organization or *governmental immunity* if operated by a governmental entity. Federal hospitals, such as Veterans Administration facilities, also may be immunized from certain allegations of negligence pursuant to the Federal Tort Claims Act (34), which bars some claims based on specifically described conduct (e.g., assault, battery, false imprisonment, slander, libel, and misrepresentation).

Standard of Care

As a general rule, a hospital, state institution, or other facility is required to exercise reasonable care in accordance with sound hospital practices to protect the health and safety of its patients "as the patient's known mental and physical condition requires" (35). Some jurisdictions require not only that the standard of care be judged by the patient's known condition but also require that the facility take reasonable steps to discover the patient's actual physical and mental status (36). The hospital's duty to the patient is independent of any duty of care owed by a private attending physician practicing within the medical care facility.

The threshold standard, *reasonable care*, is typically established by several forms of evidence. The standard of care is most typically established by expert testimony. Generally, expert testimony is presented to establish that a hospital employee (e.g., staff psychiatrist) violated an accepted standard of professional practice unless the deviation is so gross, blatant, or obvious that a layperson of "common knowledge and experience" could recognize it (37). In these cases, rare in psychiatric situations, the principle of *res ipsa loquitur* is applied. The application of res ipsa loquitur, which literally means "the thing speaks for itself," permits the inference of negligence or the rebuttable presumption of negligence through the presentation of circumstantial evidence (38). For example, a surgeon leaving a sponge in the abdomen of the patient permits the inference of negligence. In *Meier v. Ross General Hospital* (39), the court held that the doctrine of res ipsa loquitur was applicable when a psychiatric patient jumped to his death through an open window of a hospital room.

Evidence of the standard of care may also be presented in the form of voluntarily assumed regulations, policies, and bylaws. For example, hospitals may voluntarily assume standards promulgated by outside organizations (e.g., the Joint Commission on Accreditation of Healthcare Organizations [JCAHO]); federal regulations (e.g., preconditions for participation in Medicare); state regulations; and even the hospital's own policies, rules, and regulations (e.g., psychiatric ward policies). A hospital may still be held liable despite scrupulous adherence to national standards, such as JCAHO regulations, when expert testimony establishes that such standards were inapplicable to the plaintiff's situation or were erroneous (40). Conversely, violation of a hospital's own policies and regulations is not necessarily definitive evidence of actionable negligence (41).

Major Areas of Potential Liability

The following areas of liability are a sample of some of the most likely situations in which a hospital or facility providing psychiatric care might be sued for negligence or other cause of action. Table 30–1 provides a more comprehensive summary of these and other potential liability areas.

Admission

It is well established in medical jurisprudence that absent some express or implied contract, a doctor has no duty to accept a patient who simply seeks medical or psychiatric treatment (42). There are situations, however, in which an implied contractual arrangement exists, even between a physician and a patient with no previous contact. The most common illustration is the hospital emergency room doctor, who is generally acknowledged to be available to provide services to all who seek treatment. This principle may also be extended to include doctors and psychiatrists who are on call as backup or support to the emergency room staff (43). Once a patient is admitted to a hospital, whether through a voluntary or involuntary admission, a duty of reasonable care is owed to that patient.

Liability issues associated with patient admission generally occur in several instances, depending on the circumstances surrounding the admission or potential admission. For example, the most common cause of action involving an involuntary admission relates to the wrongful commitment of a person due to the psychiatrist's failure to comply in good faith with civil commitment requirements. This situation typically gives rise to a lawsuit based on the theory of false imprisonment (44), malicious prosecution, or assault (45).

Grounds for a lawsuit may exist when a voluntary patient seeks to leave a hospital and is then coerced to remain in the hospital by false threats of civil commitment. In addition, a lawsuit may be brought when actual commitment proceedings are initiated and no good-faith evidence exists for such an action (46). Another admission-related situation that could result in liability occurs when a hospital outpatient represents a foreseeable risk of danger to self or others and the hospital fails to hospitalize the patient (47).

Constitutional torts against federal hospitals and their employees based directly on violation of the U.S. Constitution raise complex litigation issues. Civil rights claims against state and county hospitals and their employees for violations of civil rights based on 42 U.S.C. §1983 (1982) are narrowly defined. For example, §1983 actions are not applicable to private hospitals and their employees, even if the hospitals receive public moneys and are regulated by state or local laws. Mental health professionals working in federal and state institutions should determine whether their malpractice insurance covers constitutional torts.

Two essential elements must be established to maintain an action under §1983 of the Civil Rights Act. The patient must establish that the conduct in question is committed by an individual acting "under color" of state or territorial law, custom, or usage and that the conduct deprived the patient of rights, privileges, or immunities secured by the Constitution or U.S. law.

Under civil rights statutes, two kinds of rights are protected: substantive and procedural rights. The Fifth Amendment creates due process procedural rights that protect against deprivations of life, liberty, or property, and this protection has been applied to the states through the Fourteenth Amendment.

Voluntary admissions make up approximately 73% of the 1.6 million admissions to psychiatric care facilities (48). Most state statutes have attempted to encourage voluntary admission in the hope of aiding treatment. Individuals who voluntarily admit themselves to hospitals generally are presumed to understand the conditions of admission as a matter of law. Only a few states have a competency requirement (49).

However, in a U.S. Supreme Court case, *Zinermon v. Burch* (50), a mentally ill patient who was unable to give a competent consent to voluntary admission was permitted to go forward with a civil rights action against state officials who committed him to a state hospital using voluntary commitment procedures. The court held that Florida must have procedures to screen all voluntary patients for competency, excluding incompetent persons from the voluntary admission process. For the few states requiring competent consent to voluntary admission, screening procedures must be created to exclude incompetent patients. Although the Court did not directly address whether a voluntary patient must be competent to consent to admission, Appelbaum (48) opined that "*Zinermon* will refocus attention on the often-neglected process of voluntary admission."

Treatment

Medication

Treatment involving psychotropic medication offers the greatest potential for a negligence action brought against a hospital or psychiatrist. This is in large part due to the frequency with which drug therapy is used in hospitals, clinics, and programs treating psychiatric patients. A variety of risks and side effects are associated with the administration of medication. Safeguards must be implemented to minimize patient injury.

A review of the relevant case law indicates a variety of mistakes, omissions, and poor treatment practices that commonly result in malpractice actions against hospitals and their staffs (e.g., attending or staff psychiatrist). The following summary, although not intended to be exhaustive, should provide a workable framework for identifying problem areas associated with medication treatment (Table 30–3).

TABLE 30–3. Common areas of negligence associated with drug malpractice claims

Failure to evaluate properly
Failure to monitor or supervise
Negligent prescription practices
Failure to disclose medication effects

Failure to evaluate properly and negligent diagnosis. The incidence of medical disorders, both diagnosed and undiagnosed, is higher in hospitalized psychiatric patients than in psychiatric outpatients. At the very minimum, a thorough physical examination, clinical history, and mental status examination should be conducted. This will not only provide useful information about the patient's complaints but also alert the physician to any physical or emotional limitations that may interfere with the obtaining of proper informed consent. Failure to evaluate a patient properly before beginning drug therapy can result in the patient's true condition being misdiagnosed and remaining untreated and may subject the patient to unnecessary side effects and risks for which informed consent was not obtained (51). For instance, a particularly serious complication of prolonged treatment with neuroleptics is the development of tardive dyskinesia (52) (Table 30–4).

Failure to monitor or supervise treatment and negligent treatment. Once psychotropic medication has been prescribed to a patient, it is the duty of the prescribing psychiatrist and support staff to monitor or supervise the patient's physical and emotional response to such treatment. This monitoring may require the use of laboratory testing, repeated physical examinations, and, of course, direct interviewing of the patient and other reliable parties (e.g., nursing staff). A failure to supervise properly a patient taking psychotropic medication can unnecessarily subject that patient to harmful side effects and can delay a change to safer or effective treatment. Malpractice lawsuits for failure to monitor drug therapy are relatively common (53).

Negligent prescription practices. The selection of a medication, initial dosage, form of administration, and other related procedures are all decisions left to the clinical discretion of the treating psychiatrist. In administering psychotropic medication, hospital psychiatrists need only conform their procedures and decision making to that which other psychiatrists ordinarily practice under similar circumstances. Certain prescribing practices,

TABLE 30–4. Recommendations for prevention and management of tardive dyskinesia

1. Review indications for neuroleptic drugs and consider alternative treatments when available.
2. Educate the patient and his or her family regarding benefits and risks. Obtain informed consent for long-term treatment, and document it in the medical record.
3. Establish objective evidence of the benefit from neuroleptics and review it periodically (at least every 3–6 months) to determine ongoing need and benefit.
4. Use the minimum effective dosage for chronic treatment.
5. Exercise particular caution with children, the elderly, and patients with affective disorders.
6. Examine the patient regularly for early signs of dyskinesia and note them in the medical record.
7. If dyskinesia occurs, consider an alternative neurological diagnosis.
8. If presumptive tardive dyskinesia is present, reevaluate the indications for continued neuroleptic treatment and obtain informed consent from the patient regarding continuing or discontinuing neuroleptic treatment.
9. If a neuroleptic is continued, attempt to lower the dosage.
10. If dyskinesia worsens, consider discontinuing the neuroleptic or switching to a new neuroleptic. At present, clozapine may hold some promise in this regard, but it is important to stay alert to new research findings.
11. Many cases of dyskinesia will improve and even remit with neuroleptic discontinuation or dosage reduction. If treatment for tardive dyskinesia is indicated, use more benign agents first (e.g., benzodiazepines and tocopherol), but keep abreast of new treatment developments.
12. If movement disorder is severe or disabling, consider obtaining a second opinion.

Source.   Reprinted from American Psychiatric Association: "Summary, Conclusions, and Recommendations for the Prevention and Management of Tardive Dyskinesia," in *Tardive Dyskinesia: A Task Force Report of the American Psychiatric Association*. Washington, DC, American Psychiatric Association, 1992, pp. 250–251. Used with permission.

however, may be associated with a higher incidence of legal liability. For example, exceeding recommended dosages that cause toxicity (54); negligent mixing of medications, or "polypharmacy" (55); prescribing medication for unapproved uses (56); and excessive administration of medication causing toxicity (57) or addiction (58) can all result in patient injury and a potential lawsuit.

Failure to disclose medication effects and informed consent.   All physicians have a duty to obtain a patient's informed consent prior to the administration of any treatment (Table 30–5). Psychiatrists frequently provide treatment to patients who may have diminished cognitive capacity due to mental illness, physical and psychological trauma, or organic impairment. In the case of a patient who lacks healthcare decision-making capacity, a psychiatrist has a duty to obtain consent from a legally authorized representative. A failure to obtain a patient's informed consent for treatment that results in an injury that would not have occurred otherwise, because of the patient's likely refusal to accept the treatment, can be ample grounds for a lawsuit (59). Similarly, the failure to apprise patients fully of medication side effects and to warn about engaging in potentially dangerous activities can be grounds for a lawsuit against the hospital and the attending physician. This is

more likely to occur when a patient receives treatment at a hospital outpatient clinic and is not warned against driving while taking certain medications (e.g., neuroleptics) (60).

Other areas of negligence involving medication effects that have resulted in legal action include failure to treat side effects once they have been recognized or should have been recognized (61), failure to monitor a patient's compliance with prescription limits (62), failure to prescribe medication or appropriate levels of medication when treatment needs called for it, failure to refer a patient for consultation or treatment by a specialist, and negligent withdrawal of a patient from a medication (63a).

Increasingly in managed care settings, psychiatrists are required to prescribe medications from a restrictive or closed formulary. For example, selective serotonin reuptake inhibitors (SSRIs) are currently considered first-line treatment for depression. However, a number of managed care companies allow only the prescribing of tricyclic antidepressants (TCAs). TCAs have a much greater lethality than SSRIs for patients who overdose. Psychiatrists, in their professional discretion, should determine which medications will be prescribed according to the patient's special clinical needs.

Psychiatrists should vigorously resist attempts to limit their choices of drugs by a restrictive or closed for-

---

TABLE 30–5. Informed consent: reasonable information to be disclosed

---

Although there is no consistently accepted set of information to be disclosed for any given medical or psychiatric situation, as a rule of thumb, five areas of information are generally provided:
  1. Diagnosis—description of the condition or problem
  2. Treatment—nature and purpose of the proposed treatment
  3. Consequences—risks and benefits of the proposed treatment
  4. Alternatives—viable alternatives to the proposed treatment, including risks and benefits
  5. Prognosis—projected outcome with and without treatment

Source. Reprinted from Simon RI: "Informed Consent: Maintaining a Clinical Perspective," in *Clinical Psychiatry and the Law,* 2nd Edition. Washington, DC, American Psychiatric Press, 1992, p. 128. Used with permission.

---

mulary. The prescribing of specific medications should be determined only by the psychiatrist and based on the patient's clinical needs. An appeal should be filed for denial of a prescription of a nonformulary approved drug.

Split Treatment

In managed care or other treatment settings, the mere prescribing of medication apart from a working doctor-patient relationship does not meet generally accepted standards of good clinical care. It is instead a prime example of fragmented care. Such a practice will diminish the efficacy of the drug treatment itself or may even lead to the patient's failure to take the prescribed medication. Fragmented care, in which the psychiatrist functions only as a prescriber of medication while remaining uninformed about the patient's overall clinical status, constitutes substandard treatment that may lead to a malpractice action.

Split treatment situations require that the psychiatrist stay fully informed of the patient's clinical status as well as of the nature and quality of treatment the patient is receiving from the nonmedical therapist (63b). In a collaborative relationship, responsibility for the patient's care is shared according to the qualifications and limitations of each discipline. The responsibilities of each discipline do not diminish those of the other disciplines. Patients should be informed of the separate responsibilities of each discipline. Periodic evaluation of the patient's clinical condition and needs, by the psychiatrist and the nonmedical therapist, is necessary to determine if the collaboration should continue. On termination of the collaborative relationship, the patient should be informed either separately or jointly. In split treatments, if negligence is claimed on the part of the nonmedical therapist, the collaborating psychiatrist will likely be sued, and vice versa (64).

Psychiatrists who prescribe medications only in split treatment arrangements should be able to hospitalize the patient, if necessary. If the psychiatrist does not have admitting privileges, then arrangements should exist with other psychiatrists who can hospitalize patients if emergencies arise. Split treatment is increasingly utilized by managed care companies and is a potential malpractice minefield.

The Omnibus Budget Reconciliation Act of 1987 regulates the use of psychotropic drugs in long-term healthcare facilities receiving funds from Medicare and Medicaid (65). The Health Care Financing Administration guidelines for neuroleptic drugs include 1) documentation of the psychiatric diagnosis or specific condition requiring neuroleptic use, 2) prohibition of neuroleptics if certain behaviors alone are the only justification, 3) prohibition of "as needed" neuroleptic use, and 4) gradual dosage reductions of neuroleptics combined with attempts at behavioral programming and environmental modification (66).

Electroconvulsive Therapy

Although electroconvulsive therapy (ECT) is considered to be a viable treatment for carefully selected patients with certain mental disorders (67), it has been estimated that no more that 3%–5% of all psychiatric inpatients in the United States have received such treatment (68). As can be expected from these figures, the potential number of ECT-related legal actions against facilities and individual psychiatrists is quite low.

Despite ECT's relatively limited use as a procedure in hospitals, it is distinguished from other psychiatric procedures by the number of guidelines and regulations that have been developed regarding its application, precautions, and therapeutic indications (69, 70). Violations of any of these guidelines (e.g., JCAHO standards) may provide a basis for at least the allegation of negligent ECT treatment. Informed consent is particularly important for ECT because of the controversy and confusion surrounding this treatment (70).

Notwithstanding this concern, malpractice liability associated with the use of ECT is typically confined to five general situations: 1) negligent administration or failure to administer premedication (e.g., muscle relaxant), 2) negligent administration of the procedure, 3) failure to obtain informed consent, 4) inadequate pretreatment examination to determine patient suitability for ECT, and 5) failure to provide adequate posttreatment supervision.

Managed Healthcare

The inpatient treatment of psychiatric disorders has changed dramatically in the managed care era. Most psychiatric units, particularly in general hospitals, have become short-stay, acute-care psychiatric facilities. Generally, only suicidal, homicidal, or gravely disabled patients with major psychiatric disorders pass strict precertification review for hospitalization. Clinical experience reveals that approximately half of these patients have comorbid substance-related disorders. Close scrutiny by utilization reviewers permits only brief hospitalization for these patients. The hospital administration may exert pressure for early discharge to maintain length-of-stay statistics within predetermined limits. The purpose of hospitalization is crisis intervention and management to stabilize patients and ensure their safety. Treatment is being provided to these patients by a variety of mental health professionals. Nonetheless, the psychiatrist must often bear the ultimate burden of liability for treatments gone awry. Limited opportunity usually exists during the hospital stay to develop a therapeutic alliance with patients. The ability to communicate with patients, the psychiatrist's stock-in-trade, is often severely curtailed. All these factors contribute to greatly increased risk of malpractice lawsuits against psychiatrists and hospitals alleging premature or negligent discharge of patients due to cost-containment policies.

In *Wickline v. State* (71), the plaintiff sued the state of California, alleging that her Medi-Cal eligibility was negligently discontinued, causing her to be prematurely discharged from the hospital. Following the patient's discharge, which was contrary to her physician's instructions, the patient developed a complete occlusion of the right iliac artery, which ultimately required amputation of her leg. The California Court of Appeals held that the state was not liable to the plaintiff because Medi-Cal, operating under a prospective utilization review system, had acted reasonably, given the information presented to it, in denying an 8-day extension but permitting 4 days. Although third-party payers may be legally accountable if medically inappropriate decisions result from defects in design or implementation of cost-containment procedures, the appellate court found that this was not the case in *Wickline.* The court concluded that the attending physician, not Medi-Cal, was responsible for the patient's discharge. In this case, the treating surgeon could have reapplied for a further extension of treatment (before the 4 days granted expired) if he thought it necessary.

In another premature release case, *Wilson v. Blue Cross of Southern California et al.* (72), a California appeals court did not follow the specific language of *Wickline*. In *Wilson*, a patient was hospitalized at College Hospital in Los Angeles for anorexia, drug dependency, and major depression. The treating psychiatrist determined that the patient required 3–4 weeks of hospitalization. After 10 days, utilization review determined that further hospitalization was unnecessary. The patient's insurance company refused to pay for further inpatient treatment. The psychiatrist filed to appeal and discharged the patient. The patient committed suicide 3 weeks later.

The Appellate Division of the California Court of Appeals held that third-party payers are not immune from lawsuits regarding utilization review activities. The court determined that the insurer and the physician may be subject to liability for harm caused to the patient by premature termination of a patient's hospitalization. The *Wickline* panel's suggestion that the physician alone is principally liable for treatment decisions is explicitly rejected in *Wilson*. Psychiatrists, however, should not take heart from these decisions. The burden of legal liability cannot be easily shifted to managed care companies, even by vigorous advocacy for the patient. If the psychiatrist recommends a longer hospital stay for a violent patient than is authorized for payment by the managed care company, immediate discharge that leads to patient self-harming or harming others will likely increase the risk of a malpractice lawsuit. Blaming the managed care company will not provide a viable defense. Both *Wickline* and *Wilson* underscore the reality that the doctor retains the ultimate responsibility for a patient's healthcare. Managed care companies generally limit or deny payment for services but not the services themselves. Accordingly, when a physician's decision and that of a third-party payer conflict, it is the doctor's duty to protest any compromise in patient care that might be presented by a third-party payer's position (73). All channels should be pursued to ensure that the psychiatrist's medical judgment (e.g., continued hospitalization) is carried out. Only after a physician has exhausted all options in an attempt to obtain what is in the patient's best medical interests can a successful argument be made that no liability attaches to the physician or affiliate hospital.

Most managed care companies and their peer reviewers are relatively immune from legal liability to state and federal law (74). Until now, the risk of lawsuits against managed care companies for the negligent performance of utilization review has been suppressed by the Employee Retirement Income Security Act of 1974 (ERISA) (75). ERISA preempts state laws and prohibits negligence claims in cases involving employer-sponsored health plans. However, cases have emerged in which courts have held that the intent of ERISA was not to abolish the right of individuals to sue for negligence. Premature release of psychiatric patients in response to pressure from managed care companies will likely be a major area of liability for psychiatrists and hospitals well into the twenty-first century (73).

Vulnerable and Special-Care Patients

Patients who present a danger to themselves or others represent the greatest malpractice risk for hospitals. These patients can be generally classified into three groups: patients requiring special care because of foreseeable mental or physical disability, suicidal patients, and potentially violent or dangerous patients. Not surprisingly, because of their unique vulnerabilities and needs, these patients receive treatment within the confines of a hospital rather than as outpatients. Because hospitalization provides a significant measure of control over a patient's behavior, a higher standard of reasonable care is expected to be provided by hospitals and their staffs. "The degree of care to be observed is measured by the patient's physical and mental ills and deficiencies as known to the officers and employees of the institution" (76).

The operative word regarding vulnerable patients is the *foreseeability* of their behavior. If a patient's words, manifest behavior, or psychiatric history suggests potential harm to himself or herself or others (e.g., staff, other patients, or parties outside the hospital), then a hospital's duty to provide reasonable care requires that it respond according to the risk that is reasonably foreseeable.

Foreseeably Disabled Patients

Patients who have readily apparent disabilities or propensities that might unwittingly endanger their lives or the lives of others require, at the very least, close supervision and appropriate precautions. The failure of hospital staff to anticipate and protect against foreseeable consequences created by a patient could be the basis for liability. Two of the most commonly encountered situations involving foreseeably vulnerable patients involve patients who are actively under the influence of drugs, especially a hallucinogen (77), and those who are actively psychotic (78).

In a New York case, the court held that a hospital had failed to supervise a mentally ill patient with a history of careless smoking and causing fires. Therefore, the hospital was liable for injuries the patient sustained when she accidentally set herself on fire (79).

Sometimes the foreseeable danger requires quick and direct action, or serious consequences may occur. For instance, in *Horton v. Niagara Falls Memorial Medical Center* (80), the plaintiff, known to be confused and disoriented, wandered out to a balcony and called for a ladder. This was brought to the attention of a doctor, who ordered a nurse to "keep an eye on him" while the physician notified the patient's wife and mother-in-law. Before either arrived, the patient fell two stories. The court found that the hospital could have at least provided continuous supervision until the mother-in-law arrived, 15 minutes after she received the doctor's call.

Suicidal Patients

Cases involving patient suicide make up, by far, the largest number of lawsuits against hospitals (81). The relatively large number of "suicide suits" is not surprising, given that suicidal patients represent a high proportion of vulnerable and unpredictable inpatients. Moreover, the standard of care by which a psychiatrist's actions will be judged makes no specific allowances for the unique situations that these patients create. In general, the suicide rate for a given psychiatric hospital is proportional to the types of patients admitted. Suicide rates are higher in facilities that admit acutely ill patients, particularly those with acute schizophrenia (82).

In assessing legal liability in suicide cases, whether it involves an inpatient or an outpatient, two questions arise. Is the suicide foreseeable? If foreseeable, did the hospital act reasonably based on that information? Accordingly, the duty of care owed to a patient by a psychiatrist or hospital is directly related to the patient's level of suicide risk, which is known or discoverable by the exercise of reasonable skill and diligence (83). Therefore, when a hospital or psychiatrist knows or reasonably should know of the patient's suicidal tendencies, the hospital or psychiatrist must exercise reasonable care to protect the patient from himself or herself (84).

The law tends to assume that suicide is preventable if it is foreseeable. However, foreseeability is a legal term of art. It does not and should not imply that clinicians are able to predict suicide. Nor should foreseeability be confused with preventability. In hindsight, some suicides that were clearly not foreseeable seem preventable.

Numerous factual variations describe the types of malfeasance and nonfeasance that could lead to suicide-related liability. The most common factual causes of action can be grouped into three categories: diagnosis, treatment, and discharge (Table 30–6).

Clinical errors involving suicidal patients generally occur when a patient is foreseeably suicidal but the psychiatrist or staff fails to assess suicide risk properly and to treat the patient accordingly. These errors can include failing to note the patient's suicidal tendencies in the patient's records (85) and failing to review the patient's medical records to obtain an accurate assessment of the patient's suicidality (86).

Failure to assess suicide risk properly is a major clinical and risk management error. Every patient should be initially asked about suicide ideation. Patients suspected of or admitting suicidal ideation should be assessed comprehensively for suicide risk rather than the prediction of suicide occurrence (87). Clinical standards exist for the assessment of suicide risk but do not exist for the prediction of a suicide occurrence. Suicide risk assessments must be balanced by consideration of the anticipated benefits in evaluating the appropriateness of clinical interventions. All such assessments must be recorded in the hospital chart. Tables 30–7 and 30–8 illustrate one method of suicide risk assessment available to clinicians. Other approaches to suicide risk assessment are also available (88, 89).

When a hospital is successfully sued for the suicide of a patient whose self-destructive tendencies were not overtly known, evidence typically exists that the suicidal tendencies should have been foreseen had a proper assessment been conducted. In one case, a paranoid and delusional patient died from deep self-inflicted razor cuts and from hanging with his belt (90). Evidence revealed that the hospital had allowed the patient to retain his belt; provided him with a razor; failed to make

TABLE 30–6. Civil liability for the suicide of a psychiatric patient: causes of action and defenses

Inpatient (hospital) liability
Diagnosis
    Unforeseeable suicide: failure to assess properly
    Foreseeable suicide:
        a) Failure to document properly
        b) Improper diagnosis or assessment
Treatment (foreseeable suicide)
    Failure to supervise properly
    Failure to restrain (high-risk patient)
    Premature release (e.g., pass)
    Negligent discharge
    Unjustified freedom of movement
Defenses
    Compliance with accepted medical practice
    Lack of reasonable knowledge of suicidality
    Justifiable allowance of freedom of movement (e.g., "open ward")
    Reasonable physician's decision regarding diagnosis or course of treatment
    Intervening acts or factors (e.g., third parties)
    Extraordinary circumstances precluding or circumventing reasonable precautions or restraint

Outpatient psychotherapist liability
Diagnosis
    Unforeseeable suicide: negligent diagnosis
    Foreseeable suicide: improper diagnosis
Treatment
    Negligent treatment (e.g., supervision, abandonment, referral)
    Failure to control (e.g., hospitalize)
Defenses
    Compliance with standard of care
    Diagnosis of suicidality not reasonable
    Intervening acts
    Extraordinary circumstances

Source. From Smith J et al: *Suicide: Caselaw Summary and Analysis.* Potomac, MD, Legal Medicine Press, 1988.

and record a mental status examination; failed to make, record, or evaluate a proper medical history; and failed to make a proper diagnosis of his condition.

In another case, a paranoid schizophrenic patient who was free to move about the hospital eventually reached the fourteenth floor and then jumped to his death (91). The patient had a history of two previous hospitalizations. In one hospitalization there was a record of at least one previous suicide attempt. The hospital, which never obtained the patient's records or interviewed him about this history, admitted liability.

TABLE 30–7. Assessment of suicide risk

Risk factors

Short-term[a]	Facilitating suicide	Inhibiting suicide
Panic attacks		
Psychic anxiety		
Loss of pleasure and interest		
Alcohol abuse		
Depressive turmoil		
Diminished concentration		
Global insomnia		
Recent discharge (within 3 months) from psychiatric hospital		

Long-term		
Therapeutic alliance—ongoing patient		
Other relationships		
Hopelessness		
Psychiatric diagnoses (Axes I and II)		
Prior attempts		
Specific plan		
Living circumstances		
Employment status		
Epidemiologic data		
Availability of lethal means		
Suicidal ideation: syntonic or dystonic		
Family history		
Impulsivity (violence, driving, money)		
Drug abuse		
Physical illness		
Mental competency		
Specific situational factors		

Note. Rating system: L = low factor; M = moderate factor; H = high factor; 0 = nonfactor. Clinically judge as high, moderate, or low the potential for suicide within 24–48 hours from assessment of suicide.
[a]Short-term indicators are risk factors found to be statistically significant within 1 year of assessment.
Source. Reprinted from Simon RI: "Clinical Risk Management of Suicidal Patients: Assessing the Unpredictable," in *American Psychiatric Press Review of Psychiatry and the Law,* Vol. 3. Edited by Simon RI. Washington, DC, American Psychiatric Press, 1992, p. 11. Used with permission.

Suicide cases alleging that the treatment was negligent are usually those in which patients were known to be suicidal but the resulting care and intervention were considered substandard. The failure to supervise a known suicidal patient is one of the most common treatment-related complaints of negligence involving patient suicide (92). Hospitals and their staffs have an affirmative duty to safeguard patients with whatever precautions are considered reasonable, given the particular circumstances. When a hospital staff is on notice that a patient is suicidal, it is held to a reasonably high standard of care. The hospital staff is in a position of control and has unique expertise in providing treatment to vulnerable patients. Courts will generally not try to second-guess a psychiatrist's medical judgment if it is reasonable, given the circumstances. For instance, in *Topel v. Long Island Jewish Medical Center* (93), the court of appeals affirmed a lower court's finding that a hospital was not liable for the suicide death of a patient in part because "a psychiatrist's decision to order a patient observed at 15-minute intervals rather than continuously was a matter of professional judgment."

The final major factual area in which liability for patient suicide typically occurs is when a foreseeably suicidal patient is inappropriately discharged or released from the facility. This can occur when a suicidal

TABLE 30–8. Assessment of suicide risk and psychiatric intervention options

Suicide risk	Psychiatric interventions
High	Immediate hospitalization
Moderate	*Consider:* Hospitalization Frequent outpatient visits Reevaluating treatment plan frequently Remaining available to patient
Low	Continue with current treatment plan

Note. Tables 30–7 and 30–8 represent only one method of suicide risk assessment and intervention. The purpose of these tables is heuristic, encouraging a systematic approach to risk assessment. The therapist's clinical judgment concerning the patient remains paramount. Given the fact that suicide risk variables will be assigned different weights according to the clinical presentation of the patient, the method presented in these tables cannot be followed rigidly.
Source. Reprinted from Simon RI: "Clinical Risk Management of Suicidal Patients: Assessing the Unpredictable," in *American Psychiatric Press Review of Psychiatry and the Law,* Vol. 3. Edited by Simon RI. Washington, DC, American Psychiatric Press, 1992, p. 12. Used with permission.

patient is prematurely released on a pass (94) or is discharged from the hospital (95) or if the patient escapes and the hospital fails to attempt reasonably to retrieve the patient (96). As with any allegation of negligence, the threshold issue is the reasonableness of the decision to release the patient or allow the patient's escape. The standard of reasonableness, however, does not require 100% accuracy or certainty. A mere mistake in diagnosis or judgment is insufficient for liability (97). Therefore, if reasonable care in observing, evaluating, and providing treatment to a patient would not have revealed the patient as suicidal at the time of release, then liability for a patient who later commits suicide will generally not be found (Table 30–9).

Violent Patients

Hospital liability related to injuries caused by violent patients generally results from the negligent release of these patients. Although duty to warn or *Tarasoff*-type outpatient cases have garnered a considerable amount of attention and media coverage in the past, cases involving the injury or death of individuals because of the negligent release or discharge of a potentially violent patient are far more common.

A hospital's decision to release a patient, whether on a pass or for final discharge, is no less important than the decisions regarding course of treatment. The decision to release a patient may be precipitated by any number of factors: the patient has benefited maximally and hospitalization is no longer required, a civil commitment order has expired, the patient is eligible for conditional release, or the therapeutic benefits of a pass outweigh considerations to maintain the patient in the hospital. Regardless of the reason, a hospital or staff psychiatrist has a duty to exercise reasonable skill, care, and judgment when deciding to release a patient. This duty is implicitly heightened when the patient has a history of violence, has been violent while in the hospital, has made threats against specific individuals or the public, or manifests certain characteristics that indicate a risk for possible future violence. Hospitals, however, generally have the power to discharge involuntarily hospitalized patients at the hospital's discretion and without court approval. In a number of states, statutes require that a patient with violent proclivities be discharged only with written consent from the appropriate hospital authorities on examination and guarantee of supervision by a reputable person (98). A criminally committed patient, a mentally retarded patient, or a juvenile committed by a court order, however, require an order for discharge from the committing court (98).

In *Semler v. Psychiatric Institute of Washington, DC* (99), the hospital violated a court order in transferring the patient to outpatient status. The patient had been previously convicted and sentenced to 20 years for abduction. As part of the sentencing agreement, the judge ordered close supervision of the patient. The court had approved weekend passes but was not asked to approve the patient's discharge. The patient killed a local schoolgirl on the premises of a private school. The court held both the psychiatrist and the institute liable for the death of the girl and awarded damages of $25,000. The court noted that by transferring the

TABLE 30–9. Suicidal patients: pass and discharge considerations

Benefits of release versus risk: analysis

Determined by direct evaluation.

Consultation with all appropriate staff.

Review of patient's current and past course of hospitalization.

Evidence of posthospitalization self-care ability

Can patient function without significant affective and cognitive impairment?

Capability of and accessibility to obtaining assistance

Is patient physically and emotionally able to employ others for support?

Remission of illness

What remains unchanged and can be dealt with as an outpatient?

Control by medication

Can side effects be tolerated and managed outside the hospital, and will patient comply with treatment?

Support system

Does family or do significant others exist and, if so, are they stabilizing or destabilizing?

Timing of proposed release

Does staff adequately know the patient?

Has the patient been acclimated adequately to the therapeutic milieu, with sufficient time allowed to develop meaningful relationships?

Has sufficient time elapsed to evaluate the effectiveness of treatment (e.g., medication)?

Therapeutic alliance

Will the patient continue to work with the psychiatrist?

Source. Reprinted from Simon RI: "The Suicidal Patient," in *Concise Guide to Psychiatry and Law for Clinicians.* Washington, DC, American Psychiatric Press, 1992, p. 112. Used with permission.

patient to outpatient status, the institute violated its duty to protect the public.

In a large majority of cases in which hospitals have been held liable for the negligent release of a violent or potentially violent patient, the liability was founded on a generalized lack of due care in issuing the decision to release the patient. For example, cases finding liability have been based on the failure of one psychiatrist to transfer records of a patient's documented violence to the discharging psychiatrist (100), the failure to conduct a reasonable discharge interview (101), the failure to investigate reports of the patient's misconduct (102), the failure to comply with a judicial order requiring notification of the court before discharging the patient (103), the failure to obtain a judicial order releasing a patient who had been committed to the hospital following a finding of "not guilty by reason of insanity" for murder (104), the decision to release based on the patient's "irritating demeanor" and poor progress in treatment (105), and the failure to maintain the patient in the hospital for the duration of a commitment order (106).

Although clinical standards exist for the assessment of risk of violence, no standard exists for predicting violent acts by patients. Clinical risk-benefit assessments should be made and entered in the medical record before releasing patients who may be potentially violent. Tables 30–10 and 30–11 illustrate one method for assessing the risk of violence.

Violent patients also may injure other patients or staff. Lion (107) observed that violence in the hospital is common. Violence within the hospital tends to be underreported, and the severity of the problem is generally denied. Criminal prosecution of patients who injure other patients or staff remains a controversial issue (108). Although psychiatrists do not have expertise in predicting violence, clinical standards do exist for the assessment of violence risk and management of these patients.

Finally, discharge decisions must be carefully documented. The record should always be kept contemporaneous with decision making. After-the-fact notes are of little value and are legally precarious. For patients who still possess potential for violence but do not meet criteria for involuntary hospitalization, a careful note explaining clinical decision making about discharge is essential.

Individuals who were specifically endangered by the patient before hospitalization should be notified of the patient's discharge well in advance, even if the patient's potential for violence is assessed as low. A significant number of patients are noncompliant with discharge treatment recommendations. A Veterans Administration study of outpatient referrals demonstrated that of 24% of inpatients referred to the Veterans Administration mental health clinic, approximately 50% failed to keep their first appointment (109). Appointments should be arranged to follow discharge as soon as possible. Thus, the clinician's obligation is to structure the follow-up so as to encourage compliance. Limitations on the powers of psychiatrists for follow-up exist and must be acknowledged by both the psychiatric and legal communities. Most discharged patients retain the right to refuse further treatment. The American

TABLE 30–10. Assessment of violence risk factors

Risk factors	Facilitating	Inhibiting
Specific person threatened[a]		
Past violent acts[a]		
Motive		
Therapeutic alliance (ongoing patient)		
Other relationships		
Psychiatric diagnoses (Axes I and II)		
Control of anger		
Situational status		
Employment status		
Epidemiologic data (age, sex, race, socioeconomic group, marital status, violence base rates)		
Availability of lethal means		
Available victim		
Syntonic or dystonic violence		
Specific plan		
Childhood abuse (or witnessing abuse of a parent)		
Alcohol abuse		
Drug abuse		
Mental competency		
History of impulsive behavior		
Central nervous system disorder		
Low intelligence		

Note. Rating system: L = low factor; M = moderate factor; H = high factor; 0 = nonfactor. Clinically judge low, moderate, or high potential for violence within 24–48 hours based on assessment of violence.
[a]When a specific person is threatened and past violence has occurred, a high risk rating for violence is achieved.
Source. Reprinted from Simon RI: "Clinical Approaches to the Duty to Warn and Protect Endangered Third Persons," in *Clinical Psychiatry and the Law,* 2nd Edition. Washington, DC, American Psychiatric Press, 1992, p. 328. Used with permission.

TABLE 30–11. Assessment of violence risk factors and psychiatric intervention options

Violence risk	Psychiatric interventions
High	Immediate hospitalization if mentally ill and likely to benefit from hospitalization
Moderate	Hospitalization Frequent outpatient visits Consider warning and calling the police Reevaluate patient and treatment plan frequently Remain available to the patient
Low	Continue with current treatment plan

Note. Tables 30–10 and 30–11 represent only one method of violence risk assessment and intervention. The purpose of these tables is heuristic, encouraging a systematic approach to risk assessment. The therapist's clinical judgment concerning the patient remains paramount. Given the fact that violence risk factors will be assigned different weights according to the patient's clinical presentation, this method of assessment should not be followed rigidly.
Source. Reprinted from Simon RI: "Clinical Approaches to the Duty to Warn and Protect Endangered Third Persons," in *Clinical Psychiatry and the Law,* 2nd Edition. Washington, DC, American Psychiatric Press, 1992, p. 329. Used with permission.

Medical Association Council on Scientific Affairs has developed evidence-based discharge criteria for safe discharge from the hospital (110).

Patient Records

One of a hospital's most important ancillary functions is the accurate compilation and retention of patient records. Records must be maintained for every individual who either is evaluated or receives treatment as an inpatient, ambulatory care patient, or emergency patient, or who receives patient services in a hospital outpatient clinic or agency. With so many persons having access to a patient's chart containing confidential communications between the patient and the psychiatrist, the ability to safeguard that information from unauthorized disclosure can be a daunting task. Certainly, there is no way to prevent the myriad professionals involved in the care of a patient from reviewing a patient's chart.

In some situations, however, the psychiatrist has control over the disclosure of confidential information in a patient's records. The psychiatrist therefore has a duty to safeguard this information from unauthorized disclosure. For example, discussions with hospital staff members regarding a patient's treatment status should be limited to that information necessary for the staff to function effectively on behalf of the patient. There is no need to divulge intimate details of the patient's mental history unless they are relevant to treatment.

Hospitals affiliated with a medical school present a unique problem. It is common for medical students to participate in diagnostic and treatment conferences despite having little or no professional involvement with a patient. In this case, if a patient's consent for clinical presentation is not obtained, a psychiatrist may be at risk of a lawsuit for breach of confidentiality. Similarly, patient participation either in person or via patient records in teaching case conferences is entirely voluntary unless a consent is obtained at the time of admission that some amount of participation may be required. Even then, it is the duty of the treating psychiatrist to see that personal information that is unrelated to case conference objectives is safeguarded from disclosure, including the patient's name.

In addition to the negligent disclosure of confidential information contained in patient records, other potential areas of liability for substandard care include alterations in record data in an attempt to cover up previous departures from standard practices (111) and the

unauthorized release of information in the hospital record (112). Unless prior consent is obtained, the unauthorized release of confidential information to third parties may subject a hospital to a lawsuit for defamation or invasion of privacy (113). The American Psychiatric Association has published policy and guideline statements concerning confidentiality and disclosure as they relate to HIV-positive patients (114, 115).

Patient Rights

Competency and Substitute Decision Makers

Only a competent person is legally permitted to make medical decisions, such as consent to treatment. The issue of competency is an important consideration in the provision of healthcare services, especially to those who are psychiatrically impaired. Patients who lack the mental capacity to make healthcare decisions require a substitute decision maker to provide consent (Table 30–12). For the psychiatric patient, evidence of impaired perception, short- and long-term memory problems, impaired judgment, language comprehension difficulties, and distortions of reality and orientation all will have a bearing on whether he or she is cognitively capable of making valid medical decisions. The lack of capacity or competency cannot be presumed from either the fact of treatment for mental illness (116) or from institutionalization of such persons (117). Moreover, mental disability or illness (e.g., psychosis) does not, in and of itself, render a person incompetent or incompetent in all areas of functioning.

TABLE 30–12. Common consent and review options for patients lacking the mental capacity for healthcare decisions

Proxy consent of next of kin[a]
Adjudication of incompetence, appointment of a guardian
Institutional administrators or committees
Treatment review panels
Substituted consent of the court
Advance directives (living will, durable power of attorney, healthcare proxy)
Statutory surrogates (spouse or court-appointed guardian)[b]

---

[a]May be excluded for treatment of mental disorders. [b]Medical statutory surrogate laws (when treatment wishes of patient are unstated).
Source. Adapted from Simon RI: "The Right to Refuse Treatment and the Therapeutic Alliance," in *Clinical Psychiatry and the Law,* 2nd Edition. Washington, DC, American Psychiatric Press, 1992, p. 109. Used with permission.

Competency is a matter of context. For instance, simply because the patient has been adjudicated incompetent for purposes of executing a will does not necessarily mean that he or she is similarly incompetent to make healthcare decisions. As a general rule, a patient with a history of mental illness must be judicially declared incompetent before he or she loses the legal power to do what other adult persons have the right to do. The patient's current or past history of physical and mental illness is but one factor to be weighed in determining whether a particular test of competency is met. In the event that a patient is judicially determined to be incompetent to make healthcare decisions, a substitute decision maker will be appointed by the court for the patient.

Right to Treatment

One of the major areas of litigation in mental disability law has been determining the rights of patients confined in institutions. The rights to treatment and rehabilitation, to the basic necessities of life, to refuse treatment, and to withhold life-sustaining measures in order to die and the volatile issue of physician-assisted suicide have all been litigated and afforded varying degrees of recognition. In 1971 an Alabama federal court in *Wyatt v. Stickney* (118) held that individuals with mental disabilities have a constitutional right to treatment, or to "habilitation." The court expressly stated that absent the opportunity to receive treatment, a person with mental disabilities in an institution was not a patient but merely a resident with an indefinite sentence. Such custodial care or punishment was not the purpose of involuntary hospitalization. Rather, the purpose of custodial care was treatment.

Although it did not find an explicit constitutional right to treatment, the U.S. Supreme Court in *Youngberg v. Romeo* (119) established the minimum civil rights that must be afforded to persons in state institutions. The Court held that mentally retarded residents of state facilities have a constitutional right to the basic necessities of life, reasonably safe living conditions, freedom from undue restraint, and the minimally adequate training needed to enhance or further their abilities to exercise other constitutional rights. Although *Youngberg* specifically dealt with a mentally retarded institutionalized patient, its holding has been applied to mentally ill or disabled patients as well.

Right to Liberty

In another landmark case, the right to liberty for committed mental patients was addressed in *O'Connor*
v. *Donaldson* (120). In *O'Connor*, the U.S. Supreme Court identified three conditions that were necessary for the release of an involuntarily hospitalized patient: 1) the patient was being warehoused in the hospital or institution, 2) the person did not present a danger to self or others, and 3) the person was capable of living in the community with the assistance of others. Although the Court did not specifically recognize a constitutional right to treatment, *O'Connor* laid the foundation for nondangerous mentally ill patients to assert their right to less restrictive environments, alternative dispositions, and other services while involuntarily hospitalized.

Right to Refuse Treatment

As of this writing, the U.S. Supreme Court has not squarely ruled on the question of whether involuntarily hospitalized mental patients have a constitutional right to refuse treatment. In fact, in its first opportunity to decide this question specifically ("right to refuse antipsychotic medication"), it declined to do so (121). The U.S. Supreme Court held in *Washington v. Harper* (122) that a state prisoner had a limited constitutional right to refuse treatment. The state's concerns, the Court concluded, will outweigh the prisoner's if the prisoner has a mental illness and is dangerous to self (including gravely disabled) or to others and if the proposed treatment will be medically beneficial. To evaluate whether these criteria are met, a committee of hospital staff convened at the time of the hearing who are not involved in the inmate's treatment should determine whether involuntary treatment (including antipsychotic medication) should be permitted. Because of the ambiguity of some portions of the decision, many commentators have speculated that although this opinion specifically dealt with a mentally ill prisoner, it also could be applied to civilly committed patients. Lower federal and state courts will now have to interpret this decision further and determine the extent to which the *Harper* opinion applies to other circumstances.

Life-Sustaining Measures ("Right to Die")

Legal decisions regarding patients' right to die fall into one of two categories: those dealing with individuals incompetent at the time that removal of life-support systems is sought and those dealing with competent patients.

In what was hoped to be the final word on this difficult and personal question of patient autonomy, the U.S. Supreme Court ruled in *Cruzan v. Director, Missouri Department of Health* (123), that the state of Missouri may refuse to remove food and water from an incompetent patient without clear and convincing evidence of her wishes. In other words, without clear evidence of a patient's decision to have life-sustaining measures withheld in a particular circumstance, the state has the right to maintain that individual's life, even at the exclusion of the family's wishes. Although this decision seemed to leave open more questions than it answered, the Court's decision buttressed the position of "right to use" treatment advocates in three significant ways.

First, and probably most important, the Court seemed to give constitutional status to a competent person's right to refuse treatment. Second, the Court did not distinguish between artificially administered food and water and other life-sustaining measures such as respirators. Third, an incompetent person who made his or her wishes known in advance, such as through a living will or a durable power of attorney, may have a constitutional right to halt life-sustaining intervention, depending on the proof of those wishes. The significance of the *Cruzan* decision for psychiatrists and physicians providing treatment to severely or terminally impaired psychiatric patients is that they must be more careful about seeking clear and competent instructions from the patient or substitute decision makers regarding foreseeable treatment decisions.

A small but growing body of case law has emerged that involves competent patients—usually those with excruciating pain and terminal diseases—who seek the termination of further medical treatment. The right to decline life-sustaining medical intervention, even for competent patients, is not absolute. In each of these situations, and depending on the circumstances, the trend has been to support a competent patient's right to have artificial life-support systems discontinued (124).

Physician-Assisted Suicide

With increasing legal recognition of physician-assisted suicide, psychiatrists are likely to be called on to act as gatekeepers. Such a role would be a radical departure from the physician's code of ethics that prohibits participation by an ethical doctor in any intervention that hastens death. Previously, the U.S. Supreme Court ruled in *Cruzan v. Director, Missouri Department of Health* (125) that terminally ill persons could refuse life-supporting medical treatment. Courts and legislators will determine whether the hastening of death is an unwarranted extension of the right to refuse treatment. Every proposal for physician-assisted suicide requires a psy-

chiatric screening or consultation to determine the person's competency to commit suicide. The presence of psychiatric disorders associated with suicide, particularly depression, will have to be ruled out as the driving factor behind physician-assisted suicide. Much controversy rages over the ethics of this gatekeeping function (126).

Patient Management

The incidence of patient abuse, either self-inflicted or by staff and other patients, is a long-standing problem in psychiatric facilities, particularly those that care for severely psychiatrically impaired patients.

Patient Abuse

Hospitals are particularly vulnerable to lawsuits if they fail to protect patients from foreseeable acts of assault, invasions of privacy, or possible violations of their civil rights. These acts may be patient initiated, such as one patient attacking another (127), or initiated by the ward staff (128) or a hospital employee (129), or involving some third party such as a visitor. The operative issue, as in any case involving acts of violence by or against a patient, is whether the violence was foreseeable. If an assault or injury could not be reasonably anticipated, then no liability will likely be found (130).

Seclusion and Restraint

The use of seclusion and restraint is a "highly respected form of treatment, of greater value to many severely disturbed patients and essential to the preservation of order and safety during psychiatric emergencies" (131). Seclusion and restraint are useful in treating a variety of mental health problems, including cases involving "violent behavior [or] behavior disruptive of the therapeutic environment," "physical attack[s] on staff or other patients," and "agitated, uncontrolled behavior" (132).

Despite the efficacy of seclusion and restraint as a short-term treatment intervention, a hospital's failure to use reasonable care and appropriate professional judgment when placing a patient in seclusion or restraint (133a, 133b) may result in a violation of federal and state statutory guidelines (134), constitutional protections (135), or JCAHO standards (136) (Table 30–13). A violation of any of these standards or laws, including the hospital's own policies, could result in civil liability (137) or court injunction (138a). Stringent federal rules and regulations now apply to the use of seclusion and restraint (138b).

TABLE 30–13. Indications and contraindications for seclusion and restraint

Indications

To prevent clear, imminent harm to the patient or others

To prevent significant disruption to treatment program or physical surroundings

To assist in treatment as part of ongoing behavior therapy

To decrease sensory overstimulation[a]

To comply with patient's voluntary reasonable request[b]

Contraindications

For extremely unstable medical and psychiatric conditions[c]

For delirious or demented patients unable to tolerate decreased stimulation[c]

For overtly suicidal patients[c]

For patients with severe drug reactions, those with overdoses, or those requiring close monitoring of drug dosages[c]

For punishment of the patient or convenience of staff

[a]Seclusion only. [b]First seclusion, then, if necessary, restraints. [c]Contraindicated unless close supervision and direct observation are provided.
Source. Adapted from Simon RI: "Seclusion and Restraint," in *Concise Guide to Psychiatry and Law for Clinicians.* Washington, DC, American Psychiatric Press, 1992, pp. 185, 187. Used with permission.

Potential Negligence of Fatigued Residents and Interns

In 1984, Libby Zion, an 18-year-old college student, was seen in a New York City hospital emergency room for evaluation of fever and an earache. The emergency room intern and resident's treatment consisted of meperidine hydrochloride and restraints. She was not seen by an attending physician. Six hours after admission, Libby Zion was dead. A grand jury investigation led to a number of recommendations, one of which was to limit the hours worked by interns and residents in teaching hospitals (139).

The Accreditation Council on Graduate Medical Education, which accredits all residency programs, has established guidelines for resident working hours and supervision through its individual subspecialty committees. Potential liability exists for hospitals, residency program directors, and residents when patients are negligently harmed by fatigued residents and interns (140).

Staff Relations

Hospital Privileges and Quality Assurance

The process governing the appointment of practitioners to the medical staff and delineation of their clinical privileges should be described in the hospital and medical staff bylaws. The issue of hospital privileges—who gets them, the scope of those privileges, and the grounds and processes for revoking privileges—is a topic of increasing importance and potential litigation for hospitals. At a minimum, hospitals must exercise due care in their decisions to admit, reject, or suspend staff privileges. Depending on the circumstances, this frequently means that the physician must be given certain due process procedures such as an opportunity to present evidence, retain counsel, and be apprised of the guidelines governing a committee's decision making. Generally, if these or similar procedures are followed, judicial intervention is unlikely (141). Nevertheless, physicians and other professionals who have had hospital privileges denied or suspended have sought relief from the courts by arguing denial of process (142).

Two cases highlight the growing significance of hospital privileges and the role of the law. The U.S. Supreme Court unanimously ruled in *Patrick v. Burget* (143) that a hospital peer review committee with the authority to grant hospital privileges was not immune from antitrust laws. The Court ruling overturned a lower court opinion that would have given hospitals and their committees absolute immunity and would have permitted them to exclude systematically nonmedical healthcare providers from hospitals pursuant to a doctrine called state action. For a peer review committee to be absolutely immune from antitrust laws under the state law doctrine, their anticompetitive acts must truly be the product of state regulation. In other words, the hospital committee must show that the restraint of competition is clearly and affirmatively a part of state policy and that the restraint of competition is actively supervised by the state.

Miller (144) noted that once exemption from anti-trust scrutiny is removed, the role of psychiatrists as the primary source of mental healthcare is dissolved by the economic arguments of nonmedical providers. They have effectively stated their position that equivalent care can be provided at lower costs.

Further opening the door of hospital privileges to nonmedical healthcare providers, the California Supreme Court in *Capp v. Rank* (145) concluded that a hospital may permit clinical psychologists on its staff to "provide psychological services within the legal scope of their licensure, without physician supervision and without discriminatory restrictions." This opinion has served as a forerunner of hospital privilege trends in other states.

Chief Executive Officer and Governing Body Liability

According to JCAHO standards, the hospital's chief executive officer is responsible to the governing board of the hospital for the overall operation of the facility and the recruitment and direction of the staff (146). Violation of specific JCAHO standards may constitute a basis for legal liability.

Hospital governing boards are primarily responsible for healthcare quality and the competency of the medical staff (147). According to Perlin (148), "psychiatric programs are subject to far greater governmental and quasi-governmental regulation than general medical facilities." JCAHO has established standards for the governing bodies of hospitals seeking accreditation (149). JCAHO standards and governmental regulations may be referred to in litigation involving hospitals.

In *Corleto v. Shore Memorial Hospital* (150), a state trial court ruled in a malpractice action that the hospital's governing board and the entire medical staff could be sued if the board knew or should have known of the incompetence of a treating physician. The mass liability threatened against the 141 members of the medical staff in *Corleto* appears to be an extension of the *Darling* doctrine noted earlier. The message from the courts is, "Clean your own house or we will do it for you."

Disciplinary Actions and the National Practitioner Data Bank

On September 1, 1990, the National Practitioner Data Bank went into effect. The data bank tracks disciplinary actions; malpractice judgments; and settlements against physicians, dentists, and other healthcare professionals (151).

Hospitals, health maintenance organizations, professional societies, state medical boards, and other healthcare organizations are required to report any disciplinary action taken against providers lasting more than 30 days (151). Disciplinary actions include limitation, suspension, or revocation of privileges or professional society membership. Immunity from liability is granted for healthcare entities and providers making peer review reports in good faith (152).

Hospitals are required to query the data bank for information concerning all physicians applying for staff privileges. Every 2 years, a query of the data bank is required concerning each physician or other practitioner on the hospital staff. Hospitals that do not comply face loss of immunity for professional peer review activities.

The public will not have access to the data bank. Plaintiffs' attorneys can have access to the data bank only if they can prove that the hospital failed to query the data bank regarding the physician in question. The information obtained can be used only to sue the hospital for negligent credentialing. Physicians can request information from the data bank about their own file without paying the $2 standard fee per name.

Conclusion

Psychiatrists who practice in hospitals, clinics, or other institutional settings generally experience increased exposure to civil liability. Some of the liability risk factors include treatment responsibilities for difficult and disturbed patients, managed care pressures adversely affecting patient care, participation on hospital committees, and vicarious liability incurred for the negligence of treatment team members. Legal liability can be minimized by placing the clinical needs of patients first and maintaining respectful relationships with colleagues. Nevertheless, psychiatrists must be sure that their malpractice insurance coverage is adequate to cover all unforeseen possibilities.

References

1. Sykes: The boundaries of vicarious liability: an economic analysis of the scope of employment rule and related legal doctrine. Harvard Law Review 101:563, 569, 1988
2. Smith JW: Hospital Liability. New York, Law Journal Seminars-Press, 1990

3. Hospital Litigation Reporter, current edition. Atlanta, Strafford

4. Simon RI: Clinical Psychiatry and the Law, 2nd Edition. Washington, DC, American Psychiatric Press, 1992

5. Smith JT: Medical Malpractice: Psychiatric Care (suppl). Colorado Springs, CO, Shephards-McGraw Hill, 1989, pp 3–5, § 9.01

6. Comment, Piercing the doctrine of corporate liability. 17 San Diego Law Review, 383, n.2 (1980)

7. Bing v Thunig, 2 NY 2d 656, 163 NYS 2d 3, 143 NE 2d 3 (1957)

8. Annotation, 12 ALR 4th, 47; ALR 3d 51: 982; see also Thompson v NASON Hospital, 591 A.2d 703 (Pa 1991)

9. Keeton WP: Prosser and Keeton Torts. St. Paul, MN, West, 1984, p 509

10. Klassette v Mecklenberg County Area Mental Health, 364 SE 2d 179 (NC 1988)

11. For example, Pamperin v Trinity Memorial Hospital, 144 Wis 2d 188, 23 NW 2d 848 (1988)

12. Paintsville Hospital Co v Rose, 683 SW 2d 255 (Ky 1985); Restatement (Second) of Agency § 269 (1958)

13. Restatement (Second) of Agency § 227 (1958)

14. Monk v Doctor's Hospital, 402 F 2d 580 (DC Cir 1968) (per curiam)

15. Mooney v Stainless, Inc, 338 F 2d 127 (6th Cir 1964), cert denied 381 US 925 (1965) (applying Illinois law)

16. Darling v Charleston Memorial Hospital, 33 Ill 2d 326, 211 NE 2d 253 (1965), cert denied 383 US 946 (1966)

17. Darling v Charleston Memorial Hospital, 33 Ill 2d 328-329 (1965)

18. Elam v College Park Hospital, 132 Cal App 3d 332, 183 Cal Rptr 156 (1982); Camacho v Mennonite Bd of Missions, 703 P 2d 598 (Colo App 1985)

19. Hull v North Valley Hospital, 159 Mont 375, 498 P 2d 136 (1972); Joiner v Mitchell County Hospital Auth, 125 Ga App 1, 186 SE 2d 307 (1971), aff'd, 229 Ga 140, 189 SE 2d 412 (1972)

20. For example, Bolen v United States, 727 F Supp 1346 (D Idaho 1989)

21. See generally King JF: The Law of Medical Malpractice in a Nutshell. St. Paul, MN, West, 1986, p 267

22. Simon RI: Clinical risk management of suicidal patients: assessing the unpredictable, in American Psychiatric Press Review of Clinical Psychiatry and the Law, Vol 3. Edited by Simon RI. Washington, DC, American Psychiatric Press, 1992, pp 3–63

23. Centeno v New York, 48 AD 2d 812, 369 NYS 2d 710 (1975), aff'd 40 NY 2d 932, 389 NYS 2d, 837, 358 NE 2d 520 (1976)

24. Johnston v Ward, 288 SC 603, 344 SE 2d 166 (1986)

25. Skar v City of Lincoln, 599 F 2d 253, 269 (8th Cir 1979)

26. Peck v Counseling Service of Addison County, Inc, 146 Vt 61, 499 A 2d 422 (1985)

27. See generally King JF: The Law of Medical Malpractice in a Nutshell. St. Paul, MN, West, 1986, p 283

28. Keeton WP: Prosser and Keeton on Torts § 135. St. Paul, MN, West, 1984, p 1072

29. Mochen v State, 53 AD 2d 484, 352 NYS 2d 290 (1974)

30. Perlin ML: Mental Disability Law: Civil and Criminal, Vol 3. Charlottesville, VA, Michie, 1989, pp 119–120

31. Paddock v Chacko, 522 So 2d 410 (Fla Ct App 1988) review denied, 533 So 2d 168 (Fla 1989) [concluding that Supreme Court lacked jurisdiction to hear appeal, thereby letting stand appeals court's ruling that psychiatrist was not liable to patient who attempted suicide]

32. Smith JT: Medical Malpractice: Psychiatric Care. Colorado Springs, CO, Shepards-McGraw Hill, 1986, pp 518–522

33. Gargiulo v Ohar, 239 Va 200, 387 SE 2d 787 (1990)

34. 28 USC § 2675 Federal Tort Claims Act

35. Hahn v Suburban Hospital Assoc Inc, 54 Md App 685, 461 A 2d 7 (1983); Zellar v Tompkins Community Hospital Inc, 124 AD 2d 287, 508 NYS 2d 84 (1986)

36. Utter v United Hospital Center, Inc, 160 WVa 703, 236 SE 2d 213 (1977); Skar v City of Lincoln, 599 F 2d 253 (8th Cir 1979) (applying Illinois law)

37. Stitts v United States, 86-Civ-6110 (2d Cir Feb 2, 1987); Washington Hospital Center v Martin, 454 A 2d 306 (DC 1982)

38. King JF: The Law of Medical Malpractice in a Nutshell. St. Paul, MN, West, 1986, pp 111–129

39. Meier v Ross General Hospital, 69 Cal 2d 420, 71, 445 P 2d 519 Cal Rptr 903 (1968)

40. Gonzalez v Nork, Cal Sup Ct Mem Dec No. 228566 (Nov 19, 1973), rev'd on other grounds, 20 Cal 3d 500, 143 Cal Rptr 240, 573 P 2d 458 (1978)

41. Swarz v Billington, 528 So 2d 1371 (Fla App 1988)

42. For example, Salas v Gamboa, 760 SW 2d 838 (Tex App 1988)

43. Dillon v Silver, 134 AD 2d 159, 520 NYS 2d 751 (1987)

44. Gonzalez v New York, 121 Misc 2d 410, 467 NYS 2d 538 (1983), rev'd on other grounds, 110 AD 2d 810 488 NYS 2d 231 (1985)

45. St. Vincent's Medical Center v Oakley, 371 So 2d 590 (Fla App 1979)

46. Plumadore v State, 75 AD 2d 691, 427 NYS 2d 90 (1980)

47. Clark v State, No. 62962 Albany Court of Claims (NY 1985)

48. Appelbaum PS: Voluntary hospitalization and due process: the dilemma of Zinermon v Burch. Hosp Community Psychiatry 41:1059–1060, 1990

49. Appelbaum PS, Gutheil TG: Clinical Handbook of Psychiatry and the Law, 2nd Edition. Baltimore, MD, Williams & Wilkins, 1991, pp 43–44

50. Zinermon v Burch, 110 S Ct 975 (1990)

51. Blanchard v Levine, No. D 014550 Fulton Cty Super Ct (GA 1985); Shaughnessy v Spray, No A7905-02395 Multnomah Cty Cir Ct (Ore Feb 16, 1983)

52. Faigenbaum v Cohen, Wayne County Circuit Court No 79-904-736, NW Michigan, May 1982; Faigenbaum v Oakland Medical Center, 143 Mich App 303, 373 NW2d 161 (Mich Ct App 1985), aff'd Hyde v University of Michigan Board of Regents, 426 Mich 223, 393 NW2d 847 (1986), revised in accord with Ross v Consumer Power Company, 420 Mich 567, 363 NW2d 641 (1986)

53. Chaires v St. John's Episcopal Hospital, No. 20808/75 NY Cty Sup Ct (NY Feb 21, 1984); Clifford v United States, No 82-5002 USDC (SD 1985); Kilgore v County of Santa Clara, No 397-525 Santa Clara Cty Super Ct (Cal 1982)

54. Fitrak v United States, No. CU81-0950 USDC (SD NY 1986); Estate of Verenna v Commonwealth of Pennsylvania, No 82-C-486 Harrison Cty Ct Comm Pleas (PA June 1985)

55. French v Corbett, No. 84-4063 (USDC NJ 1985); Hand v Krakowski, 89 AD 2d 650, 453 NYS 2d 121 (1982); Karasik v Bird, 98 AD 2d 359, 470 NYS 2d 605 (1984)

56. Shaughnessy v Spray, No. A7905-02395 Multnomah Cty Cir Ct (Ore Feb 16, 1983)

57. Clemens v St. Mary Hospital, No 82017-1140 Ct Comm Pleas, Phila Cty (PA Sept 24, 1986)

58. Reese v Health Centers Inc., No 6369 Ct Comm Pleas Phila Cty (PA July 1988)

59. Wright v State, No. 83-5035 Orleans Parish Civ Dist Ct (LA April 1986)

60. Kirk v Michael Reese Hospital Medical Center, 136 Ill App 3d 945, 483 NE 2d 906 (1985) rev'd 117 Ill 2d 507, 513 NE 2d 387, cert denied, 485 US 905 (1988); also see Schuster v Altenberg, 144 Wis 2d 223, 424 NW 2d 159 (1988)

61. LaTour v St. Luke's Hospital, No 147547 St. Louis Cty Dist Ct (MO Sept 22, 1983)

62. Clifford v United States, No 82-5002 USDC (SD 1985)

63a. Bloch v Alhambra Community Hospital, No C 385,300 Pasadena Super Ct (CA 1986)

63b. Meyer DJ, Simon RI: Clarity between psychiatrists and psychotherapists. I, Psychiatric Annals 29:241–245, 1999; II, Psychiatric Annals 29:327–332, 1999

64. Woodward B, Duckworth K, Gutheil TG: The pharmaco-therapist-psychotherapist collaboration, in Annual Review of Psychiatry, Vol 12. Edited by Oldham J. Washington, DC, American Psychiatric Press, 1993

65. Hendrickson RM: New federal regulations, psychotropic and nursing homes. Drug Therapy (suppl), August 1990, pp 101–105

66. Health Care Financing Administration: Medicare and Medicaid: requirements for long-term care facilities. Final rule with request for comments. Federal Register 54(February 12):5316–5336, 1989

67. Weiner RD, Coffey CE: Indications for use of electroconvulsive therapy, in American Psychiatric Press Review of Psychiatry, Vol 7. Edited by Frances AJ, Hales RE. Washington, DC, American Psychiatric Press, 1988, p 458

68. Weiner RD: The psychiatric use of electrically induced seizures. Am J Psychiatry 136:1507–1517, 1979

69. The Practice of Electroconvulsive Therapy: Recommendations for Treatment, Training and Privileging (A Task Force Report of the American Psychiatric Association). Washington, DC, American Psychiatric Association, 1990

70. Winslade WJ, Liston EH, Ross JW, et al: Medical, judicial, and statutory regulation of ECT in the United States. Am J Psychiatry 141:1349–1355, 1984

71. Wickline v State, 183 Cal App 3d 1175, 228 Cal Rptr 661 (1986), remanded, 239 Cal Rptr 805, 741 P 2d 613 (1987)

72. Wilson v Blue Cross of Southern California et al., 222 Cal App 3d 660 (1990)

73. Simon RI: Duties in discharging sicker and potentially violent psychiatric inpatients in the managed care era. Psychiatr Serv 49:62–67, 1998

74. Impact of verdict in California utilization review case disputed. The Psychiatric Times, July 1992, p 18

75. Stone AA: Paradigms, pre-emption, and stages: understanding the transformation of American psychiatry by managed care. Int J Law Psychiatry 18:353–387, 1995

76. Zajaczkowski v State, 189 Misc 299, 71 NYS 2d 261 (Ct Cl 1947)

77. Bucklew v Washington Adventist Hospital, No 80-196 Maryland Health Arbitration Panel (Mar 27, 1984)

78. LaTour v St. Luke's Hospital, No 147547, St. Louis Cty Dist Ct (Mo Sept 22, 1983)

79. Bianco v New York, No. 59769 Court of Claims (NY Dec 27, 1977)

80. Horton v Niagara Falls Memorial Medical Center, 51 AD 2d 152, 380 NYS 2d 116 (1976)

81. Smith JT: Medical Malpractice: Psychiatric Care. Colorado Springs, CO, Shephards-McGraw Hill, 1986

82. Lion JR: Violence and suicide within the hospital, in Modern Hospital Psychiatry. Edited by Lion JR, Adler WN, Webb WL. New York, WW Norton, 1988, pp 291–299

83. Emory Univ v Lee, 97 Ga App 680, 104 SE 2d 234 (1958); Weglarz v State, 312 AD 2d 595, 295 NYS 2d 152 (1968)

84. Annotation: Suicide: liability of mental care facility for suicide of patient or former patient. 19 ALR4th 7 (1983)

85. Rivera v New York City Health & Hospital Corp, 72 NY 2d 1021, 534 NYS 2d 923, 531 NE 2d 644 (1988)

86. Barrett v State, No. 65243 Court of Claims (NY Mar 1985)

87. Simon RI: Clinical risk management of suicidal patients: assessing the unpredictable, in American Psychiatric Press Review of Clinical Psychiatry and the Law, Vol 3. Edited by Simon RI. Washington, DC, American Psychiatric Press, 1992, pp 3–63

88. Maris RW, Berman AL, Maltsberger JT, et al: Assessment and Prediction of Suicide. New York, Guilford, 1992

89. Chiles JH, Strohsall K: The Suicidal Patient: Principles of Assessment, Treatment and Case Management. Washington, DC, American Psychiatric Press, 1995

90. Evernham v Immanuel Medical Center, No 86-0040 USDC (D Neb May 1987)

91. Wormbly v United States, No 85 C-983 (ND Ill Jan 1987)

92. Abille v United States, 482 F Supp 703 (ND Cal 1980); Brown v State, 84 AD 2d 644, 444 NYS 2d 304 (1981); Brown v St. Mary's Health Center, 713 SW 2d 15 (Mo App 1986); Mahoney v Lensink, 17 Conn App 130, 550 A 2d 1088 (1988) rev'd in part, 213 Conn 548, 569 A 2d 518 (1990); Cortez v United States, 854 F 2d 723 (5th Cir 1988)

93. Topel v Long Island Jewish Medical Center, 55 NY 2d 682, 431 NE 2d 293 (1981)

94. Uphoff v DePaul Hospital Corp, CD #83-18047 New Orleans Dist Ct (La 1987)

95. Bell v New York City Health & Hospital, 90 AD 2d 270, 456 NYS 2d 787 (1982)

96. Lando v State, 47 AD 2d 972, 366 NYS 2d 679 (1975) modified 39 NY 2d 803, 385 NYS 2d 759, 351 NE 2d 426 (1976)

97. Dimitrijevic v Chicago Wesley Memorial Hospital, 92 Ill App 2d 251, 236 NE 2d 309 (1968)

98. Slovenko R: Psychiatry and the Law. Boston, MA, Little, Brown, 1973, p 213

99. Semler v Psychiatric Institute of Washington, DC, 538 F2d 121 (4th Cir), cert den, Folliard v Semler, 429 US 827 (1976)

100. Underwood v United States, 356 F 2d 92 (5th Cir 1966)

101. Bell v City of New York City Health & Hospital Corp, 90 AD 2d 270, 456 NYS 2d 787 (1982)

102. Merchant's National Bank & Trust Co. v United States, 272 F 2d 409 (DND 1967)

103. Hicks v United States, 511 F 2d 407 (DC Cir 1975)

104. Valenti v United States, No 78C-5198 (ND Ill July 2, 1982)

105. Deacy v State of New York, No 66789 Binghamton Cty Court of Claims (NY 1985)

106. Pangburn v Saad, 73 NC App 336, 326 SE 2d 365 (1985)

107. Lion JR: Violence and suicide within the hospital, in Modern Hospital Psychiatry. Edited by Lion JR, Adler WN, Well WL. New York, WW Norton, 1988, pp 291–299

108. Eichelman BS, Hartwig A: Choices in administrative psychiatry: risk and liability in decision making, in American Psychiatric Press Review of Clinical Psychiatry and the Law, Vol 3. Edited by Simon RI. Washington, DC, American Psychiatric Press, 1992, pp 99–113

109. Zeldow PB, Taub HA: Evaluating psychiatric discharge and aftercare in a VA medical center. Hosp Community Psychiatry 32:57–58, 1981

110. Report of the Council on Scientific Affairs. Evidence-Based Principles of Discharge and Discharge Criteria (CSA Report 4-A-96). Chicago, IL, American Medical Association, 1996

111. Piseo v Stamford Hospital, 41 Conn Law Journal, 43, (1980)

112. Watts v Cumberland County Hospital System, Inc, 74 NC App 769, 330 SE 2d 256 (1985) aff'd in part and rev'd in part, 317 NC 110, 343 SE 2d 879; MacDonald v Clinger, 84 AD 2d 482, 446 NYS 2d 801 (1982)

113. Feretich v Parsons Hospital, 88 AD 2d 903, 450 NYS 2d 594 (1982)

114. APA Official Actions: AIDS policy: position statement on confidentiality, disclosure, and protection of others. Am J Psychiatry 150:852, 1993

115. AIDS Policy: Guidelines for inpatient psychiatric units. Revised statement approved by APA board of trustees. Washington, DC, American Psychiatric Association, December 15, 1996

116. Wilson v Lehmann, 379 SW 2d 478, 479 (Ky 1964)

117. Rennie v Klein, 462 F Supp 1131 (D NJ 1978)

118. Wyatt v Stickney, 325 F Supp 781 (MD Ala 1971) aff'd 503 F 2d 1305 (5th Cir 1974)

119. Youngberg v Romeo, 457 US 307 (1982)

120. O'Connor v Donaldson, 422 US 563 (1975)

121. Mills v Rogers, 457 US 291 (1982)

122. Washington v Harper, 110 SCt 1028 (1990)

123. Cruzan v Director, Missouri Department of Health, 110 S Ct 284 (1990)

124. Tune v Walter Reed Army Medical Hospital, 602 F Supp 1452 (DDC 1985); Bartling v Superior Court, 163 Cal App 3d 186, 209 Cal Rptr 220 (1984); Bouvia v Superior Court, 225 Cal Rptr 297 (1986); In re Farrell, 529 A 2d 404 (NJ 1987); In re Peter, 529 A 2d 419 (NJ 1987); In re Jobes, 529 A 2d 434 (NJ 1987); In re Conroy, 486 A 2d 1209 (NJ 1985)

125. Cruzan v Director, Missouri Department of Health, 497 US 261 (1990)

126. American Medical Association: Physician-assisted suicide. Code of Medical Ethics Reports 5(2):269–275, 1994

127. Irelan v Community Psychiatric Center of Florida, No 85-7085 Duval Cty Cir Ct (Fla 1987)

128. Moss v Central State Hospital, 179 Ga App 359, 346 SE 2d 580 (Ga 1986)

129. Newman v Glendale Adventist Medical Center, No NCC 15537 G Los Angeles Cty Super Ct (Cal Feb 1986)

130. Cavitt v University of Chicago Hospitals, No 77L-14101 Ill Cty Cir Ct (Ill 1985)

131. Amicus brief of Massachusetts Psychiatric Association, No 79-1649, in Rogers v Okin, 634 F 2d 650 (1st Cir 1980)

132. Mattson MR, Sacks S: Seclusion: use and complications. Am J Psychiatry 135:1210, 1978

133a. American Psychiatric Association: The Psychiatric Uses of Seclusion and Restraint (Task Force Report No 22). Washington, DC, American Psychiatric Association, 1985

133b. Gutheil TG, Tardiff K: Indications and contraindications for seclusion and restraint, in The Psychiatric Uses of Seclusion and Restraint. Edited by Tardiff K. Washington, DC, American Psychiatric Press, 1984, pp 11–17

134. For example, Ariz Rev Stat Ann 36-513 (1983); DC Code Ann § 6-1970 (1989); NJ Rev Stat § 30:4-24.2(d)(3) (1981); NY Mental Hyg Law § 33.04 (1988)

135. Youngberg v Romeo, 457 US 307 (1982)

136. Joint Commission on Accreditation of Healthcare Organizations: Comprehensive Accreditation Manual for Behavioral Health. Chicago, Joint Commission on Accreditation of Healthcare Organizations, 2001

137. Annotation: Civil liability for physical measures undertaken in connection with treatment of mentally disordered patient. 8 ALR 4th 464-518

138a. O'Sullivan v Secretary of Human Services, 402 Mass 190, 521 NE 2d 997 (1988)

138b. Simon RI: Concise Guide to Psychiatry and Law for Clinicians, 3rd Edition. Washington, DC, American Psychiatric Publishing, 2001

139. Grand Jury Report, Supreme Court of the State of New York. Report concerning the care and treatment of a pateint and the supervision of residents and interns and junior residents at a hospital in New York County 2 (Dec 1986)

140. McNoble DJ: Expanded liability of hospitals for the negligence of fatigued residents. J Leg Med 11:427–449, 1990

141. Adkins v Sarah Bush Lincoln Health Center, 129 Ill 2d 497, 544 NE 2d 733 (1989)

142. Callahan MR, Vocke DN: Current legal developments in medical staff credentialing disputes, in Legal Implications of Hospital Policies and Practices. Edited by Miller RD. San Francisco, CA, Jossey-Bass, 1989, pp 81–93

143. Patrick v Burget, 486 US 911 (1988)

144. Miller RD: Recent developments in antitrust: challenges to medical autonomy, in Legal Implications of Hospital Policies and Practices. Edited by Miller RD. San Francisco, CA, Jossey-Bass, 1989, pp 69–80

145. Capp v Rank, No. B020113, C 502929 (Cal Sup Ct Aug 1990)

146. Joint Commission on Accreditation of Healthcare Organizations. Comprehensive Accreditation Manual for Behavioral Health. Chicago, Joint Commission on Accreditation of Healthcare Organizations, 2001

147. Stern v Lucy Webb Hayes Nat Training School, 381 F Supp 1003 (D DC 1974)

148. Perlin ML: Mental Disability Law: Civil and Criminal, Vol 3. Charlottesville, VA, Michie, 1989, p 24

149. Joint Commission on Accreditation of Healthcare Organizations. Comprehensive Accreditation Manual for Behavioral Health. Chicago, Joint Commission on Accreditation of Healthcare Organizations, 2001

150. Corleto v Shore Memorial Hospital, 138 NJ Super 302, 350 A 2d 534 (1975)

151. Johnson ID: Reports to the National Practitioner Data Bank. JAMA 265:407–411, 1991

152. Walzer RS: Impaired physicians: an overview and update of legal issues. J Leg Med 11:131–198, 1990

❖ 31 ❖

Criminal Law

Robert D. Miller, M.D., Ph.D.

Clinical administrators, whether of inpatient or outpatient facilities, must increasingly be aware of laws governing their behavior and that of their patients (Miller 1996). In this chapter we discuss issues related to criminal law and criminal patient populations with which administrators should be familiar. Issues and regulations in civil law are discussed in Chapter 30.

Because of economic and legal pressures that have restricted admissions to psychiatric facilities (both inpatient and outpatient) and reduced inpatient lengths of stay dramatically (Miller 1987, 1991), an increasing number of people with mental disorders are forced to receive what mental healthcare they can get through the criminal justice system. In addition, the character of even civil populations has changed significantly, away from the chronically mentally ill toward those diagnosed with personality disorders and characterized by their perceived dangerousness (Oldham and Skodol 1991). Although chronically mentally ill patients are less likely than the general population to become involved in serious criminal activity, those with personality disorders, especially Cluster B disorders, are significantly more likely to commit serious crimes and thus to encounter the criminal justice system. Because this patient population is more likely to be involved with the criminal justice system, administrators must become

more familiar with its operation, particularly aspects that are relevant to the patient populations with which they work.

Pretrial Evaluations

Once a person is arrested, his or her mental condition may be relevant to further criminal proceedings, and mental health professionals may be called on to provide evaluations for the courts. Previously these evaluations were performed almost exclusively in forensic hospitals, but they are increasingly being performed on an outpatient basis (i.e., on defendants either in jails or out on bond) (Miller and Germain 1989). Administrators of public outpatient facilities need to become familiar with the evaluations and with the differences between legal and clinical evaluations.

Criminal Competency

Once a person has been arrested, his or her capacity to participate in the criminal justice process may be questioned. Most common (and most discussed in the legal and forensic literature) is *competency to proceed.* Derived from the English common law requirement that defendants must be present at their trials (Gobert 1973), this concept has evolved to include cognitive and physical presence. In the United States the definition of competency to proceed was handed down by the U.S. Supreme Court in *Dusky v. United States* (1960): "[T]he test must be whether [the defendant] has sufficient present ability to consult his attorney with a reasonable degree of rational understanding and a rational as well as factual understanding of proceedings against him." The test thus contains both volitional (capacity to consult) and cognitive (rational and factual understanding) tests for competency.

Subsequent decisions have made it clear that defendants' competency to proceed must be evaluated and adjudicated at a formal hearing if there is any reason to suspect that they may not be competent (*Pate v. Robinson* 1966). Also, if a defendant's competency changes during the trial process, further formal evaluations and hearings may be required (*Drope v. Missouri* 1975). Neither defendants nor their attorneys may prevent such evaluations of competency, although many jurisdictions permit defendants to refuse to cooperate with them.

In addition to competency to stand trial, questions can be raised concerning defendants' competencies to waive their Miranda rights, to enter a plea, to waive representation by counsel, to stand trial, to be sentenced, to waive appeals, to have their probation or parole revoked, and to be executed (Miller 1994). Although there is some case law (court decisions) in this area, mental health professionals asked to perform these evaluations will find little in statutes or court decisions to guide them. Although trial judges make the ultimate decisions about criminal competencies, they also have little guidance in making those decisions and are usually quite dependent in practice on the mental health professionals who perform the evaluations. Clinical facilities that provide services to patients charged with a criminal offense must develop expertise in performing such evaluations.

A number of attempts have been made to devise tests of competency to proceed (Grisso 1986). Even the more sophisticated of them, however, remains basically a structured interview that addresses the relevant points and is not adequate in the hands of an interviewer inexperienced in evaluating criminal defendants.

If found incompetent to proceed *and* treatable, defendants may be committed for treatment to restore competency. Before 1975 such commitments were indeterminate—until competency was restored—and

often amounted to life sentences without trial. In 1975 the U.S. Supreme Court held that "a person charged by a state with a criminal offense who is committed solely on account of his incapacity to proceed to trial cannot be held more than the reasonable period of time necessary to determine whether there is a substantial probability that he will retain the capacity in the foreseeable future" (*Jackson v. Indiana* 1972). After *Jackson,* most states limited the duration of commitment to restore competency to the maximum length of the sentence for the crime charged. Prosecutors, who had been the most frequent petitioners for competency evaluations before *Jackson,* largely lost interest, and the overwhelming majority of petitions are now brought by defense attorneys (Miller and Kaplan 1992).

Restoration of competency has both clinical and legal aspects. The majority of defendants found incompetent have major psychiatric disorders such as schizophrenia or major affective disorders; therefore, the clinical approach begins with appropriate psychopharmacologic treatment. In the majority of cases, this treatment alone is sufficient to restore adequate cognitive capacity to allow defendants to meet the criteria for competency. Competency requires only such capacity to understand the proceedings and to cooperate with counsel. In order to determine if capacity has been restored, however, evaluators must have sufficient knowledge of and experience with legal proceedings to provide adequate evaluations for the courts.

The task is different with defendants who have developmental disabilities or organic brain injuries. Psychotropic medications are not effective, and in most cases no treatment exists that will increase cognitive capacity. In these cases a psychoeducational approach is necessary, if not always effective (Webster et al. 1985) Unfortunately, few psychiatric facilities have staff experienced in working with either population, and even fewer facilities specializing in treating either population have staff experienced with forensic practice. Administrators who accept the responsibility of working with these populations must ensure that their staffs have the clinical and legal knowledge necessary to restore competency where possible and that they are able to perform adequate evaluations to determine when that restoration has occurred.

A major difference exists between clinical and legal evaluations. Clinicians have little reason to question their patients' histories or symptoms and rarely go beyond obtaining previous medical records in seeking external corroborating information. It is crucial not to jeopardize the development of trust in the therapeutic relationship by challenging, or even attempting to verify, a potential patient's reports. Forensic evaluators, in contrast, cannot afford to accept at face value what the patients tell them and must attempt to obtain as much external information as possible (e.g., police reports, witness and victim statements, criminal history). All patients being evaluated for the courts, either criminal or civil, have clear reasons to distort their histories or symptoms, and those reports must be verified as much as possible. The American Psychiatric Association (1994) emphasizes this need by making a court-requested evaluation the first criterion for suspecting malingering in any patient.

Administrators who accept the responsibility of having their staff provide forensic evaluations must ensure that those evaluations are comprehensive and must recognize that in those cases the client is the court, not the individual patient. Because a forensic evaluation may significantly interfere with the development of a trusting therapeutic relationship, it is always best, if possible, to assign the treatment and evaluation responsibilities to clinicians different from those providing the direct treatment (Miller 1990).

Insanity

The other major psychiatric evaluation in the criminal justice system is that of criminal responsibility. Of these evaluations, the best known by far is that of *insanity*. Insanity is a legal concept, the finding of which relieves defendants of all guilt for their otherwise criminal behavior, while permitting the state to confine the acquitted individual for treatment and for protection of the public. Many people (including some attorneys and judges) confuse competency (which is a contemporary and prospective evaluation) with criminal responsibility, which is a retrospective evaluation and refers to a defendant's mental state at the time of an alleged crime.

The earliest generally established test of insanity in Anglo-American law was devised by the English Law Lords in the M'Naghten Case (1843). According to that case, "To establish a defense on the ground of insanity, it must be clearly proved that at the time of the committing of the act, the party accused was laboring under such defect of reason, from disease of the mind, as not to know the nature and quality of the act he was doing, or if he did know it, that he did not know he was doing what was wrong." This is a cognitive test of criminal responsibility.

Although now considered the most restrictive test of insanity in the United States, the M'Naghten test replaced even more narrow tests in England. In 1265, Lord Bracton, archdeacon of Barnstable, held that "an insane person is one who does not know what he is doing, is lacking in mind and reason and is not far removed from the brutes" (quoted in Bromberg 1979). In 1671, Lord Matthew Hale ruled that "[s]uch a person is laboring under melancholy distempers hath yet ordinarily as great understanding as ordinarily a child of fourteen years hath, is such a person as may be guilty of treason or felony" (Hale 1847). Finally, in *Rex v. Arnold* (1724), Judge Tracy held that for the defendant to be found insane, "It must be a man totally deprived of his understanding and memory and doth not know what he is doing, no more than an infant, than a brute, or a wild beast."

The M'Naghten test came to the United States with the rest of English common law and was initially the legal test for insanity in every state. Several states subsequently adopted a so-called product test of insanity (*Parsons v. State* 1887; *State v. Jones* 1871), under which defendants are insane if their criminal acts are the product of mental disorder. The most famous of these tests was the Durham Rule (*Durham v. United States* 1960) created by Judge Bazelon of the District of Columbia Court of Appeals in response to psychiatric criticisms that the M'Naghten test did not permit them to provide the court with sufficient information. The Durham experiment lasted for 12 years; after several unsuccessful attempts to prevent psychiatrists from offering conclusory opinions, the court finally abandoned the test (*United States v. Brawner* 1972). Only New Hampshire retains a product test.

Although the product test went too far for the law, continued criticisms of the M'Naghten test's exclusive focus on a defendant's cognitive capacities led to several modifications. Several states added a volitional prong to M'Naghten, called the irresistible impulse test. It was criticized by those who favored a broadening of the criteria, who argued that not all insane behavior was impulsive and that the test thus did not go far enough. The test has largely disappeared today, although several states retain it as an adjunct to the M'Naghten test.

In 1955, the American Law Institute (1955) proposed a test that contained both cognitive and volitional prongs: "A person is not responsible for criminal conduct if at the time of such conduct as a result of mental disease or mental defect he lacks substantial capacity either to appreciate the criminality of his conduct or to conform his conduct to the requirements of law." Over the next 20 years, three-fourths of the states and federal law changed from M'Naghten to the American Law Institute test.

In the 1980s, with the political shift to the right and the growing emphasis on law and order, the insanity defense came under increasing attack, even though the defense is raised in less than 1% of criminal cases and is successful in far fewer than half of those. After John Hinckley's successful insanity defense, those attacks intensified. Four states (Utah, Montana, Idaho, and Nevada) have abolished the formal defense of insanity, although all four states permit evidence of a defendant's mental state to be introduced to reduce a defendant's degree of culpability or to affect the disposition of the case. More frequent have been changes to the insanity test itself. A number of states and Congress removed the volitional prong of the American Law Institute test, reverting to the M'Naghten formula. These changes were supported by the American Bar Association (1983) and the American Psychiatric Association (1983); the latter justified its position on an assertion that volition is harder to evaluate than cognition. Rogers (1987) strongly criticized this conclusion as being without empirical support and as a political rather than a scientific position.

In the past, defendants found not guilty by reason of insanity were committed indefinitely, "until cured." With the civil rights movement in the 1970s, indefinite commitments of all kinds came under attack, and most states adopted lengths of commitment not to exceed the sentences that acquitted individuals could receive if they had been found guilty of the crimes charged. In addition, the civil rights movement pushed for more liberal release criteria for those found insane. As the law and order movement gained momentum in the 1980s, however, the pendulum began to swing toward longer commitments. Unlike civil commitments, in which psychiatrists have not only the authority but also the responsibility to release patients as soon as they no longer satisfy the commitment criteria, the criminal courts continue to retain jurisdiction over release decisions involving insanity acquittees in most states, although recommendations from the treating facility continue to have great influence.

When an individual has been civilly committed, it is usually far easier to prove continued mental illness than continued dangerousness; with insanity acquittees the reverse situation often holds, in which the difficulty is often in demonstrating a legally sufficient mental ill-

ness. Many of these individuals have both a major mental disorder and a personality disorder (frequently antisocial personality). The major disorder is often responsive to treatment, but the personality disorder is usually not. The U.S. Supreme Court has twice ruled definitively that the state must prove both mental illness and dangerousness in order to continue to hold an insanity acquittee (*Foucha v. Louisiana* 1992; *Jones v. United States* 1983). Because of the public's misperceptions about the dangers posed by mentally ill persons, significant political pressure is put on directors of forensic facilities not to recommend release for acquittees. Such pressure has the potential to turn clinical treatment facilities into the warehouses of the 1950s and 1960s; and nonclinical administrators (who are now in the majority in state mental hospitals) tend to be more sensitive to such pressures than are the clinicians who have to provide the treatment. These administrators in turn put pressure on clinicians to argue that personality disorders are mental illnesses for the purpose of continued commitment.

Other Forms of Criminal Responsibility

A defendant's mental state may affect the consequences of a criminal prosecution outside the insanity defense in several ways. The oldest way is through the concept of *diminished capacity,* in which the presence of a mental illness can reduce a defendant's culpability, as from murder to manslaughter. The defendant is still found guilty of a criminal act and will go to prison instead of a hospital. The concept was pioneered by the California Supreme Court (*People v. Gorshen* 1959; *People v. Wells* 1949) and adopted by a number of other states. Since the 1980s, however, public reaction to the defense has been as negative as to the insanity defense. Public outrage at the infamous "Twinkie Defense" in the Dan White case in San Francisco, California (*People v. White* 1981) provided the excuse to abolish the defense; it has lost favor in other states as well.

Although the concept of diminished capacity was created to reduce the severity of consequences for mentally ill defendants who did not meet criteria for the insanity defense, the *guilty but mentally ill* (GBMI) verdict was created as an alternative to the insanity defense, in the hopes that many defendants would be found GBMI instead of insane. The verdict is not well defined, essentially meaning only that at the time of the crime the defendant had a mental disorder that does not qualify for either an insanity or a diminished capacity defense. Defendants found GBMI go to prison. Most states with such statutes provide for required psychiatric evaluations, but data from Michigan, the first state to create the verdict, reveal that GBMI inmates receive no more services than other inmates and are likely not to be paroled as soon as inmates found simply guilty of the same crimes (Smith and Hall 1982). A comprehensive study by the National Center for State Courts concluded that the GBMI verdict has not accomplished what its advocates had hoped (Keilitz et al. 1984).

Steadman et al. (1993) found that few legislative reform efforts have had much success in reducing the numbers of defendants found insane. For example, abolition of the defense altogether in Montana resulted in an increase in the number of defendants found permanently incompetent to proceed; this increase equaled the previous number of insanity acquittals.

Mentally Disordered Sex Offenders

Many states passed "mentally disordered sex offender" (MDSO) laws in the 1950s and 1960s; those laws were written to provide treatment, rather than punishment, for sex offenders, who were at that time viewed as having treatable mental disorders. For a variety of reasons, including civil libertarian challenges as well as insufficient treatment resources and selection on grounds other than treatability, both leading to poor treatment results, most of those laws were repealed or fell into disuse in the 1970s and 1980s (Weiner 1985).

Another consequence of the conservative social trend in the United States is a growing demand that something definitive be done about sex offenders. The first result of this trend is the creation of a new generation of MDSO laws, now generally called sexual predator laws. Previous laws were typically sentencing alternatives to imprisonment, whereas the new laws go into effect only at the completion of a full prison sentence. Offenders are "civilly" committed indefinitely, based on predictions that they would otherwise continue to commit violent sexual crimes. Purely civil commitments would be unlikely to be ordered under such criteria, but state supreme courts in Washington, Minnesota, and Wisconsin have upheld them, and the U.S. Supreme Court has found them constitutional (*Kansas v. Hendricks* 1997).

The state rationale for such preventive detention, which has been accepted by the courts, is the same as

for ordinary civil commitment—the provision of treatment. The major differences are easily seen, however, when three factors are compared. The first factor is length of commitment. The average duration of truly civil involuntary hospitalization is 2–3 weeks. The new sexual predator laws are too recent to have many long-term data, but no one has been released yet, and some of the laws have been in effect for several years. The second factor is the reality of treatment provision. A significant majority of state civil mental hospitals are accredited by the Joint Commission on Accreditation of Healthcare Organizations, which ensures at least minimally adequate staff and other treatment resources. By contrast, the Wisconsin legislature that enacted that state's sexual predator law appropriated less than $200,000 a year for the program, which grew within a year to 90 offenders and to more than 200 the second year (Gregory Van Rybroek, personal communication, April 21, 1997).

The third factor is that states with sexual predator laws are filling up their forensic treatment beds with frequently untreatable (the Kansas law *defines* its population as untreatable!) offenders, at the expense of the more traditional, and far more treatable, forensic patients. Sex offenders now occupy more than two-thirds of the beds in one of the two state forensic facilities in Wisconsin, obviously causing serious problems for clinicians and administrators alike.

Another political approach to sex offenders is the chemical castration legislation that passed in California in 1996 and in 4 other states in the next 2 years. similar bills were introduced in 22 other states but failed to pass (Miller 1998). Antiandrogens (medroxyprogesterone acetate in the United States) have been known for years to help certain sex offenders control their abnormally high sex drives or fantasies (Money 1970). More recently, the selective serotonin reuptake inhibitors (SSRIs) have been shown to have similar effects (Bradford 1996). Rather than encourage and support the clinically appropriate use of such medications, however, these laws require that all members of certain legally defined classes of offenders (most typically repeat child molesters) take antiandrogen medication as an absolute condition of any parole. Only 6 of the 27 bills (and only 2 of those that passed) even mention any type of medical evaluation, and none requires judges to follow medical advice, with respect to either indications or contraindications. Only 6 of the bills (and again, only 2 of those that passed) recognize the dilemma in which such laws place physicians by providing that courts cannot force them to prescribe the medications against their professional judgment. Only the Wisconsin statute provides funding and structure for medical follow-up.

None of the bills deals with the major problem of finding physicians knowledgeable about treating sex offenders with either antiandrogens or SSRIs. Psychiatric training programs do not usually provide any training in this area, and few psychiatrists outside state forensic facilities choose to work with sex offenders. Because such bills may be introduced in the future, administrators may need to develop expertise in their staffs to provide both the medication (if appropriate) and the ongoing psychotherapy that has been shown to be an essential part of treatment plans for sex offenders.

Criminal Laws Leading to Liability for Clinicians

Criminal codes are increasingly being used to regulate the conduct of clinicians, unfortunately mostly in the direction of turning them into investigators and police. Since the 1960s, every state has required a variety of professionals, including mental health professionals, to report suspected child abuse. This has become accepted practice among clinicians who provide treatment to the victims. Adult psychiatrists and psychologists, however, are more likely to provide treatment to perpetrators. To be required to report these individuals to law enforcement or social services, which usually destroys any possibility of a therapeutic relationship, prevents clinicians from providing the treatment for which they have been trained (Miller and Weinstock 1987). Many states provide for criminal penalties for the specified professionals if they fail to make required reports, although prosecution is quite rare in practice. Many states have applied the same principles to domestic and elder abuse, with required reporting at least by physicians and in some cases criminal penalties for failure to report.

A growing number of states have also criminalized therapist-patient sexual contact, and prosecution is no longer rare. Several states have required subsequent therapists to report previous sexual abuse by previous therapists, again with criminal penalties for failure to do so. Because some of these laws require patients to make reports, and even testify against their alleged abusers, before they have dealt effectively with the emotional consequences of the abuse, critics feel that such laws may in effect victimize patients twice (Strasburger

et al. 1990). Nevertheless, where such laws exist, therapists who are subject to the reporting requirements, and administrators of mental health facilities, need to be aware of the laws and make sure they are followed.

Differences Between Criminal and Civil Systems

In general, people with mental disorders who are involved in the criminal justice system have the same disorders as those in the civil or private systems (with the exception of a higher incidence of personality disorders). Effective clinical evaluation and treatment of these individuals requires knowledge and experience with the law enforcement and correctional systems.

Clinical administrators in primary correctional facilities (jails and prisons) are in a very different situation from those in healthcare facilities. The overriding goals of correctional facilities are punishment and security. The provision of healthcare (including mental healthcare) is a secondary goal, which in most cases has been imposed on the system by federal courts under the Eighth Amendment and is thus a service that many correctional facilities provide grudgingly.

Mental healthcare is based on individualized treatment plans and services tailored to inmates' specific needs and capacities, whereas correctional systems are solidly based on forcing inmates to behave identically, with the same consequences for the same behaviors, regardless of individual inmates' differences. Clinicians working with inmates must learn to operate within these parameters and to be sparing with requests for anything that might be considered special treatment.

Inmates frequently try to convince clinicians to order special privileges for them, particularly individual cells (which are in extremely short supply in jails and prisons). Clinicians and their administrators need to learn to resist such requests, without becoming so coopted into the correctional mentality that they ignore legitimate requests such as ordering lower bunks for inmates experiencing orthostatic hypotension side effects of medication or additional medication-dispensing times to fit inmates' schedules (e.g., giving sedating antidepressants before supper for inmates who have to get up very early to work in the kitchen).

Until recently, few community mental health centers were willing to provide treatment services to local jails, operating under the assumption that such inmates were no longer in their catchment areas. Prisons and larger jails have sufficient numbers of inmates with mental disorders to justify providing regular services (the Los Angeles jail system, for example, admits over 20,000 chronically mentally ill inmates each year). Small jails, which make up the significant majority of facilities, cannot afford to have their own mental health staff, and most did not until lawsuits began to be filed after suicides and other adverse events involving inmates with mental disorders.

With jails under legal pressure to provide mental health services, and community mental health centers under economic pressures to develop new funding sources, there would seem to be a convergence of interests that could lead to more centers providing services to jail inmates. This has in fact happened in a growing number of cases (Steadman et al. 1989).

Prison inmates with mental disorders and insanity acquittees are often not released until they can prove to the parole board or court that they will continue treatment in the community. Community facilities have been even less willing to provide services to such patients, both because of misconceptions and lack of knowledge about forensic patients and because of concerns about liability, some of which are realistic. If patients who have been proved in court to have committed serious criminal acts are released and subsequently commit further criminal acts, those responsible for their treatment in the community are more likely to be found liable than they would if the same acts were committed by patients without the criminal history (*Cain v. Rijken* 1986).

Another major difference between civil and criminal patients is that the latter usually have extensive experience with attorneys and have learned to use grievances and litigation as weapons against staff (Miller 1992). Although few grievances or suits result in findings of staff liability, many patients have discovered the harassment value of such complaints and can be expected to continue such behavior as long as it has the desired effect on staff. It is important, however, for staff not to assume that all complaints are frivolous or malicious; they may represent psychological defenses, which may be effectively interpreted in therapy (Miller et al. 1986).

Because patients who come into treatment through the criminal justice system are more likely to display dangerous behavior and are more likely to have that behavior based on characterological rather than psychotic disorders, treatment plans must actively in-

corporate methods to deal with aggressive behavior. The literature makes it clear that such incidents are significantly underreported for a variety of reasons (Lion and Reid 1983).

One major cause of underreporting is denial on the part of clinicians; such denial must be actively addressed if clinical facilities and treatment programs are to provide effective treatment for aggressive patients and provide protection for other patients. Most programs that used to avoid such patients at all costs can no longer afford to do so and need to avail themselves of the developing knowledge in treating and managing such patients (Maier et al. 1987).

One technique that clinicians have been reluctant to employ is prosecution of competent patients who commit criminal acts in treatment facilities. Though clearly inappropriate for patients who break the law as a result of hallucinations or delusions, for those whose behavior is characterologically based, it not only is necessary from a safety standpoint but also may be therapeutic by increasing patients' sense of responsibility for their behavior (Miller and Maier 1987).

Adapting to treating patients involved with the criminal justice system requires major changes in staff behaviors. Traditional staff orientation and training programs have ignored these problems almost entirely and need to be revised to deal with them (Miller et al. 1988). Administrators need to take the initiative in developing such training programs.

A final difference between working with civil and criminal patients lies in the differences between civil and criminal judges. Judges who preside over civil commitment hearings have become familiar with the laws and rules of commitment over the years and often specialize in those areas. By contrast, few criminal judges have much experience with defendants who have mental disorders, and many are woefully ignorant of the governing laws. In over 25 years of working in the public system, I have never had a major problem with judges misusing or ignoring the laws to accomplish what they want, but I have had numerous problems with criminal judges, from unauthorized orders to hospitalize defendants to contempt citations handed down when I declined to obey manifestly illegal orders. Individual clinicians cannot be expected to resist such transgressions on their own—they need support from their administrators, who therefore must become sufficiently familiar with the relevant laws, rules, and regulations to be able to support their staff against unreasonable and illegal judicial actions.

References

American Bar Association: Position Statement on the Insanity Defense. Washington, DC, American Bar Association, 1983

American Law Institute: Model Penal Code sec. 401.1(1), Tentative Draft #4, 1955

American Psychiatric Association: Position paper on the insanity defense. Am J Psychiatry 140:681–688, 1983

American Psychiatric Association: Diagnostic and Statistical Manual of Mental Disorders, 4th Edition. Washington, DC, American Psychiatric Press, 1994, p 683

Bradford JMW: The role of serotonin in the future of forensic psychiatry. Bulletin of the American Academy of Psychiatry and the Law 24:57–72, 1996

Bromberg W: The Uses of Psychiatry in the Law: A Clinical View of Forensic Psychiatry. Westport, CT, Quorum Books, 1979

Cain v Rijken, 717 P 2d 173 (Or 1986)

Drope v Missouri, 95 S Ct 896, 980 (1975)

Durham v United States, 214 F 2d 862 (DC Cir 1960)

Dusky v United States, 363 US 402 (1960)

Foucha v Louisiana, 112 S Ct 1780 (1992)

Gobert JJ: Competency to stand trial: a pre- and post-Jackson analysis. Tenn L Rev 40:659–688, 1973

Grisso T: Evaluating Competencies: Forensic Assessments and Instruments. New York, Plenum, 1986

Hale M: Pleas of the Crown, 1847 Edition 1:14

Jackson v Indiana, 406 US 715, 737-8 (1972)

Jones v United States, 103 S Ct 3043 (1983)

Kansas v Hendricks, Nos. 95-1649, 95-9075 (Sup Ct, decided June 23, 1997)

Keilitz I, Farthing-Capowich D, McGraw D, et al: The Guilty But Mentally Ill Verdict: An Empirical Study. Williamsburg, VA, National Center for State Courts, 1984

Lion JR, Reid WH (eds): Assaults Within Psychiatric Facilities. New York, Grune & Stratton, 1983

Maier GJ, Van Rybroek GJ, Doren D, et al: A comprehensive model for understanding and managing aggressive inpatients. American Journal of Continuing Education in Nursing 2(4):89–104, 1987

Miller RD: Involuntary Civil Commitment of the Mentally Ill in the Post-Reform Era. Springfield, IL, Charles C. Thomas, 1987

Miller RD: Ethical issues involved in the dual role of treater and evaluator, in Ethical Practice in Psychiatry and the Law. Edited by Rosner R, Weinstock R. New York, Plenum Press, 1990

Miller RD: Economic factors leading to diversion of the mentally disordered from the civil to the criminal commitment systems. Int J Law Psychiatry 15:1–12, 1991

Miller RD: Grievances and lawsuits against public mental health professionals: cost of doing business? Bulletin of the American Academy of Psychiatry and the Law 20:395–408, 1992

Miller RD: Forensic evaluation and treatment in the criminal forensic system, in Principles and Practice of Forensic Psychiatry. Edited by Rosner R. New York, Chapman & Hall, 1994, pp 171–224

Miller RD: Legal issues for hospital administrators, in Creating a Secure Workplace: Effective Policies and Practices in Health Care. Edited by Lion JR, Dubin WR, Futrell DE. New York, American Hospital Publishing, 1996, pp135–152

Miller RD: The forced administration of sex-drive reducing medications to sex offenders: treatment or punishment? Psychology, Public Policy, and the Law 4:175–199, 1998

Miller RD, Germain EJ: Inpatient evaluation of competency to stand trial. Health Law in Canada 9(3):74–78, 92, 1989

Miller RD, Kaplan LV: Representation by counsel: right or obligation? Behav Sci Law 10:395–406, 1992

Miller RD, Maier GJ: Factors affecting the decision to prosecute mental patients for criminal behavior. Hosp Community Psychiatry 38:50–55, 1987

Miller RD, Weinstock R: Conflict of interest between therapist-patient confidentiality and the duty to report child sexual abuse. Behav Sci Law 5:161–174, 1987

Miller RD, Maier GJ, Blancke FW, et al: Litigiousness as a resistance to therapy. Journal of Psychiatry and Law 14:109–123, 1986

Miller RD, Maier GJ, Kaye M: Orienting the staff of a new maximum security forensic facility. Hosp Community Psychiatry 39:780–781, 1988

Money J: Use of an androgen-depleting hormone in the treatment of male sex offenders. Journal of Sex Research 6:165–172, 1970

M'Naghten's Case, 10 Clark and Fin 200 8 Eng Rep 718 (1843)

Oldham JM, Skodol AF: Personality disorders in the public sector. Hosp Community Psychiatry 42:481–487, 1991

Parsons v State, 2 So 854 (Ala 1887)

Pate v Robinson, 86 S Ct 836,841 (1966)

People v Gorshen, 336 P 2d 492 (Cal 1959)

People v Wells, 202 P 2d 53 (Cal 1959); cert. denied, 337 US 919

People v White, 117 Cal App 2d 270, 172 Cal Rptr 612 (1981)

Rex v Arnold, 16 How St Tr 695 (1724)

Rogers R: APA's position on the insanity defense: empiricism versus emotionalism. Am Psychol 42:840–848, 1987

Smith GA, Hall JA: Evaluating Michigan's guilty but mentally ill verdict: an empirical study. University of Michigan Journal of Law Reform 16:77–114, 1982

State v Jones, 50 NH 369 (1871)

Steadman HJ, McCarty DW, Morrissey JP: The Mentally Ill in Jail. New York, Guilford, 1989

Steadman HJ, McGreevy MA, Morrissey JP, et al: Before and After Hinckley: Evaluating Insanity Defense Reform. New York, Guilford, 1993

Strasburger LH, Jorgenson L, Randles R: Mandatory reporting of sexually exploitative psychotherapists. Bulletin of the American Academy of Psychiatry and the Law 18:379–384, 1990

United States v Brawner, 471 F 2d 969 (DC Cir 1972)

Webster C, Jenson F, Stermac C, et al: Psycho-educational assessment programmes for forensic psychiatric patients. Canadian Psychologist 26:50–53, 1985

Weiner B: Sexual psychopath laws, in The Mentally Disabled and the Law, 3rd Edition. Edited by Parry J, Weiner B, Brakel J. Chicago, American Bar Foundation, 1985, pp 739–743

❖ 32 ❖

American Prisons

Donald H. Williams, M.D.

Thomas S. Gunnings, Ph.D.

Franklyn L. Giampa, Ph.D.

The inmate population in American prisons and jails has expanded greatly since the 1970s. According to the U.S. Bureau of Justice Statistics, the incarceration rate has more than tripled since 1980. At year end 1999, 3.1% of allU.S. adult residents (6.3 million) were on probation, in jail or prison, or on parole (Bureau of Justice Statistics 2001). Experts attribute this increase in the inmate population to the enactment of nondiscretionary sentencing, "the war on drugs," harsher and longer sentencing for crack cocaine use and sale, race, poverty, unemployment, and inadequate community treatment of mental illness and substance abuse (Center for Mental Health Services 1995; Hatsukami and Fischman 1996; Kappeler et al. 1996; Torrey et al. 1992).

Mauer and Huling (1995) agreed that public policies ostensibly written to control drug abuse and crime have increased racial disparity in the criminal justice system while having little impact on illicit drug use. They reported that as of 1995,

- Almost one in three (32.2%) young black men in the 20- to 29-year-old age group is under criminal justice supervision on any given day—in prison or jail, on probation, or on parole.

- African American women have experienced the greatest increase in criminal justice supervision of all demographic groups; the rate of criminal justice supervision of African American women rose by 78% from 1989 to 1994.

- Drug policies constitute the single most significant factor contributing to the rise in criminal justice populations in recent years; the number of incarcerated drug offenders has risen by 510% since 1983. The number of black, non-Hispanic women incarcerated in state prisons for drug offenses increased more than eightfold—828%—from 1986 to 1991.

- Although arrest rates for African Americans accused of violent crimes—45% of arrests nationally—are disproportionate to the percentage of African Americans in the general population, this proportion has not changed significantly since the 1970s. For drug offenses, the proportion of arrests among African Americans increased from 24% in 1980 to 39% in 1993, well above the proportion of African American drug users nationally.

African Americans and Hispanics constitute almost 90% of offenders sentenced to state prison for drug possession.

During this same period, mentally ill persons came to occupy greater proportions of the jail and prison populations. Many drug-abusing mentally ill adults have been imprisoned as a result of the so-called war on drugs. The decreasing availability of adequate community treatment for persons with dual diagnoses; increasing homelessness as the stocks of low-income housing disappear; lack of employment opportunities; falling welfare benefits; the closing of long-term facilities for chronically ill patients; and the public's wish to rid the community of the bizarre, the unemployed, and the homeless have contributed to the incarceration of this population. Williams et al. (1980) noted the reluctance of Americans to share scarce resources with the have-nots in economic recessions. Social benefits are used to shore up the system rather than to aid those who have not yet benefited from it.

Estimates of the prevalence of mental illness in prison populations vary. Neighbors et al. (1987) found an 80% lifetime prevalence rate of alcohol and substance abuse; lifetime prevalence rates of psychotic mood, anxiety, and organic brain disorders are significantly greater than in comparable community samples.

Psychiatry and other mental health professions must now address the problems of providing care to some of the nation's most seriously mentally ill in correctional settings that are mandated to contain and punish their inmates for criminal offenses often related to substance abuse and other severe mental disorders. The development and maintenance of correctional clinical mental health programs that conform to national professional accrediting and community standards and that are cost effective in the current political climate are among the most complicated challenges facing psychiatric administrators today.

In this chapter we provide an administrative model for psychiatric administration in the American prison system. This model is based in part on historical analysis of the failures of rehabilitation programs in American prisons. It is also based on the knowledge the authors gained using the open-systems theory of organizations in their collaborative efforts to help establish and manage a prison psychiatric service.

Historical Perspectives

Colonial Americans regarded criminal behaviors as inherent in humans and not a result of societal flaws.

Punishments were dispensed to deter the offender from committing future crimes in that particular community by frightening the offender into the lawful behavior. The punishments included monetary fines, whippings, public shaming (e.g., stocks, public branding, public cages), banishment from the community, and hanging. Punishments depended as much on the offender's social status as on the seriousness of the crime. Town residents tended to receive lighter sentences than outsiders. Prosperous town residents were fined; poor town residents were shamed. Outsiders were more likely whipped and banished. The criminal recidivists, no matter the nature of their crimes, were most likely hanged. On becoming an independent nation, America set about changing the British colonial model of criminal justice. Capital punishments were replaced by the certainty of long terms of incarceration in prisons. The more serious the crimes, the longer the sentences. These legal reforms, however, had little discernible impact on crime rates. By the 1820s, prisons were centers of rampant disorder, escapes, and riots. Over the next 30 years, major reforms of the prison system took place as America underwent social and economic transformations (Rothman 1995).

The early nineteenth century was marked by territorial expansion and settlement beyond the Appalachian Mountains, industrialization, urbanization, and large-scale immigration in the North, expansion of the slave-based agricultural economy in the South, and significant political and social upheaval. The old tightly knit colonial village society was supplanted by rapidly growing industry-based cities with their transient populations divided along socioeconomic, religious, ethnic, and racial lines. The possibility that America would be transformed into a copy of class-ridden and undemocratic European society alarmed many post-revolutionary Americans who believed that our democratic institutions, abundant unsettled lands, and untapped natural resources would lead to a society free of poverty and oppression—a society in which each person would have a chance to fulfill his or her inherent human potential. Accompanying the revolutionary fervor was a diminution of belief in the established Protestant church teachings that a person's fate was preordained and in God's hands. People now believed that human problems were no longer beyond human capabilities to solve. Because human societies could now solve human problems, Jacksonian reformers set about addressing the crime problem, which they saw as a threat to the social order. Criminal behaviors, alcoholism, and mental illness were thought to arise from violations of the natural laws that govern human behaviors. In the past, families and the churches had taught and enforced conformance with the natural laws. Industrialization, urbanization, territorial expansion, and immigration had weakened the influence and authority of family and churches. New institutions were needed to correct individuals' violations of natural laws. Insane asylums were developed to treat the mentally ill. Likewise, new penitentiaries were built to rehabilitate criminals. State insane asylums were built in rural areas to remove mentally ill persons from the pathogenic influences of the city. The local native-born Anglo-American asylum staffs were expected to provide moral treatment to acutely disturbed patients from all classes (Rothman 1971, 1995; Williams et al. 1980).

State penitentiaries were also built in rural areas. Their staffs were expected to punish and rehabilitate "good boys gone bad" and return them to the community as productive law-abiding citizens. Prisons were organized on a quasi-military model, in which the inmates were to be both punished and transformed into good citizens using practices similar to those used by the military to transform motley groups of men into disciplined, well-trained soldiers. Prison wardens were often retired military officers. Penitentiary guards were drawn from the local native-born Anglo-American communities. The guards had little formal education and received little or no formal job training to become prison guards. The tasks of prison confinement were to punish offenders for their crimes; protect the community from the offenders' criminal activities; and then return the offenders to the community as hard-working, law-abiding citizens. These goals were to be met by totally regimenting the prisoners' lives. Prisoners were denied contact with family or community members. Prisoners lived in single cells and were forbidden to talk or fraternize with other prisoners. Convicts were to maintain unbroken silence, be obedient, and perform useful manual labor. These regimens were intended to instill a sense of order, discipline, and good work habits in the prison population. Guards were authorized to use corporal punishments to enforce strict discipline and prisoner compliance.

The massive influx of non-English, non-Protestant immigrants (and their associated problems) into northern, rapidly industrialized urban areas alarmed and threatened the established native-born Anglo-Americans, who responded to the new immigrants with hostility and rejection. Prison rehabilitative programs were soon rendered ineffective by overcrowding, insufficient funding, and ethnic and religious hostilities. By the 1850s, most penitentiaries had two or three inmates living in cells built for one person. The prisoners were no longer first-time offenders, but hardened criminals serving long sentences. The inmates increasingly consisted of poor recent immigrants whom the native-born Anglo-Americans (including prison staff) considered to be morally and socially inferior, prone to crime, and incapable of acquiring American traditions and rules. The prisons' task shifted from rehabilitation to the long-term incarceration of hardened, poor, ethnically and religiously despised prisoners. Guards invented increasingly harsh and brutal corporal punishments to maintain order and discipline. At the same time, inmates bribed corrupt, poorly paid guards to obtain special privileges. Reflecting public attitudes, staff punishments became a means of societal retaliation, revenge, and retribution (Rothman 1995).

Prison conditions continued to deteriorate after the Civil War. States tried to confine the largest numbers of prisoners at the lowest cost. Living space became so small that both physical and mental health were endangered. Contagious diseases and drug abuse spread through the inmate population. Wardens were given wide latitude to secure their prisons as long as they avoided adverse publicity. They in turn gave guards unlimited power over inmates' bodies and lives. The American public was aware of the deplorable prison conditions but considered the prisons good enough for the mainly immigrant prisoner population. Native-born Americans considered the recent immigrants to be dangerous and preferred them imprisoned rather than free in the community. Southern whites used the criminal justice system to reinforce the political and economic subjugation of the newly freed black population. Blacks constituted 75% of the prison population in southern states. These inmates were contracted out to work for private employers. The inmates' working conditions were described as comparable with the worst conditions of slavery (Rothman 1995).

Despite the prevailing political climate, some Americans did advocate prison reform. Reformers argued for larger prisons, better pay and training for prison guards, and centralized administration of state prisons. They also advocated rehabilitation of inmates by instituting inmate educational programs; prison libraries; indeterminate sentencing; and parole for good conduct, schooling, and industry. Reformers persuaded the New York state government to establish a reformatory at Elmira, New York, that embodied the new rehabilitation programs and paroles based on inmates obtaining an education. Prison order and discipline was based on reward. Programs were designated for young first-time offenders between ages 16 and 31 years (i.e., the so-called good boys gone bad). Unfortunately, the reformatory could not control its admissions. The institution quickly became overcrowded; one-third of the inmate population was made up of hard-core recidivists. As a result of the overcrowding and inmate mix, the staff returned to the use of corporal punishment to maintain discipline. The institution's rehabilitative programs were rendered ineffective. Overall, late nineteenth century reform programs had an insignificant effect on the nation's prisons.

The Progressive movement of the early twentieth century instituted the next prison reform effort. These reformers addressed the nation's problems of social, ethnic, and economic disparities by attempting to educate and extend social programs to the poor European immigrant populations. (Although the southern white Progressive movement ignored the overall plight of African Americans in southern prisons, the Progressives did officially abolish the convict leasing system [Allen 1975, p. 109].) Progressives believed that science and medicine coupled with active government interventions would resolve societal and individual conflicts. Progressives believed that prisons must give inmates positive lessons in good citizenship and provide opportunities to influence the conditions of their confinement and become more responsible for their behavior. Wardens and guards would lose their absolute power over prisoners' lives. Prisons were renamed correctional facilities and were built with different levels of security. Corporal punishment was forbidden as a method to enforce discipline and was replaced by solitary confinement and the placing of more dangerous or troublesome inmates in higher security prisons. The criminally insane were separated from the general population and placed in special units. Physical separation of prisoners, enforced silence, and regimentation were eliminated. Inmates were allowed recreational time together, and they were allowed to have personal items. Indeterminate sentencing, parole, and reduced time for good behavior were instituted. Reformers believed that the personal factors that helped cause an inmate's criminal behaviors must be addressed by individual treatments based on medical and psychological sciences. Reformers established educational, vocational training, and psychotherapy programs. Psychiatrists,

psychologists, and social workers were hired to develop and administer classification systems to direct inmates to the appropriate services and to provide the appropriate treatments. Too few psychiatrists and psychologists were hired (one or two per large prison) to provide effective treatments. Most important, the mental health professionals lacked the scientific knowledge and therapeutic skills needed to successfully treat the deviant behaviors found in the inmate population. Rothman (1979, p. 22) summarized the prison psychiatrist's activities as follows: "The psychiatrist's devotion to the details of classification did not carry over into a careful and meticulous description of the actual content of rehabilitative programs. Psychiatrists were most comfortable in talking about vocational education and schooling, to the consistent neglect of psychological counseling or therapeutic interventions."

Historians have concluded that the Progressive prison reform initiatives (self-government, inmate educational and vocational programs, prison work programs, and mental health treatment programs) were inconsequential and ineffective. Rothman (1979) wrote that all of these reform initiatives were overwhelmed by the primary goal of incarceration. He observed that it is extremely difficult to run a program that is both custodial and rehabilitative, or a custodial program that is at once secure and humane.

The history of the Massachusetts Norfolk Prison Colony exemplifies these observations. This institution was founded in 1927 by Howard Gill, an economist and strong advocate of prison reform. The Colony was organized on the Progressive principles of reforming inmates by placing them in settings that prepared them for return to the community by giving them joint responsibility with staff for institutional governance and by providing each inmate with an individualized physical, mental, vocational, and recreational program. The staff tried to select inmates thought to be amenable to treatment. The staff consisted of social workers and male custody guards. The social workers and guards argued over decision-making authority. The social workers saw the guards as ignorant and cruel; the guards viewed social workers as too soft and coddling of prisoners. The guards had little respect for the effectiveness of the social workers' treatment programs. In fact, the methods of casework classification and treatment were not notably effective. Although Gill supported the social workers, the guards exercised considerable day-to-day authority over inmates and were in a position to undermine the marginally effective rehabilitation program.

Contrary to the original agreement, the state overloaded the Norfolk institution with hard-core and difficult prisoners. These prisoners further subverted the rehabilitation program. They challenged the institutional order and shifted the program emphasis to security rather than rehabilitation. Gill was dismissed in 1934 after several inmate escapes. Prison administrators perceived that the Norfolk program was soft on criminals. The experiment was then terminated (Rotman 1995).

The last political support for the Progressive ideal of prisoner rehabilitation evaporated following the 1974 publication of an article evaluating outcomes of correctional treatment. Martinson (1974) and colleagues reviewed evaluations of prisoner rehabilitative treatments and concluded that there were no convincing findings that correctional treatment programs reduced recidivism. The authors noted that some programs were effective for particular types of offenders. Ignoring these specific findings, politicians, advocating getting tough on crime, cited the study's overall conclusions as evidence that all rehabilitation programs were ineffective. This study was then used to justify reducing and eliminating prison vocational, educational, and other rehabilitative services and related research activities (Tonry 1995).

Public funding for prison research is sporadic and contains political limitations on the types and possible outcomes of such research. Lacking a scientific base, correctional policy is often driven by political agendas or by political reactions to adverse publicity about prisons or inmates. Correctional officials have no valid methodology to help them establish authoritative professional findings to counter draconian legislative policies that may ultimately undermine prison safety and security.

Until the 1970s, jail and prison inmates had no right to health or mental healthcare. In a 1976 decision (*Estelle v. Gamble*), the U.S. Supreme Court ruled that jail and prison inmates were constitutionally entitled to health and mental healthcare because incarcerated persons are unable to seek or obtain treatment on their own (Anno 1994). The Court held that "deliberate indifference" by corrections officials to the serious medical needs of prisoners was "willful and wanton" infliction of pain, which the Eighth Amendment prohibits. Jails and prisons have a duty to protect and to treat serious medical or psychiatric disorders. However, no specific judicial standards indicate the types and amounts of care that must be minimally provided.

Corrections and health professional groups have developed national standards for correctional health-

care. Three of these groups offer accreditation of correctional facilities based on their standards—the American Correctional Association (1990, 1991), the Joint Commission on Accreditation of Healthcare Organizations (1991), and the National Commission on Correctional Health Care (1992 a, 1992b, 1992c). Representatives of the American Psychiatric Association and the American Psychological Association helped develop the standards for the National Commission on Correctional Health Care. The American Psychiatric Association (1989) has also developed standards that specifically address the role of the psychiatrist in correctional settings. The American Nurses' Association (1985) has issued standards of nursing practice in correctional settings. Courts can use these standards and institutional accreditation as mechanisms in determining constitutionally adequate care. Given the public hostility toward the current group of minority offenders (African Americans and Latinos), state governments have rarely adopted these standards without a court order.

Open-Systems Theory of Organizations

Rothman's observation concerning the difficulty of running prison programs that are both custodial and rehabilitative, or a custodial program that is at once secure and humane, can be understood within the context of the open-systems theory of organizations (Miller and Rice 1973; Rice 1971). This theory holds that an enterprise exists by exchanging material with its environment. An enterprise imports material, transforms it, and then exports the converted product. All organizations have a primary task—the task the organization must perform to survive. Performance of the primary task is constrained by the political, economic, legal, and social constraints of the environment in which the organization exists and by the constraints particular to the organization, such as the human, physical, scientific, and technological resources available for the task performance. Human resources bring inherent constraints on the efficiency of any work activity. These constraints involve the employees' experiences of satisfaction or deprivation in their work arising from the following four areas (Miller and Rice 1973):

1. The formal and informal interpersonal and group relationships involved in performing the work activities.

2. The harmonies or disharmonies of these relationships with the workers' other group memberships—these other groups include the workers' internal group identifications (e.g., internalized objects and part-objects derived from relationships they have made, family, gender, ethnicity, class, race), external group identifications (e.g., political, professional, union, social, religious), sentient groups (a group that demands and receives loyalty from its members), and unconscious group dynamics (basic assumption groups).

3. Satisfaction or deprivation experienced in the work activities themselves.

4. Work activities can also provide satisfaction or deprivations through reciprocation with the workers' inner worlds of unconscious drives and needs for defense against anxiety.

External societal constraints interact with the organization's internal constraints and become part of the enterprise's internal culture and reinforce the organization's internal constraints. It is thus difficult to introduce new knowledge or fresh experiences into the organization's culture.

The effectiveness of the work group is constrained because the group operates not only at the manifest level to perform specific tasks but also at an unconscious level. On the unconscious level, the work group operates as if it had met to carry out one of three discrete assumptions (basic assumption groups): 1) to reproduce itself and produce a new magical leader (pairing group assumption), 2) to obtain security from one person upon whom group members can depend (dependent group assumption), or 3) to preserve itself by attacking someone or something or by running away (fight-flight group assumption). Effective work groups utilize and express the emotions and attitudes associated with one basic assumption and suppress and control the emotions and attitudes associated with the other two basic assumptions. Basic assumption thinking and feelings are activated when group task structure and performance break down. Factors that affect work performance can foster the shifting of the work group to another basic assumption. For example, the physician-patient work group evokes the emotions of the dependent group basic assumption. Many physicians are concerned that managed care will alter the physician-patient relationship to a more adversarial physician-customer relationship. Such an alteration may evoke the emotions and attitudes of a fight-flight group.

Fight-flight basic assumptions underlie much of the task performance of military and paramilitary organizations (e.g., police, prison guards). Bion (1961) described the following characteristics of the fight-flight basic assumption group: Group members are united against external enemies. Members expect the group leader to direct the group against external threats, prevent internal group conflicts, and lead the group into retreat if indicated. Opposition to the group ideology is not tolerated. However, the group easily splits into subgroups that fight each other. One subgroup is subservient to the idealized leader; another subgroup is either fighting the first group or in flight from it. Fight-flight groups try to absorb other groups. The group tries to suppress new ideas that are perceived to threaten the status quo. Group members express a sense of incapacity to understand or experience loving feelings without which understanding cannot exist. Attention to the passage of time or to the process of group development is lacking. The group's predominant defenses are projection of aggression on outside groups, splitting, and projective identification. The group evidences conflicts related to aggressive control, suspiciousness, and dread of annihilation. Bion found that panic, uncontrolled anger, and flight are equivalents. Panic does not arise in a situation unless the situation is one that would easily give rise to rage. If the work group process is unable to provide an outlet for fear or rage, fight-flight group members will become frustrated and engage in attacking or flight behaviors. Such consequences occur when the situation falls outside the realm of the work group functions. Groups operating at the level of the fight-flight basic assumption can evidence a psychotic anxiety associated with primitive oedipal conflicts working on a base of part-object relationships and utilizing the defense mechanisms of splitting and projective identification.[1]

The primary task of organizational leadership is to manage the boundary relationships between the organization and its external and internal environments to facilitate the optimal performance of its primary tasks. Complex organizations often have more than one pri-

---

[1] In the text, we call work groups that are operating close to the level of their activated basic assumption a *basic assumption group* (e.g., a fight-flight basic assumption group).

mary task. For example, teaching hospitals have the primary tasks of patient care, medical education, and medical research. Miller and Rice (1973) listed four kinds of boundary control:

1. Regulation of the boundaries of the organization's constituent work units and systems of work units, and regulation of the work units to the external environment
2. Regulation of sentient group boundaries
3. Regulation of the organization's boundaries to the external environment
4. Regulation of the relations between work groups, sentient groups, and the organizational boundaries

We can now reformulate Rothman's observation.

When first established, prisons had three primary goals: to punish, to incarcerate inmates to protect the community, and to rehabilitate. Initially, inmates were regarded both as felons to be punished and as recruits to be inducted and transformed into hard-working, disciplined, law-abiding citizens by using strict discipline, physical and social isolation, and hard work. ("Good boys gone bad" are transformed by "tough love.") Although expression of the fight-flight group basic assumption included most of the work groups in this quasi-military organizational culture, the training and rehabilitation processes require understanding and mentoring activities. Effective training groups require the expression of a dependent group basic assumption, in which the guard/teacher is the group leader from whom the inmate members seek intellectual and psychological supports.

The change of public policy toward the now overwhelming numbers of immigrant inmates eliminated the primary task of rehabilitation and converted the prisons into overcrowded, poorly funded custodial institutions whose inmates were to be punished and prevented from escaping. Prison staff were also to avoid adverse publicity. Prisoners had become permanent societal outcasts—society's and the prison guards' permanent external enemies. In the prison the fight-flight basic assumption underlay all work activity. The guards and prisoners were locked into a lifetime battle with no permanent victory or defeat-only uneasy truces. The lack of understanding and organizational resources made staff work groups only partially effective in managing the staff's rage and fears of annihilation. The only development these staff work groups evidenced was increasingly sophisticated methods of physical pun-

ishment and torture of inmates. These activities only increased the warring groups' defenses of splitting, projection of aggressive motives on each other, and projective identifications.

Prison staff groups, operating under the fight-flight basic assumption, would interpret the Progressives and their reforms as increasing the power of the inmates to destroy them. The Progressive prison rehabilitative programs lacked professional knowledge, treatments, and sufficient professional staff to effectively treat the heterogeneous prison populations.

These outsiders also wanted to replace the guards' methods of control and safety with theories and treatments that were ineffective in dealing with the more troublesome and dangerous inmates. These reforms, with the exception of classification and levels of security, increased staff fears of annihilation. Given their fears and beliefs, the custody staff sabotaged and then destroyed these rehabilitation programs.

Current Perspectives

As was true over 150 years ago, prison systems today are overcrowded, inadequately funded custodial institutions. Feared minorities are African American and Latino men and women. Racial and ethnic tensions exist between guards and inmates and within each group. State legislatures continue to reduce the reward system for good behavior. Illicit drug use is reported in a number of prison systems, as are organized social and ethnic gangs. The prison's major task of punishment, preventing escapes, and avoidance of adverse publicity are the same. Wardens have the major day-to-day responsibility for fulfilling these tasks. Prisoners have the day-to-day power to create a disturbance. Thus, wardens maintain a quiet and secure prison by balancing their powers to control and punish inmates against their need to maintain prisoner cooperation by providing inmates with recreation, visitation, and movement about the facility. In some prisons, wardens have made alliances with inmate gangs to help maintain order.

Prisoners considered less prone to escape and less violent are housed in dormitories in low- and medium-security prisons. These prisons are more open and have more recreational and vocational opportunities than do higher level security prisons. However, Rotman (1995) reported that prisoner assault rates are higher in dormitory facilities than in any other type of prison. Ostfeld (1987) found that prisoners living in dormitories had significantly higher hypertension levels than prisoners in high-security prisons. These findings suggest that dormitory living is stressful for prisoners. White-collar criminals and European American prisoners tend to be placed at these security levels.

Inmates who are considered violent, prone to escape, or disciplinary problems are housed in higher security levels. These prisons have one or two inmates per cell. Prisoners spend more time in their cells, up to 23 hours per day. Their freedom of movement is greatly restricted and supervised. Few recreational or vocational facilities are available. Prisoners at this level have described their lives as one of boredom, idleness with little work or recreational opportunities, and suffused with a constant sense of danger from attack by other prisoners. African American and Latino minorities are greatly overrepresented at this level. Carroll (1974) studied disciplinary proceedings in an American maximum-security prison. He found that black prisoners were cited more frequently than white prisoners for disciplinary infractions. The guards saw black prisoners as dangerous and conspiring revolutionaries. As a result, guards kept closer surveillance and control of black prisoners. The black prisoners, believing that many of the guards' orders were arbitrary and unfair, reacted with hostility. This reaction then reinforced the guards' perceptions of the dangerousness of black males—a self-fulfilling prophecy.

The Michigan prison mental illness survey found a bimodal distribution of severe and moderately mentally ill inmates (Neighbors et al. 1987). European American mentally ill inmates were housed in lower security prisons; African American mentally ill inmates were in higher security prisons. This finding suggests that custody staff judge the African American inmates' symptoms of mental illness as evidence of criminal behaviors that must be punished rather than as signs of mental illness that should be tolerated or treated (i.e., "bad not mad"). However, regardless of the security level, overtly symptomatic mentally ill prisoners are ostracized, exploited, and harmed by other inmates. Prison staff will sometimes house the mentally ill in higher security units to protect them from other inmates.

As throughout the history of prisons, custody remains with predominantly rural, native-born, low-income European American males. Women and African American and Latino minorities now are part of the work force. Significant intergroup conflict exists between these work subgroups. The majority of prison guards have little or no knowledge of the cultures, nor

previous personal relationships with African American and Latino minorities. Guards often have stereotypes of minority prisoners as subhuman and violent. Formal guard training varies by state. However, most programs teach little about mentally ill offenders. Many guards believe that the sentencing court determines whether a prisoner is mentally ill. Guards then interpret psychiatric symptoms in inmates not judged insane to be signs of malingering or manipulation to avoid punishment. Few formal training programs address the techniques of nonphysical de-escalation of potentially violent incidents with inmates.

Prison guards work in a highly stressful environment in which they, like the prisoners, have a constant sense of danger of being physically assaulted or killed. Guards must deal with the risk of being exposed to infectious disease (e.g., hepatitis, AIDS, tuberculosis) and bodily fluids or of being covered with urine and feces. Most prisons lack procedures for routine debriefing of staff after they experience violent or traumatic events. The prison system gives few rewards for high-quality work; emphasis is placed on punishing (sometimes scapegoating) staff for staff errors or mistakes.

Ostfeld (1987) evaluated the prevalence of hypertension in prison guards working various security settings. He found the highest prevalence of hypertension among guards working in high-security settings, and he concluded that higher security settings were more stressful for guards than lower security settings. Not surprisingly, guards captured by rioting prison inmates have experienced the greatest stress. They experienced posttraumatic stress symptoms, marital discord and divorce, and substance abuse and sometimes were unable to work (Jenish 1996; Porter 1995).

Few studies have examined occupational stress in prison guards. A Canadian prison guard union official estimated that 10% of union members were on long-term leave—due mainly to stress. Some guard union officials believe that governments do not fund such studies out of fear of increased liability for prison work conditions and workers' compensation. People work as prison guards an average of 10 years: Some states have annual prison guard turnover rates of 5%; others have 33% turnover rates (Kappeler et al. 1996).

Although prisons forbid heterosexual and homosexual activities, sexual activity occurs within the context of violent and exploitative relationships. Women guards and prisoners must constantly be on guard against sexual assaults. Showers are particularly dangerous and stressful. In older male prisons, shower areas are built with obstructions that prevent observation from outside. Physical assaults of inmates, homosexual intercourse, and rapes are not uncommon. Guards assigned to monitor showering inmates to prevent such activity are also fearful of being assaulted because other guards cannot see them from the hallway. Women guards assigned to monitoring showers are afraid of being raped by inmates before help comes. They fear that if they refuse the shower monitoring assignment, they will prove that women are not qualified for prison guard jobs in male prisons. Concerned for their own safety, guards monitoring showers often stay outside the shower area.

Many women prisoners have histories of physical and sexual abuse and of sexual exploitation by men. Women prisoners feel intimidated and degraded by the male guards assigned to monitor their showers. Some male guards report that they enjoy the fact that the women feel intimidated by their monitoring. Guards also enjoy the sexual stimulation of observing women showering. There are continuing reports of sexual assaults on women prisoners by male guards.

Developing a Correctional Mental Health System

In our opinion, a psychiatric management team is necessary if an effective, efficient and humane prison mental health treatment program is to be established and maintained. Team members should occupy the leadership positions within the mental health program. The team should be composed minimally of three to four mental health professionals, all of whom have prior clinical and administrative experience. The team should have a minimum of one psychiatrist to direct the clinical programs. At least one team member should have clinical experiences that include treating minority individuals with co-occurring mental illnesses. It is helpful to have one team member who has worked in the state's public mental health and/or criminal justice systems, is familiar with state policies and politics, and has personal relationships with various state government officials. Before entering into a service contract with the state, the management team must learn as much as possible about the political environment in which the prison mental health services is immersed. A partial list follows:

- The team should learn the history of prison health and mental health services.
- The team must learn about issues of state mental health service control and financing, as well as any plans to contract prison health services.
- It is important that the team determine the relationship between the state department of mental health and the state department of corrections.
- The team must evaluate the correction department's commitment of resources to create and maintain a nationally accredited prison mental health program.
- The team must determine the role played by incarceration and jail diversion in the political agendas of political parties and government officials.
- Finally, the team should identify the decision makers that determine the fate of the prison mental health program.

The organizational structure in which the psychiatric team works is crucial to the successful development and implementation of a prison mental health program. Currently there are two basic models.

In the first model, the state government directly funds, administers, and provides prison mental health services. The mental health services are provided either by an administrative component of the corrections department's health bureau or by a dedicated component of the state mental health department. Currently, there are a number of problems with this model. First, many state governments are downsizing. State government jobs are now less attractive than nongovernmental positions. State-run programs are frequently unable to recruit and retain competent professional staff to work in prison mental health programs. Staff recruitment, hiring, and retention are often made more difficult by civil service and state employee union contracts. Occasional budget deficits and the resulting hiring freezes further complicate adequate mental health program staffing. Staff turnovers, staff vacancies, and the necessity of employing high-cost temporary professional workers contribute to programmatic turmoil and ineffective, costly care. Partly as a result of deinstitutionalization, state governments no longer have the need for personnel with extensive professional and direct clinical mental health experience in the higher management levels of the state bureaucracy. States now hire individuals primarily on the basis of their business and management skills. Currently, there are often no professional senior-level state officials to provide ongoing professional and clinical input into the daily bureaucratic work of implementing policies and allocating resources. Thus bureaucratic decisions can be made without an understanding by the decision makers of the effects of the decisions on the functioning of prison mental health programs.

A number of states are considering a second model: contracting with for-profit or nonprofit managed care organizations to provide prison mental health services. In past decades, states have contracted with nonprofit academic medical centers or medical school departments of psychiatry to staff and operate public mental hospitals and mental health centers. In some instances, these collaborations have provided high quality clinical care, professional training, and clinical research. In other instances, such collaborations were unsuccessful, especially in predominantly minority urban communities.(Williams 1981). It is unlikely that academic medical centers will now aggressively seek contracts for prison mental health services. Such contracts can carry significant financial risk to these institutions, which are already losing money on health and mental health indigent patient care. Additionally, few prison contracts are likely to adequately cover associated teaching and research costs. Currently there are relatively few sources of outside funding for teaching and research in prison settings.

Additionally, in an effort to further prevent adverse publicity, some state prison systems are eliminating prison training sites for professional students and increasing their restrictions on the release of information. These policies and the strict guidelines on inmate involvement in clinical research will further limit both research and training opportunities. Finally, academic medical centers are also concerned that the stigma and possible negative publicity associated with treating prison inmates will adversely affect patient referrals and income, diminish community charitable support, and harm the medical centers' relations with state government.

Some states are considering hiring national managed care organizations to provide health and mental health services to their prison inmate populations, for several reasons. National managed care organizations have the potential to provide mental healthcare that conforms to national standards at costs that are equal to or less than the costs of service provision by the state itself. Managed care organizations have more professional, administrative, and financial resources than states have to run their prison programs. It is likely that for-profit managed care companies will have greater financial resources to cover treatment program losses or state reimbursement delays than will nonprofit providers. The buying power of the large multistate patient

population served by managed care providers enable them to purchase medications at costs lower than those of state-run programs. These organizations can be more successful in recruiting and retaining healthcare professionals than state programs because of having more flexible personnel policies and possessing access to national provider pools. Managed care organizations can avoid the constraints of state civil service bureaucracies and state employee unions. These organizations can spread the cost of their professional staff in-service training programs over all their multistate contractual service sites. These training programs can be more extensive and more readily responsive to deficiencies identified in the contractors' quality care auditing programs. These organizations believe that extensive and continuing training and staff development programs promote standardized care throughout all their multistate treatment sites and lower mental healthcare costs. Some companies try to further increase the level of their staffs' professional competence and identity by seeking affiliation with mental health professional schools, hiring faculty to conduct staff training, and offering their treatment programs as training sites for professional mental health students. As a result of a variety of factors, state-run mental health programs often have recurring difficulties in maintaining national standards of care. Such difficulties expose the current state government to political attacks.

Interestingly, states are likely to benefit politically by holding their contracted managed-care organizations to national standards of correctional mental health. Contracting state governments are no longer directly responsible for mental healthcare. The contracting service provider is now responsible for addressing any problems with the provision of care to inmates. The state government can demand that the contractor correct the problems. In doing so, state government demonstrates effective managerial oversight of the contractor. Finally, the contractor can build support for prison mental health services. As a private entity, the contractor can directly or indirectly lobby and contribute financially to state politicians who support prison mental health programs. The contractor can also purchase as many program goods and services within the state as possible. This purchase strategy builds political support by demonstrating that the contractor is trying to keep state monies within the state. This strategy also gains the political support of the program's suppliers.

There are also significant disadvantages to contracting for prison mental health services. A for-profit corporation's first responsibility is to its shareholders. For-profit managed care corporations must maintain an adequate return on capital. There have been reports of for-profit mental health programs significantly reducing mental health services in order to maintain profits. In other instances, corporations have terminated service contracts because of unexpected costs and inadequate state reimbursements. The provision of mental healthcare has often been disrupted.

State governments have also contributed to the instability of contracted services and their quality. Some state governments continue to decrease payments through the contractual years in the belief that the contractor will continue to find additional ways to reduce costs. Then the contractor, fearing poor profits, legal liabilities for poor care, and negative publicity, will withdraw. Other states continually shop for the low bidder for mental health services. Such a policy forces the current service provider to follow treatment practices that ensure maximum short-term profits. The contractor sees no benefit in making long-term cost-saving programmatic commitments such as mental health prevention strategies and early treatment interventions. Some mental healthcare providers try to circumvent state low-bid strategies by making the state an active partner: both the contractor and state share program profits and losses.

The psychiatric administrative team must develop and maintain a system of managed mental health services, whether the system is state-run or contracted to nonprofit or for-profit care providers. Like public community mental health systems, prison mental health's system should include the following:

- Crisis stabilization programs
- Acute inpatient treatment units
- Long-term residential treatment programs for mentally ill inmates unable to function in the general prison population
- Outpatient treatment teams to screen, refer, and/or treat mentally ill inmates who can reside in the general prison population

The latter two services are located throughout the system in facilities administered by the corrections administration (prisons, training camps, halfway houses, etc.). The mental healthcare system may also be responsible for providing targeted diagnostic and treatment services to inmate populations with special needs (e.g., geriatric, developmentally disabled, self-mutilat-

ing, and AIDS patient populations). The self-mutilating population has high morbidity and mortality rates, and self-mutilating inmates are one of the most disruptive groups in the prison system in custodial costs, psychological stress on custody and healthcare staffs, and health and mental health services costs (Giampa 1998). The mental healthcare system may also be given responsibility for the psychological screening and triage of inmates entering the prison system.

Mental health system management must develop and put in place clearly defined clinical policies, procedures, and diagnostic and treatment protocols. Establishing and maintaining ongoing staff education and clinical supervision are crucial to the staffs' ability to implement the system's policies, procedures, and protocols. As previously noted, it is difficult to recruit and retain competent mental health professionals to staff correctional mental health treatment units. Most prisons are located in rural areas. Most mental health professionals live and work in metropolitan areas and have no wish to live in what they perceive as isolated, culturally poor rural areas. It is particularly difficult to recruit and retain minority professionals to work in these rural areas. Many professionals view working in prisons as frightening and unrewarding, and noncompetitive pay scales and benefits and rigid personnel policies can also be disincentives.

Newly hired mental health staffs are likely to have had insufficient training or experience in treating severely mentally ill persons. The psychiatric administrative team must establish a comprehensive in-service educational program for the mental health staff, including psychiatric diagnosis, interviewing skills, the management of potentially violent patients, models of psychotherapy and their uses, psychopharmacology, and the evaluation and treatment of minority patients. Whenever possible, the education program should include mental health professional students from local colleges and universities. Not only do the students help create a learning environment, but if they find the educational experience worthwhile, some are likely to seek employment in the prison psychiatric service upon graduation.

At the conclusion of formal training, mechanisms must be in place to monitor staff for their quality of care and efficiency, including mechanisms such as authorization of services, ongoing clinical supervision, chart auditing, and continuous quality improvement programs. Centralized authorizations of services create a systemwide feedback mechanism to ensure that clinical standards of practice and practice protocols are being used. Some staff will respond to these guidelines and protocols by adopting a routinized, cookbook approach to mental health diagnosis and treatment. Ongoing in-service training and supervision can address this problem.

The psychiatric administrative team must also develop educational programs for the custody staff. Program topics should include the definition of severe and persistent mental illness and the signs and symptoms of mental disorders. It is important to seek opportunities for joint training of the custody and mental health staffs. Joint training topics might include 1) the responsibilities of each group for the care of mentally ill inmates in the general population and 2) the categories of inmate referral for mental health evaluation: routine, emergent, and urgent.

Psychiatric Administration Inside a Prison

This section discusses the role of the psychiatrist as clinical director in a prison setting.

Entering prison is frightening. You fear being locked in and never getting out, even though you consciously think you will walk out at the end of your work period. As you pass through the admission point, you are entering an institution suffused with the fight-flight group basic assumption. You are wary of physical attack, injury, and death; and you are guarded and suspicious about both inmates and guards. Those daily thoughts and feelings are evoked not only by the realities of prison life but also by the underlying fight-flight basic assumption.

Members of such prison fight-flight assumption groups experience being inside the beast (prison) as well as the beast's being within them. The primary task of the psychiatric administrative team is to create and maintain programs of good-quality psychiatric care for mentally ill offenders, using dependent group assumptions, in which group members who are needy seek care from the psychiatrist. This must all be done within an organizational setting characterized by constant anxiety, fears of annihilation, and warring groups and subgroups.

Given the complexities of the task, we believe that management of psychiatric services is best accomplished by a management group whose members are

able to control the various organizational boundaries noted earlier in this chapter. Group membership might consist of unit managers from central prison administration (e.g., warden, deputy warden, personnel director), custody guard leadership (e.g., shift commanders), medical leadership, the chief pharmacist, and mental health discipline chiefs. The mental health program director chairs the group. The group is responsible for establishing program policies and procedures and their implementation within the system's protocols of acceptable clinical practice. These protocols standardize care across the prison system and ensure the delivery of uniform care.

Psychiatric programs must address the concerns of both inmates and custody staff about increased safety and security in the context of the underlying fight-flight assumption. Effective psychiatric care can reduce the incidence of violent and disordered behaviors in the mentally ill prison population. Such reductions will increase the security of both inmates and staff. The psychiatric administrator can also reduce stress and the potential for violence by expanding the interpersonal skills of custody staff. The custody staff can be trained in verbal and nonverbal techniques to de-escalate potentially violent confrontations with prisoners and to promote conflict resolution. The psychiatric administrator can assist the prison administration in developing staff debriefing sessions following stressful or violent incidents with inmates. These sessions can help staff to deal with their emotional reactions to these incidents and/or to develop more skilled management of future occurrences. The psychiatrist, in order to encourage custody staff to control the violent behaviors of some of the guards toward inmates, can point out that such violence can provoke inmates to retaliate by attacking other guards, thus increasing the danger to all staff. Mental health professionals can also function as consultants to the staff's designated leaders and group members. The psychiatric administrator should encourage informal consultations from custodial staff and administration concerning their own or family mental health problems and facilitate their referral to employee assistance programs or to a mental health professional.

We recommend that an educational management group be established to administer the educational and staff training programs for the professional staff and students. This group should also direct custody staff educational programs and any other training programs conducted by the mental health staff for the custody staff. Group membership should consist of leaders of units that will interact with the educational program—for example, central prison administration, custody staff leadership, medical leadership, and mental health discipline chiefs.

Each mental health discipline has its own issues that also affect the successful operation of psychiatric services.

Psychiatrists

Psychiatrists are the most difficult group to recruit and retain in the prison system. They may lack experience working with severely mentally ill minority patients and may reflect the attitudes and beliefs of the custody staff. Some psychiatrists behave in an idiosyncratic manner toward their patients and colleagues, and some practitioners raise questions as to their clinical competence. Psychiatrists may find it hard to operate as a professional group and may instead operate as individual practitioners, whereas all the other mental health disciplines operate as hierarchically organized groups. Long-employed psychiatrists have worked out a relationship with custody staff and other professionals and are reluctant to change their behaviors or affiliations to accommodate a new psychiatric administrator who they believe is transitory. The transient nature and varied clinical competencies of psychiatrists have often required that other mental health professionals perform the psychiatrists' clinical leadership roles. These professionals are then reluctant to return these authoritative roles to a newly hired psychiatrist. Some mental health professionals prefer that the psychiatrist—like the British monarch—reign, not rule.

The psychiatrist's interactions with the custody staff are complex and emotionally charged. Staff perceive the psychiatrist as a powerful figure with "magical" powers who, like a magician, is capable of both helping and harming them. Participation in the care of mentally ill offenders evokes the staff's awareness of their needs for care. They also experience psychological and medical problems associated with working in the prison environment. The thoughts and feelings associated with the staff's needs for care can shift the basic assumption of the custody staff work group from fight-flight to dependent group assumption.

However, creating the psychiatrist as the dependent-group leader increases group anxiety and vulnerability. Custody staff voice concerns about whether the psychiatrist understands, respects, or shares their community values and lifestyles. Staff question whether the psychiatrist is either concerned or aware that his or her patient-care decisions may cause staff to experience emotional or physical injuries. Given prison realities, custody staff feel fewer fears of annihilation when interacting with the psychiatrist as a work group activated by the fight-flight group assumption. In this mode, the psychiatrist is no longer a potential leader but is either a powerful ally to be coopted and controlled or a powerful enemy who has joined the inmates and whose power to make and implement clinical decisions must be limited. The psychiatrist's race can further increase the splitting. African American psychiatrists are often viewed by custody staff as "prisoner lovers" and as clinically incompetent.

These complexities become activated when the psychiatrist or custody staff decide to place mentally ill prisoners in seclusion and restraint. Custody staff view seclusion and restraint as their major legitimate mechanism for enforcing order, ensuring safety, and administering punishment. Custody staff sentence inmates to seclusion and restraint for a specified period of time. Psychiatrists have different views: seclusion and restraint are the last option to be used to control patients who are a danger to themselves or others, and these methods are not to be used to punish patients. Patients are to be released as soon as they are able to function in a less restrictive setting. Custody staff perceive the psychiatrist's use of seclusion and restraint as undermining staff authority and control and as increasing the likelihood of inmate assault on custody staff. The effective regulation of the psychiatrist–custody staff relationship is crucial to the success of the prison psychiatric program.

Psychologists

Psychologists make up the largest group of prison mental health professionals. For several decades, they have conducted psychological testing and classification of incoming prisoners. Psychologists also conduct specialized group and individual therapy programs for sex offenders, assaultive offenders, substance abusers, and other special-needs groups, and they provide psychological evaluations of suicidal and self-mutilating inmates. Few prison psychologists have been degreed as clinical psychologists, and they tend to have little clinical experience beyond their work with prisoners. A majority of psychologists are European American men, and they tend to occupy mental health administrative positions throughout the prison system. Prison administrators, who are often psychiatrists' administrative superiors, view psychologists overall as more competent than psychiatrists. However, prison psychologists may feel intimidated by clinically competent psychiatrists (or by psychologists from the community). The psychiatric administrator is most likely to openly conflict with psychologists: they are often clinical treatment team leaders and are seen as alternative mental health leaders. They may ally themselves with custody staff, dissident psychiatrists, and other professionals in opposing psychiatric leadership.

Social Workers

Bachelor's- and master's-level social workers currently staff many of the clinical administrative positions in community mental health centers. As prison mental health services expand, it is likely that social workers will also occupy most clinical administrative positions in the prison mental health system. The clinical training of social workers is quite varied. Well-trained psychiatric social workers are likely to be in private practice, and there are relatively few social workers who have psychiatric social work training or experience before joining prison staff. Ongoing in-service education and clinical supervision are essential to developing the clinical skills of social workers to work effectively with the complex mental disorders of prison inmates.

Nurses

Nurses have the most difficult job of all mental health professionals. Most nurses have no prior psychiatric nursing experience beyond nursing school, yet they must quickly acquire the skills needed to provide nursing care to complex and potentially violent psychiatric patients, to supervise a mostly male security staff, to manage the milieu, and to relate to the psychiatrist and other treatment team members. The nursing shifts are often short of staff, which increases the remaining nurses' workloads. Charting and medication errors occur. Lacking prior psychiatric experience, nurses may turn to the security staff for patient management advice. Nurses rely on the custody staff for protection from patient violence and sometimes defer to their wishes for patient seclusion. Nurses often are from the community and have personal ties to some of the custody staff. Shortages of nurse shift supervisors are ongoing. Few supervisors have had previous psychiatric experience, and they therefore lack psychiatric clinical skills. Super-

visors tend to follow the recommendations of custody staff in the absence of the psychiatrist. The nurse-psychiatrist partnership is difficult to maintain.

Conclusions

In the historical review section of this chapter, we described how the failures of prison rehabilitative programs were due partly to a lack of program resources, inadequate scientific understanding of the problems of inmates and custody staff, lack of control over program admissions, and ineffective treatment interventions. Although the scientific basis for treating severe and persistent mental illness has greatly increased, the prison psychiatric administrative team is still faced with inadequate staff resources to convert current mental health scientific knowledge into effective treatments. State officials may want to expand mental health services too quickly with too few resources and too little training, in order to give a semblance of care throughout the prison system. Such expansions will reduce mental health-care to custodial care.

We recommend that the beginning psychiatric administrator develop psychiatric programs only to the extent that allotted resources (including the clinical competence of mental health professional staff) and the strong support of the correctional administration will allow. In our experience, acute inpatient treatment units offer the best initial opportunities to develop effective clinical care and training programs for professional staffs, professional students, and assigned custody staff. Acute inpatient units have the distinct psychiatric treatment task and have organizational boundaries with other prison units. They are a hospital within a prison setting and are governed by correctional mental health standards and by professional standards of practice. Inpatient units afford the best opportunity of building effective mental health treatment teams based on a dependent group assumption.

As noted earlier, one of the administrator's most important tasks is to regulate admissions and discharges. The admission process should be based on standardized admission criteria and assessment instruments. The interviewing process should be recorded to ensure reliability and for teaching purposes. The admission criteria should have low thresholds: we recommend admitting inmates whom custody staff consider to be mentally ill, even if they don't meet admission criteria, since it is likely that some inmates have unusual forms of psychiatric illnesses not detected by screening instruments. The psychiatric administrator should monitor the patterns of referrals to ensure that mentally ill inmates who have a history of violence and are placed in high-security settings are not screened out in favor of less threatening patients. Similarly, there is a risk that potentially violent or minority patients may be discharged before receiving full treatment benefits.

Acute treatment units can be the training sites for mental health treatment teams to be assigned to outlying triage, evaluation, crisis, and after-care units. Often these teams will represent the mental health services within prison units controlled by custody staff. The team members will experience divided loyalty—working with the issue of whether to remain representatives of the psychiatric organization or to adapt the values and attitudes toward inmates that are held by the custody staff and the community they reside in. Again, the psychiatric administrative team should consider local or regional management groups, composed of both custody staff and mental health supervisors, to supervise these representatives. The use of standardized diagnostic and treatment protocols, central authorization of services, case auditing, and monitoring and supervising by teleconferencing can all help maintain uniform standards of care in these outlying units.

Psychiatric administration of prison mental health programs can be challenging, stressful, overwhelming, and sometimes very rewarding. We have found that our attempts to understand the organizational complexities of this setting by using the processes discussed in this chapter increased our abilities to manage. We hope readers will find these comments useful as they continue their work of understanding this most complex area of psychiatric administration.

References

Allen RL: Reluctant Reformers. Garden City, NY, Anchor Press/Doubleday, 1975

American Correctional Association: Standards for Adult Correctional Institutions, 3rd Edition. Laurel, MD, American Correctional Association, 1990

American Correctional Association: Standards for Adult Local Detention Facilities, 3rd Edition. Laurel, MD, American Correctional Association, 1991

American Nurses' Association: Standards of Nursing Practice in Correctional Facilities. Kansas City, MO, American Nurses' Association, 1985

American Psychiatric Association: Psychiatric Services in Jails and Prisons, Report of the Task Force on Psychiatric Services in Jails and Prisons. Washington, DC, American Psychiatric Association, 1989

Anno BJ: Standards for the delivery of mental health services in a correctional setting, in Principles and Practice of Forensic Psychiatry. Edited by Rosner N. New York, Chapman & Hall, 1994, pp 375—379

Bion WR: Experience in Groups. New York, Basic Books, 1961

Bureau of Justice Statistics. Washington, DC, U.S. Department of Justice, 2001

Carroll L: Hacks, Blacks and Cons. Lexington, MA, Lexington Books, 1974, pp 115–145

Center for Mental Health Services: Double Jeopardy: Persons with Mental Illness in the Criminal Justice System. Rockville, MD, Substance Abuse and Mental Health Services Administration, 1995

Giampa F: The Self Mutilating Prisoner, in Frontiers of Justice, Vol 2: Coddling or Common Sense? Edited by Whitman C, Zimmerman J, Miller T. Brunswick, Maine, Biddle Publishing, 1998

Hatsukami DK, Fischman MW: Crack cocaine and cocaine hydrochloride—are the differences myth or reality? JAMA 276:1580–1588, 1996

Jenish D: A troubled watch. Maclean's, November 11, 1996, pp 46, 64, 66

Joint Commission on Accreditation of Healthcare Organizations: Consolidated Standards Manual. Oakbrook Terrace, IL, Joint Commission on Accreditation of Healthcare Organizations, 1991

Kappeler VE, Blumberg M, Potter GW: The Mythology of Crime and Criminal Justice, 2nd Edition. Prospect Heights, IL, Waveland Press, 1996

Martinson D: What works—questions and answers in the male prison. Journal of Offender Rehabilitation 16:1–25, 1974

Mauer M, Huling T: Young Black Americans and the Criminal Justice System: Five Years Later. Washington, DC, The Sentencing Project, 1995

Miller EJ, Rice AK: Systems of Organization. New York, Tavistock, 1973

National Commission on Correctional Health Care: Standards for Health Services in Jails. Chicago, National Commission on Correctional Health Care, 1992a

National Commission on Correctional Health Care: Standards for Health Services in Juvenile Detention and Confinement Facilities. Chicago, National Commission on Correctional Health Care, 1992b

National Commission on Correctional Health Care: Standards for Health Services in Prisons. Chicago, National Commission on Correctional Health Care, 1992c

Neighbors HW, Williams DH, Gunnings TS, et al: The Prevalence of Mental Disorder in Michigan Prisons. Lansing, MI, Michigan Department of Corrections, 1987

Ostfeld A: Stress, Crowding and Blood Pressure in Prison. Hillsdale, NJ, Erlbaum, 1987

Porter B: Terror on an Eight Hour Shift. The New York Times Magazine, November 26, 1995, pp 42

Rice AK: The Enterprise and Its Environment. New York, Tavistock, 1971

Rothman DJ: The Discovery of the Asylum. Boston, Little, Brown, 1971

Rothman DJ: Incarceration and Its Alternatives in 20th Century America. Washington, DC, U.S. Government Printing Office, 1979, p 72

Rothman DJ: Perfecting the Prison: United States 1789–1865, in The Oxford History of the Prison. New York, Oxford University Press, 1995, pp 111–129

Rotman E: The Failure of Reform, in The Oxford History of the Prison. Edited by Morris N, Rothman DJ. New York, Oxford University Press, 1995, pp 169–197

Tonry M: Malign Neglect—Race, Crime and Punishment in America. New York, Oxford University Press, 1995

Torrey EF, Stieber J, Ezekiel J, et al: Criminalizing the Seriously Mentally Ill: The Abuse of Jails as Mental Hospitals. Washington, DC, Public Citizen's Health Research Group and National Alliance for the Mentally Ill, 1992

Williams DH, Bellis EC, Wellington SW: Deinstitutionalization and social policy: historical perspectives and present dilemmas. American Journal of Orthopsychiatry 50:54–64, 1980

Williams DH: The empty lot: passage of mental health center through a black urban community. Social Psychiatry 16: part I, 97–103; part II, 163–170, 1981

❖ 33 ❖

Ethics

Jeremy A. Lazarus, M.D.

There have been administrative psychiatrists since the beginning of organized psychiatry, and medical ethics have always provided guidance to those psychiatrists. Why then a special chapter on ethics in this text? When one examines the published codes of ethics from either the American Psychiatric Association (APA) or the American Medical Association (AMA), from which the APA's code is derived, very little can be found delineating any special issues for administrative physicians. Although the APA's Opinions (American Psychiatric Association 1995a; American Medical Association 1995) and the AMA's Code of Medical Ethics (American Medical Association 1994) contain some directives, no organized AMA or APA publication has covered administrative ethics. After a request was made to the APA Ethics Committee in 1991, the committee pulled together a source book of APA positions and references (American Psychiatric Association 1992) to serve as a guide for administrative psychiatrists. Although this source book has served an important purpose, it is neither comprehensive nor widely disseminated.

In addition, the major changes in healthcare in the 1990s led many psychiatrists to take new administrative positions in both the public and the private sectors. This has created new administrative ethical problems, especially in the for-profit or managed care arenas.

The challenges of this chapter, then, are first to consider the background of psychiatric ethics, the application of an ethic for all psychiatrists, and how that ethic applies to administrative psychiatrists; and then to set the framework for future ethical dilemmas for administrative psychiatrists. The chapter presents background information regarding medical and psychiatric ethics and discusses possible ethical areas of study in the context of the seven principles of medical ethics articulated in the AMA's principles of medical ethics.

Background on Ethics in Psychiatry

The first recognized ethical code for physicians was that of Hippocrates, which was used for centuries until the modern medical ethical code of Thomas Percival was published in 1803. The first code of medical ethics published in 1847 by the AMA has been changed on numerous occasions, resulting in its current version (American Medical Association 1994). The APA bases its principles of medical ethics on the AMA code but has added annotations that apply to psychiatry (American Psychiatric Association 1995b). The APA has also published opinions based on questions the APA Ethics Committee receives (American Psychiatric Association 1995a). The annotations and opinions of the APA have been changed over the years to respond to current ethical questions. Although the APA code of ethics does not purport to be the only voice regarding psychiatric medical ethics, it does serve as the code for members of the APA, who represent about 85% of all psychiatrists in the United States.

The field of biomedicine has had a profound impact on thinking in medical ethics. An ethical approach based on an expanded set of ethical principles, which include beneficence, nonmaleficence, autonomy, and justice, has broadened ethical thinking (Beauchamp and Childress 1994).

The APA also enforces its code of ethics through a comprehensive process initiated at the district branches of the APA and reviewed at several levels of the APA. It has been estimated that the APA spends between $1 million and $2 million per year in direct and indirect costs (mostly through volunteer hours of APA members) in pursuit of ethics enforcement (Lazarus and Sharfstein 1992). The APA has also been involved in educational activities, including developing a model ethics training curriculum and making numerous educational materials available to all members and district branches.

Although considerable effort has been put into developing and enforcing the code of ethics, massive changes in healthcare delivery have brought into question the core values of the medical profession. New problems have evolved as care for patients has moved into various organized systems of care, mainly managed care. The ownership of healthcare entities and healthcare delivery systems by for-profit corporations has presented new challenges and concerns for physicians.

The new roles for psychiatrists that have been created have led to concerns about potential conflicts between the psychiatrist's role as advocate for individual patients and his or her role as the person responsible for whole populations of patients. The ethical position of the AMA/APA has been that a physician's primary obligation is to advocate for the individual patient and that this obligation should be the same no matter what system a physician might work in. The AMA/APA's position regarding allocation discussions is that they should not be done at the bedside (American Medical Association 1994). The ethical dilemmas that have existed for decades and the newer ethical dilemmas that have arisen are the background for the remainder of this chapter.

Seven Principles of Medical Ethics

"A physician shall be dedicated to providing competent medical service with compassion and respect for human dignity."

The AMA has stated clearly that administrative physicians must put the needs of patients first. The Council on Ethical and Judicial Affairs of the AMA goes on to state, "The ethical obligations of physicians are not suspended when a physician assumes a position that does not directly involve patient care" (American Medical Association 1994, p. 105). Thus, when any conflict exists between an administrative psychiatrist's obligation to an employer and any decision that affects patient care, the conflict must be resolved in favor of patient care. This principle has placed administrative psychiatrists in binds since the 1970s because of underfunding for mental illness services, because of political motivation for administrative actions taken in public or private systems, or because psychiatrists are being asked to make administrative decisions that can be harmful to individual patients.

Considerable controversy exists about managed systems of care that may divert a significant portion of the healthcare dollar into corporate profit. Some observers think that if this diversion of funds leads to no detriment to healthcare outcomes it can be seen as the market working to benefit both patients and stockholders. Others believe that either decreased access or decreased availability of treatment for patients leads to a basically unjust system.

The ethical conflict is between the physician's beneficent role as healer and his or her role as a potential decision maker who allocates healthcare dollars across a population of patients. This dilemma and its potential solutions have been presented elsewhere (Sabin and Daniels 1994). The administrative psychiatrist is often one or more steps removed from the treatment relationship and may feel less of the beneficent advocacy burden articulated by the APA. Clearly, a principled medical ethics attitude should support the patient advocate role of a psychiatrist in any administrative position.

Case Vignette I

You are a medical director for a large managed care organization responsible for psychiatric and substance abuse services in the northwestern part of the United States. The chief executive officer (CEO), who is not a physician, spells out, through an intermediary, certain utilization targets that he expects you to achieve in the region. Based on your best assessment of the situation, you determine that in order to meet those utilization targets, significant cuts will be needed in services that you deem necessary and effective. You are aware that a previous medical director in another region was demoted when utilization targets were not achieved. What should you do?

Opinion. As the physician ultimately responsible for the treatment of a potentially large group of patients, your primary responsibility must be to advocate for adequate services for that group of patients. If you agree to attempt to aim for unrealistic utilization targets, unsupported by outcome information, your behavior could be considered unethical. If any decisions regarding utilization of resources are beyond your control, your position should continue to be that of patient advocate.

Case Vignette 2

After serving as medical director in a managed care company for many years, you are also given a job as CEO of the company. At times, decisions you would make as medical director might conflict with your obligations as CEO. How should you resolve this conflict?

Opinion. The conflict must first be discussed with all involved parties. If in your judgment your primary obligation is as CEO, you should consider resigning the medical directorship so that another physician can advocate for patients in a manner unfettered by conflict. If, however, you continue to identify yourself as a physician, your ethical obligations as patient advocate do not end, and you should not be party to any decision that is in conflict with medical ethics.

Case Vignette 3

You are the medical director for a not-for-profit health maintenance organization (HMO) and bear final responsibility for making utilization decisions. The patient group that has purchased the HMO coverage is aware of and concurs with how its premium dollars are allocated and has agreed to the utilization review process. By following the agreed-on allocation guidelines, you will be approving more services at lower cost for those patients with severe mental illness and fewer services at higher cost for patients with less severe mental illness. Is this ethical?

Opinion. Assuming that the patient group has agreed to the manner of resource allocation, you are acting ethically. If you believe that resources are not sufficient to provide services that have been agreed on, it continues to be your ethical duty to advocate for increased resources.

"A physician shall deal honestly with patients and colleagues, and strive to expose those physicians deficient in character or competence, or who engage in fraud or deception."

Just as trust is paramount in the doctor-patient relationship, honesty between administrative psychiatrists and patients or colleagues is crucial to ethical behavior. Patients or patient groups should assume that a physician administrator is a physician first and an administrator second. As mentioned earlier, a physician cannot abrogate the role of patient advocate. Likewise, ethical behavior requires administrative physicians to deal honestly with colleagues. This is not only to preserve a good working or collegial environment but also because it should benefit patient care.

If an administrative psychiatrist has knowledge that another psychiatrist under his or her supervision, or through other means of receiving information, is incompetent or unethical, the administrative psychiatrist must take action to prevent patient harm. This may require reporting another mental health professional to a medical staff, licensing board, or ethics committee. The underlying ethical principle is that a physician's first duty is to protect patient care. Such decisions are difficult and have been discouraged for decades of medical teaching. Indeed, the Hippocratic Oath provided a pledge to protect colleagues. Today, in an age of accountability and public awareness, there can be little excuse for avoiding one's responsibility to protect the public. Any reporting of colleagues must be based on knowledge of incompetent or unethical behavior and not on legitimate disagreement over diverse treatment approaches or styles of practice.

Case Vignette 1

As an administrative psychiatrist in a large public psychiatric system, you oversee the work of numerous other clinical psychiatrists. You become aware that one of the psychiatrists routinely prescribes combinations of medications for patients who have medical conditions in which these combinations would be contraindicated. It is clear that other combinations are equally effective and that the combinations this psychiatrist uses are not necessary, considering the risk to patients. Although you have provided education for the psychiatrist regarding prescribing practices, he refuses to alter his prescription style, claiming that he personally has not witnessed any adverse reactions in his patients. What should you do?

Opinion. Because your first duty is to patient care, termination or suspension of the psychiatrist from clinical work should be considered. In addition, referral to the medical licensing board and ethics committee in the state would be appropriate.

Case Vignette 2

You are working as a utilization reviewer for a managed care company. In reviewing the case of a young female patient, you become aware that she has complained to an administrator in the company that her treating psychiatrist has engaged in flirtatious behavior, including asking her out for a date shortly after the termination of her treatment. What should you do?

Opinion. You should make every attempt to get additional facts yourself from the patient and to encourage the patient to file an ethics complaint with the local psychiatric society or with the medical licensing board. Internal action within the managed care company should also be considered, with proper legal and confidentiality safeguards for all involved.

"A physician shall respect the law and also recognize a responsibility to seek changes in those requirements which are contrary to the best interests of the patients."

The administrative psychiatrist is often in the unique position of being aware of all of the influences that affect patient care. By approaching those influences using patient care as the primary focus, the administrative psychiatrist can support legislation that will improve patient care. Ethical dilemmas arise when the administrative psychiatrist recognizes that advocating for changes in the law to improve patient care may have an adverse impact on the psychiatrist's organization. This may be through need for increased administrative oversight, decreased profit, or a combination of both.

Case Vignette

You assume the role as medical director of a large managed care company. You become aware that the treatment algorithms approved by the company discourage the use of combined psychotherapy and medications in situations you believe could benefit from consideration of the combination. You also become aware that the company's payment structure

provides incentives to treating psychiatrists to avoid the use of combined treatment. Psychiatrists in your company have also been discouraged from informing patients about the possible benefits of combined treatments. Proposed legislation in your state mandates full disclosure of all treatment options available for patients. You have previously supported this type of legislation but now realize it may affect your current job. What should you do?

Opinion. Because your primary obligation should always be to patient care, you must continue to support legislation you believe will improve patient care. At the same time, you should advocate immediate changes within your organization to achieve those goals even without legislation. It is ethical to continue in a position through which you hope to influence better patient care; however, at times, the appropriate ethical decision may be to opt out of the system.

"A physician shall respect the rights of patients, of colleagues, and of other health professionals, and shall safeguard patient confidences within the constraints of the law."

The administrative psychiatrist often has responsibilities to oversee the rights of patients, including issues such as informed consent to treatment, involuntary treatment, informed consent for research, and the right to refuse treatment. Also, some administrative psychiatrists may be involved in activities that require them to work with other mental health professionals in team approaches to patient care or in other administrative tasks. The administrative psychiatrist should be aware of the appropriate scope of practice and of the competencies of the other mental health professionals in the organization. Those competencies should be respected and utilized for the benefit of patients. If concerns exist about the competency of another mental health professional, the administrator must regard as paramount the overarching considerations regarding patient safety.

Confidentiality is the bedrock of psychiatric treatment and should be of equal concern to any administrative psychiatrist. Organizations should have the strictest confidentiality standards for both mental health professionals and nonprofessional staff. The patient places trust in the treating doctor, and the administrative doctor must make sure that treatment trust is not breached. Unfortunately, modern healthcare may require the disclosure of various kinds of patient information to numerous personnel. Concerns about breaches of confidentiality are real, and, whether by accident or intent, release of confidential patient information could have a deleterious effect on patients' willingness to enter into psychiatric treatment.

In this era of accountability, reporting of patient information to outside agencies or for internal review has become commonplace. There is no problem when aggregate data without patient identifiers are used. However, identifiable patient information released to any outside third parties presents the possibility for breach of patient confidentiality. Accrediting and reviewing organizations may ask for patient charts during the course of review. The APA has taken the position that such information should not be released without contemporaneous patient consent; if that cannot be obtained, identifying information should be removed (American Psychiatric Association 1996).

Clearly, special problems are associated with the computer age, and administrative psychiatrists need to be familiar with the potential for technological override of confidentiality firewalls. Concerns have been raised about large data banks of patient information that can be used or sold for purposes other than improved patient care. For these reasons, President Clinton appointed a Commission on Confidentiality to make recommendations about technological confidentiality, including in healthcare systems. It is hoped that all involved will recognize the long-term importance of maintaining the confidentiality of patient information.

Case Vignette

You are the medical director for a large HMO that has experienced large financial losses over the past year. The HMO has been approached by a large supplier of healthcare products to enter into an agreement to pay a significant fee to the HMO for lists of patients receiving treatment for various illnesses. The CEO of the HMO thinks this will help keep the HMO from going into bankruptcy and needs your consent to turn over the list of patients. What should you do?

Opinion. You should refuse the CEO's request for the patient names, as this would be a breach of confidentiality. A secondary issue to look at relates to the conflict of interest created if the HMO receives a fee for marketing a health supplier's products to patients receiving HMO services. It would be appropriate for the HMO to reveal such a fee arrangement to patient groups if a way could be found to advertise or promote the health supplier's products ethically.

"A physician shall continue to study, apply, and advance scientific knowledge, make relevant information available to patients, colleagues, and the public, obtain consultation, and use the talents of other health professionals when indicated."

Medical ethics has had a strong tradition of teaching colleagues and providing beneficial information to the public. In the current market-based healthcare climate, however, countervailing forces may impede the unrestricted sharing of information that could benefit other colleagues or patients. This may be in areas considered proprietary by a healthcare system that could provide a competitive advantage for the system. The ethical high ground should be that any information obtained by a system that can improve the health of patients should be shared with other professionals, systems, and the public. Psychiatrists have an ethical obligation to advocate for the unfettered flow of scientific information that will benefit patients. It is less clear whether information systems or billing systems that improve the efficiency of patient treatment should be shared with others or appropriately can be considered proprietary. If the healthcare environment were not as competitive as it is, such information would surely be shared to improve the healthcare and cost efficiency of all healthcare systems.

Administrative psychiatrists are in the unique position of working with other health professionals who may be in other mental health disciplines as well as other physicians and non–mental health professionals. All professionals must be treated with respect for their unique contributions to the healthcare of patients. The administrative psychiatrist must make certain that duties beyond his or her competence are not given to or shared with other health professionals. Conversely, the administrative psychiatrist must not allow his or her unique training to be utilized in any way that is adverse to the best interests of patients.

Case Vignette

A group of psychologists working within an HMO ask you (the administrative psychiatrist) to allow them to provide written prescriptions (signed by a physician) for antidepressant and antianxiety medications. The psychologists indicate that they have had training in such prescribing and will follow your instructions on the manner in which these prescriptions should be dispensed. Is this ethical?

Opinion. No. This would be a breach of ethics because it grants competence to those who are not licensed to prescribe. Also, it is currently illegal in all states for psychologists to prescribe, and for you to allow this would be a breach of the state's laws regulating the practice of medicine.

❖

"A physician shall, in the provision of appropriate patient care, except in emergencies, be free to choose whom to serve, with whom to associate, and the environment in which to provide medical services."

Administrative positions often entail responsibilities that do not allow for the absolute freedom to choose whom to serve, with whom to associate, and the environment in which to provide medical services. Often those determinations are built into the administrative position and are understood when one takes the position. For example, taking on the responsibility to contract for the care of a group of patients necessitates taking on full responsibility for those patients. While not obligating an individual to care directly for particular patients, the administrative psychiatrist must make available appropriate care for any patient in that group. To do otherwise would be unethical patient abandonment. This places an increased burden on the administrative psychiatrist to have available for such a group, whether public or private, competent professionals to care for the patients within that group. If patient services are required that no one in the group is competent to deliver, the administrative psychiatrist must make sure those services are provided elsewhere.

There have been long-standing concerns in underfunded public (and now private) systems that psychiatrists were being asked to provide less-than-competent services and therefore might be acting unethically. Although administrative psychiatrists could leave these systems, it might be ethically more appropriate to remain in the system and try to improve the conditions and healthcare for patients.

Case Vignette

You are working as an administrative psychiatrist for a prison system and are asked to do competency evaluations on prisoners awaiting execution. Personally you do not believe that it is ethical for a psychiatrist to perform such examinations, but it is a requirement of your job. What should you do?

Opinion. Because opinions vary about psychiatrists' involvement in this phase of the execution process, you would have the right to exercise your ethical belief by not participating. It is hoped that the system would recognize the differing ethical positions of physicians in this situation and find a substitute for that aspect of your job. It is ethical for you to refuse to perform such an evaluation.

❖

"A physician shall recognize a responsibility to participate in activities contributing to an improved community."

A psychiatrist has an ethical obligation to patient, self, and society. The manner in which an individual administrative psychiatrist exercises the obligation to contribute to an improved community is an individual decision. All psychiatrists have an obligation to improve the healthcare of the community, to speak out on public health and psychiatric issues, and to attempt to influence the community in a manner consistent with improving patient care. Psychiatrists can also participate in the community in areas totally outside of psychiatry. When so participating, psychiatrists should not blur their professional roles with their roles as dedicated citizens. In addition, psychiatrists should make it perfectly clear whether an opinion is a personal one or whether it represents the profession of psychiatry.

Case Vignette

As the administrator of the largest psychiatric facility in your state, you are asked to comment on the recent increase in AIDS-related illnesses in your state. You are not an expert in AIDS and do not feel competent to answer the question. The reporter presses you to give some opinions nevertheless. What should you do?

Opinion. Respectfully decline the interview and refer the reporter to an expert in the field. Utilize the opportunity to discuss AIDS-related psychiatric illnesses that have resulted in treatment at your facility and offer to comment on a subject about which you feel more knowledgeable.

Conclusion

Although there is both complexity and nuance in the ethical dilemmas of the administrative psychiatrist, the similarities with the dilemmas of the clinical psychiatrist are obvious when one clearly understands the ethical principles all physicians should follow. Advocating for the patient, an extension of the ethical principle of benevolence, is primary and is not altered by the role a physician assumes. Paying close attention to the wishes and needs of patients applies the ethical principle of autonomy and must be respected. Making certain that any actions taken do not harm patients follows the principle of nonmaleficence. Attending to the fair and honest distribution of psychiatric services follows the principle of justice. Although ethical dilemmas usually indicate conflicts between two or more of these primary principles, the solution lies in the overall benefit to the patient(s). Whenever an administrative psychiatrist senses a blurring in role or identify that does not allow that primary focus to be on the patient, an ethics consultation would be appropriate. Some healthcare organizations that employ psychiatrists and other physicians as administrators have formed their own internal ethics committees to review ethical concerns. With proper and unimpeded ethics consultation, the psychiatrist administrator could make clear-cut and fair ethical decisions within healthcare systems. If, however, the dilemmas surrounding medical ethics become intermingled with those of business ethics, powerful competing forces may result that cannot be reconciled. In the end, all psychiatrists and other physicians in any role must put the patient first.

References

American Medical Association Council on Ethical and Judicial Affairs: Code of Medical Ethics, Current Opinions With Annotations. Washington, DC, American Medical Association, 1994

American Medical Association: Ethical issues in managed care. JAMA 273:330–335, 1995

American Psychiatric Association: Ethics Source Book. Washington, DC, American Psychiatric Association, 1992

American Psychiatric Association: Opinions of the Ethics Committee on the Principles of Medical Ethics. Washington, DC, American Psychiatric Association, 1995a

American Psychiatric Association: The Principles of Medical Ethics With Annotations Especially Applicable to Psychiatry. Washington, DC, American Psychiatric Association, 1995b

American Psychiatric Association: Position Statement on Accrediting and Auditing Organizations. Washington, DC, American Psychiatric Association, 1996

Beauchamp TL, Childress JF: Principles of Biomedical Ethics. New York, Oxford University Press, 1994

Lazarus JA, Sharfstein SS: APA acts against ethics violators. Psychiatric News, October 16, 1992, p 14

Sabin J, Daniels N: Determining medical necessity in mental health practice. Hastings Center Report 24:5–14, 1994

Conclusion

Future Issues for Administrative Psychiatry

John A. Talbott, M.D.

Textbooks of administrative psychiatry tend to chronicle the issues, problems, and opportunities facing the field at the time of their publication, despite their unstated wish to provide information that is not time-bound. For example, the first such textbook, the estimable *Administration in Psychiatry* (W. E. Barton 1962), dwelt largely on administrative issues encountered in state hospitals, which at that time were the primary treatment sites for the mentally ill. *Mental Health Administration* (W. E. Barton and G. M. Barton 1983) dealt more with community psychiatric issues. Likewise, the two editions of *The Administration of Mental Health Services* (Feldman 1973, 1980) reflected administrative issues at the height of the era of community mental health and community mental health centers.

In addition to this current volume, I have been the editor of two earlier textbooks of administrative psychiatry (Talbott and Kaplan 1983; Talbott et al. 1992). Each also reflected the times in which we lived. In 1983, the era of community care—what some have called the post-deinstitutionalization era—was in full swing, and efforts to patch up the failures of that movement were reflected in that edition. Likewise, in 1992, issues of cost-containment and managed care began to be discussed.

It is no surprise that this edition of the *Textbook of Administrative Psychiatry* reflects the changing times we now live in. In this concluding chapter, I summarize and synthesize some of the trends, themes, and issues that have surfaced repeatedly in this textbook, without repeating the details so ably provided by the chapter authors. In addition, I discuss some of the implications of these trends for psychiatric administrators.

Patient Trends

Patient trends are powerful predictors of services and systems efforts. The trends that have most affected psychiatric administration include demographic, diagnostic, and economic ones as well as the location where patients are treated and the changing roles of those patients, from passive recipient through collaborator to advocate and provider.

Demographic Trends

We continue to experience a further "graying" of America, with the life extension of the American population leading to more senior citizens, more frail elderly, and more elderly people with medical and psychiatric problems and a higher incidence of comorbid chronic conditions. In addition, the population described by Bachrach (1984) as the "young adult chronic patient" is now no longer young, and the insufficient care and treatment these persons received is further complicating their movement into the older age group. The implication of this trend is that psychiatric administrators need to become even more heavily involved with primary care specialists and gerontologists and in settings where the elderly are housed (e.g., nursing homes, retirement communities, assisted living settings) (Talbott 1998). While continuing to train geropsychiatrists, we must also train general psychiatrists to better treat the elderly who have both psychiatric and medical problems.

Diagnostic Trends

Comorbidity of medical and psychiatric conditions is common among the elderly, and comorbidity of psychiatric and addictive disorders is common in younger age groups. Across the age spectrum, we are seeing many more patients with co-occurring psychiatric, medical, and developmental disability problems. Surely the most vexing example is that posed by co-occurring mental illnesses and addictions, which, as we have learned from the National Comorbidity Study, are extraordinarily common. The implication of this trend is that psychiatric services must be broader, more inventive, and increasingly modeled after dual-diagnosis programs that combine addiction and psychiatric philosophies of treatment (e.g., lay-directed self-help as well as professionally prescribed medication) and practices (e.g., 12-step programs as well as cognitive therapy) (Ridgely et al. 1989).

The Severity Issue

Overlapping the demographic and diagnostic trends is the issue of the increased severity of the illnesses we are seeing, combined with the fact that patients are now seen for shorter lengths of time with different goals for treatment episodes than just a few years earlier. Whether in the hospital, in outpatient clinics, or in private offices, the rule regarding patients and their hospital stays is certainly "sicker and quicker." The implication of this trend is that we must be better equipped to diagnose, treat, and follow-up patients who have severe mental illness in less time and with fewer resources, while maintaining our effectiveness.

Economics

The two economic trends that have had and will continue to have the most impact on patients are the burden of caring for the uninsured and cost control/cost cutting, carried out currently through the aegis of managed care. The implication of the move to managed care is probably the most discussed issue in this textbook. It includes almost every topic, from leadership to staffing, from cultural issues to ethical ones, and from the private sector to the public one. The implications of our society's continuing unwillingness to provide all Americans with health insurance is that we must advocate for a political solution to the problem while struggling with the ethical and clinical dilemmas of providing what we often think is substandard care or suffering economic consequences in a highly competitive market.

Issues Related to Where Patients Are Seen

Especially for psychiatric administrators working in the public sector, the vast shift in where patients are located presents challenges for the present and future. For example, in the late 1950s the preponderance of the severely mentally ill were in hospitals; now they are in a host of community settings, including "homes" that vary in quality and accessibility as well as some places that are even more difficult to reach (e.g., the correctional system and homeless shelters). The implication of this trend is that if we are ethically and/or contractually mandated or required to provide care for all the mentally ill wherever they are, the way we provide services and our ability to track patients must be improved.

Participation

A trend that has become more significant in the past few years is the increasing incidence of citizen/patient/consumer participation in decision making. Whereas in the 1960s, citizen participation was part of the community psychiatry ideology, now it is a necessary ingredient of public managed care initiatives and a potentially decisive force if consumers of private managed care exert their influence rather that let insurance executives and benefit managers continue their unmodified. A disturbing development is the increasing tension between primary consumers and secondary ones (e.g., family members), which makes some decisions hard to reach when consumer input is sought. The implication of this trend is that these citizens/patients/consumers hold tremendous power and can have a profound impact on the way services are shaped, cut, or provided. For whatever reasons, however, most effective citizen power has been exerted primarily through legislation ensuring access to nonpsychiatric care (e.g., mastectomies, childbirth). The stigma of mental illness in the private corporate world and the lack of a critical mass in the public world seem to be the rate-limiting factors to the exercising of this potential power.

Treatments

Since the publication of the first edition of this textbook, services have been instituted, expanded, or modified as a result of scientific, demographic, epidemiologic, organizational, economic, and administrative factors.

New Services in Response to Scientific Developments

Services derived from research have more scientific credibility than those advocated because of other factors, including economic, political, or administrative reasons. Thus, cognitive-behavioral therapy and other short-term therapies for a variety of illnesses, combined with drugs and psychosocial treatment for depression and schizophrenia, group interventions and psychoeducational approaches for the chronically ill, and the new antipsychotics and selective serotonin reuptake inhibitors (SSRIs) are clearly shaping the clinics and service lines set up to deliver them. The implication of this trend is that treatments that have recently been proved effective will continue to dictate the way services develop unless formulary restrictions prevent it or payment is denied.

New Services in Response to Demographic and Epidemiologic Developments

Many services have developed or thrived because of the demographic and epidemiologic trends detailed earli-

er in this conclusion, in the section on patient trends. Thus, the provision of services for some groups of patients has been driven by these groups' prevalence in the population—for example, services for the dually diagnosed, those for the elderly with both medical and mental illnesses, those for mentally ill offenders, those for the homeless mentally ill, those for nursing home residents, and those for the chronically mentally ill in need of resocialization-rehabilitation. The implication of this trend is that we must be prepared to serve not only existing groups of patients but also those created by future unpredictable events.

New Services in Response to Organizational Developments

As a result of the trend toward the development of service and product lines that are marketable in the current competitive environment, services are often shaped by organizational pressures rather than scientific, demographic, or epidemiologic ones. Thus, behavioral health programs incorporate psychiatry and the addictions, geriatric and children's health services incorporate geropsychiatry and child psychiatric services, and women's health services incorporate psychiatric and psychological services. The implication of this trend is that in the future, as now, market niches, popular and competitive services, and packaging opportunities will have to be closely followed.

New Services in Response to Economic and Administrative Developments

Economic and administrative pressures can also bring about the development of new services. For example, managed care has been singularly important in helping to stimulate the initiation or expansion of services such as triage and rapid treatment, short-term hospitalization, employee assistance programs (EAPs), culturally competent services, and women's health services. However, as Hollingsworth and Sweeney (1997) pointed out, some pressures to reduce services may be penny wise and pound foolish, such as the decision to trim services for the chronically mentally ill under public managed care, notably rehabilitation, community support, and nonmedical counseling. The implication of this trend is that economic and administrative pressures will continue to shape service provision, and psychiatric administrators must be sensitive to market forces and demands. Undoubtedly, the next great wave of services will come as a result of technological advances (as Freeman argued in the introduction to this textbook and I discuss later in this conclusion). Telemedicine represents one area of enormous need and opportunity; another area comprises chat rooms and Internet-based information for patients and families.

Systems Issues

Several trends are related to the systems of health and mental healthcare as a whole. These trends include integrated delivery systems, the relationship between primary care and psychiatry, the behavioral health carve-out, networks of providers, and the privatization of the public system.

Development of Integrated Delivery Systems

Integrated delivery systems mean different things to different people but in all cases bring about a greater necessity on the part of psychiatric administrators to interact with others and other systems. For instance, if a delivery system offers primary, secondary, tertiary, and quaternary care, its practitioners and administrators must interact with an active expanded cast of medical, nonmedical professional, and administrative staff. Likewise, if a system encompasses hospital intensive care, step-down, alternatives, and ambulatory care, interaction with team managers, patient coordinators, and case or care managers becomes essential. In a carve-in situation, psychiatrists and other mental health providers have increased commerce with all primary and specialty care providers.

Increasing Ties Between Primary Care and Psychiatry

As primary caregivers do more of the gatekeeping and provide what were once tertiary care services, psychiatrists will find increased opportunities to do formal outpatient consultation-liaison psychiatry, elbow-to-elbow consultation in primary care satellites, and teaching of "how-to and when-to" (refer or treat). The implication of this trend is that we have to find staff members who are willing and able to perform these new roles, who are comfortable with teaching others, who are able to keep their hands off service provision, and who are skilled at interacting effectively with primary caregivers.

The Behavioral Health Carve-Out

Although there has been a de facto behavioral health carve-out in the United States since the creation of mental hospitals that were separate from general hospitals, the carve-out of mental health and addiction services and of patients needing those services to behavioral healthcare organizations is a relatively recent phenomenon. For psychiatric administrators who have functioned in private hospitals and public systems, life goes on but under different rules. For those working in general hospitals, those in integrated delivery systems, and those dealing with primary and tertiary care initiatives, "life" now means maintaining or developing the capacity to perform both carved-in and carved-out work. The implication of the trend is that we must develop the entire spectrum of services, including EAPs and sports team products, as well as administrative, outcomes measurement, sophisticated information management, quality assurance, and quality improvement services.

The Trend Toward Networks of Providers

The ability to deliver services on greater than the local level, often on a regional or statewide basis, requires a network of providers or partnerships. This represents a challenge for psychiatric administrators who are accustomed to closed staffs; small, elite, academic faculties; or providers employed by the public sector. The implication of this trend is that psychiatric administrators need to develop systems, staffs, and monitoring capacities—internally, through contracts, or through partnerships.

Privatization of the Public System

As the public system privatizes, whether through traditional public entitlement programs such as Medicaid and Medicare or through sales to or partnerships with private entities (e.g., hospitals, clinics, and other community services), psychiatric administrators involved in such initiatives will see marked changes. Such changes include the adoption of standards, methods to improve efficiency, and management techniques pioneered in the private sector, as well as the adoption of market-driven behavior, a greater spirit of entrepreneurship and competitiveness, and thinking that is "out of the box" that the public entity has been in. The implication of this trend is that psychiatric administrators require skills and training and knowledge about a host of activities that may seem foreign, for example, those acquired first by persons working in the managed care industry and later by those in large private provider groups.

From Reimbursement to Revenues

Since the early 1990s we have gone from depending on and talking about reimbursement to depending on and talking about revenues. This shift involves a number of areas.

Assumption of Risk in Private Managed Care

From the beginning, managed care companies have operated in a fixed-income, prospective, essentially capitated economic system. Providers—whether individual practitioners, provider groups, or larger systems of care—continue to receive much of their income retrospectively. Only as we move more steadily toward providers taking risk will we see them turn toward prospective revenue and away from retrospective reimbursement. The implication of this trend is that budgets will be more predictable if costs can be controlled, outcomes maintained, and satisfaction ensured. But assuming risk means that one must have the ability to act rapidly, contract rapidly, and hire and fire rapidly as well as control costs, manage care of populations oneself, and have the information systems and the like needed to handle the job.

Contracts

A relatively new way that large entities or provider groups have survived or thrived is by becoming contractors of services, for instance, contracting to provide addiction or emergency services for other hospitals, delivering crisis intervention services for geographic areas, and providing care in long-term care facilities (e.g., nursing homes). Such contracts, like capitation, lead to the creation of more predictable budgets, without the risk of capitation or the uncertainty of maintaining volumes of fee-for-service activities. The implication of this trend is that psychiatric administrators must have the skills needed to negotiate fair contracts, to ensure fulfillment of each contract, to monitor all their own activities, and to manage pressures at the margins (e.g., to serve patients not strictly covered by the contract).

Medicaid

The rapid acquisition by state governments of 1115 waivers granted by the Health Care Financing Administration for Medicaid expenditures has been dramatic. Consequences of such new systems are now commonplace, despite the differences in methods and regardless of whether behavioral healthcare is carved in, carved out, or in some instances both (e.g., in Maryland, substance abuse is carved in; services for the mentally ill, not usually performed by a primary care physician, are carved out). In most cases, the moneys allocated are less than was the case historically, start-up problems and indeed massive screw-ups are frequent, and psychiatric administrators on the state or managed behavioral healthcare organization (MBHO) side see things much rosier than do those on the provider side. The latter is the case with private managed care as well; the difference here is that we expect government to be less efficient than industry but to care more about the populations for which they have historically cared for. The implications of this trend are that those working in systems that traditionally serve such populations are at risk of losing both their populations and their care systems; that a whole new set of skills and tools is necessary (as mentioned earlier); and that, like the U.S. Postal Service, converting to a private model requires vast shifts in cultural contexts, operating modalities, and staff attitudes and behaviors.

One or Two Systems

I have discussed elsewhere whether managed care or managing care would lead to a single system of care or perpetuate the two current systems, although not necessarily with its two-class difference (Talbott 1998) (Figure 1).

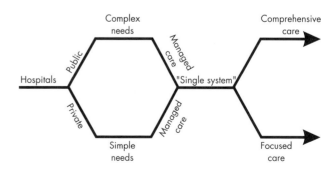

FIGURE 1. One or two systems of care?

Looking at it one way, we could hope that the historical split between the public and private populations (at least since the establishment of state versus private mental hospitals) would finally disappear under a single system of management (e.g., managed care). Alternatively, you could argue that the differences between the private acutely ill population and the public chronically ill one—in illnesses, symptoms, disabilities, service need, monitoring, and outcomes—are so vast that the two populations will always require different systems. For example, the employed, generally adequately functioning citizen living in a family with shelter, benefits, and health insurance will require a different system than will the unemployed or underemployed, lower functioning citizen from an often dysfunctional family with shaky shelter and uncertain or only government safety-net benefits and insurance. The implication of this difference in these two possible futures is vast. Under a single system we could be training, working, and managing in a consistent manner, but we would be trying to fit all patients into rigid molds or we could continue to operate ambidextrously—e.g., training, working, and managing in different ways for different patients and services.

Technology

No area has such explosive growth and vast potential to change the way we function as does technological change.

Computers

In just a few years, the availability, power, and reasonable cost of computers and computer services have revolutionized our world. Personal computers, whether in the hands of providers or patients, permit access to the Internet, chat rooms, information services, and the like, a level of access to information and advice that has yet to be fully exploited. Patients, now able to use MEDLINE at no charge or seek help regarding SSRIs or talk to other patients, are truly empowered. Likewise, providers have access to data sets, MEDLINE, drug information, and chat rooms to consult with others in real-time.

Large computers enable insurance companies, managed care organizations (MCOs), MBHOs, and provider groups to perform provider profiling, billing, outcome measurement, and the like. Although the thorny issues of patient confidentiality and misuse of some provider or outcome data will never be fully resolved, one can only hope that well-protected patient registers will permit ethical providers to know instantly what medications, treatments, and case management each patient is receiving. The implication of this trend is that investments in computer technology, training, and maintenance will continue to increase and that staying ahead of the curve will become increasingly important.

Telemedicine

For years we have struggled to provide services and manpower to underserved areas, largely in rural or inner-city areas. Now, through the power of technology, we are able to deal interactively with each other as well as with patients and citizens in general. Except for teaching, research, and consultation, psychiatry has been seen as a less fertile ground than other medical specialties for development of this technology. However, a tremendous push is under way to exploit telemedicine in psychiatry. Interesting cost-benefit questions arise. For instance, a trauma anesthesiologist colleague is assessing whether it is better to train 16,000 military medical technicians in critical airway support, an event they will be faced with at most once in their careers, or to supply each with miniaturized cameras linked to experts who can talk them through the procedure. The implication of this trend is that, as with outpatient consultation-liaison psychiatry or elbow-to-elbow consulting with primary caregivers, psychiatric administrators must become more skilled in giving advice, supervising others from a distance, and conducting so-called virtual therapy.

Outcome Measurements and Report Cards

Eventually cost will no longer be the only determinant of choice of treatment, plan, or provider—quality will be incorporated into the equation. Outcome measurement for individual patients and outcome and cost-outcome analyses for individual or combined treatments will become increasingly critical. On the flip side, report cards on the performance of MCOs, MBHOs, insurance companies, and provider groups will also become more available and better utilized. The primary obstacle here is the difficulty in cleaning the research data so that apples are being measured against apples or, stated contrariwise, so that the treatment of inner-city dually diagnosed HIV patients is not compared with the treatment of phobias in suburban soccer moms.

Nevertheless, the implication of this trend is that the measurement of everything will become more commonplace and our ability to articulate key questions and to explain the data and their differences will become crucial.

Protocols, Treatment Guidelines, and Disease Management

The proliferation of protocols, treatment guidelines, and tools to assist in disease management is proof that both industry and professional bodies agree about the need to standardize treatment, improve outcomes, and utilize research data on effectiveness. Services research is a relatively new discipline, and only recently have results appeared that enable us to translate research into practice. However, the implication of this trend is that psychiatric administrators will be increasingly able to use hard data to drive clinical practice. The danger is that confusion will result about which guidelines to follow if the trend continues toward the development of multiple sets of guidelines. This trend is the result of intense competition between the instruments' authors, who are affiliated with different professional associations, private groups, and the pharmaceutical industry.

Quality Assurance and Quality Improvement

In my mind, a difference exists between the attempts on the part of clinical administrators to improve the quality of care by measuring outcomes or comparing treatments in patient subgroups in various settings and the slickly packaged campaigns by business administrators and marketing experts, using almost incomprehensible jargon, in thinly veiled attempts to appear scientific while intending primarily to compete more effectively in the marketplace. The implication of this split in efforts is that psychiatric administrators must encourage attempts to truly improve quality of care that coincidentally can be used in marketing, not vice versa.

Virtually Everything

The combination of technologies, including computers, the Internet, CD-ROMs, television, cellular telephones, and the like, is rapidly producing what will become a practice and administrative world in which almost all activities can go on interactively in real-time. A danger in this "virtual everything" is that as rapidly as events are occurring now, the situation will soon get even worse and there will be no escaping the pressure to answer questions instantly or to solve problems in seconds. With cellular phones, modems, faxes, and Federal Express, there is almost no way that one can say, "Let me think about that." Why does one need time to think when the patient and provider are on your video screen; the data sets are on the Internet; and help, tests, and services are available 24 hours a day, 7 days a week. The implication of this trend is a bit frightening. Maybe we will have to avoid over-virtualizing reality through team management, shift work, and splitting work up into small tasks. Otherwise, no one may be willing to become a psychiatric administrator.

Language

It is said that part of the definition of a field or profession is that it has developed its own language or jargon. In the years since the first edition of this textbook, the language we use has exploded exponentially. Whereas at that time we talked about the language of the "alphabet soup" (e.g., HMOs, PPOs, IPAs) that we were using, now we have an "alphabet life" and a jargon-filled day. Some words we use in everyday professional conversations are reflective of our wish or need to talk "business-speak" (e.g., bottom-line or one-stop shopping), and some words are from the computer world (e.g., user-friendly services). Others are true neologisms (e.g., gatekeeping). Bachrach (1995), our field's William Safire, has written extensively about the words we use, but few others have discussed this issue.

The biggest shift has been in our titles or roles. For example, we have gone from being physicians or psychiatrists to being providers—and persons with illnesses have gone from being patients through being clients and consumers to being customers. Then there is the use of so-called compressed words: The leading examples are *healthcare* and *behavioral healthcare*. My own institution has created a service called ExpressCare, which, with its compression, presumably implies fast, seamless, businesslike care. While I am discussing behavioral healthcare, let me note that this term not only replaces *psychiatry* and *addiction services* but also has been seen by some as implying the deprofessionalization and replacement of higher qualified staff by lower qualified staff.

Surely we still have the alphabet soup of organizations that we had when the first edition of this textbook was published, but we now have new ones. The most recent additions are PHOs, MCOs, MBHOs, and NCQA.

For readers needing assistance in wending their way through this soup, we have provided a glossary at the end of the book.

We have also adopted a great deal of business lingo and are heavily involved with "downsizing" and "rightsizing," mergers and acquisitions, and markets and capital markets (not to be confused with marketing). In addition, we no longer refer to bed days, bed occupancy, or admissions but to volumes of service. Also, we have swept away departments and divisions and centers and replaced them with product lines and service lines. Some of the business language also reflects our adoration of *re* and *retro* (e.g., retrofit, re-engineer, and reinvent).

The computer industry has provided us with a lot of words that we have borrowed or adapted; we are now on-line and interfacing with others. An administrative assistant in our institution became so swept up in computer terminology that when she announced a phone call, she would say that so-and-so was on-line.

Finally, the neologisms to which I referred earlier: In classical psychiatry these were largely the productions of persons with schizophrenia. No longer! We have created words such as *carve-in* and *carve-out* or *integrated delivery systems* out of necessity more than psychosis, although, in truth, that too may play a role.

Psychiatric Administration: Past, Present, and Future

In this concluding section I try to tie together the themes and trends mentioned in this textbook and derive some implications for the education and training of psychiatric administrators (i.e., ourselves and our successors).

Past

In the past, psychiatric administrators had a modicum of certainty: They had a body of knowledge, often derived from classical management theory, from McGregor (1969) to Drucker (1973–1974), and from business experience (often published in the *Harvard Business Review*); a set of values shared by most psychiatric administrators (such as fiduciary responsibility and "above all, do no harm"); a series of agreed-on desirable skills (including the POSDCORB ones of planning, organizing, budgeting, and so on) (Talbott 1988); and a common history.

Present

At present we are in the midst of a whirlwind, and the experiences we share are related to that situation. For example, uncertainty exists about the shape or even continuance of certain types of systems, treatments, and practices; threats are experienced from above (be it government or academia), below (resentful troops), or outside (society, all levels of government, industry in general, and the insurance and managed care industries in particular); and there are enormous changes in funding (risk and shifts and reductions), enormous changes in the structure of the enterprises we administer, and enormous changes brought about by technology.

Future

A major task in the future will be to take those skills, experiences, and knowledge bases that are applicable in any administrative setting, in any era—such as budgeting, a knowledge of systems, people skills, and the context of our psychiatric and medical training—and blend into them the new elements essential to modern management. These new elements may be new treatments; new administrative concepts (e.g., networks, partnering, capitation, telemedicine); new economic forces; new devices and methods; or new methods of measuring ourselves, our systems, and our patients.

Implications for Education and Training (Ourselves and Our Successors)

In medical education, residency, and fellowship training—as well as in postgraduate education, continuing medical education, and on-the-job training—we must do three things: 1) continue to educate ourselves about basic, core issues as they relate to our changing times and situations (e.g., the "new accountability," new planning methods, new budgeting techniques), 2) teach ourselves new skills to handle changing systems, such as technological ones (e.g., information systems), scientific ones (e.g., measurement of true quality of care), and administrative ones (e.g., partnering, merging and acquiring, cost-efficiency, rapid firing/hiring, incentive systems), and 3) perhaps most important, train ourselves and others how to handle change through preparation, education, experience, supervision, consultation, peer-advice, acquisition of new lingo, and blind luck.

Light at the End of the Tunnel

Everyone predicts that we will pass through this period of turmoil into a brighter future, and most agree that managed care companies have a time-limited future. But care will still be managed (by psychiatric administrators, it is hoped), and the hope for a return to the past is wishful thinking. Nonetheless, as an old Vietnam veteran, I am suspicious of those who already see the light at the end of the tunnel; however, preserving our spirit of inquiry, innovation, and creativity in the face of pervasive fear, gloom, and despair will get us through. We hope that this textbook, through its presentations of old and new challenges, will help keep psychiatric administration strong and able.

References

Bachrach LL: The young adult chronic psychiatric patient in an era of deinstitutionalization. Am J Public Health 74:382–384, 1984

Bachrach LL: The chronic patient: managed care: I. delimiting the concept. Psychiatr Serv 46:1229–1230, 1995

Barton WE: Administration in Psychiatry. Springfield, IL, Charles C. Thomas, 1962

Barton WE, Barton GM: Mental Health Administration: Principles and Practice, Vol 1–2. New York, Human Sciences Press, 1983

Drucker PF: Management: Tasks, Responsibilities, Practices. New York, Harper & Row, 1973–1974

Feldman S: The Administration of Mental Health Services. Springfield, IL, Charles C. Thomas, 1973

Feldman S: The Administration of Mental Health Services, 2nd Edition. Springfield, IL, Charles C. Thomas, 1980

Hollingsworth EJ, Sweeney JK: Mental health expenditures for services for people with severe mental illnesses. Psychiatr Serv 48:485–490, 1997

McGregor D: The human side of enterprise, in Behavioral Science: Concepts and Management Application. New York, The Conference Board, 1969, pp 11–16

Ridgely MS, Talbott JA, Goldman HH: Treatment of chronic mentally ill young adults with substance abuse problems: emerging national trends. Annals of the American Society for Adolescent Psychiatry 16:288–313, 1989

Talbott JA: The perspective of John Talbott. New Directions for Mental Health Services, No 37. San Francisco, Jossey-Bass, 1988

Talbott JA: Il futuro dei servizi psichiatrici negli Stati Uniti: ovvero: cosa verra dopo la Managed Care? [The future of psychiatric services in the United States: What comes after managed care?] Rivista Sperimentale di Freniatria 122:16–24, 1998

Talbott JA, Kaplan SR (eds): Psychiatric Administration: A Comprehensive Text for the Clinician-Executive. New York, Grune & Stratton, 1983

Talbott JA, Hales RE, Keill SL (eds): Textbook of Administrative Psychiatry. Washington, DC, American Psychiatric Press, 1992

Glossary

Access The ability to obtain desired healthcare. Access is more than having Medicaid or commercial insurance coverage or the ability to pay for services. It is also determined by the availability of services, acceptability of services, cultural appropriateness, location, hours of operation, transportation, and cost.[1]

Administrative service organization (ASO) A management service contracted to control a health plan's costs, conduct utilization review, and pay providers. Same as a management service organization (MSO) and a third-party administrator (TPA).[2]

Adverse selection Enrollment that disproportionately creates adverse risk, such as a more impaired population with higher healthcare utilization.[3]

Any willing provider Laws that permit any provider willing to abide by terms and conditions of a certain network contract and holding certain credentials to be admitted to that network.[2]

Armed Services' Medical Corps The military's medical services network. Each branch has its own network.[3]

At-risk Any financial arrangement or contract in which a provider or health plan assumes exposure for the costs of services through a fee-for-service model; used to determine Medicare rates for HMOs.[2]

Average adjusted per capita cost (AAPCC) The estimated amount it would cost to provide services through a fee-for-service model; used to determine Medicare rates for HMOs.[2]

Benefit management An early form of managed care that relied on the structure and language of benefit allotments to contain and manage services provided.[3]

Benefit package A contractually defined set of healthcare benefits that are covered under an insurance, HMO, or capitation plan.[2]

Capitation The practice whereby an entity receives a fixed amount of money per member per month to provide specific health services.[3]

Capitation rate For insurers, the monthly revenue requirement from premiums per member per month to cover the health plan's costs. For providers, the rate paid per month under capitation arrangement to provide care to a fixed population. See Per member per month.[2]

Carve-in The tendency to revert the carve-out to the originally capitated group, giving them the responsibility and income on whatever service had previously been carved out.[1] See Carve-out.

Carve-out A managed care system in which some of the services and benefits (e.g., mental health and substance abuse) are uniformly managed or provided by another entity (e.g., a behavioral managed care company) and are not the responsibility of the physician group receiving the capitation.[3]

Superscript numbers are for the references at the end of the Glossary.

Case management   The handling or directing of a patient's treatment as to which services are needed and how they should be provided.[2]

Case mix   The blend of diagnoses or treatment types (e.g., inpatient and outpatient) for a particular provider, facility, group practice, or health plan.[2]

Case rate   A flat rate fee schedule based on a fixed amount per patient, often by diagnosis, and especially for inpatient care. See Fixed rate and Diagnostic-related group.[2]

Certificate of need (CON)   A certificate issued by a government body to an individual or organization proposing to construct or modify a health facility, acquire major new medical equipment, or offer a new or different health service. Such issuance recognizes that a facility or service, when available, will meet the needs of those for whom it is intended.[4]

Closed panel   A fixed group of clinicians from which enrollees must choose.[2]

Community rating   The method of setting premiums, mandated for federally qualified HMOs, in which the HMO uses a community-wide premium rate or equivalency formula to determine premium rates for members in a defined service area, based on the average family size, mix of single versus family contracts, and community standards.[2]

Concurrent review   A form of utilization review conducted during the provision of services (such as during an inpatient treatment period) to determine if the services meet the insurer's or third party's requirements to justify payment for the services provided.[2]

Consolidated Omnibus Budget Reconciliation Act (COBRA)   A federal law requiring that in specific circumstances when an employee loses his or her insurance coverage (e.g., through employment termination), the employer must give the employee the option to continue his or her insurance for a specified period (usually 18 months).[2]

Continental United States (CONUS)   Used to distinguish domestic services from worldwide military duty and location.[3]

Co-payment   A cost-sharing arrangement whereby the insured beneficiary pays a fixed fee at the time of service, augmenting the amount paid to the provider by the health plan. The co-payment does not vary with the provider's charge for the service.[2]

Cost sharing   A provision of a health plan that requires the insured to pay some portion of the costs for services. Deductibles and co-payments are forms of cost sharing.[2]

"Cream-skimming"   Attempts of health plans or provider groups to selectively enroll patients with a less severe illness or lower likelihood of using health services. Strategies to accomplish this goal include targeted marketing, development of programs that appeal to health populations, or neglect of programs that appeal to the more severely ill.[3]

Diagnostic-related group (DRG)   A prospective payment arrangement under which services are paid on a case rate or fixed rate, based on retrospective data about costs for treating certain diagnoses.[2]

Debriefing   The process by which survivors of a disaster review and assess the situation and design a preventive plan of action.[3]

Drug formulary   A list of prescription drugs for which a health plan will pay. If a drug is not on the formulary, some health plans have procedures to obtain special authorization for its use.[1]

Due diligence review   An employer's or insured's review of a provider panel to determine if the panel is adequate to meet expected healthcare needs and if providers meet community standards.[2]

Dyadic model (of medical care)   Treatment paradigms based on the assumption that a patient's needs can be best served through a one-to-one relationship with a treating clinician, drawing on the healing potential of that relationship.[3]

Employee Retirement Income Security Act of 1974 (ERISA)   An act that exempts the health plans of self-insured employers from many state laws (including freedom-of-choice laws).[2]

Experience rating   A system of setting insurance premiums so that they reflect the cost and utilization experience of a particular group or employer.[2]

Federally qualified   An HMO that has met the standards determined by the HMO Act of 1973 or its many amendments. Plans are no longer mandated to be federally qualified.[2]

Fee for service   The practice whereby a provider or entity receives payment for each service rendered according to a schedule of fees.[3]

Financial risk   A payment methodology in which the payments are fixed, regardless of the number of services utilized.[3]

First-dollar coverage   A health plan coverage that has no deductible amount; in some cases, a co-payment may be required.[2]

Gatekeeper   A person, usually a clinician, who is responsible for triage and authorization of initial requests to receive services.[2]

Health Care Financing Administration (HCFA) The agency within the U.S. Department of Health and Human Services that oversees the Medicaid and Medicare programs. Regional HCFA offices, located throughout the country, are each responsible for working with a group of states.[1]

Health maintenance organization (HMO) A term used to describe healthcare services provided by a sponsored group (i.e., labor unions, employers, hospitals) wherein all services (inpatient, outpatient, ancillary) are provided through a prepaid premium per person (see Capitation). There are four models of HMOs: group model, individual practice association, network model, and staff model.[3]

Horizontal integration Functional integrity of a system of care at a given level or intensity of service, as reflected in coordination among treaters or institutions.[3]

Hospital-physician organization (HPO) A joint venture between a hospital and group of providers to market or contract with one or more health plans. See Physician-hospital organization (PHO).[2]

Incurred but not reported (IBNR) Costs associated with a medical service that has been provided but for which a claim has not yet been received by the carrier. IBNR reserves are recorded by the carrier to account for estimated liability based on studies of prior lags in claim submissions.[4]

Independent practice association (IPA) A group of healthcare providers who are often in solo private practices, organized together by contract to facilitate participation in more than one healthcare plan. Also called independent practice organization (IPO).[2]

Integrated mental health system (IMHS) An HMO-like health plan for the chronically mentally ill.[2]

Integrated service network (ISN) Proposed networks of providers and payers that would provide care and compete with other systems for enrollees in their region. Systems could include hospitals, primary care physicians, specialty care physicians, and other providers and sites that could offer a full range of preventive and treatment services. Also referred to as accountable health plans (AHPs), coordinated care networks (CCNs), community care networks (CCNs), integrated health systems (IHSs), and organized delivery systems.[4]

Integration A healthcare delivery system that receives funds for physical healthcare, mental healthcare, and chemical dependency services from a payer.[3]

IPA model A health plan organized to provide services through one or more independent practice associations (IPAs), which are contracted to the health plan and paid on a fixed rate, fee-for-service, incentive, or capitation basis.[2]

Joint Commission on Accreditation of Healthcare Organizations (JCAHO) A private, not-for-profit organization that evaluates and accredits hospitals and other healthcare organizations that provide home care, mental healthcare, ambulatory care, and long-term care services.[3]

Last-dollar coverage An insurance coverage without a maximum or lifetime limit to the benefits payable.[2]

Limited duty medical board A disability determination document formally compiled by military medical officers during review of the service status of individual military personnel for diminished ability to perform their duties.[3]

Line command The name used for operational military forces to distinguish them from the medical and other service corps.[3]

Managed behavioral healthcare organization (MBHO) An organized system of behavioral healthcare delivery usually to a defined population of members of HMOs, preferred provider organizations, and other managed care structures; also known as a carve-out organization.[3]

Managed care A general term used to describe a variety of arrangements in healthcare financing, organization, and delivery, in which an entity other than the direct treating physician is managing or overseeing payment for medical services.[3]

Managed care organization (MCO) Any group conducting or implementing healthcare through managed care concepts of service preauthorization, utilization review, and a fixed network of providers. In mental healthcare, the term is often used to refer to a utilization review organization.[2]

Management information system (MIS) The computer and data management system.[2]

Management service organization (MSO) An organization that provides practice management, administration, and support services to individual physicians or group practices. Same as an administrative service organization (ASO) and a third-party administrator (TPA).[4]

Medicaid A health insurance program for eligible disabled and low-income people, administered by the federal government and participating states.[4]

Medicaid waiver A provision of federal law that allows the Health Care Financing Administration (HCFA) to permit a state Medicaid program design that does not comply with all requirements of federal law as long as HCFA approval is obtained. States no longer need a waiver to require most Medicaid recipients to enroll in managed care, but a research and demonstrated waiver (a 1115) is still required for states to expand Medicaid eligibility.[1]

Medical necessity   Need for services, defined both diagnostically and functionally. Treatment is required because of the presence of a mental or substance use disorder as evidenced by a valid (documentable) DSM-IV diagnosis and resultant impairments in the level of clinical stability or functioning or both. Treatment services are medically necessary insofar as they can be demonstrated to be efficacious in reversing or mitigating these impairments.[4]

Medicare   A nationwide, federally administered health insurance program that covers the costs of hospitalization, medical care, and some related services for eligible people. Eligible people are either age 65 years and over or disabled.[4]

Medigap   The coverage difference between Medicare and supplemental insurance.[2]

Moral hazard   A form of direct financial risk resulting from enrollee dishonesty, carelessness, or lack of judgment.[2]

Morbidity risk   A form of direct financial risk resulting from the actual degree or amount of psychopathology and psychiatric morbidity in the population.[2]

Network model   A health plan that provides healthcare services through a network of independent practitioners and group practices contracted to the HMO and paid on a salary, fee-for-service, incentive, or capitation basis.[2]

Omnibus Budget Reconciliation Act of 1986 (OBRA 86)   A congressional act taking effect in 1991 that prohibits HMOs from making payments directly or indirectly to providers as an inducement to reduce or limit services to Medicare or Medicaid patients.[2]

Open enrollment   A period of time during which new subscribers or employees of a particular employer may elect a new health plan or switch plans.[2]

Open panel   A large group of clinicians from which subscribers can select for their healthcare.[2]

Outcomes   The consumer's clinical status, level of functioning, quality of life, and satisfaction with care subsequent to the receipt of health services.[4]

Outlier   An enrollee requiring or using distinctly more or less services than is typical for patients with a given condition or illness. Usually defined as two standard deviations from the mean.[2]

Out-of-area benefits   The benefits an insurance plan provides when members are outside the geographical-

ly defined limits of the plan. These always include emergency services.[2]

Out-of-plan benefits   When services are authorized to be provided by a clinician or facility outside of a plan's closed panel, or beyond the standard limits of the plan benefits.[2]

Penetration   In marketing managed care plans, the percentage of possible subscribers actually enrolled in a particular plan or set of plans. In the provision of care or capitation, the percentage of possible enrollees accessing care.[2]

Performance measures   Data intended to summarize the quality of care delivered by providers.[4]

Per member per month (PMPM)   The fixed rate used to prepay a capitation contract monthly, based on the number of enrollees.[2]

Physician-hospital organization (PHO)   A joint venture between a hospital and a group of providers to market or contract with one or more health plans. See Hospital-physician organization (HPO).[2]

Physician's current procedural terminology (CPT)   A list of medical services and procedures performed by physicians and other providers. Each service or procedure is identified by its own unique five-digit code. CPT has become the healthcare industry's standard for reporting of physician procedures and services, thereby providing an effective method of nationwide communication.[4]

Point-of-service plans   Plans that combine traditional health coverage with HMO-type benefits. At each point of service (whenever a participant receives medical care), the participant may choose in-network services or go outside the network for treatment at a significantly higher deductible or co-payment. If the participant goes to an in-network physician, the participant will receive a higher level of benefits.[3]

Practice guidelines   Recommendations, developed by physician-directed private or public organizations, that suggest the most appropriate diagnostic and treatment approaches for an individual with a medical problem.[1]

Preadmission certification (PAC)   A review of the need for inpatient hospital care, done prior to the admission. Established review criteria are used to determine the appropriateness of inpatient care.[3]

Preauthorization   An authorization made under utilization review by an insurer or third party, before the provision of services, designating the services to be paid by the insurer or third party. Also called prior authorization, precertification, or predetermination.[2]

Precertification See Preauthorization.[2]

Preferred provider network (PPO) A network of healthcare providers that provide a discount on the fee for service to patients that remain within the network for care. Patients can go outside of the network but pay increased co-payments or deductibles. The network has structured quality assurance and utilization management.[3]

Prepaid group practice (PGP) A group practice paid on a capitation basis.[2]

Prepaid health plan (PHP) An insurance arrangement in which subscribers pay the insurer in advance for access to a specified set of healthcare benefits. HMOs are prepaid health plans.[2]

Price elasticity The relationship between price and utilization of services, for example, the higher the cost of co-payments, the lower the use of services. Also called price responsiveness.[2]

Price risk A form of direct financial risk, especially under capitation, which is the variance between the capitation bid price and the cost of providing services.[2]

Primary care The set of health services delivered by clinicians who define themselves, or who are defined by payers or regulators, as generalist providers. Primary care clinicians are often defined to be those physicians (including allopathic, chiropractic, osteopathic, and naturopathic doctors) and allied health professionals (especially nurse practitioners and physician assistants) who work in the areas of family practice, general internal medicine, obstetrics and gynecology, and pediatrics.[3]

Primary care physician (PCP) A subscriber's designated physician for basic medical care; usually a family practitioner, pediatrician, internist, or OB/GYN.[2]

Private sector Participants in the planning, provision, and evaluation of services that are not part of government.[3]

Processes Healthcare services.[3]

Providers Individual clinicians or agencies that deliver direct clinical services.[3]

Public Participants in the planning, provision, and evaluation of services that are not part of government.[3]

Purchasers The entities responsible for buying services.[3]

Quality assurance A set of measures, requirements, and tasks used to determine the quality of services. These items include the hiring process, chart reviews, complaint and grievance procedures, clinical supervision, in-service training, practice guidelines, team meetings, and critical incident reviews.[3]

Reasonable and customary (R&C) The commonly charged or prevailing fees for health services within a geographic area. A fee is considered to be reasonable if it falls within the parameters of the average or commonly charged fee for the particular service within that specific community.[3]

Resource-based relative value scale (RBRVS) A fee schedule introduced by the Health Care Financing Administration to reimburse physicians' Medicare fees based on the amount of time and resources expended in treating patients, with adjustments for overhead costs and geographic differences.[4]

Risk A situation in which the managed care plan provider or provider group takes a chance, a risk, that the monthly capitation payment (see earlier) won't be enough to pay for needed care. If a person's care costs more than the prepaid, fixed monthly amount, the plan provider or provider group must pay the extra amount out of its own pocket, and it loses money. But, when the person's healthcare costs less than the prepaid monthly amount, the plan provider or provider group makes money. To stay in business, the plan provider or provider group needs to control the amount it spends on healthcare so that the capitation payments received cover the cost of providing care and administering the managed care plan.[3]

Risk adjustment Methods for predicting health service utilization and adjusting reimbursement according to measurable characteristics of the covered population. These methods often rely on available computerized data (e.g., age, sex, insurance coverage group, and prior claims history).[3]

Risk band Utilization strata fixing changes in capitation payments for very high or low utilization. Also called risk corridor.[2]

Social health maintenance organization (S/HMO) An HMO that provides social and preventive services to a geriatric or other special-needs population with unique long-term care requirements.[2]

Staff model A health plan that employs its own providers.[2]

State mental health agency (SMHA) State mental health agencies are currently the principal organizational structure for mental health services in the public sector.[3]

State hospitals State-owned and operated hospitals.[3]

Stop-loss In a capitation contract, the maximum expense the provider can incur before the capitation rate structure changes; like a risk band except that it addresses only the upper limits of expenses. For subscribers, the upper amount for which a co-payment is due before the health plan assumes full coverage for costs incurred.[2]

Subcapitation   The practice whereby an entity receiving capitated dollars for enrollees sets a per member per month contract with another entity, usually within its own system, to provide specific services (e.g. an independent physician group receives $50 per member per month for all professional services and then subcapitates to the psychiatry group within the group to provide all mental health and substance abuse treatment for $1.75 per member per month).[3]

Tax Equity and Fiscal Responsibility Act of 1982 (TEFRA)   Among other medical insurance provisions, this law allows HMOs to contract with Medicare on a capitated basis.[2]

Termination without cause   Removal of a provider from a behavioral health network by invoking a stipulation in the contract that provides for termination of the contractual relationship without citing the reason(s) such action is being taken.[3]

Third-party administrator (TPA)   A fiscal intermediary or agent that pays claims on behalf of a payer. Same as an administrative service organization (ASO) and a management service organization (MSO).[2]

Uniform Code of Military Justice   The formal body of rules used to adjudicate military conduct and behavior.[3]

Usual, customary, and reasonable (UCR)   A fee structure for services based on assessment of prevailing fees in a particular community or region.[2]

Utilization management   A phase of managed care characterized by the management of service utilization through assessing the necessity for services prior to, during, and/or following service provision and authorizing reimbursement for such services only when they meet (or have met) criteria of appropriateness and medical necessity.[3]

Utilization review (UR)   A mechanism used by managed care plans to evaluate treatment options on the basis of appropriateness, necessity, and quality. For inpatient care, utilization review can include preadmission approval, concurrent review during the hospital stay, discharge planning, and retrospective review.[2]

Utilization Review Accreditation Commission (URAC)   A Washington-based, not-for-profit corporation formed in 1990 and dedicated to improving the quality of utilization review in the healthcare industry by providing a method of evaluation and accreditation of utilization review programs.[4]

Utilization review organization (URO)   A business entity that provides utilization review for insurers or employers. Utilization review may be prospective, concurrent, or retrospective.[2]

Vertical integration   Functional integrity of a system of care between or among levels or intensities of service, as reflected in the seamless transition of patients in moving from one level or intensity to others during an episode of care.[3]

Waivers   The chief mechanism by which states have implemented managed care systems within their state-financed Medicaid populations is through 1115 (research and demonstration) and 1915(b) (Medicaid managed care) waivers. Waivers allow states to waive requirements in the Medicaid law to develop innovations in the financing and delivery of services to Medicaid recipients.[3]

Withhold   A portion of a provider's fee retained by a health plan as part of a risk-sharing arrangement. The provider receives all or a portion of the withhold periodically, based on the financial performance of the health plan.[2]

Wraparound services   Services that enable persons to access health services. They include transportation, child care services, legal assistance, domestic violence services, and even cash assistance.[2]

References

[1]Hall LL, Edgar ER, Flynn LM: Stand and Deliver: Action Call to a Failing Industry: The NAMI Managed Care Report Card. Reprinted with permission from the National Alliance for the Mentally Ill

[2]Zieman GL: The Complete Capitation Handbook: How to Design and Implement At-Risk Contracts for Behavioral Healthcare. Tiburon, CA, CentraLink Publications, in cooperation with Jossey-Bass, 1995. Reprinted with permission from CentraLink Publications, copyright 1995

[3]Authors of this textbook

[4]United HealthCare: Abbreviations and Acronyms, 1996. Reprinted with permission of United HealthCare, MN008-W220, 9900 Bren Road E., Minneapolis, MN 55434

Index

*Page numbers printed in **boldface** type refer to tables or figures.*

403

healthcare organizations and culture
of service to, 44–45
legal issues in management of, 346
medical director and, 90
population-based care and, 123–124
rights of and legal responsibilities of
hospital, 344–346
trends and future of administrative
psychiatry, 387–389
Patrick v. Burget, 347
PDCA (plan, do, check, act) cycle, 63,
63, 64, **65,** 70
*Peck v. Counseling Service of Addison
County, Inc.,* 332
Peer counseling programs, 204
Peer Review Improvement Act (1982),
240
Peer review organizations (PROs), 241
Pennsylvania Hospital (Philadelphia),
10, 181, 228
Percival, Thomas, 379
Performance appraisal, and leadership,
50
Performance measures, 400
Performance review and monitoring, of
behavioral health networks,
110–111
Per-member per-month (PMPM)
capitation rates, 297, 400
Personal Health Improvement
Program, 164
Personality disorders, and criminal
activity, 353, 356
Personal mastery, 40
Petersdorf, Robert G., 255
Pharmacies, and confidentiality, 148.
See also Prescriptions and
prescription practices
Physical abuse, and prisons, 371. *See also*
Domestic violence
Physician-assisted suicide, 346
Physician executives, 196–197
Physician-hospital organizations
(PHOs)
behavioral group practices and,
308
definition of, 400
development of, 295
factors in emergence of, 293–294
formation of, 294–295
integration and, **225**
mental health professionals and
implementation of, 296–298
strategic planning and, 59

Physicians. *See also* Physician-hospital
organizations (PHOs); Primary
care physicians
autonomy of, 171
career changes and, 193–198
changing roles of, 158
health maintenance organization
contracts and, **282**
legal liability of hospitals and classes
of staff members, 330
profession of medicine and, 170
Physician's current procedural
terminology (CPT), 400
Physician-systems integration, 224
Piaget, J., 314
Pierce, Franklin, 271
Pinel, Phillippe, 181
Planning. *See also* Strategic plans
continuous quality improvement
and, 63–64, 69
definition of, 53
in environment of rapid change,
53–54, 60
product-line management and,
41–42
in stable environments, 59–60
systems thinking and, 54–58
Play space, and child services, 315
Point-of-service plans (POS)
behavioral health networks and,
100–101
capitation and, 131–132
definition of, 400
Policy
confidentiality and, 150–152, 153
medical director and, 91
prison system and, 367, 369
Politics. *See also* Federal government;
State governments
insanity defense and, 356
prison reforms and, 365–366
Polypharmacy, and prescription
practices, 335
Population-based care
capitation and, 123–125, 132
development of, 125–126
redesign of, 127–130
Posttraumatic stress disorder (PTSD),
251, 252, 262
Practice guidelines, 111, 400
Pratt, Joseph Hersey, 161, 162
Preadmission certification (PAC),
400
Preauthorization, 400

"Pre-existing condition" exclusions,
and health insurance, 149
Preferred provider organizations
(PPOs)
behavioral health networks and, 100,
107
care management and, 109
definition of, 401
Prepaid group practice (PGP), 401
Prepaid health plan (PHP), 401
Prescriptions and prescription
practices. *See also*
Psychopharmacology
confidentiality and, 148
legal negligence and, 334–335
President's Commission on Mental
Health, 18, 271, 272
Pretrial evaluations, and criminal law,
353–357
Prevention
future of private sector and, 15
military psychiatric services and,
261–262
training in administrative psychiatry
and, 78–79
Price elasticity and price risk, 401
Primary behavioral healthcare
administrative strategies for,
164–166
capitation and, 165
definition of, 159–160, 401
emerging primacy of, 160
improved treatment of medical
disorders and, 160–162
somatization and, 163–164
treatment of psychiatric disorders
and, 162–163
Primary Care Education Program
(Veterans Administration), 255
Primary care managers, and managed
care, 189
Primary care physicians (PCPs). *See also*
Physicians
definition of, 401
future of psychiatry and, 390
managed care and roles of, 187
psychiatric disorders and, 162–163,
174–175
referrals to specialists by, 160
somatization and, 163–164
Prioritization, and continuous quality
improvement, 66
Priority clinical areas, and population-
based care, 127

Psychotherapy. *See also* Cognitive-
behavioral therapy; Group therapy;
Treatment
family and, 215
hospitals and lawsuit damage awards,
329
patient preferences and, 129–130
as potential area of liability for
hospitals, **328**
research on effectiveness of, 135
Psychotic disorder, 126
Public health psychiatry, 175
Public sector. *See also* State agencies;
State mental hospitals
capitation, 132
future of, 25, 83–84, 275–279
history of, 18–19, 270–271
managed care and, 76
present status of, 19–25
private sector and, 233
privatization of, 390–391
reform of, 271
role of in mental healthcare, 17–18
role of psychiatrists in, 175–178
strategic planning and, 55–57, 58

Quakers, and history of mental
healthcare, 10
Quality. *See also* Continuous quality
improvement; Quality assurance;
Quality management
behavioral group practices and,
310–311
behavioral health networks and, 102,
110–112
definition of, 61
health maintenance organizations
and, 287–288
improvement of and future of
administrative psychiatry, 393
managed care and, 173, 189
managers' orientations toward, **66**
medical director and clinical, 86–88
network management and, 70–71
as objective of organization, 56
private psychiatric hospitals and,
235
satisfaction data and improvement
of, 70
steps for improving, 64
Quality assurance. *See also* Quality
continuous quality improvement
and, **63**
definition of, 401

future of administrative psychiatry
and, 393
health maintenance organizations
and, 284–285
hospital privileges and legal liability
of hospital, 347–348
Quality of care, 61–62
Quality management, and quality
management programs, 62, 65
Queuing, and capitation, 132

Race, and prison populations, 363, 365,
369, 370. *See also* Ethnicity
Rand Corporation, 24, 287, 288
Rationing, of psychiatric services, 325
Reasonable care, and legal liability of
hospitals, 332–333, 341
Reasonable and customary (R&C),
401
Reasonable professional judgment, and
legal defense, 331
Records, patient, as potential area of
liability for hospitals, **328,** 342, 344.
See also Confidentiality;
Information systems
Re-engineering
military psychiatric services and,
264
organizational theory and, 39–40
primary behavioral healthcare and,
165
as strategy to remain current, 224
Referrals, to psychiatrists
family and, 216–217
managed care and, 184–185
prisons and mental healthcare, 377
Reform and reform movements. *See*
Healthcare reform; Prisons;
Welfare reform
Refusal, of treatment as patient right,
345
Regression, and leadership, 50
Regulation and regulatory agencies. *See
also* Federal government; State
government
child and adolescent services and,
322
managed care and, 186
Rehabilitation, and prisons, 365, 367,
369
Rehabilitative perspective, and
psychiatry, 170
Report cards, 392–393
Reporting laws, and psychiatrists, 358

Requests for proposals (RFPs), and
continuous quality improvement,
70
Research
on career changes by physicians,
193–194
future of private sector and, 15
new services in response to, 389
prisons and, 367, 372
Veterans Administration and, 256
Residency Review Committee in
Psychiatry, 77–78
Residential treatment, and private
psychiatric hospitals, 232
Res ipsa loquitur, legal principle of, 333
Resource-based relative value scale
(RBRVS), 401
Resources
continuous quality improvement
and, 65
population-based systems and use of,
127
Respite programs, and children,
316–317
Respondeat superior, legal doctrine of, 330
Restoration, of competency, 354
Restraint, of patient as legal issue, 346,
347
Restrictive or closed formularies, and
prescription practices, 335–336
Resumes, of physicians, 198
Rex v. Arnold (1724), 355
Risk and risk management
behavioral health networks and, 108,
112–113
capitation and adjustment methods,
130–131
child and adolescent services and,
317–319
confidentiality and, 146–148
definition of, 401
legal theory of assumption of, 332
managed care and, 391–392
physician-hospital organizations
and, 295
planning and, 54
suicide and, 339, **340, 341, 342**
violent behavior and, **343**
Roberts Rules of Order (Robert 1990),
50
Robert Wood Johnson Foundation
Program on Chronic Mental
Illness, 21
Rush, Benjamin, 10, 181–182